NEUROMUSCULAR JUNCTION DISORDERS

HANDBOOK OF CLINICAL NEUROLOGY

Series Editors

MICHAEL J. AMINOFF, FRANÇOIS BOLLER, AND DICK F. SWAAB

VOLUME 91

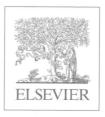

ELSEVIER

EDINBURGH LONDON NEW YORK OXFORD PHILADELPHIA
ST LOUIS SYDNEY TORONTO 2008

NEUROMUSCULAR JUNCTION DISORDERS

Series Editors

MICHAEL J. AMINOFF, FRANÇOIS BOLLER, AND DICK F. SWAAB

Volume Editor

ANDREW G. ENGEL

VOLUME 91

3rd Series

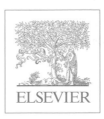

ELSEVIER

EDINBURGH LONDON NEW YORK OXFORD PHILADELPHIA
ST LOUIS SYDNEY TORONTO 2008

ELSEVIER B.V
Radarweg 29, 1043 NX, Amsterdam, The Netherlands
© 2008, Elsevier B.V. All rights reserved.

First published 2008

ISBN: 978 0 444 52008 1

British Library Cataloguing in Publication Data
A catalogue record for this book is available from the British Library

Library of Congress Cataloging in Publication Data
A catalog record for this book is available from the Library of Congress

Notice
Knowledge and best practice in this field are constantly changing. As new research and experience broaden our knowledge, changes in practice, treatment and drug therapy may become necessary or appropriate. Readers are advised to check the most current information provided (i) on procedures featured or (ii) by the manufacturer of each product to be administered, to verify the recommended dose or formula, the method and duration of administration, and contraindications. It is the responsibility of the practitioner, relying on their own experience and knowledge of the patient, to make diagnoses, to determine dosages and the best treatment for each individual patient, and to take all appropriate safety precautions. To the fullest extent of the law, neither the Publisher nor the Editors and Authors assume any liability for any injury and/or damage to persons or property arising out of or related to any use of the material contained in this book.

The Publisher

Working together to grow
libraries in developing countries

www.elsevier.com | www.bookaid.org | www.sabre.org

ELSEVIER | BOOK AID International | Sabre Foundation

 ELSEVIER | your source for books, journals and multimedia in the health sciences
www.elsevierhealth.com

Printed in China

The publisher's policy is to use **paper manufactured from sustainable forests**

For Elsevier:
Commissioning Editor: Timothy Horne
Development Editor: Michael Parkinson
Project Manager: Anne Dickie
Design Direction: George Ajayi

Handbook of Clinical Neurology 3rd Series

Available titles
Vol. 79, The human hypothalamus: basic and clinical aspects, Part I, D.F. Swaab ISBN 9780444513571
Vol. 80, The human hypothalamus: basic and clinical aspects, Part II, D.F. Swaab ISBN 9780444514905
Vol. 81, Pain, F. Cervero and T.S. Jensen ISBN 9780444519016
Vol. 82, Motor neuron disorders and related diseases, A.A. Eisen and P.J. Shaw ISBN 9780444518941
Vol. 83, Parkinson's disease and related disorders, Part I, W.C. Koller and E. Melamed ISBN 9780444519009
Vol. 84, Parkinson's disease and related disorders, Part II, W.C. Koller and E. Melamed ISBN 9780444528933
Vol. 85, HIV/AIDS and the nervous system, P. Portegies and J.R. Berger ISBN 9780444520104
Vol. 86, Myopathies, F.L. Mastaglia and D. Hilton-Jones ISBN 9780444518996
Vol. 87, Malformations of the nervous system, H.B. Sarnat and P. Curatolo ISBN 9780444518965
Vol. 88, Neuropsychology of behavioral neurology, G. Goldenberg and B. Miller ISBN 9780444518972
Vol. 89, Dementias, C. Duyckaerts and I. Litvan ISBN 9780444518989
Vol. 90, Disorders of consciousness, G.B. Young and E.F.M. Wijdicks ISBN 9780444518958

Forthcoming titles
Vol. 92, Stroke Part I: Basic and epidemiological aspects, M. Fisher ISBN 9780444520036
Vol. 93, Stroke Part II: Clinical manifestations and pathogenesis, M. Fisher ISBN 9780444520043
Vol. 94, Stroke Part III: Investigation and management, M. Fisher ISBN 9780444520050

Foreword

We are pleased and proud to present this volume on disorders of the neuromuscular junction in the *Handbook of Clinical Neurology* series, and congratulate the editor, Professor Andrew Engel, and the outstanding group of authors whom he brought together as contributors to the book.

In an excellent chapter on historic aspects of neuromuscular junction disorders, John Keesey reviews how knowledge of the neuromuscular junction developed from the 1743 illustration by Herman Boerhaave, the founder of Dutch medicine, who showed the nerve as flowing directly into the substance of the muscle, leading eventually to recognition of the molecular defects of presynaptic, synaptic, and postsynaptic proteins in congenital myasthenic syndromes, to which Dr. Engel has himself contributed so much. A varied assortment of people has contributed to our current insights, including Emperor Napoleon III, who donated the South American arrow poison, curare, to Claude Bernard. Important insights came also from clinical descriptions, such as the first one in 1672, by Thomas Willis in *De Anima Brutorum*, of a "prudent and honest woman" with fluctuating muscle weakness "not only in the members but also in her tongue" and epidemics such as the sausage poisoning *(Wurstvergiftung)* in Germany, now known to have been due to botulism. The road from curare to immunotherapy, via muscle antibodies, took 330 years.

Recent progress has been at higher speed. Volumes 40 and 41 of the *Handbook*, which appeared in 1979, contained a chapter by Andrew Engel on myasthenia gravis. The rapid advances in our understanding of the neurobiology of neuromuscular transmission, and of the molecular background of the various forms of neuromuscular junction disorders that have been made since then, make publication of the present volume very timely. New insights have been obtained into the immunopathogenesis of myasthenia gravis, not only in relation to anti-acetylcholine receptor antibodies but also to different antibodies, such as those against the voltage-gated calcium channels on the presynaptic membrane. Considerable knowledge has also been gained recently into the molecular mechanisms underlying the links between activity and patterns of gene expression, particularly in muscle, and we have a much better idea of the factors regulating the adaptive plasticity of the neuromuscular junction, which may in turn lead to new therapeutic strategies for enhancing the restoration of normal function in neuromuscular disorders. The clinical features and electrodiagnosis of neuromuscular junction disorders, and the optimal treatment of myasthenia gravis, receive exquisite attention in this volume. Novel and important information is also provided to enhance understanding of the pathophysiology of the heterogeneous group of peripheral nerve hyperexcitability syndromes, and the toxicity of pesticides such as the acetylcholinesterase-inhibiting organophosphates and carbamates.

We are greatly indebted to the volume editor and to the authors who have put together this outstanding volume, which will be of great interest to both practising neurologists and scientists working in this field. As always, we are also very grateful to the team at Elsevier for their expert assistance in the development and production of this book.

Michael J. Aminoff
François Boller
Dick F. Swaab

Preface

In 1992, when the second series of the *Handbook of Clinical Neurology* was published, a single 65-page chapter summarized the then current knowledge of diseases of the neuromuscular junction. Commensurate with advances in the field, the third series of the *Handbook* devotes an entire volume comprised of 14 chapters to these disorders.

The book begins with an account by John Keesey on the historic aspects of diseases that commonly involve neuromuscular transmission. Chapters 2–4 acquaint the reader with the structure and function of the neuromuscular junction and with the relevant clinical electrodiagnostic methods. Thus, Chapter 2 by Clarke Slater reviews the safety margin of neuromuscular transmission. Chapter 3 by Andrew Engel describes the basic anatomy and the functional significance of each structural component of the neuromuscular junction. Chapter 4 by C. Michel Harper explains how electrophysiologic techniques identify defects of neuromuscular transmission and provide information related to the mechanism and severity of the disorder.

Chapters 5–8 focus on autoimmune myasthenia gravis. In Chapter 5, Norbert Sommer, Björn Tackenberg and Reinhard Hohlfeld review the immunological principles relevant to myasthenia gravis, survey the autoantibodies and their target antigens, discuss the associated cellular immune responses, and consider the contribution of genetic factors and the thymus gland to the pathogenesis of the disease. In Chapter 6, Angela Vincent describes different antibodies directed against the acetylcholine receptor (AChR) and how these antibodies can be assayed. She also explains how antibodies against the fetal form of AChR in maternal sera can cause multiple joint contractures at birth and compromise the survival of the offspring. She also relates the intriguing discovery that autoantibodies directed against the muscle specific tyrosine kinase (MuSK) underlie the pathogenesis of autoimmune myasthenia in a proportion of patients who harbor no anti-AChR antibodies. Chapter 7 by Donald Sanders and Janice Massey details the semiology of myasthenia gravis, and discusses different subtypes of the disease and their diagnosis. Chapter 8 by Dan Drachman is an elegant and authoritative exposition of the principles of therapy based on many decades of personal experience. This chapter will serve as a valuable guide to therapy of myasthenic patients whose disease ranges from mild ocular symptoms to recurrent life-threatening crises.

Chapters 9 and 10 deal with myasthenic syndromes. In Chapter 9, Donald Sanders and Vern Juel provide a full account of the clinical presentation, pathophysiology, immunopathology, diagnosis, association with malignancy, and therapy of the Lambert–Eaton syndrome. Unlike in myasthenia gravis, where antibodies directed against AChR or MuSK attenuate the synaptic response to acetylcholine, in the Lambert–Eaton syndrome antibodies directed against the presynaptic voltage-gated calcium channel decrease the number of transmitter quanta released by nerve impulse. In Chapter 10, Andrew Engel describes the clinical and basic science features and therapy of the congenital myasthenic syndromes and discusses how defects in different components of the neuromuscular junction, namely choline acetyltransferase, the collagenic tail of acetylcholinesterase, the acetylcholine receptor, rapsyn, the voltage-gated sodium channel, MuSK, and Dok-7, the recently identified muscle-intrinsic activator of MuSK, impair the safety margin of neuromuscular transmission. The commonest congenital syndromes are caused by defects in AChR that either reduce the expression or profoundly alter the kinetic properties of the receptor.

Chapters 11–13 survey neuromuscular transmission disorders caused by the exogenous agents that include bacterial and marine toxins, numerous drugs, and organophosphates. Perhaps the commonest of the intoxications worldwide is botulism, and Chapter 11 by Eric Johnson and Cesare Montecucco provides a scholarly and definitive account of the various types of botulinus toxins, and the diagnosis and therapy of the various forms of human botulism.

The final chapter by Steven Vernino discusses the clinical features and pathophysiology of genetic, toxic, and immune-mediated diseases that cause neuromyotonia. The majority of these disorders stem from hyperexcitability of the distal motor nerve, or motor nerve terminal, so they are appropriately considered neuromuscular junction disorders.

PREFACE

Diseases of the neuromuscular junction are, and are likely to remain, of keen interest to clinicians and basic scientists alike. Although many are highly disabling, most are treatable; and understanding their basis has yielded sharp insights into basic immunology, neurotoxicology, and the neurobiology of synaptic transmission.

I wish to thank Michael J. Aminoff for reading and critiquing each chapter and the production staff of Elsevier for their expert assistance in bringing this volume of the *Handbook of Clinical Neurology* to fruition.

Andrew G. Engel

List of contributors

J.L. De Bleecker
Neurology Department, University Hospital, Ghent, Belgium

D.B. Drachman
Department of Neurology and Neuroscience, Johns Hopkins School of Medicine, Baltimore, MD, USA

A.G. Engel
Department of Neurology, Mayo Clinic, Rochester, MN, USA

C.M. Harper
Department of Neurology, Mayo Clinic, Rochester, MN, USA

R. Hohlfeld
Institute for Clinical Neuroimmunology, Klinikum der LMU München, Campus Grosshadern and Department of Neuroimmunology, Max-Planck-Institute of Neurobiology, Martinsried, Germany

J.F. Howard, Jr.
Laboratory for Myasthenia Gravis Research, Department of Neurology, The University of North Carolina at Chapel Hill, Chapel Hill, NC, USA

E.A. Johnson
Department of Bacteriology, Food Research Institute, University of Wisconsin, Madison, WI, USA

V.C. Juel
Duke University Medical School, Durham, NC, USA

J. Keesey
Department of Neurology, University of California School of Medicine, Los Angeles, CA, USA

J.M. Massey
Division of Neurology, Department of Medicine, Duke University Medical School, Durham, NC, USA

C. Montecucco
Dipartimento di Scienze Biomediche Sperimentali, University of Padova, Padova, Italy

D.B. Sanders
Division of Neurology, Department of Medicine, Duke University Medical School, Durham, NC, USA

C.R. Slater
Institute of Neuroscience, Faculty of Medical Sciences, University of Newcastle upon Tyne, Newcastle upon Tyne, UK

N. Sommer
Clinical Neuroimmunology Group, Philipps-University, Marburg, and Department of Neurology, Christophsbad, Göppingen, Germany

B. Tackenberg
Clinical Neuroimmunology Group, Philipps-University, Marburg, Germany

S. Vernino
Department of Neurology, University of Texas Southwestern Medical Center, Dallas, TX, USA

A. Vincent
Department of Clinical Neurology, University of Oxford, Oxford, UK

Contents

CONTENTS

Handbook of Clinical Neurology, Vol. 91 (3rd series)
Neuromuscular junction disorders
A.G. Engel, Editor

Chapter 1

The most vulnerable synapse: historic aspects of neuromuscular junction disorders

JOHN KEESEY *

Department of Neurology, University of California School of Medicine, Los Angeles, CA, USA

1.1. Introduction

The site where a motor nerve meets a skeletal muscle fiber, termed either the "neuromuscular" or the "myoneural" junction, was a very poorly understood structure until the 20th century. Herman Boerhaave, the 18th century founder of Dutch medicine, illustrated the nerve as flowing directly into the substance of the muscle (Boerhaave, 1743) and these structures were still pictured as fused 100 years later (Doyére, 1840). Willy Kühne, one of the finest light microscopists of the 19th century, although able to visualize the "motor endplate" of skeletal muscle *en face* (Kühne, 1863), was unable to resolve whether it was a part of the terminal innervation or a part of the skeletal muscle fiber (Keesey, 2002).

Despite this uncertainty, in 1850 the great French physiologist Claude Bernard reasoned from ingenious experiments on frogs that the South American arrow poison, curare (a gift from Emperor Napoleon III), acted only at the terminal fibers of motor nerves (Bernard, 1857). Emil Du Bois-Reymond, the pre-eminent electro-physiologist of his time, speculated in 1877 that transmission between the nerve and the muscle was either electrical or else occurred by liberation from the motor nerve of a substance, such as ammonia or lactic acid, capable of exciting the muscle (Du Bois-Reymond, 1877). During the first half of the 20th century, pharmacological evidence for acetylcholine in that latter role became compelling (Brown, 1937). When electron microscopes became commercially available, the nerve terminal and the specialized region of muscle where the nerve terminated were shown to be separate, highly organized structures with a space in between (Robertson,

1956). At about the same time biophysicists, using saline-filled glass microelectrodes in muscle fibers near nerve terminals, were able to describe in detail the electrical events occurring during normal neuromuscular transmission (Fatt and Katz, 1952).

It was only by using these new tools in the second half of the 20th century that the pathophysiology of an assortment of previously unrelated conditions could be localized to the neuromuscular junction. These include the most common neuromuscular disorders worldwide—those caused by particular snake and spider venoms—as well as illnesses caused by some bacterial and marine toxins and by numerous drugs, all of which may be regarded as "exogenous" neuromuscular disorders (Swift and Greenberg, 1984). This chapter will focus on one of these, botulism. It will also describe the history of myasthenia gravis and its relatives, major representatives of what Swift and Greenberg (1984) termed "endogenous" neuromuscular disorders. The eventful histories of botulism and myasthenia gravis began long before it was realized that the neuromuscular junction, "the most vulnerable synapse known" (Estable, 1959), was involved.

1.2. History of human botulism

The word "botulism" is derived from *botulus*, the Latin word for "sausage," suggested by the German physician Müller in 1870 (Erbguth and Naumann, 1999) to describe a peculiar type of food poisoning, the only known cause of which at that time was the ingestion of spoiled sausages. Others preferred to describe it by the term "allantiasis," derived from the Greek word for sausage, *allantiko*.

---

*Correspondence to: John Keesey, MD, 1144 Iliff Street, Pacific Palisades, CA 90272, USA. E-mail: jkeesey@ucla.edu, Tel: 1-310-454-7910, Fax: 1-310-459-6197 (not automatic).

1.2.1. Sausages, 1820

At the beginning of the 19th century sausage poisoning was particularly frequent in southern Germany, especially in the spring. Authorities in the Kingdom of Württemberg at the time realized that the sausages usually involved were large fatty sausages in hog stomach casings containing blood, liver or milk that during preparation probably had been boiled inadequately for fear of their bursting (Grüsser, 1986). Numerous speculations about causation were proposed, including contamination by toxic saliva (*agua tofana*) from the cruelly butchered hogs, metal contamination from cooking vessels, or poisonous seeds used as spices (Dickson, 1918). These sausages were typically hung in chimneys to be smoked, and frozen during the winter. On subsequent thawing in spring, the inner portions of the sausage were considered to produce the poorly understood toxic symptoms such as "some incidental nervous conditions" including blindness (Grüsser, 1986).

In 1820 Justinus Kerner, the 34-year-old town physician (*Oberamtsarzt*) of Weinsberg in Württemberg (Fig. 1.1), published a 120-page monograph on the symptoms of sausage poisoning, *Wurstvergiftung*, based on the evaluation of 76 patients, 37 of whom died (Kerner, 1820). This gave an astute clinical description of the peripheral motor and autonomic symptoms recognized today as characteristic of the disease, such

as dry mouth and skin, lack of tears, bladder atony, fixed wide pupils, double vision, ptosis, trouble eating and speaking, and death from paralysis of the respiratory musculature. Kerner even noticed decreased production of ear wax and cessation of dreams, attributing the latter to peripheral nerve damage, since he was unable to observe any other symptoms that in his opinion demonstrated involvement of the central nervous system. As he stated in his second monograph two years later, "Hypotheses pass away, but careful observation remains a given, useful in all changes in the system, a gain for all the days ahead" (Kerner, 1822). By 1822 Kerner was able to describe a total of 155 patients with sausage poisoning, 84 of which had been fatal.

Kerner boldly administered a watery extract from spoiled sausages to himself and to a variety of animals, and he concluded in his second monograph that the sausage poison was a "fatty acid" that developed under anaerobic conditions (air pockets in the sausages seemed to prevent toxicity) and was lethal even in small doses (Kerner, 1822). Remarkably, in light of modern developments, Kerner suggested that the sausage poison in extremely small doses might sooth motor over-stimulation, such as St Vitus' Dance. However, Kerner is remembered mainly as a leading poet of Swabian Romanticism (Grüsser, 1986). After 1822 he pursued sausage poisoning only as it related to his interests in animal magnetism and the medical occult (Schiller, 1993).

Although Kerner's work made sausage-poisoning a reportable disease, Kerner was discouraged that 20 years later, in 1842, no progress had yet been made in treating sausage poisoning (Grüsser, 1986). His suggestions regarding prevention, however, had led to a lessening incidence of the condition in southern Germany, and his clinical descriptions are still relevant today.

1.2.2. Ham, 1897

Further progress in understanding botulism had to wait for the advances in the understanding of bacteria and bacterial toxins provided in the second half of the 19th century by Louis Pasteur in France and Robert Koch in Germany. One of Koch's students in 1883 in Berlin was a highly cultured Belgian, Émile Van Ermengen, who spoke six languages and had already studied in London, Edinburgh, Vienna and Paris (with Ranvier and Claude Bernard). In 1888 at the age of 37 he became *Professeur ordinaire* of Microbiology at the University of Ghent (Fig. 1.2).

After a peculiar epidemic of food poisoning in 1895 at an inn in the Belgian village of Ellezelles, in which 23 members of a music club became ill after

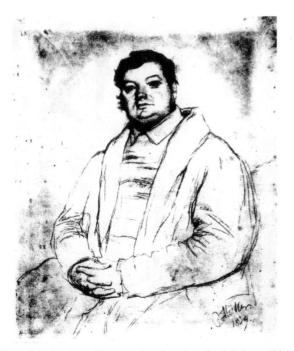

Fig. 1.1. Justinus Kerner, drawing by O. Müller, 1834. Deutsches Literaturarchiv Marbach, Schiller-Nationalmuseum.

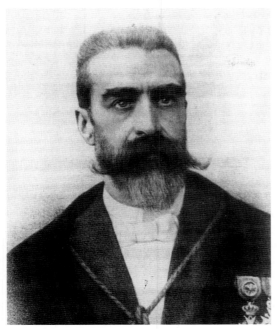

Fig. 1.2. Émile Van Ermengen. Archives of the University of Ghent.

eating raw smoked ham and three of the young men died (Devriese, 1999), portions of the unspoiled ham and organs from the dead victims were sent to Van Ermengen for investigation (as well as another spoiled ham that had caused no illness although it had been on top of the submerged toxic one in the same barrel of brine). He published full reports of his findings in French and German in 1897 (Van Ermengen, 1897a, b).

Van Ermengen compared this episode to previous cases of meat or fish poisonings, with some of which he already had been involved, and reviewed the difficulties others had had reproducing these illnesses in animals. In contrast, by extensive experiments, Van Ermengen was able to reproduce the characteristic neuromuscular and autonomic signs (which he remarked in passing "have their origin very probably in lesions of the central nervous system") by feeding or injecting the suspected ham or cultures from the ham into monkeys, cats, rabbits and pigeons. Dogs, chickens, frogs and fish seemed almost completely refractory to poisoning by the ham.

After demonstrating that the illness was not an infection but an intoxication by an exceedingly potent preformed toxin that was not inactivated by digestion, Van Ermengen nevertheless isolated from the spleen of one of the victims, using newer culture methods, an anaerobic spore-bearing bacterium and named it *Bacillus botulinus*. Salt concentrations above 5%

inhibited the production of the toxin, and unlike the heat-resistant spores, the toxin was easily inactivated by heat. Van Ermengen commented, "If the Ellezelles ham had been roasted or boiled before being eaten, instead of being eaten raw, no illness would have resulted" (Van Ermengen, 1897b).

1.2.3. Beans, 1904

In 1904 an outbreak resembling botulism killed 11 of 21 people in Darmstadt, Germany, who had eaten a salad containing unheated home-canned white beans. At the time only meat products were accepted as causing botulism, so the person at Merck laboratories in Darmstadt who had found that the beans contained a bacillus resembling that isolated by Van Ermengen, which produced a similar toxin, suggested that maybe a small amount of pork must have been present in the beans (Landman, 1904). Because of skepticism that this really was botulism, bacteria isolated from the Ellezelles ham and from the Darmstadt beans were compared by Leuchs at the Royal Institute of Infectious Disease in Berlin in 1910. Toxins produced by the two strains were very similar, but serologically they were distinct; antitoxins prepared from the two strains did not crossneutralize (Leuchs, 1910). Georgina Burke at Stanford University designated the two types of toxin "type A" and "type B" (Burke, 1919). Although by then the original strains had been lost, Van Ermengen's strain was considered to be type B and Landman's strain type A (Smith, 1977). Spores of *B. botulinus*, associated with type A toxin, were more heat resistant than those associated with type B. In the United States, 9 of 14 strains found ubiquitously in soils west of the Mississippi were type A (5 were type B), whereas all of 9 strains east of the Mississippi were type B (Burke, 1919). European strains that produced type B toxin were non-proteolytic, whereas American bacterial isolates that produced type A or type B toxins were proteolytic, raising the possibility that affected food in America might more likely seem spoiled than toxic food in Europe.

The first well-studied epidemic in the United States caused by growth of botulinum organisms in vegetable tissues (without meat) occurred in 1913 when 12 of 24 girls at a sorority supper at Stanford University became severely ill and one died from eating home-canned string beans in a salad (Wilbur and Ophüls, 1914). The salad was not retrieved, but Ernest C. Dickson at Stanford Medical School in San Francisco (Fig. 1.3) showed that *B. botulinus* injected into commercially canned beans grew anaerobically over several months, producing the typical toxin (Dickson, 1918).

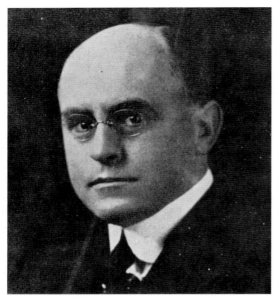

Fig. 1.3. E.C. Dickson, Stanford University. (From Dolman, 1964, p. 12.)

1.2.4. Commercial canning crisis, 1925

Fatal cases of botulism in America from commercial canned beets, spinach, olives (Fig. 1.4) and other foods rose to double-digit levels between 1919 and 1925. There were 29 deaths in 1919 and 23 deaths in 1920 from commercially canned foods. Botulism was giving canned foods a bad name in the United States (Young, 1976). The National Canners Association created a Botulism Commission—consisting of Professor Dickson, Professor Karl Meyer of the University of California (Fig. 1.5), and Jacob Geiger of the US Public Health Service—who determined experimentally that while boiling for as long as 22 hours did not kill the spores, a temperature of 121°C would kill one thousand billion *Clostridium botulinum*[1] type A spores in 2.4 minutes (Foster, 1993). After institution of these procedures, not a single outbreak attributable to US-produced commercially canned foods occurred between 1926 and 1941. After 1941, rare outbreaks attributed to under-processing or leakage of commercial cans continued to occur, but the major source of food-borne botulism became home-canned

low acid foods—primarily vegetables in the United States, Italy and Spain; meats in Germany, France and Poland; and fermented bean products the usual source in China. An increasing number of outbreaks attributed to a previously-unidentified type of botulism associated with marine and freshwater fish occurred in cooler northern countries.

1.2.5. Fish and seafood, 1936

In the 1930s a toxin was found in sturgeon from the Sea of Azov that caused at least 40 outbreaks in the Ukraine involving 350 persons and 93 deaths (Dolman, 1964). Representative cultures were sent to Dr Meyer at the University of California in San Francisco, who, with his colleagues Janet Gunnison and E.C. Cummings, found that this toxin was not neutralized by any of the previously known types of antitoxin. They proposed that this *C. botulinum* be designated type E (Gunnison et al., 1936).[2] "Fish poisoning," termed *ichthyism*, had been recognized in Russia since 1818, long before the bacteriological era, but even after the discovery of the botulinum toxins the relation of ichthyism to botulism was controversial. In 1937 Elizabeth Hazen of the New York State Department of Health confirmed that a 1934 outbreak of botulism caused by canned sprats imported from Germany had also been caused by this new type E toxin (Hazen, 1937). The durable spores of non-proteolytic bacteria producing type E toxin are only moderately resistant to heat, but the bacteria multiply and produce toxin at unusually low temperatures, making them a frequent cause of lethal food-borne botulism in the colder northern areas of the northern hemisphere, where *C. botulinum* type E is found in soil in contact with either fresh or marine water (Dolman and Iida, 1963). Implicated foods were not canned and were generally unheated. The first reported outbreak of botulism in Japan was in 1951 on the northern island of Hokkaido and was attributed to

---

[1]Since the genus *Bacillus* is restricted to aerobic spore-forming rods, Ida Bengston of the US Public Health Service intentionally placed all anaerobic toxin-producing bacteria into the genus *Clostridium* as a single toxic species, *C. botulinum* (Bengston, 1924). This has become a conglomerate of four quite distinct groups of bacteria, however, and since 1979 two other previously named Clostridium species, *C. baratii* and *C. butyricum*, have been found capable of producing botulinum-like neurotoxins (Hatheway, 1993).

[2]Types C and D had already been described. Type C was isolated simultaneously in 1922 from greenfly larvae involved in "limberneck," a paralytic disease of chickens (Bengston, 1922) and from cattle in Australia with bulbar paralysis (Seddon, 1922). Major outbreaks of botulism among wild waterfowl are often caused by type C. In 1929 type D was isolated from a cow in South Africa that had died from a common paralytic cattle disease called *lamsiekte* (Meyer and Gunnison, 1928). Perhaps because toxigenicity is phage-mediated in types C and D and transport across the human gut is limited, association of these types with human disease is extremely rare. [Type F, first recognized in 1960, is also extremely rare, as is type G, found in soil in Argentina in 1970 (Smith, 1977).]

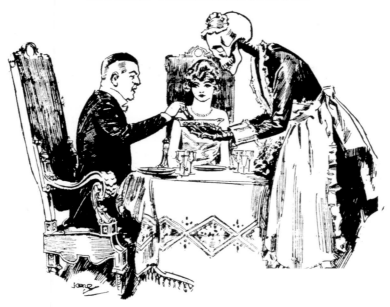

Fig. 1.4. Cartoon from San Francisco Examiner, 7 December 1919. Library of Congress (from Young, 1976, p. 388). Caption read, "It Was in the Olives Which were served as a Relish at Mrs. Sale's Dinner That the Little Newly Discovered Bacillus Botulinus Had Deposited Virulent Poison Which in Less Than a Week sent Five to Their Graves."

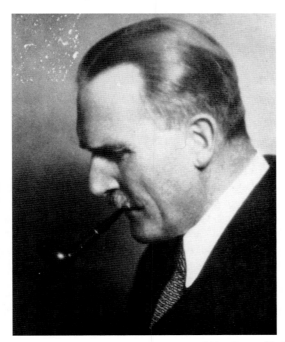

Fig. 1.5. Karl Friederich Meyer, about 1930. (From Clark, 1961, opposite p. 306.)

type E poisoning by a mixture of rice and fermented raw fish called *izushi* (Dolman, 1964).

1.2.6. Wounds, 1951

Clostridium botulinum does not compete well with other bacteria. Food-borne botulism occurs in part because ordinary spoilage bacteria and molds have been killed or inhibited in the improperly preserved food. Normal microflora of the intestine, including non-toxic *Clostridium sporogens*, may therefore be a critical factor in vivo in repressing growth and production of toxin by *C. botulinum*. This competition also may be the reason that (unlike *C. tetanus*) *C. botulinum* spore germination and toxin production in infected wounds in vivo, although produced experimentally (Coleman, 1929), was until recently a rarity in clinical practice. The first three cases of human wound infections by *C. botulinum* were reported in 1951. They described undiagnosed fatal cases of a 15-year-old Pennsylvania girl in 1943 (Davis et al., 1951), a 13-year-old Iowa boy in 1948 (Thomas et al., 1951), and a middle-aged California man in 1951 (Hampson, 1951). By 1975 only 14 cases of wound botulism had been reported in the medical literature (Cherington and Ginsburg, 1975). However, in 1982 the Center for Disease Control in Atlanta, Georgia, began receiving reports of botulism and botulism-like illnesses in chronic drug abusers who employed subcutaneous infiltration, called "skin-popping" (MacDonald et al., 1985). Sinusitis from intranasal cocaine was also implicated (Kudrow et al., 1988). By 1990 another 47 laboratory-confirmed cases of wound botulism had been reported (Weber et al., 1993) and the number of wound botulism cases steadily increases, especially in California with the use of "black-tar" heroin (Maselli et al., 1997).

1.2.7. Infants, 1976

Besides food-borne and wound botulism, a third form of botulism, called "infant botulism" when first recognized in 1976 by Thaddeus Midura and Stephen Arnon of the California State Department of Health Services (Midura and Arnon, 1976), had actually been encountered previously in infants as early as 1931, but at that time the limited diet of infants and the predominance of food-borne botulism inhibited consideration of the possibility of an intestinal toxemia in which ingested spores in the lumen of the large intestine could, under special circumstances, produce botulinum neurotoxin, which then would be absorbed systemically (Arnon et al., 1979). Botulism poisoning due to ingestion of spores had been demonstrated experimentally in guinea pigs in 1922, but the possibility of such occurrence in man was considered "very rare, if it occurs at all" (Orr, 1922). However, Dr Karl Meyer, contacted in 1971 about the case that occurred in California in 1931, speculated correctly that "in the intestinal tract of the baby some spores germinated, multiplied, and produced just enough toxin to cause the symptoms and prolonged illness" (Arnon et al., 1979).

Infant botulism has become the most common form of human botulism recognized in the United States, about half of the approximately 100 cases annually being reported from California (Arnon, 1986). Presumably the normal intestinal flora of adults prevents *C. botulinum* spore germination and colonization of the large intestine, but the simpler diet of infants leads to a simpler flora in which *C. botulinum* spores can germinate, as shown by antibiotic treatment in experimental mouse models (Moberg and Sugiyama, 1979). The first well-documented case of botulism from intestinal toxemia in an adult was reported in 1986, in which predisposing factors of recent gastrointestinal surgery and antibiotic treatment were suggested to explain why the patient but not her husband developed botulism after ingesting cream of coconut that contained type A *C. botulinum* spores but no preformed toxin (Chia et al., 1986). Cases of "unclassified" adult botulism in which no food or wound source can be found are frequently associated with presumed abnormal intestinal flora from surgery and/or antibiotics that may predispose to toxemia originating from botulinum spores in the large intestine.

1.2.8. Site of action, 1949

Justinus Kerner in 1820 attributed the symptoms of botulism to peripheral motor and visceral nerve damage, as did Pürckhauer (also on clinical grounds) in 1877 (Pürckhauer, 1877), whereas in 1897 Van Ermengen remarked that lesions of the central nervous system were probably responsible, based upon pathological examination of his experimental animals. The latter was the generally held opinion of several European histological studies (summarized by Dickson and Shevky, 1923a) until the work of Dale (1914) and Gaskell (1916) suggested to Dickson at Stanford that acetylcholine stimulated the same parts of the nervous system, namely peripheral involuntary "non-sympathetic" fibers and voluntary motor fiber endings, that seemed to be depressed in botulism (Dickson and Shevky, 1923a, b). In investigations from the University of Michigan, the actions of various isolates of toxins from victims of botulism injected into a variety of animals were localized to "the connection mechanism" at the junction between nerve and muscle (Edmunds and Long, 1923), but there was considerable early confusion about whether botulinum toxins affected the terminal nerve endings or the muscle receptors.

Reproducing Langley's now-famous experiments with nicotine and curare (Langley, 1905), Edmunds and Long concluded, using a "botulinus cock," that the "receptive substance" on muscle was "probably normal and that the botulinus toxin had exerted its action on the histologic nerve endings" (Edmunds and Long, 1923). At least nerve conduction and muscle contraction were not affected (Bishop and Bronfenbrenner, 1936). However, using impure cultures of botulinus toxin, Bishop and Bronfenbrenner postulated a "curare-like" action on muscle receptors, but Richard Masland and George Gammon at the University of Pennsylvania accurately described the small initial muscle action potential of a botulinum-poisoned muscle that, unlike curare poisoning, became progressively larger during a subsequent tetanus (Masland and Gammon, 1949).

Lieutenant Arthur Guyton and Captain Marshall MacDonald at the US Army's Camp Detrick, using electrophoretically homogeneous type A toxin, concluded that acetylcholine was not "produced" at vagus nerve endings and the motor endplate (Guyton and MacDonald, 1947). These investigators also demonstrated that the toxin's effects were not reversible by antitoxin, and recovery "must await re-growth of a new element." Using an "about 5% pure" type A toxin on isolated rat phrenic nerve-diaphragm preparations, Burgen and colleagues at Middlesex Hospital in London noted a latent period of 25–40 minutes, during which no effects of the toxin were visible, and they also measured a greatly reduced output of acetylcholine on nerve stimulation (Burgen et al., 1949). This latter important finding was attributed variously to interference with impulse conduction in terminal nerve filaments (Brooks, 1954), decreased acetylcholine synthesis (Torda and

Wolff, 1947), or decreased release of acetylcholine (Stover et al., 1953). As had Guyton and MacDonald earlier (Guyton and MacDonald, 1947), Stephen Thesleff from Lund, Sweden, likened botulinus poisoning to muscle denervation (Thesleff, 1960), poisoned muscle fibers showing persistent fibrillation potentials (Josefsson and Thesleff, 1961).

1.2.9. Toxin type A purification, 1946, and clinical use, 1989

The risk that this "most poisonous poison" (Lamanna, 1959) might be used as a biological warfare agent against the United States stimulated basic research, beginning during World War II, to develop effective toxoid vaccines and antitoxins at Camp Detrick (later named Fort Detrick) in Frederick, Maryland, supported by the US Army Chemical Corps (Middlebrook, 1993). This research included purification of botulinum toxin type A. Building upon the initial work of Herman Sommer at the University of California in San Francisco (Snipe and Sommer, 1928), Carl Lamanna and colleagues at Fort Detrick obtained type A toxin in "crystalline" form (Lamanna et al., 1946). Edward Schantz was charged with producing the purified type A toxin in large amounts at Fort Detrick, and he subsequently provided small amounts of the purified toxin to investigators such as Vernon Brooks (Brooks, 1954) at McGill University in Montreal, Canada, and Daniel Drachman (Drachman, 1971) at Johns Hopkins University in Baltimore, Maryland, for use in experimental animal research (Schantz, 1995). When Fort Detrick closed in 1972, Schantz moved to the University of Wisconsin in Madison.

Meanwhile, in 1970–1971 Alan Scott of the Smith-Kettlewell Eye Research Institute in San Francisco, California, had been examining pharmacological approaches towards correcting strabismus, including injection of local anesthetics, alcohol, cholinesterase inhibitors, and snake toxins into extraocular muscles. Stimulated by Drachman's work with botulinum toxin (Drachman, 1971), Scott used purified toxin type A from Schantz to weaken the extraocular muscles of monkeys successfully for months without side effects (Scott et al., 1973). However, several years passed before the US Food and Drug Administration (FDA) approved Investigational New Drug human volunteer clinical trials for strabismus of what Scott then called "Oculinum." Between 1977 and 1981 these showed that "Oculinum" injections safely and effectively improved strabismus, nystagmus, blepharospasm and hemifacial spasm in humans (Scott, 1981). Eight years later the FDA finally licensed use of "Oculinum" for strabismus and blepharospasm in December 1989.

In 1991 Oculinum, Inc. was sold to the drug company Allergan and in 1992 the name of the product was changed to "Botox." Most of the drug used for humans in the United States came from Batch 79-11 that Schantz prepared in November, 1979. The lot used in Europe for Botox (88-4) had a much higher potency and probably fewer antibodies developed (Scott, 2004).

Recently botulinum toxin type B ("Myobloc") has also become available clinically. The use of small doses of these toxins for focal dystonias, cerebral palsy, facial cosmetics, headache and numerous other forms of excessive muscle contraction represents a brilliant example of the imaginative and courageous clinical application of basic research. One expert has remarked, "I believe I can safely say that more people in this country now are receiving the botulinum toxin by injection than by ingestion" (Foster, 1993).

1.2.10. Mechanism of action, 1992

When Burgen and colleagues made their important discovery in 1949 that botulinum toxin, after a latent period, caused a greatly reduced output of acetylcholine from nerve terminals (Burgen et al., 1949), they said that decreased release of acetylcholine "seems to us unlikely" as a possible explanation, "but cannot confidently be excluded owing to the lack of knowledge of the final mechanism of acetylcholine release" (Burgen et al., 1949). Subsequent investigations indicated that botulinum toxins consisted of heavy and light chain polypeptides, the heavy chain responsible for high-affinity binding to unspecified molecules on the plasma membrane of nerve terminals and subsequent internalization, the light chain then dissociating to block transmitter release (Simpson, 1981). This last step was particularly perplexing until the various toxin types were sequenced. Then it was discovered that botulinum light chains acted as zinc-dependent endopeptidases, those from B, D, F and G types being specific for different parts of a synaptic vesicle membrane protein called *synaptobrevin* or vesicle-associated membrane protein (VAMP) (Schiavo et al., 1992, 1993a, 1994), types A and E specific for *SNAP-25*, a "soluble NSF-attachment protein" (Blasi et al., 1993a; Schiavo et al., 1993b), and type C specific for the active-zone protein called *syntaxin* (Blasi et al., 1993b). These proteins are involved with docking and release of vesicles throughout the body, and have their counterparts even in yeast (Bennett and Scheller, 1993). By destroying one of these proteins, each type of zinc endo-peptidase prevents release of neurotransmitter. Specific membrane-permeable inhibitors of these enzymes might be potential therapeutic agents for the treatment of botulism.

1.3. History of myasthenia gravis and related disorders

The development of ideas regarding the pathogenesis of myasthenia gravis (MG) and related conditions was illustrated in a recent monograph (Keesey, 2002), and the history of treatments for MG in a recent review (Keesey, 2004). This section will attempt to summarize both these aspects of the history of MG.

1.3.1. Clinical recognition, 1879–1899

The 1672 description by Thomas Willis in *De Anima Brutorum* of a "prudent and honest woman" with fluctuating muscle weakness "not only in the members but also in her tongue" (Willis, 1672) is often cited by English-speaking authors as the first description of a case of MG. Willis' brief comment, first in Latin and then translated into English by Pordage (1685), was not associated with MG until 1903 (Guthrie, 1903), 20 years after the clinical aspects of that condition had been described in standard German medical journals and had been differentiated from typical progressive bulbar paralysis or "la paralysie glosso-labio-laryngée" of Duchenne (1860). In 1879 Wilhelm Erb, Professor Extraordinarius in Nikolaus Friedreich's clinic in Heidelberg, described "a new bulbar symptom complex" in three patients with bilateral drooping eyelids, severe neck weakness and trouble chewing, in which the muscle atrophy characteristic of progressive bulbar palsy was absent (Erb, 1879). One of the three patients whom Erb described with this form of "bulbar palsy" recovered after over 60 galvanic treatments to his mastoid bone and neck muscles, a form of electrical therapy pioneered by Erb (1883). A second patient got worse during such electrical treatments. These two patients were also given potassium iodide and iron, while Erb's third patient was treated with quinine, now known to make MG worse, and died suddenly in the night after 18 months of remissions and relapses. No autopsy was performed, but Erb presumed that the origin of the disease was a toxic cause in the brainstem.

Hermann Oppenheim, Privatdocent in Carl Westphal's clinic at the Charité hospital in Berlin, suggested that Erb's "work did not, however, give the impulse to the investigation of this disease and to the establishment of our conception of it" (Oppenheim, 1911). In March 1887 Oppenheim published a paper about a maidservant with prominent bulbar symptoms whom "I had for a long time under clinical observation and had thoroughly investigated pathologically" (Oppenheim, 1887). For Oppenheim "the most remarkable point" was that "most careful microscopical examination of the nervous system gave a negative result." He therefore termed the illness a "chronic progressive and fatal neurosis" (Oppenheim, 1911). Six months later, Carl Eisenlohr, one of Erb's pupils working in Hamburg, was the first to emphasize the extraocular muscle weakness in this syndrome and the remarkable fluctuation of muscle strength during the day (Eisenlohr, 1887). Herman Hoppe, an American working in Oppenheim's polyclinic, published the pathology of a case that Oppenheim had diagnosed during life, and collected all the reported similar cases in an attempt to establish a symptom-complex (Hoppe, 1892; Keesey, 2003). However, it is Samuel Goldflam of Warsaw who is credited with "the most important (paper) ever written in the history of the disease" (Viets, 1953). In 1893 Goldflam described in detail "an apparently curable bulbar paralytic symptom-complex with involvement of the extremities" in three patients with fluctuating weakness of extraocular muscles, jaw muscles and limbs as well as attacks of dyspnea (Goldflam, 1893). All three of Goldflam's "apparently curable" patients improved with galvanic stimulation, iron and quinine, but 19 years later, Goldflam reported that all three of his patients had subsequently died (Goldflam, 1902).

Friedrich Jolly, Professor of Nervous Disease at the University of Berlin, objected to terms that emphasized the bulbar aspects because, he argued, more of the nervous system than the bulb or brainstem might be involved. In 1895 he coined the term "myasthenia gravis pseudoparalytica (generalisata)" to describe the condition in two teenage boys characterized by progressive weakness of muscle contraction on repetitive stimulation that improved with rest (Jolly, 1895). In a discussion at a meeting of the Berlin Society for Psychiatry and Nerve Disease in 1899 about what to call this peculiar condition, Jolly's term won out over ten alternative names (Cohn, 1897), including "asthenic bulbar paralysis" proposed by Adolph Strümpell, Professor of Medicine in Erlangen (Strümpell, 1896). Strümpell's paper contains what may be the first photograph of a patient with MG (Fig. 1.6).

1.3.2. Early symptomatic treatments for MG, 1900–1954

In their 1900 review in the journal Brain, summarizing the 60 then-known cases of "myasthenia gravis," Harry Campbell and Edwin Bramwell stressed rest and avoidance of muscle fatigue, excitement and cold (Campbell and Bramwell, 1900). The following year Oppenheim, in the first monograph on this distinct syndrome, translated as "The Myasthenic Paralysis (Bulbar Paralysis Without Anatomical Findings)," stated that stimulating electrical treatments such as Erb

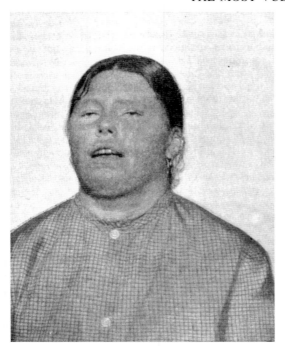

Fig. 1.6. Perhaps the first photograph of a patient with myasthenia gravis. (From Strümpell, 1896, p. 25.)

were considered ineffective by most physicians. For the next decade MG was also treated with "organotherapy" (extracts of suprarenals, thyroid, pituitary and ovarian glands) on the supposition that MG might be an endocrine disorder. Until the 1930s the treatment of MG was "a source of discouragement to the patient and a cause of nightmare for the physician" (Kennedy and Moersch, 1935).

By the use of alkaloids from plants, however, two women permanently changed this dismal outlook. The first woman was Harriet Edgeworth, who herself had myasthenia. After numerous failed regimens, she noted sustained improvement of her MG symptoms with ephedrine, a derivative of the ancient Chinese herb *ma huang* (Edgeworth, 1930, 1933). The second woman was Mary Broadfoot Walker, a house officer at St Alfege's Hospital in Greenwich, England (Fig. 1.7). Prompted by an analogy that her neurology consultant, Derek Denny-Brown, made between MG and curare poisoning, Walker discovered that the antidote to curare, physostigmine, injected subcutaneously, temporarily relieved her MG patients' symptoms of eyelid, jaw and arm muscle weakness and difficulty swallowing (Walker, 1934; Keesey, 1998). Soon after, Walker also showed that the safer synthetic physostigmine analogue, neostigmine methylsulfate (Roche "Prostigmin"), also temporarily relieved the symptoms of MG (Walker, 1935). Walker's two brief reports, each on a single patient, not only offered symptomatic treatment for MG that has stood the test of time, but also provided the most convincing evidence at the time that the neuromuscular junction was the focus of the disease.

and Goldflam used were to be avoided, and instead the patient should rest in bed, speak little, and avoid muscle fatigue, especially during meals (Oppenheim, 1901). "As to drugs," Campbell and Bramwell admitted, "little can be said." Tonics of potassium iodide, iron, mercury, arsenic, and especially large doses of the stimulant strychnine had been tried but

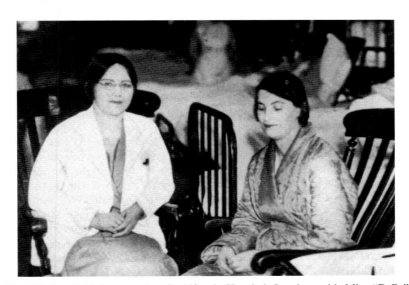

Fig. 1.7. Mary Broadfoot Walker (left) in a ward at St Alfege's Hospital, London, with Miss "D.C.," one of her first MG patients treated with Prostigmin, 1935. (From Keeney and Keeney, 1997, with permission of Springer Science and Business Media.)

While Prostigmin became "the undisputed drug of choice" (Osserman et al., 1954) for the treatment of MG, its short duration of action, the possibility of tolerance, and its pronounced cholinergic adverse effects stimulated a search for other cholinergic drugs that might be effective, long-lasting and nontoxic. Long-acting alkyl phosphates proved too long-lasting, their effects lasting weeks in some cases. Numerous alterations of the neostigmine molecule were also tried, including edrophonium ("Tensilon") by Martha Westerberg of the University of Michigan in 1951 (Westerberg et al., 1951). Pyridostigmine bromide ("Mestinon") was used unsuccessfully at the same milligram dosage as neostigmine in 1948, but seven clinical reports in Europe in 1952 and 1953, and four 1954 reports in the United States, established that four-times-higher doses of pyridostigmine, although weaker than neostigmine and not longer-acting, produced a more even response with less toxicity and was subjectively better tolerated by most MG patients (Osserman et al., 1954; Keesey, 2004). Several other drugs for MG were proposed between 1954 and 1966 (for references, see Keesey, 2004), including ambenonium chloride ("Mysuran" or "Mytelase") in 1954, but from all these attempts pyridostigmine emerged as the new drug of choice for the short-term treatment of the symptoms of MG.

1.3.3. Thymus involvement, from thymoma to thymectomy, 1901–1950

In 1899 Oppenheim reported as an incidental finding the presence of a tumor "the size of a mandarin orange" growing from the thymic remnant of a patient who died from MG (Oppenheim, 1899). Two years later, Carl Weigert of Frankfurt described an invasive lymphoid tumor of thymic origin in the anterior mediastinum of another MG patient. Weigert interpreted it to be a lymphosarcoma because conspicuous collections of lymphoid cells were also found in deltoid, diaphragm and heart muscles (Weigert, 1901). He presumed these to be metastases from the lymphosarcoma, but E. Farquhar Buzzard of London showed that these lymphoid deposits, which he termed "lymphorrhages," were present in muscles, adrenals, thyroid, and liver at autopsies of MG patients who did not have thymic abnormalities (Buzzard, 1905). Elexious T. Bell of the University of Minnesota concluded that only about half of the 56 MG autopsies in his review had thymic lesions, so "thymic lesions cannot be regarded as the cause of myasthenia" (Bell, 1917).

By comparison, almost 20 years later Edgar Norris, then also at the University of Minnesota, concluded from his review that "pathologic changes may be found in the thymus in cases of myasthenia gravis in direct ratio to the care with which they are sought" (Norris, 1936). Surprisingly, Norris nevertheless concluded that lymphorrhages were more characteristic of MG than changes found in the thymus. Ernst Ferdinand Sauerbruch, Professor of Surgery at the University of Zurich, was the first to remove successfully—by a cervical approach—the thymus in a 20-year-old woman with MG, but he did so to treat her concomitant hyperthyroidism (Schumacher and Roth, 1913). Her physicians were surprised that after surgery there was more improvement of the patient's myasthenic symptoms than of the symptoms of hyperthyroidism. Sauerbruch also removed large thymomas (the name suggested by James Ewing in 1916) from two MG patients in the 1930s, but both patients died from infection a few days post-operatively. Sauerbruch designed cumbersome negative pressure chambers in which to perform his thoracic surgery without collapse of the lungs. Similarly, cuirass or tank respirators employing negative pressure, such as the "iron lung" (Drinker and McKhann, 1929), were extensively used subsequently for MG patients with breathing problems. However, intermittent positive pressure ventilation eventually proved to be more effective and lifesaving than negative pressure (Secher, 1987).

In 1936, the year in which Lièvre wrote that he knew of no published report of the successful removal of a thymoma (Lièvre, 1936), Alfred Blalock of Vanderbilt University in Nashville, Tennessee, using a midline sternal approach and positive pressure ventilation via intra-tracheal intubation, successfully removed from a 21-year-old woman with generalized MG the cystic remains of a necrotic thymoma that had been treated previously with two courses of thymic radiation (Blalock et al., 1939). No thymus tissue was identified. Shortly after he assumed the Chair of Surgery at Johns Hopkins University in 1941 (Fig. 1.8), Blalock also performed the first transternal thymectomy on an MG patient without a thymic tumor, and in the next six weeks performed six such operations, claiming improvement in MG had resulted in most of the cases (Blalock et al., 1941). By 1944 he had performed 20 thymectomies for MG, of which 13 were said to have improved. Examination of the pathological specimens from these surgeries revealed characteristic germinal centers in MG thymuses (Sloan, 1943). However, by 1947 Blalock had lost interest, commenting, "I thought we had an answer to this problem of the relationship to the thymus and MG, but such does not appear to be the case" (Clagett and Eaton, 1947). This comment was made after a surgical paper from the Mayo Clinic, where thymectomy results combining MG patients

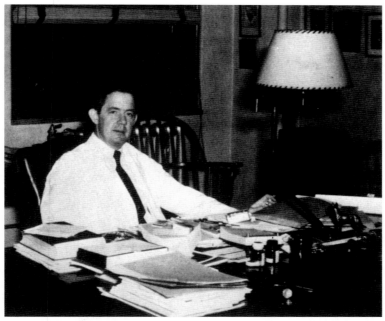

Fig. 1.8. Photograph taken by Dr David Goddard of Alfred Blalock at his desk in his first office at Johns Hopkins Hospital in the early 1940s. (From Ravitch, 1966.)

with and without thymomas were equivocal (Eaton and Clagett, 1950). However, Geoffrey Keynes in London reported that 65% of 120 MG patients without tumors showed complete or almost complete remission of symptoms (Keynes, 1949). He did not operate on thymomas. Problems of heterogeneity, non-randomization and unmatched or no controls have plagued the MG thymectomy literature for over 50 subsequent years, although almost all results of numerous uncontrolled, retrospective reports of thymectomies by a variety of techniques claim that hymectomy is effective as a treatment for MG. Skeptics still call for evidence-based results.

1.3.4. Something in the blood, from curare to muscle antibodies, 1934–1966

From the beginning, speculation about the cause of MG centered on the possibility that some debilitating factor circulated in the blood. Because his first three cases presented within three years of each other, Erb postulated a toxic cause (Erb, 1879). However, he did not see another such case for the next 20 years! In Berlin both Oppenheim (1887) and Jolly (1895) were impressed that MG resembled curare poisoning. Goldflam thought that the disease was the result of an infectious toxin upon the brain (Goldflam, 1893), and Campbell and Bramwell (1900) evoked "a poison probably of microbic origin acting upon the lower

motor neurons." Buzzard (1905) believed that lymphorrhages in MG muscles came from blood vessels because of some "toxic, possibly autotoxic, agent which has a special influence on the protoplasmic constituent of voluntary muscle." All of this was mere speculation until Walker successfully treated MG symptoms with the curare-antidote physostigmine and later demonstrated that fatigue of forearm muscles in an MG patient could induce additional weakness of extraocular muscles. She argued that "myasthenic muscles liberate a chemical agent" (perhaps a normal constituent) "which passes into the blood-stream and blocks neuromuscular transmission at the motor end-plates of skeletal muscle elsewhere" (Walker, 1938). As a result, from 1938 onward into the 1960s numerous short-term experimental studies using MG blood, serum or thymic extracts attempted to prove or disprove, by the response of a neuromuscular preparation from a frog or a cat in an organ bath, the presence of what Mary Walker had called the "curarizing" agent in the blood of myasthenics. Most of these studies were negative, and the few positive ones were unreproducible (for summaries, see Bergh, 1953).

However, the discovery of transient neonatal myasthenia in a few newborns born to myasthenic mothers (Wilson and Stoner, 1944) kept alive the interest in characterizing a circulating substance presumed to pass from mother to infant. William Nastuk at the College of Physicians and Surgeons at Columbia

University in New York City, during similar frog organ bath experiments that produced variable results which he said "could be used as an argument *against* the circulating inhibitor hypothesis," in addition noticed cloudiness of many surface muscle fibers, suggesting the presence of "a cytologic agent of poor penetrating power" (Nastuk et al., 1959). This phenomenon sometimes also occurred with normal sera and was therefore "not a property the appearance of which depends solely on the presence of myasthenia gravis in the donor." Some thermolabile system present in normal serum was apparently essential for cytolytic activity, prompting Nastuk and colleagues (Nastuk et al., 1960) to look at serum complement activity serially in MG patients. They found that complement activity varied much more widely in MG patients than controls (Fig. 1.9) and appeared to follow the activity of the disease, falling during exacerbations and rising even above normal during periods of improvement or stability.

An accompanying paper by Arthur Strauss and colleagues, also at Columbia, described the alternating fluorescent staining pattern on muscle biopsies produced by complement-fixing globulins from pooled sera from 10 MG patients, at least half of whom had thymomas (Strauss et al., 1960). This was confirmed by Ernst Witebsky and associates from the School of Medicine at the University of Buffalo, New York (Beutner et al., 1962). In the Netherlands Hugo van der Geld and colleagues also confirmed the presence of anti-striated muscle antibodies in some sera of MG patients (van der Geld et al., 1964) and in addition showed that over a third of MG sera (and all those associated with a thymoma) also reacted with large "epithelial cells" in sections of calf thymus (Fig. 1.10). The intriguing possibility that the thymic "epithelial cells" that cross-reacted with skeletal muscle antibodies might actually be rounded-up "myoid cells" (Strauss et al., 1966a) was prompted by the concurrent rediscovery of striated myoid cells in embryonic and adult thymuses (Henry, 1966). However, the sera from 24% of patients with thymomas who had no clinical evidence of MG also contained similar antibodies against both thymus and muscle, suggesting that autoantibodies to thymus and muscle in MG patients should be viewed "as indicators rather than as causes of disease" (Strauss et al., 1966b). Their presence nevertheless bolstered the new hypothesis that MG was a disorder with autoimmune features (Simpson, 1960).

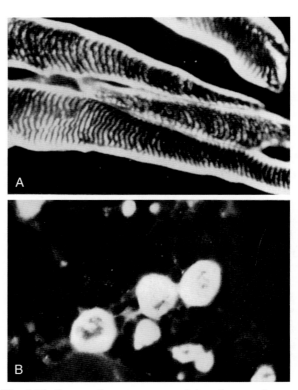

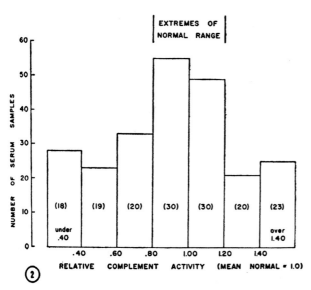

Fig. 1.9. Distribution of relative serum complement (C') activity in serum samples obtained from 68 patients with myasthenia gravis, compared to the average serum C' activity (1.00) of 32 samples from 13 normal individuals (range 0.8–1.2). The numbers in parentheses in each bar indicate the number of MG patients whose C' activities fell in the range indicated. (Nastuk et al., 1960, with permission of the Society for Experimental Biology and Medicine.)

Fig. 1.10. Immunofluorescence reactivity of serum from a patient with myasthenia gravis. The serum reacts with alternate striations of (A) rat skeletal muscle and (B) the cytoplasm of epithelial (myoid?) cells in calf thymus. (Van der Geld and Strauss, 1966, with permission of Elsevier.)

1.3.5. Medical treatments, from adrenal extracts to immunotherapy, 1896–2001

MG is unique in responding to adrenocorticosteroids by sometimes worsening initially, especially at higher doses, before improvement, if any, occurs. Therefore it is not surprising that much controversy characterized the variable results of adrenal extracts given for MG at the end of the 19th century (Marsh, 1974), of anterior pituitary extracts in the 1930s (Simon, 1935; Schlezinger, 1940), cortisone in the 1950s (Millikan and Eaton, 1951; Grob and Harvey, 1952), adrenocorticotropic hormone (ACTH) over a period of 15 years (Torda and Wolff, 1949; Freydberg, 1960; von Reis et al., 1965), and prednisone or prednisolone in the 1970s (Kjaer, 1971; Jenkins, 1972; Warmolts and Engel, 1972).

The above treatments were considered "hormonal therapy" initially (Harvey et al., 1954) and little if any consideration was given to possible immunological aspects of these therapies until after 1960 when Nastuk, Strauss, and colleagues demonstrated the presence of muscle antibodies in sera of patients with MG (Strauss et al., 1960) and Simpson presented his hypothesis that MG might be an autoimmune disease (Simpson, 1960). The discovery of the importance of lymphocytes in the immunological function of the thymus by J.F.A.P. Miller the following year (Miller, 1961) encouraged the use for MG of drugs that had been developed initially for their cytotoxic effects on lymphomas and leukemias but had then been found useful to suppress lymphocytes and immune reactions following renal transplantation. Generally positive results using azathioprine for MG were obtained in Belgium (Delwaide et al., 1967), France (Guille-Minault, 1968), Germany (Mertens et al., 1969; Hertel et al., 1979), and Sweden (Matell et al., 1976), while cyclophosphamide was effective for MG in Czechoslovakia (Nouza and Šmat, 1968) and the Phillipines (Perez et al., 1981). More recently, biological immunosuppressive agents such as cyclosporine (Goulin et al., 1986; Tindall et al., 1987) and mycophenolate mofetil (Chaudhry et al., 2001; Ciafaloni et al., 2001) have also been found useful to treat MG.

While irradiation of the thymus gland for nonthymomatous MG had its advocates throughout the 20th century (Schulz and Schwab, 1971), splenic and total lymphoid irradiation (Engel et al., 1981) and total body irradiation (Durelli et al., 1993) have more recently been proposed as treatments for severe intractable MG. Thoracic duct lymph drainage was also found to be of great value in the acute treatment of myasthenic crisis in Sweden (Bergström et al., 1975). Once serum immunoglobulins were implicated in the pathogenesis of MG (see below), the drawing off of plasma (plasmapheresis or plasma exchange) also became an accepted temporary MG treatment (Pinching et al., 1976; Dau et al., 1977), as did administration of gamma globulin intravenously (IVIG) (Gajdos et al., 1984; Arsura et al., 1986). All of these immunosuppressive treatments were first tried empirically during organ transplantation and other autoimmune diseases before being tried in MG.

1.3.6. But why is the MG patient weak? (1934–1972)

Physicians in the late 19th century who first differentiated MG as a separate disease were surprised to find no pathological explanation in the central nervous system (CNS) of autopsied cases for the characteristic clinical signs of fluctuating skeletal muscle weakness during life. Samuel Wilks commented in 1877 about his case of myasthenic bulbar palsy, "The medulla oblongata was very carefully examined, and no disease was found. It appeared quite healthy to the naked eye, and the microscope discovered no manifest change in the tissue" (Wilks, 1877). Hermann Oppenheim titled his 1901 monograph "Bulbarparalyse ohne anatomischen Befund" (bulbar paralysis without anatomical findings). Even in the 1920s some people remained convinced that the site of pathogenesis could be found in the CNS (Mott and Barrada, 1923; McAlpine, 1929), although the attention of most people in their search for pathology had shifted to muscle (Buzzard, 1905) or to the thymus (Bell, 1917).

It became clear by the middle of the 20th century that the most likely explanation for most of the clinical features of MG was some abnormality of the neuromuscular junction (Walker, 1934; Harvey and Masland, 1941), but there was still considerable disagreement for decades about whether the site of the problem was on the nerve side (presynaptic), the muscle side (postsynaptic), or in between (synaptic). Sir Henry Dale and Wihelm Feldberg demonstrated the possible role of acetylcholine at the neuromuscular junction (Dale and Feldberg, 1934) at about the same time as Mary Walker discovered the positive effect of physostigmine on MG symptoms. So in MG was there a presynaptic deficiency of acetylcholine synthesis by the nerve, excess of cholinesterase breaking down acetylcholine in the synaptic junction, or a block of acetylcholine activity at the postsynaptic muscle endplate? Mary Walker and her pharmacologist, Philip Hamill, offered the hypothesis in 1935 that "in myasthenia gravis there is a defective production at the nerve terminals of acetylcholine or some allied substance, and under the influence of the drug (Prostigmin) destruction of the substance is delayed" (Hamill and Walker, 1935). But in addition to this anti-cholinesterase action, physostigmine and "Prostigmin" also seemed to have an additional anti-curare action at the muscle endplate, an opinion that was again proposed in 1954 when pyridostigmine was introduced into the United States (Osserman et al., 1954). Therefore even the medicines used to treat myasthenia did not provide a specific answer to the question of why MG patients were weak. The neuromuscular pathology in MG continued to elude definite localization even with the availability of the electron microscope after World War II. A careful quantitative study of neuromuscular junction ultrastructure in intercostal muscles from normal controls and patients with MG (Santa et al., 1972) revealed that in MG both the mean *presynaptic* nerve terminal area and the *postsynaptic* membrane folds and clefts were decreased, and the *synaptic* cleft widened (Fig. 1.11).

Indirect evidence for a *postsynaptic* lesion included the demonstration by A.E. Bennett of the University of Nebraska in Omaha that myasthenics were much more sensitive than others to curare (Bennett and Cash, 1943), corroborating the clinical similarities of MG to curare pointed out by Oppenheim (1901) and the similar electrical responses evoked by Harvey and Masland (1941). Curare was considered to compete with acetylcholine for the muscle endplate and thereby block acetylcholine stimulation of muscle. In contrast to their susceptibility to curare, some myasthenic muscles were several times more tolerant to a new "acetylcholine-like" drug, decamethonium, which was not destroyed by cholinesterase and thus depolarized the muscle endplate for several minutes (Churchill-Davidson and Richardson, 1953). However, other myasthenic muscles became rapidly paralyzed by decamethonium but, unlike normal muscles, this paralysis could be reversed by anti-cholinesterases in myasthenic muscles. This was interpreted as a myasthenic "dual response" of the motor endplates to acetylcholine.

A somewhat similar "dual response" was also obtained from myasthenic muscle by intra-arterial injection of acetylcholine, interpreted as decreased responses of myasthenic motor endplates to depolarization (Grob et al., 1956). Other electrical and pharmacological responses of myasthenic muscles that differed from the normal muscle response to curare suggested to John Desmedt at the University of Brussels in Belgium that a *presynaptic* defect was (also) present in MG (Desmedt, 1957), and he was bolstered in this opinion by the myasthenic-like features that occurred after administration of hemicholinium, a chemical compound that strongly inhibits synthesis of acetylcholine by interfering with the supply of choline (Desmedt, 1958). Meanwhile, Dan Elmqvist and colleagues at the University of Lund in Sweden (Elmqvist et al., 1964) reported that the mean amplitude of miniature endplate potentials measured in muscle biopsies with glass electrodes near the endplates of myasthenic muscles was only one-fifth that of normal muscle (Fig. 1.12). While this could be the result of any lesion "upstream" from the endplate, the sensitivity of myasthenic muscle endplates in these biopsies when bathed with acetylcholine-like drugs and decamethonium seemed similar to normal, so these researchers concluded (wrongly, it turned out) that "in myasthenia there is a deficiency in the amount of acetylcholine in the transmitter quantum, probably brought about by a defect in the quantum formation mechanism or by the presence of a 'false transmitter.'"

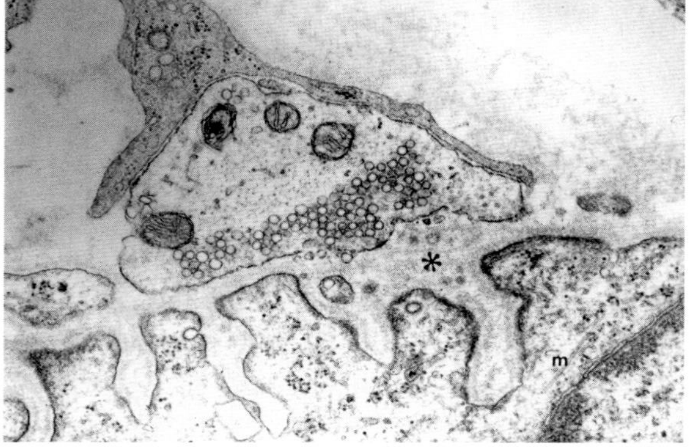

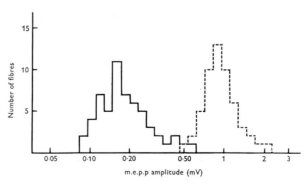

Fig. 1.11. Electron micrograph of a neuromuscular junction of a patient with myasthenia gravis. The postsynaptic folds are wide and secondary synaptic clefts are sparse. The asterisk marks the widened synaptic cleft. (From Santa et al., 1972, with permission of Lippincott Williams & Wilkins.)

Fig. 1.12. Distributions of mean miniature endplate potential amplitudes obtained from 57 muscle fibers of myasthenic patients (full line) and 54 normal muscle fibers (broken line) corrected to a membrane potential of 85 mV. (From Elmqvist et al., 1964, with permission of The Physiological Society, Cambridge, UK.)

1.3.7. Acetylcholine receptor breakthrough, 1963–1977

In just three weeks in the summer of 1939 at Arcachon Marine Biological Station on the west coast of France, Wilhelm Feldberg, Alfred Fessard and David Nachmansohn showed that acetylcholine was the sole physiological stimulus able to excite the *Torpedo* electric organ and cause its discharge (Feldberg et al., 1939), the final demonstration that electric organs of fish (including *Electrophorus electricus*) were actually modified motor endplates of muscles (Keesey, 2005). Nachmansohn, an enzyme chemist, used electric organs of fish to characterize acetylcholinesterase and the enzyme that synthesizes acetylcholine, choline acetyltransferase (Nachmansohn, 1972). In the 1950s Nachmansohn also talked about a hypothetical protein distinct from enzymes, an allosteric "receptor" that could recognize acetylcholine and change configuration (Changeux, 1985). The concept of a receptor was originally a pharmacological one originated in the early days of chemical transmission research (Langley, 1905). Nachmansohn realized that electric organs, because of their abundant cholinergic innervation, might be a rich source of the acetylcholine receptor protein (Whittaker, 1992). However, early attempts at isolation by Chagas, Ehrenpreis, DeRobertis and others were unsuccessful because the "labels" chosen, such as radioactive curare or decamethonium, could bind only reversibly to the receptor.

Working on snake venoms in Taiwan under difficult conditions (Chu, 2005) Chuan-Chiung Chang and Chen-Yuan Lee of National Taiwan University discovered α-bungarotoxin, a neurotoxin that bound specifically and nearly irreversibly to the motor endplate (Chang and Lee, 1963). Now, using α-bungarotoxin labeled with radioactivity, the acetylcholine receptor protein could be labeled and then purified from the electric organs of both *Electrophorus* (Changeux et al., 1970) and *Torpedo* (Miledi et al., 1971), and as a bonus, also separated from the enzyme acetylcholinesterase, which had been thought formerly to be part of the receptor.

In Baltimore, Maryland, in 1972 Douglas Fambrough of the Carnegie Institution and Criss Hartzell of Johns Hopkins University compared the specific locations of radioactive α-bungarotoxin and the endplate marker acetylcholinesterase in single muscle fibers from rats and revealed that virtually all of the acetylcholine receptors, labeled with α-bungarotoxin, were localized in the postsynaptic endplate (Fambrough and Hartzell, 1972). Using human muscle fibers, these tools were applied immediately by Fambrough, Daniel Drachman and S. Satyamurti to the

elucidation of the pathogenesis of MG, in which the number of junctional acetylcholine receptors in myasthenic muscles was found to be reduced to 11–30% of that in normal control muscles (Fambrough et al., 1973). These authors speculated that this reduction in receptors might account for the defect of neuromuscular transmission in MG (Fig. 1.13).

Meanwhile, at the Salk Institute in La Jolla, California, two basic scientists interested in the structure of highly purified *Electrophorus* acetylcholine receptor injected it into rabbits in order to produce antibodies to the eel receptor. Unexpectedly, several of the rabbits died and others developed a flaccid paralysis and respiratory distress (Patrick and Lindstrom, 1973). The rabbit muscles showed a decremental response to repetitive nerve stimulation, similar to MG, and both the weakness and the decremental responses could be alleviated by acetylcholinesterase inhibitors, as suggested by Vanda Lennon (Fig. 1.14). The rabbits produced serum antibodies not only against eel acetylcholine receptor but also against their own muscle acetylcholine receptors. Jim Patrick and Jon Lindstrom postulated that human MG might be an immune response to *human* acetylcholine receptor, and this was demonstrated soon after, 85% of patients with MG demonstrating serum antibodies to human acetylcholine receptor (Lindstrom et al., 1976). Reduction of these antibodies by plasma exchanges of MG patients ameliorated the disease (Pinching et al., 1976; Dau et al., 1977) and passive transfer of immunoglobulin antibodies from MG patients to mice reproduced disease features in the mice (Toyka et al., 1977). These demonstrations indicated that MG was an antibody-mediated autoimmune disease, although the specific antibodies that might be causing weakness were not actually identified by these latter two procedures. Nevertheless, by 1977 the autoimmune pathogenesis of MG, at least at the neuromuscular junction, seemed to have been clearly established by a remarkable series of scientific and clinical contributions.

1.3.8. Lambert–Eaton myasthenic syndrome, 1951–1989

In 1951 physicians at St Thomas's Hospital in London encountered a patient whose severe weakness disappeared almost immediately after removal of a bronchial neoplasm, suggesting to them "that such neoplasms might give rise to an unusual form of peripheral neuropathy, possibly similar to myasthenia gravis" (Anderson et al., 1953). They investigated another case in 1953, a man with a bronchial neoplasm and leg weakness, fatigue and decreased deep tendon reflexes but without ptosis or dysarthria whose response to decamethonium,

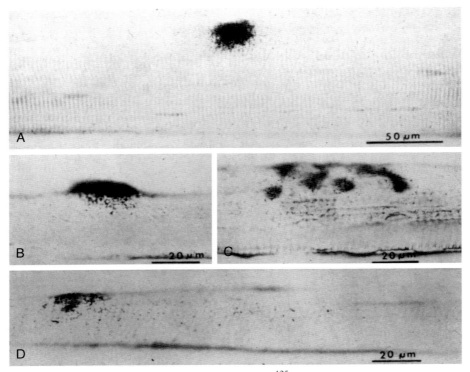

Fig. 1.13. Autoradiographs of human muscle fibers after incubation in ^{125}I-labeled α-bungarotoxin and staining for acetylcholinesterase to reveal neuromuscular junctions. In normal fibers (A and B) there is a dense accumulation of silver grains over a limited junctional area and a paucity of grains outside that region. Fibers from myasthenic patients (C and D) show a markedly reduced number of silver grains, mostly localized over cholinesterase-stained areas in C but localized over an adjacent extra-junctional region in D. (From Fambrough et al., 1973, with permission of American Association for the Advancement of Science.)

d-tubocurarine, succinylcholine and neostigmine was "similar to that seen in myasthenia gravis" (Anderson et al., 1953).

The following year a pathological review from London Hospital of 19 patients with "carcinomatious neuropathy and myopathy" described five patients with carcinoma of the bronchus who exhibited neostigmine-responsive fatigue like that of MG but were different in having sensory complaints, decreased or absent deep tendon reflexes and early muscle wasting (Henson et al., 1954). The adjacent article in the same issue of Brain described five more cases of "peripheral neuropathy and myopathy associated with bronchogenic carcinoma" from St Bartholomew's Hospital in London, among which was a man who was discovered to have a carcinoma of the lung 18 months *after* he developed decreased tendon reflexes and neostigmine-responsive hip and thigh weakness (Heathfield and Williams, 1954). The definitive electrophysiological delineation of this myasthenic syndrome from other carcinomatous neuropathies and from myasthenia gravis was provided by

Edward Lambert and colleagues of the Mayo Clinic, Rochester, Minnesota, who reported at the fall meeting of the American Physiological Society in September, 1956, "an unusual defect in neuromuscular conduction" observed in six patients with evidence of a malignant chest tumor (Lambert et al., 1956). The characteristic electrophysiological findings of this syndrome were a greatly decreased compound muscle action potential to a single stimulus and pronounced facilitation of this decreased response to stimulation rates greater than 10 Hz. The first full description of the new syndrome in 1959 called it "Myasthenic Syndrome S.C.Ca," meaning "myasthenic syndrome sometimes associated with small cell bronchogenic carcinoma" (Lambert et al., 1961), but the suggested name was so awkward that it was soon replaced by Eaton–Lambert syndrome and eventually by Lambert–Eaton myasthenic syndrome or LEMS (Keesey, 2002). Intracellular microelectrode studies of muscle biopsies from patients with this syndrome showed insufficient release of acetylcholine quanta (Elmqvist and Lambert, 1968). This could be increased

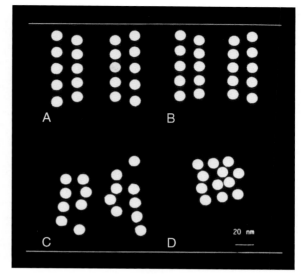

Fig. 1.15. Stereometric reconstruction of the spacing and arrangement of particles in normal active zones of control mice (A) and in active zones of mice treated with LEMS IgG (B, C and D). Disruption (C) and clustering (D) of active zone particles occurred in treated mice. (From Fukuoka et al., 1987a, with permission of John Wiley & Sons, Inc.)

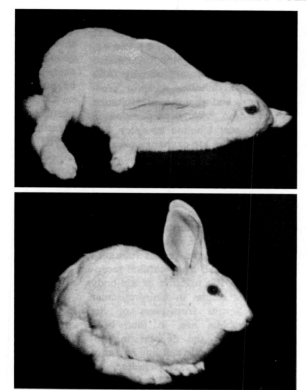

Fig. 1.14. The upper photograph shows a rabbit five days after the third injection of purified eel acetylcholine receptor protein. The lower photograph is of the same animal one minute after receiving 0.3 mg edrophonium intravenously. (From Patrick and Lindstrom, 1973, with permission of American Association for the Advancement of Science.)

by increasing extracellular calcium, indicating that calcium entry into motor nerve terminals might be reduced. Association of LEMS with autoimmune disorders (Gutmann et al., 1972) and benefit from plasmapheresis (Denys et al., 1979) suggested that LEMS might be an autoimmune disease of presynaptic motor nerve terminals (Lang et al., 1981). This hypothesis was strengthened (Fukunaga et al., 1982) by the visualization by electron microscopy of the paucity and disorganization of active zone particles on presynaptic neuromuscular membranes (Fig. 1.15).

The two leading laboratories investigating LEMS at that time, one at the Mayo Clinic and the other at the Royal Free Hospital in London, collaborated in 1987 on two important papers, the first showing that several days of "passive transfer" of serum IgG from LEMS patients into mice produced similar disruption and clustering of active zones of mouse motor nerve endings (Fukuoka et al., 1987a). The second paper showed that ferritin particles attached to immunoglobulin from LEMS

patients could be localized by electron microscopy to this same presynaptic target (Fukuoka et al., 1987b). Physiologically, LEMS immunoglobulin produced a 30–40% reduction in the number of functional presynaptic voltage-gated calcium channels (Lang et al., 1987). Radioimmune antibody assays employing cone shell toxins and spider venom suggest that LEMS antibodies bind preferentially to several subunits of different types of voltage-gated calcium channels.

1.3.9. Congenital myasthenic syndromes, 1937–1990

Children who develop myasthenia have always been of special interest, ever since the first case of probably autoimmune myasthenia in a child—that of a previously healthy two-year-old boy who died suddenly after a month's illness—was described by Max Mailhouse, a neurologist at the Vanderbilt Clinic in New York City (Mailhouse, 1898). A special situation seemed to apply when the myasthenia occurred at birth and was "congenital" and permanent (Fig. 1.16). When more than one child in a family was affected, this was termed "familial myasthenia." Paul Levin of Dallas, Texas, emphasized the "perfect symmetry" of the muscular weakness in congenital myasthenia and the stability of its course (Levin, 1949).

The true difference between these cases of congenital or familial myasthenia and other cases of MG,

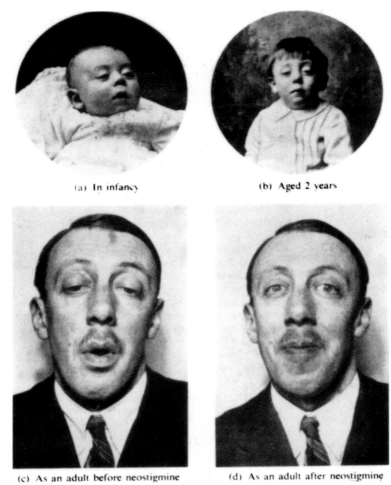

(a) In infancy   (b) Aged 2 years

(c) As an adult **before** neostigmine   (d) As an adult after neostigmine

Fig. 1.16. Congenital myasthenia that occurred at birth and persisted as an adult. The lower right photograph shows the response to neostigmine. (From Greene, 1969, with permission of Heinemann Publishers, Oxford, UK.)

however, could not be appreciated until the specific autoimmune nature of most MG was elucidated in the 1970s. Cases of congenital myasthenia never had elevated titers of serum acetylcholine receptor antibody, nor did they respond to thymectomy or immunosuppression. The possibility that congenital myasthenia was genetic rather than autoimmune was examined, particularly at the Mayo Clinic by Andrew Engel using quantitative electron microscopy and cytochemistry of muscle biopsies from patients with congenital myasthenia, and by Lambert using microelectrodes to analyze the electrophysiology of the same muscle biopsies in vitro.

When thoroughly studied in this way, several congenital myasthenic syndromes could be grouped into genetic defects of presynaptic, synaptic and postsynaptic proteins. Presynaptic syndromes included choline acetyltransferase mutations that produced episodic apnea (Greer and Schotland, 1960; Conomy et al.,

1975; Ohno et al., 2001) and a congenital myasthenic syndrome resembling the Lambert–Eaton syndrome (Bady et al., 1987). Mutations of the collagen-like tail subunit of the endplate species of acetylcholinesterase provided examples of synaptic defects, first described in 1977 (Engel et al., 1977; Engel et al., 1999). Most postsynaptic congenital myasthenic syndromes were associated with a kinetic abnormality or decreased expression of the acetylcholine receptor. These included the dominantly inherited "slow channel syndromes" (Engel et al., 1982) with increased affinity for acetylcholine and prolonged open times of the acetylcholine-induced ion channel (Engel et al., 1999), and the recessively inherited "fast channel syndromes," in which there seems to be decreased affinity for acetylcholine (Engel et al., 1990). Each of these "experiments of nature" has provided unique information about the importance of the multiple steps required for effective communication between nerve and muscle.

1.3.10. Seronegative myasthenia and muscle-specific receptor tyrosine kinase antibodies, 1981–2001

The sera of 10–25% of patients with MG have no elevated antibodies to human muscle acetylcholine receptor and were initially called "seronegative" (Sanders et al., 1997). The clinical features of seronegative MG patients were initially thought to be very similar to those of antibody-positive MG patients (Soliven et al., 1988), although the seronegative patients were more likely to have milder disease or purely ocular myasthenia (Sanders et al., 1997). The possibility of an antibody different from that directed toward the acetylcholine receptor was suggested by the facts that some seronegative MG patients improved when they were treated with plasma exchange (Miller et al., 1981), and immunoglobulins from some seronegative MG patients could passively transfer a distinct disease to mice although acetylcholine receptor loss was minimal (Mossman et al., 1986).

A possible candidate for such an antibody was proposed by Hoch et al. (2001) in Oxford, UK, when 70% of 24 serum samples from "seronegative" generalized MG patients were reported to contain an antibody again muscle-specific receptor tyrosine kinase (MuSK), a protein on the muscle side of the neuromuscular junction that during synapse formation mediates agrin-induced clustering of acetylcholine receptors. The function of MuSK in mature neuromuscular synapses is not clear, but the presence of MuSK antibodies has been confirmed repeatedly in a varying percentage of MG patients previously thought to be seronegative. The clinical features of these MuSK-positive MG patients may be different from those of MG patients with serum antibodies to acetylcholine receptor, and the therapeutic responses to conventional MG therapies may also be different (Vincent and Leite, 2005). Changes in the thymus of MuSK-positive MG patients are minimal (Lauriola et al., 2005). At this time there is still considerable doubt about the role of serum MuSK-antibodies in clinical MG (Lindstrom, 2004).

References

Anderson HJ, Churchill-Davidson HC, Richardson AT (1953). Bronchial neoplasm with myasthenia, prolonged apnoea after administration of succinylcholine. Lancet 2: 1291–1293.

Arnon SS (1986). Infant botulism: anticipating the second decade. J Infect Dis 154: 201–206.

Arnon SS, Werner SB, Faber HK, et al. (1979). Infant botulism in 1931, discovery of a misclassified case. Am J Dis Child 133: 580–582.

Arsura EL, Bick A, Brunner NG, et al. (1986). High-dose intravenous immunoglobulin in the management of myasthenia gravis. Arch Intern Med 146: 1365–1368.

Bady B, Chauplannaz G, Carrier H (1987). Congenital Lambert–Eaton myasthenic syndrome. J Neurol Neurosurg Psychiatry 50: 476–478.

Bell ET (1917). Tumors of the thymus in myasthenia gravis. J Nerv Ment Dis 45: 130–143.

Bengtson IA (1922). Preliminary note on a toxin-producing anaerobe isolated from the larvae of Lucilia Caesar. Public Health Rep 37: 164–170.

Bengtson IA (1924). Studies on Organisms Concerned as Causative Factors in Botulism. Hygienic Lab Bull No.136, Government Printing Office, Washington, pp. 1–101.

Bennett AE, Cash PB (1943). Myasthenia gravis-curare sensitivity, a new diagnostic test and approach to causation. Arch Neurol Psychiatry 49: 537–547.

Bennett MK, Scheller RH (1993). The molecular machinery for secretion is conserved from yeast to neurons. Proc Natl Acad Sci U S A 90: 2559–2563.

Bergh NP (1953). Biological assays in myasthenia gravis for any agents causing a neuromuscular block. Scand J Clin Lab Invest 5(Suppl 5): 1–47.

Bergström K, Franksson C, Matell G, et al. (1975). Drainage of thoracic duct lymph in twelve patients with myasthenia gravis. Eur Neurol 13: 19–30.

Bernard C (1857). Leçons sur les effect des substances toxiques et médicamenteuses. J-B Baillière et fils, Paris, pp. 238–353.

Beutner EB, Witebsky E, Ricken D, et al. (1962). Studies on autoantibodies in myasthenia gravis. JAMA 182: 156–168.

Bishop GH, Bronfenbrenner JJ (1936). The site of action of botulinus toxin. Am J Physiol 117: 393–404.

Blalock A, Mason MF, Morgan HJ, et al. (1939). Myasthenia gravis and tumors of the thymic region: report of a case in which the tumor was removed. Ann Surg 110: 544–561.

Blalock A, Harvey AM, Ford FR, et al. (1941). The treatment of myasthenia gravis by removal of the thymus gland: preliminary report. JAMA 117: 1529–1533.

Blasi J, Chapman ER, Link E, et al. (1993a). Botulinum neurotoxin A selectively cleaves the synaptic protein SNAP-25. Nature 365: 160–163.

Blasi J, Chapman ER, Yamasaki S, et al. (1993b). Botulinum neurotoxin C blocks neurotransmitter release by means of cleaving HPC-1/syntaxin. EMBO J 12: 4821–4828.

Boerhaave H (1743). Institutiones Medicae, Leyden, p. 91, cited in Brazier MAB (1984). A History of Neurophysiology in the 17th and 18th Centuries, From Concept to Experiment. Raven Press, New York, p. 114.

Brooks VB (1954). The action of botulinum toxin on motor-nerve filaments. J Physiol 123: 501–515.

Brown GL (1937). Transmission at nerve endings by acetylcholine. Physiol Rev 17: 485–513.

Burgen ASV, Dickens F, Zatman LJ (1949). The action of botulinum toxin on the neuro-muscular junction. J Physiol 109: 10–24.

Burke GS (1919). Notes on Bacillus botulinus. J Bacteriol 4: 555–565.

Buzzard EF (1905). The clinical history and post-mortem examination of five cases of myasthenia gravis. Brain 28: 438–483.

Campbell H, Bramwell E (1900). Myasthenia gravis. Brain 23: 277–336.

Chang CC, Lee CY (1963). Isolation of neurotoxins from the venom of Bungarus multicinctus and their modes of neuromuscular blocking action. Arch Int Pharmacodyn Ther 144: 241–257.

Changeux JP (1985). David Nachmansohn (1899–1983): a pioneer of neurochemistry. In: Molecular Basis of Nerve Activity. Walter de Gruyter, Berlin, pp. 1–32.

Changeux JP, Kasai M, Lee C-Y (1970). Use of a snake venom toxin to characterize the cholinergic receptor protein. Proc Natl Acad Sci U S A 67: 1241–1247.

Chaudhry V, Cornblath DR, Griffin JW, et al. (2001). Mycophenolate mofetil: a safe and promising immunosuppressant in neuromuscular diseases. Neurology 56: 94–96.

Cherington M, Ginsburg S (1975). Wound botulism. Arch Surg 110: 436–438.

Chia JK, Clark JB, Ryan CA, et al. (1986). Botulism in an adult associated with food-borne intestinal infections with Clostridium botulinum. N Engl J Med 315: 239–241.

Chu NS (2005). Contribution of a snake venom toxin to myasthenia gravis; the discovery of α-bungarotoxin in Taiwan. J Hist Neurosci 14: 138–148.

Churchill-Davidson HC, Richardson AT (1953). The action of decamethonium iodide (C.10) in myasthenia gravis. J Neurol Neurosurg Psychiatry 15: 129–133.

Ciafaloni E, Massey JM, Tucker-Lipscomb B, et al. (2001). Mycophenolate mofetil for myasthenia gravis: an open-label pilot study. Neurology 56: 97–99.

Clagett OT, Eaton LM (1947). Surgical treatment of myasthenia gravis. J Thorac Surg 16: 62–80.

Clark PF (1961). Pioneer Microbiologists of America. University of Wisconsin Press, Madison, Wisconsin.

Cohn T (1897). Ueber myasthenia pseudoparalytica gravis. Dtsch Med Wochenschr 23: 785–789.

Coleman GE (1929). Intramuscular infection of guinea pigs with spores of Cl. botulinum. Am J Hygiene 9: 47–55.

Conomy JP, Levinsohn M, Fanaroff A (1975). Familial infantile myasthenia gravis: a cause of sudden death in young children. J Pediatr 87: 428–430.

Dale HH (1914). The action of certain esters and ethers of choline, and their relation to muscarine. J Pharmacol Exp Therap 6: 147–190.

Dale HH, Feldberg W (1934). Chemical transmission at motor nerve endings in voluntary muscle? J Physiol 81: 39P–40P.

Dau PC, Lindstrom JM, Cassel CK, et al. (1977). Plasmapheresis and immunosuppressive drug therapy in myasthenia gravis. N Engl J Med 297: 1134–1140.

Davis JB, Mattman LH, Wiley M (1951). Clostridium botulinum in a fatal wound infection. JAMA 146: 646–648.

Delwaide PJ, Salmon J, van Cauwenberger H (1967). Premiers essais de traitement de la myasthenia par azathioprine. Acta Neurol Psychiatr Belg 67: 701–712.

Denys EH, Dau PC, Lindstrom JM (1979). Neuromuscular transmission before and after plasmapheresis in myasthenia gravis and the myasthenic syndrome. In: PC Dau (Ed.), Plasmapheresis and the Immunology of Myasthenia Gravis. Houghton Mifflin, Boston, pp. 248–257.

Desmedt JE (1957). Nature of the defect of neuromuscular transmission in myasthenic patients: "post-tetanic exhaustion." Nature (London) 179: 156–157.

Desmedt JE (1958). Myasthenic-like features of neuromuscular transmission after administration of an inhibitor of acetylcholine synthesis. Nature (London) 182: 1673–1674.

Devriese PP (1999). The discovery of Clostridium botulinum. J Hist Neurosci 8: 43–50.

Dickson EC (1918). Botulism, a clinical and experimental study. Monographs of the Rockerfeller Institute for Medical Research. No. 8, Rockerfeller Institute, New York, p. 8.

Dickson EC, Shevky R (1923a). Studies on the manner in which the toxin of Clostridium botulinum acts upon the body, I. The effect upon the autonomic nervous system. J Exp Med 37: 711–731.

Dickson EC, Shevky R (1923b). Studies on the manner in which the toxin of Clostridium botulinum acts upon the body, II. The effect upon the voluntary nervous system. J Exp Med 38: 327–346.

Dolman CE (1964). Botulinism as a world problem. In: KH Lewis, D Cassel (Eds.), Botulism, Proceedings of a Symposium. Public Health Service, Cincinnati, Ohio, pp. 5–30.

Dolman CE, Iida H (1963). Type E botulism: its epidemiology, prevention and specific treatment. Can J Public Health 54: 293–308.

Doyére M (1840). Mémoire sur les tardigrades. Ann Sci Nat 14: 269–351.

Drachman DB (1971). Botulinum toxin as a tool for research on the nervous system. In: LL Simpson (Ed.), Neuropoisons. Plenum Press, New York, pp. 325–346.

Drinker P, McKhann CF (1929). The use of a new apparatus for the prolonged administration of artificial respiration. JAMA 92: 1658–1660.

Du Bois-Reymond EH (1877). Gesammelte Abhandlungen zur allgemeinen Muskel- und Nervenphysik. Vol. 2. Veit, Leipzig.

Duchenne GBA (1860). Paralysie musculaire progressive de la langue, du voile, du palais et des lèvres; affection non encore décrite comme espèce morbide distincte. Arch Gén Méd (5 ser) 16: 283, 431.

Durelli L, Ferrio MF, Urgesi A, et al. (1993). Total body irradiation for myasthenia gravis; a long-term follow-up. Neurology 43: 2215–2221.

Eaton LM, Clagett OT (1950). Thymectomy in the treatment of myasthenia gravis. Results in seventy-two cases compared to one hundred and forty-two control cases. JAMA 142: 963–967.

Edgeworth H (1930). A report of progress on the use of ephedrine in a case of myasthenia gravis. JAMA 94: 1136.

Edgeworth H (1933). The effect of ephedrine in the treatment of myasthenia gravis: second report. JAMA 100: 1401.

Edmunds CW, Long PH (1923). Contribution to the pathologic physiology of botulism. JAMA 81: 542–547.

Eisenlohr C (1887). Ein Fall von Opththalmolplegia externa progressive und finaler Bulbärparalyse mit negativem

Sectionsbefund. Neurologisches Centralblatt 6: 337–341, 361–365, 389–390.

Elmqvist D, Lambert EH (1968). Detailed analysis of neuromuscular transmission in a patient with the myasthenic syndrome sometimes associated with bronchogenic carcinoma. Mayo Clinic Proc 43: 689–713.

Elmqvist D, Hofmann WW, Kugelberg J, et al. (1964). An electrophysiological investigation of neuromuscular transmission in myasthenia gravis. J Physiol 174: 417–434.

Engel AG, Lambert EH, Gomez M (1977). A new myasthenic syndrome with end-plate acetylcholinesterase deficiency, small nerve terminals and reduced acetylcholine release. Ann Neurol 1: 315–330.

Engel AG, Lambert EH, Mulder DM, et al. (1982). A newly recognized congenital myasthenic syndrome attributed to a prolonged open time on the acetylcholine-induced ion channel. Ann Neurol 11: 553–569.

Engel AG, Walls TJ, Nagel A, et al. (1990). New recognized congenital myasthenic syndromes: I. Congenital paucity of synaptic vesicles and reduced quantal release, II. High-conductance fast-channel syndrome, III. Abnormal acetylcholine receptor (achr) interaction with acetylcholine, IV. Achr deficiency and short channel-open time. Prog Brain Res 84: 125–137.

Engel AG, Ohno K, Sine SM (1999). Congenital myasthenic syndromes. In: AG Engel (Ed.), Myasthenia Gravis and Myasthenic Disorders. Oxford, New York, pp. 251–297.

Engel WK, Lichter AS, Dalakas M (1981). Splenic and total-body irradiation treatment of myasthenia gravis. Ann N Y Acad Sci 377: 744–754.

Erb W (1879). Sur Cauistik der bulbären lähmungen. Arch Psychiatr Nervenkr 9: 336–350.

Erb W (1883). Handbook of Electrotherapeutics. L Pützel (Trans.). William Woods, New York.

Erbguth FJ, Naumann M (1999). Historical aspects of botulinum toxin, Justinus Kerner (1786–1862) and the "sausage poison." Neurology 53: 1850–1853.

Estable C (1959). Curare and synapse. In: D Bovet, F Bovet-Nitti, GB Marini-Bettòlo (Eds.), Curare and Curare-like Agents. Elsevier, Amsterdam, pp. 356–373.

Fambrough DM, Hartzell HC (1972). Acetylcholine receptors: number and distribution at neuromuscular junctions in rat diaphragm. Science 176: 189–190.

Fambrough DM, Drachman DB, Satyamurti S (1973). Neuromuscular junction in myasthenia gravis: decreased acetylcholine receptors. Science 182: 193–195.

Fatt P, Katz B (1952). Spontaneous subthreshold activity at motor nerve endings. J Physiol 117: 109–128.

Feldberg W, Fessard A, Nachmansohn D (1939). The cholinergic nature of the nervous supply to the electrical organ of the torpedo (Torpedo marmorata). J Physiol 97: 3P–4P.

Foster EM (1993). Reflections on a half-century of food-borne botulism. In: BR DasGupta (Ed.), Botulinum and Tetanus Neurotoxins. Plenum Press, New York, pp. 505–513.

Freydberg LD (1960). The place of corticotrophin in the treatment of myasthenia gravis. Ann Intern Med 52: 806–818.

Fukunaga H, Engel AG, Osame M, et al. (1982). Paucity and disorganization of presynaptic membrane active zones in the Lambert–Eaton myasthenic syndrome. Muscle Nerve 5: 686–697.

Fukuoka T, Engel AG, Lang B, et al. (1987a). Lambert–Eaton myasthenic syndrome I. Early morphological effects of IgG on the presynaptic membrane active zones. Ann Neurol 22: 193–199.

Fukuoka T, Engel AG, Lang B, et al. (1987b). Lambert–Eaton myasthenic syndrome II. Immunoelectron microscopy localization of IgG at the mouse motor endplate. Ann Neurol 22: 200–221.

Gajdos P, Outin H, Elkharrat D, et al. (1984). High-dose intravenous gammaglobulin for myasthenia gravis. Lancet 1: 406–407.

Gaskell WH (1916). The Involuntary Nervous System. Monographs on Physiology. Longmans Green, London, p. 178.

Goldflam S (1893). Ueber einen scheinbar heilbaren bulbärparalytischen Symptomencomplex mit Betheiligung der Extremitäten. Dtsch Z Nervenheilkd 4: 312–352.

Goldflam S (1902). Weisteres uber die asthenische lahmung nebst einem obductionsbufund. Neurologishes Zentralblatt 21: 97–107, 490–496.

Goulin M, Elkharrat D, Gajdos P, et al. (1986). Preliminary results in myasthenia gravis treated with cyclosporin. Ann N Y Acad Sci 505: 857–860.

Greene R (1969). Myasthenia Gravis. Heinemann, London.

Greer M, Schotland M (1960). Myasthenia gravis in the newborn. Pediatrics 26: 101–108.

Grob D, Harvey AM (1952). Effect of adrenocorticotropic hormone (ACTH) and cortisone administration in patients with myasthenia gravis, and report on onset of myasthenia gravis during prolonged cortisone administration. Bull Johns Hopkins Hosp 91: 124–136.

Grob D, Johns RJ, Harvey AM (1956). Studies in neuromuscular function IV. Stimulating and depressant effects of acetylcholine and choline in patients with myasthenia gravis, and their relationship to the defect in neuromuscular transmission. Bull Johns Hopkins Hosp 99: 153–181.

Grüsser O-J (1986). Die ersten systematischen Beschreibungen und tierexperimentellen Untersuchungen des Botulismus. Sudhoffs Arch Z Wissenschaftsgesch 70: 167–187.

Guille-Minault C (1968). Premiers essais de traitement de la myasthenia par azathioprine. Gaz Med Fr 75: 6545.

Gunnison JB, Cummings JR, Meyer KF (1936). Clostridium botulinum type E. Proc Soc Exptl Biol Med 31: 278–280.

Guthrie LG (1903). "Myasthenia gravis" in the seventeenth century. Lancet 1: 330–331.

Gutmann L, Crosby TW, Takamore M, et al. (1972). The Lambert–Eaton syndrome and autoimmune disorders. Am J Med 53: 354–356.

Guyton AC, MacDonald MA (1947). Physiology of botulinus toxin. Arch Neurol Psychiatry 57: 578–592.

Hamill P, Walker MB (1935). The action of "Prostigmin" (Roche) in neuro-muscular disorders. J Physiol 83: 36P–37P.

Hampson CR (1951). A case of probable botulism due to wound infection. J Bacteriol 61: 647.

Harvey AM, Masland RL (1941). The electromyogram in myasthenia gravis. Bull Johns Hopkins Hosp 69: 1–13.

Harvey AM, Shulman LE, Tumulty PA, et al. (1954). Systemic lupus erythematosus: review of the literature and clinical analysis of 138 cases. Medicine 33: 291–437.

Hatheway CL (1993). Bacteriology and pathology of neurotoxigenic Clostridia. In: BR DasGupta (Ed.), Botulinum and Tetanus Neurotoxins. Plenum Press, New York, pp. 491–502.

Hazen EL (1937). A strain of B. botulinus not classified as A, B or C. J Infect Dis 60: 260–264.

Heathfield KWG, Williams JRB (1954). Peripheral neuropathy and myopathy associated with bronchogenic carcinoma. Brain 77: 122–137.

Henry K (1966). Mucin secretion and striated muscle in the human thymus. Lancet 1: 183–185.

Henson RA, Russell DS, Wilkinson M (1954). Carcinomatous neuropathy and myopathy, a clinical and pathological study. Brain 77: 122–137.

Hertel G, Mertens HG, Reuther P, et al. (1979). The treatment of myasthenia gravis with azathioprine. In: PC Dau (Ed.), Plasmapheresis and the Immunobiology of Myasthenia Gravis. Houghton Mifflin, Boston, pp. 315–328.

Hoch W, McConville J, Helms S, et al. (2001). Autoantibodies to the receptor tyrosine kinase musk in patients with myasthenia gravis without acetylcholine receptor antibodies. Nat Med 7: 365–368.

Hoppe HH (1892). Ein Beitrag zur Kenntniss der Bulbär-Paralyse. Berliner Klinische Wochenschrift 29: 332–336.

Jenkins RB (1972). Treatment of myasthenia gravis with prednisone. Lancet 1: 765–767.

Jolly FI (1895). Ueber myasthenia gravis pseudoparalytica. Berl Klin Wochenschr 32: 1–7.

Josefsson JO, Thesleff S (1961). Electromyographic findings in experimental botulinum intoxication. Acta Physiol Scand 51: 163–168.

Keeney AH, Keeney VT (1997). Mary B. Walker M.D. and the pioneering use of prostigmin to treat myasthenia gravis. Doc Ophthalmol 93: 125–134.

Keesey JC (1998). Contemporary opinions about Mary Walker, a shy pioneer of therapeutic neurology. Neurology 51: 1433–1439.

Keesey JC (2002). Myasthenia Gravis, an Illustrated History. Publishers Design Group, Roseville, California, pp. 24–25.

Keesey JC (2003). The role of Herman Hoppe of Cincinnati in the initial clinical recognition of myasthenia gravis. J Hist Neurosci 12: 167–174.

Keesey JC (2004). A history of treatments for myasthenia gravis. Semin Neurol 24: 5–16.

Keesey JC (2005). How electric fish became sources of acetylcholine receptor. J Hist Neurosci 14: 148–164.

Kennedy FS, Moersch FP (1935). Myasthenia gravis: a clinical review of eighty-seven cases observed between 1915 and the early part of 1932. CMAJ 37: 216–223.

Kerner J (1820). Neue Beobachtungen über die in Würtemberg so häufig vorfallenden tödlichen Vergiftungen durch den Genuss geräucherter Wurste. Osiander, Tübingen, p. 120.

Kerner J (1822). Das Fettgift oder die Fettsäure und ihre Wirkungen auf den theirischen Organismus, ein Beytrag zur Untersuchung des in verdorbenen Würsten giftig wirkenden Stoffes. Cotta, Stuttgart und Tübingen, p. 368.

Keynes G (1949). The results of thymectomy in myasthenia gravis. BMJ 1: 611–616.

Kjaer M (1971). Myasthenia gravis and myasthenic syndromes treated with prednisone. Acta Neurol Scand 47: 464–474.

Kudrow DB, Henry DA, Haake DA, et al. (1988). Botulism associated with Clostridium botulinum sinusitis after intranasal cocaine abuse. Ann Intern Med 109: 984–985.

Kühne W (1863). Uber die peripherischen Endogane der motorischen Nerven, Mit 5 Tafeln. W. Engelmann, Leipzig.

Lamanna C (1959). The most poisonous poison. Science 130: 763–772.

Lamanna C, Eklund HW, McElroy OE (1946). Botulinum toxin (type A), including a study of shaking with chloroform as a step in the isolation procedure. J Bacteriol 52: 1–13.

Lambert EH, Eaton LM, Rooke ED (1956). Defect of neuromuscular conduction associated with malignant neoplasms. Am J Physiol 187: 612–613.

Lambert EH, Rooke ED, Eaton LM, et al. (1961). Myasthenic syndrome occasionally associated with bronchial neoplasm: neurophysiologic studies. In: HR Viets (Ed.), Myasthenia Gravis, The Second International Symposium Proceedings. CC Thomas, Springfield, Illinois, pp. 362–410.

Landman G (1904). Ueber die Ursache der Darmstadter Bohnenvergiftung. Hyg Rundschau 10: 449–452.

Lang B, Newsom-Davis J, Wray D, et al. (1981). Autoimmune aetiology for myasthenic (Eaton–Lambert) syndrome. Lancet 2: 224–226.

Lang B, Newsom-Davis J, Peers C, et al. (1987). The effect of myasthenia syndrome antibody on presynaptic calcium channels in the mouse. J Physiol 390: 257–270.

Langley JN (1905). On the reaction of cells and of nerve-endings to certain poisons, chiefly as regards the reaction of striated muscle to nicotine and to curare. J Physiol 33: 376–413.

Lauriola L, Ranelletti F, Maggiano N, et al. (2005). Thymus changes in anti-musk – positive and negative myasthenia gravis. Neurology 64: 536–538.

Leuchs J (1910). Beitrage zu Kenntnis des Toxins und Antitoxins des Bacillus botulinus. Atschr Hyg Infection 65: 55–84.

Levin PM (1949). Congenital myasthenia in siblings. Arch Neurol Psychiatry 62: 745–758.

Lièvre JA (1936). Peut-on tenter un traitement chircurgical de la myasthénia? Presse Med 44: 991–992.

Lindstrom JM (2004). Is "seronegative" MG explained by autoantibodies to musk? Neurology 62: 1920–1921.

Lindstrom JM, Seybold ME, Lennon VA, et al. (1976). Antibody to acetylcholine receptor in myasthenia gravis. Neurology 26: 1054–1059.

MacDonald KL, Rutherford GW, Friedman SM, et al. (1985). Botulism and botulism-like illness in chronic drug abusers. Ann Intern Med 102: 616–618.

Mailhouse M (1898). A case of myasthenia pseudo-paralytica gravis (Jolly) or asthenic bulbar paralysis (Strumpell). Boston Med Surg J 138: 439–441.

Marsh DO (1974). Adrenal therapy for neuromuscular disease including myasthenia gravis from 1896. NY State J Med 74: 1974–1976.

Maselli RA, Ellis W, Mandler RH, et al. (1997). Cluster of wound botulism in California: clinical, electrophysiologic, and pathologic study. Muscle Nerve 20: 1284–1295.

Masland RL, Gammon GD (1949). The effect of botulinus toxin on the electromyogram. J Pharmol Exp Therap 97: 499–506.

Matell G, Bergström K, Franksson C, et al. (1976). Effects of some immunosuppressive procedures on myasthenia gravis. Ann N Y Acad Sci 274: 659–676.

McAlpine D (1929). A form of myasthenia gravis with changes in the central nervous system. Brain 52: 6–22.

Mertens HG, Balzereit F, Leipert M (1969). The treatment of severe myasthenia gravis with immunosuppressive agents. Eur Neurol 2: 321–339.

Meyer KF, Gunnison JB (1928). Cl. botulinum type D sp. N. Proc Soc Exptl Biol Med 26: 88–89.

Middlebrook JL (1993). Contributions of the U.S. Army to botulinism toxin research. In: BR Dasgupta (Ed.), Botulinism and Tetanus Neurotoxins. Plenum Press, New York, pp. 515–519.

Midura TF, Arnon SS (1976). Infant botulism, identification of Clostridium botulinum and its toxins in faeces. Lancet 2: 934–936.

Miledi R, Molinoff P, Potter LT (1971). Isolation of the cholinergic receptor protein of Torpedo electric tissue. Nature 229: 554–557.

Miller JFAP (1961). Immunological function of the thymus. Lancet 2: 748–749.

Miller RG, Milner-Brown HS, Dau PC (1981). Antibody-negative acquired myasthenia gravis: successful therapy with plasma exchange. Muscle Nerve 4: 255.

Millikan Ch, Eaton LM (1951). Clinical evaluation of ACTH and cortisone in myasthenia gravis. Neurology 1: 145–152.

Moberg LJ, Sugiyama H (1979). Microbial ecologic basis of infant botulism as studied with germfree mice. Infect Immun 25: 653–657.

Mossman S, Vincent A, Newsom-Davis J (1986). Myasthenia gravis without acetylcholine-receptor antibody: a distinct disease entity. Lancet 1: 116–119.

Mott FW, Barrada YA (1923). Pathological findings in the central nervous system in a case of myasthenia gravis. Brain 46: 237–241.

Nachmansohn D (1972). Biochemistry as part of my life. Annu Rev Biochem 41: 1–28.

Nastuk WL, Strauss AJL, Osserman KE (1959). Search for a neuromuscular blocking agent in the blood of patients with myasthenia gravis. Am J Med 26: 394–409.

Nastuk WL, Plescia OJ, Osserman KE (1960). Changes in serum complement activity in patients with myasthenia gravis. Proc Soc Exp Biol Med 105: 177–184.

Norris EH (1936). The thymoma and thymic hyperplasia in myasthenia gravis with observations on the general pathology. Am J Cancer 27: 412–433.

Nouza K, Šmat V (1968). The favourable effect of cyclophosphamide in myasthenia gravis. Rev Fr Etud Clin Biol 13: 161–163.

Ohno K, Tsujino A, Brengman JM, et al. (2001). Choline acetyltransferase mutations cause myasthenic syndrome associated with episode apnea in humans. Proc Natl Acad Sci U S A 98: 2017–2022.

Ophüls W (1914). Botulism, a report of food poisoning apparently due to eating canned string beans, with pathological report of a fatal case. Arch Intern Med 14: 589–604.

Oppenheim H (1887). Ueber einen Fall von chronischer progressiver Bulbärparalyse ohne anatomischen Befund. Virchow's Archiv für pathologische Anatomie und Physiologie und für klinische Medicine 108: 522–530.

Oppenheim H (1899). Weitere beitrag sur lehre von den acuten, night-eitrigen encephalitis und der polioencephalomyelitis. Deutsche Z Nervenheilkunde 15: 1–21.

Oppenheim H (1901). Der Myasthenische Paralyse (Bulbarparalyse ohne anatomischen Befund). S Karger, Berlin.

Oppenheim H (1991). Text-book of Nervous Diseases for Physicians and Students, 5th Ed., A Bruce (Trans.). Otto Schulze, Edinburgh, pp. 1029–1038.

Orr PF (1922). Pathogenicity of Bacillus botulinus. J Infect Dis 30: 118–127.

Osserman KE, Teng P, Kaplan LI (1954). Studies in myasthenia gravis. Preliminary report on therapy with Mestinon bromide. JAMA 155: 961–965.

Patrick J, Lindstrom J (1973). Autoimmune response to acetylcholine receptor. Science 180: 871–872.

Perez MC, Buot WL, Mercado-Danguilan C, et al. (1981). Stable remission in myasthenia gravis. Neurology 31: 32–37.

Pinching AF, Peters DK, Newsom-Davis J (1976). Remission of myasthenia gravis following plasma exchange. Lancet 2: 1373–1376.

Pordage S (1685). The London Practice of Physick, or the Whole Practical Part of Physick Contained in the Works of Dr. Willis. Printed for Thomas Bassett & William Crooke, London, England, pp. 431–432.

Pürckhauer H (1877). Zur casuistik der allantiasis. Aerztliches Intelligenz-Blatt 24: 245–248.

Ravitch MM (1966). The Papers of Alfred Blalock. Johns Hopkins Press, Baltimore, Maryland.

Robertson JD (1956). The ultrastructure of a reptilian myoneural junction. J Biol Biochem Cytol 2: 381–393.

Sanders DB, Andrews I, Howard JF, et al. (1997). Seronegative myasthenia gravis. Neurology 48(Suppl 5): S40–S45.

Santa T, Engel AG, Lambert EH (1972). Histometric study of neuromuscular junction ultrastructure I. Myasthenia gravis. Neurology 22: 71–82.

Schiavo G, Benfenati F, Poulain B, et al. (1992). Tetanus and botulinum-B neurotoxins block transmitter release by a proteolytic cleavage of synaptobrevin. Nature 259: 832–835.

Schiavo G, Shone CC, Rossetto O, et al. (1993a). Botulinum neurotoxin serotype F is a zinc endopeptidase specific for VAMP/synaptobrevin. J Biol Chem 268: 11516–11519.

Schiavo G, Rossetto P, Catsicas S, et al. (1993b). Identification of the nerve-terminal targets of botulinum neurotoxins serotypes A, D and E. J Biol Chem 268: 23784–23787.

Schiavo G, Malizio C, Trimble WS, et al. (1994). Botulinum G neurotoxin cleaves VAMP/synaptobrevin at a single Ala/Ala peptide bond. J Biol Chem 269: 20213–20216.

Schiller F (1993). Doctor Justinus C.A. Kerner (1786–1862) and his own case of juvenile hyperemesis. J Hist Neurosci 2: 217–230.

Schlezinger NS (1940). Evaluation of therapy in myasthenia gravis. Arch Intern Med 65: 60–77.

Schulz MD, Schwab RS (1971). Results of thymic (mediastinal) irradiation in patients with myasthenia gravis. Ann N Y Acad Sci 183: 303–307.

Schumacher CH, Roth P (1913). Thymektomie bei einem Fall von Murbus Basedowi mit Myasthenia. Mitteilungen aus den Grenzgebieten der Medizin und Chirurgie 25: 746–765.

Scott AB (1981). Botulinum toxin injection of eye muscles to correct strabismus. Trans Am Ophthalmol Soc 79: 734–770.

Scott AB (2004). Development of botulinum toxin therapy. Dermatol Clin 22: 131–133.

Scott AB, Rosenbaum A, Collins CC (1973). Pharmacologic weakening of extraocular muscles. Invest Ophthalmol 12: 924–927.

Secher O (1987). The polio epidemic in Copenhagen 1952. In: RS Atkinson, TB Boulton (Eds.), The History of Anesthesia. Parthenon Publishing Group, Park Ridge, New Jersey, pp. 425–432.

Seddon HR (1922). Bulbar paralysis in cattle due to the action of a toxicogenic bacillus, with a discussion on the relationship of the condition to forage poisoning (botulism). J Comp Pathol Therap 35: 147–190.

Shantz EJ (1995). Historical perspective. In: J Jankovic, M Hallett (Eds.), Therapy with Botulinum Toxin. Marcel Dekker, Inc., New York, pp. xxiii–xxvi.

Simon HE (1935). Myasthenia gravis, effect of treatment with anterior pituitary extract: preliminary report. JAMA 104: 2065–2066.

Simpson JA (1960). Myasthenia gravis: a new hypothesis. Scot Med J 5: 419–426.

Simpson LL (1981). The origin, structure, and pharmacological activity of botulinum toxin. Pharmacol Rev 33: 155–188.

Sloan HE (1943). The thymus in myasthenia gravis with observations on the normal anatomy and histology of the thymus. Surgery 12: 154–174.

Smith LDS (1977). Botulism, the Organism, its Toxin, the Diseases. CC Thomas, Springfield, Illinois, p. 10.

Snipe PT, Sommer H (1928). Studies on botulinus toxin 3. Acid precipitation of botulinus toxin. J Infect Dis 43: 152–160.

Soliven BD, Lange DJ, Penn AS, et al. (1988). Seronegative myasthenia gravis. Neurology 38: 514–517.

Stover JH, Fingerman M, Roester RH (1953). Botulinum toxin and the motor end plate. Proc Soc Exp Biol 84: 146–147.

Strauss AJL, Seegal BC, Hsu KC, et al. (1960). Immunofluorescence demonstration of a muscle binding, complement-fixing serum globulin fraction in myasthenia gravis. Proc Soc Exper Biol Med 105: 184–191.

Strauss AJL, Kemp PG, Douglas SD (1966a). Myasthenia gravis. Lancet 1: 772–773.

Strauss AJL, Smith CW, Cage WS, et al. (1966b). Further studies on the specificity of presumed immune associations of myasthenia gravis and consideration of possible pathogenic implications. Ann N Y Acad Sci 135: 557–579.

Strümpell A (1896). Ueber die asthenische Bulbärparalyse (Bulbärparalyse ohne anatomischen Befund, Myasthenia gravis pseudoparalytica). Dtsch Z Nervenheilkd 8: 16–40.

Swift TR, Greenberg MK (1984). Miscellaneous neuromuscular transmission disorders. In: RA Brumback, J Gerst (Eds.), The Neuromuscular Junction. Futura, New York, pp. 285–340.

Thesleff S (1960). Supersensitivity of skeletal muscle produced by botulinum toxin. J Physiol 151: 598–607.

Thomas CG, Keleher MF, McKee AP (1951). Botulism, a complication of *Clostridium botulinum* wound infection. Arch Pathol 51: 623–628.

Tindall RSA, Rollins J, Phillips JT, et al. (1987). Preliminary results of a double-blind, randomized, placebo-controlled trial of cyclosporine in myasthenia gravis. N Engl J Med 316: 719–724.

Torda C, Wolff HG (1947). On the mechanism of paralysis resulting from toxin of *Clostridium botulinum*. J Pharmacol Exp Therap 89: 320–324.

Torda C, Wolff HG (1949). Effects of adrenocorticotrophic hormone on neuro-muscular function in patients with myasthenia gravis. Proc Soc Exp Biol Med 71: 145–152.

Toyka KV, Drachman DB, Griffith DE, et al. (1977). Study of humoral immune mechanisms by passive transfer to mice. N Engl J Med 296: 125–130.

Van der Geld HWR, Strauss AJL (1966). Myasthenia gravis, immunological relationship between striated muscle and thymus. Lancet 1: 57–60.

Van der Geld HWR, Feltkamp TEW, Oosterhuis HJGH (1964). Reactivity of myasthenia gravis serum gammaglobulin with skeletal muscle and thymus demonstrated by immunofluorescence. Proc Soc Exp Biol Med 115: 782–785.

Van Ermengen E (1897a). Contribution à l'étude des intoxications alimentaires. Recherches sur des accidents à caractères botuliniques provoqués par du jambon. Arch Pharmacodyn 3: 213–350.

Van Ermengen E (1897b). Ueber einen neuen anaëroben Bacillus und seine Beziehungen zum Botulismus. Z Hygiene Infectionskrankheiten 26: 1–56 (partial English translation in Rev Infect Dis 1: 701–719, 1979).

Viets HR (1953). A historical review of myasthenia gravis from 1672 to 1900. JAMA 153: 1273–1280.

Vincent A, Leite MI (2005). Neuromuscular junction autoimmune disease: muscle specific kinase antibodies and treatments for myasthenia gravis. Curr Opin Neurol 18: 519–525.

von Reis G, Liljestrand Å, Matell G (1965). Results with ACTH and spironolactone in severe cases of myasthenia gravis. Acta Neurol Scand Suppl 13: 463–471.

Walker MB (1934). Treatment of myasthenia gravis with physostigmine. Lancet 1: 1200–1201.

Walker MB (1935). Case showing the effect of Prostigmin on myasthenia gravis. Proc R Soc Med 28: 759–761.

Walker MB (1938). Myasthenia gravis: a case in which fatigue of the forearm muscles could induce paralysis of the extra-ocular muscles. Proc R Soc Med 31: 722.

Warmolts JR, Engel WK (1972). Benefit from alternate-day prednisone in myasthenia gravis. N Engl J Med 286: 17–20.

Weber JT, Goodpasture HC, Alexander H, et al. (1993). Wound botulism in a patient with a tooth abscess; case report and review. Clin Infect Dis 16: 635–639.

Weigert C (1901). Pathologisch-anatomischer Beiträg zur Erb'schen Krankheit (Myasthenia gravis). Neurologisches Zentralblatt 20: 597–601.

Westerberg MR, Magee KR, Shideman FE (1951). Effect of 3-hydroxy phenyldimethylethyl ammonium chloride (Tensilon) in myasthenia gravis. Med Bull (Ann Arbor) 17: 311–316.

Whittaker VP (1992). The Cholinergic Neuron and its Target: The Electromotor Innervation of the Electric Ray Torpedo as a Model. Birkhäuser, Boston.

Wilbur RL, OPhils W (1914). Botulinism, a report of food poisoning apparently due to eating canned string beans, with pathological report of a fatal case. Arch Inter Med 14: 589–684.

Wilks S (1877). On cerebritis, hysteria, and bulbar paralysis. Guys Hosp Rep 22: 7–55.

Willis T (1672). De anima brutorum quae hominis vitalis ac sensitive est, exercitations duae. Londini, Typis EF, impensis Ric Davis, Oxford, England.

Wilson A, Stoner HB (1944). Myasthenia gravis: a consideration of its causation in the study of fourteen cases. QJM 13: 1–18.

Young JH (1976). Botulism and the ripe olive scare of 1919–1920. Bull Hist Med 50: 372–391.

Handbook of Clinical Neurology, Vol. 91 (3rd series)
Neuromuscular junction disorders
A.G. Engel, Editor

Chapter 2

Reliability of neuromuscular transmission and how it is maintained

CLARKE R. SLATER *

Institute of Neuroscience, Faculty of Medical Sciences, University of Newcastle upon Tyne, Newcastle upon Tyne, UK

2.1. An introduction to neuromuscular transmission

An important function of all nervous systems is to control muscle contraction so that movements of the body are appropriate to promote survival. In most species specialized motor neurons convey the signals that represent the neural commands for contraction from the central nervous system to the muscle fibers. These signals are transmitted to the individual muscle fibers at highly differentiated neuromuscular junctions (NMJs). In vertebrates, the process of neuromuscular transmission involves the rapid release of multimolecular "quanta" of acetylcholine (ACh) from the nerve, the binding of the ACh to ligand-gated cation channels (ACh receptors, AChRs) in the surface of the muscle fiber, the opening of those channels and the flow of current into the muscle fiber leading to depolarization and opening of voltage-gated sodium channels causing initiation of an action potential (AP) and contraction of the muscle cell.

In most vertebrates, each motor neuron provides the sole innervation for each of many muscle fibers. A fundamental design principle of neuromuscular systems in higher vertebrates, including humans, is that every nerve impulse in a motor neuron should evoke contraction of every muscle fiber innervated by it. Thus each motor neuron and the muscle fibers it innervates operates as a "motor unit". For this principle to be realized in practice, it is essential that the process of neuromuscular transmission should be reliable, operating unfailingly over a wide range of functional demands.

The reliability of transmission at the NMJ sets it apart from most other chemical synapses. In the central nervous system (CNS) the impact of individual synapses on the postsynaptic cell must generally be small, to allow many inputs to influence the final output. At the NMJ just the opposite is true. To ensure that each nerve impulse triggers muscle contraction, its impact on the muscle fiber is usually significantly greater than required to trigger an AP. For this reason, the process of neuromuscular transmission is said to have a big "safety factor". This results from specializations of both pre- and postsynaptic components. While the immediate molecular processes of neuromuscular transmission are qualitatively similar to those at central synapses, the distinctive functional organization of the NMJ is what accounts for its essential reliability. To understand the basis of the reliability of neuromuscular transmission, it is therefore just as important to know how NMJs differ from central synapses as how they resemble them. This understanding provides the necessary foundation for any effort to interpret how impaired transmission arises in human disease.

A detailed account of the cellular, subcellular and molecular organization of the NMJ is given in Chapter 3. This chapter describes the process of neuromuscular transmission. It emphasizes how the properties of the NMJ normally ensure the reliability of transmission in a wide range of biological circumstances and how changes to those properties may lead to impaired transmission in disease. After a brief review of the main features of neuromuscular transmission (Section 2.1), the essential presynaptic (Section 2.2) and postsynaptic (Section 2.3) aspects of neuromuscular transmission are considered in more detail. Section 2.4 describes how the safety factor has been defined and measured. Section 2.5 considers

*Correspondence to: Professor (Emeritus) Clarke R. Slater, Institute of Neuroscience, Faculty of Medical Sciences, University of Newcastle upon Tyne, Framlington Place, Newcastle upon Tyne NE2 4HH, UK. E-mail: c.r.slater@ncl.ac.uk, Tel: 44-191-222-5732, Fax: 44-191-222-5227.

some of the many modulating influences on the safety factor during normal use. Section 2.6 describes several important aspects of the "biology" of the NMJ; how it varies within and between muscles and species, and how its efficacy arises during development and is maintained in old age. Section 2.7 describes the remarkable adaptive plasticity of the NMJ, triggered by trauma or intoxication, which promotes maintenance of the effective neural control of muscle. Finally, Section 2.8 shows how the principles of the functional organization of the NMJ, developed in the earlier sections, can inform efforts to understand impaired neuromuscular transmission in disease. This account of neuromuscular transmission and its reliability is based primarily on studies of a small number of laboratory species. The emphasis is on mammals, including humans. While neuromuscular transmission in different species has much in common, there are also many important differences. It is therefore always necessary to use caution when trying to interpret findings in one species on the basis of knowledge of another.

2.1.1. The organization of muscle innervation

2.1.1.1. The muscle fiber

The aim of neuromuscular transmission is to cause muscle contraction. The contractile cells, or muscle fibers, that make up muscles are highly specialized to generate mechanical force under the control of the nervous system. At a molecular level, muscle contraction results from the interaction between myosin and actin molecules. These are organized into distinct thick (myosin) and thin (actin) filaments, which are further organized into overlapping arrays, the sarcomeres. These form the functional units of contraction in skeletal muscles.

Muscle contraction is regulated by the level of free Ca^{++} in the cytoplasm. This, in turn, is controlled by the sarcoplasmic reticulum (SR), a specialized form of ER, which contains energy-dependent Ca^{++} transporters that allow it to maintain the free Ca^{++} at a very low level. Ca^{++} is released from the SR if the surface membrane of the muscle fiber is adequately depolarized. In vertebrates, this membrane is generally excitable and, like neurons, can generate APs. This membrane property results from the presence of a distinct class of voltage-gated Na^+ channels. The specific class of these channels in adult mammalian (including human) muscle is known as $Na_V1.4$ (Goldin et al., 2000). During an AP, the depolarization of the surface membrane is carried into the cell interior along invaginations of the surface membrane known as T-tubules. These make contact with the SR at sites called triads.

At these sites, voltage-dependent Ca^{++} channels in the T-tubules (dihydropyridine receptors) interact with Ca^{++}-release proteins in the SR (ryanodine receptors) to trigger Ca^{++} release into the cytoplasm, thus triggering contraction.

Skeletal muscle fibers possess many nuclei. This is a result of the fusion of many mononucleated myoblasts during myogenesis to make individual muscle fibers. The diversity of mature muscle fibers reflects distinctive patterns of gene expression by the nuclei in muscle fibers of different functional types. Within each muscle fiber, the great majority of nuclei away from the NMJ express the same pattern of genes. However in mammals, including man, the 5–10 nuclei closest to the NMJ express a distinctive set of genes that encode key proteins of the NMJ, e.g., AChRs. The manner in which this specialization of gene expression is controlled plays an important part in ensuring the efficacy of neuromuscular transmission (see below).

Each muscle fiber is surrounded by a sheath of basal lamina (BL). This is a thin, but mechanically strong, layer of extracellular matrix. Within the BL sheath are a number of mononucleated myogenic cells known as satellite cells. Following damage to the muscle, the satellite cells may become activated and divide and then fuse to form new muscle fibers within the original BL sheaths.

There is considerable diversity in the properties of different vertebrate skeletal muscle fibers, even within the same muscle in the same animal. Some muscle fibers are specialized to produce relatively slow, well-maintained contractions while others produce fast but brief contractions. This diversity results from the expression of specialized isoforms of many of the proteins that give rise to and regulate contraction. It allows patterns of contraction ranging from the sustained contractions needed to maintain posture to the rapid forceful contractions needed to cause sudden movements of limbs.

2.1.1.2. The motor neuron

Motor neurons are among the largest neurons in the nervous system. Their cell bodies are located in the ventral horn of the spinal cord or the cranial nerve nuclei in the brainstem. Each motor neuron receives synaptic contact from many sensory and interneurons. When the summed depolarization resulting from the activity in these cells reaches the threshold, action potentials are initiated in the most proximal part of the axon. Each motor neuron has a single myelinated axon. After leaving the CNS, the motor axons generally remain unbranched until they reach their target muscle. There, within the intramuscular nerve bundles, they send off branches to the numerous muscle fibers they innervate.

Like muscle fibers, motor neurons have different functional properties (Kernell, 2006). In particular, different motor neurons tend to generate APs with characteristic temporal patterns. These are determined by the "intrinsic excitability" of the neuron, which reflects its size and the particular ion channels in its membrane (Gardiner and Kernell, 1990). Motor neurons innervating slow muscle fibers tend to be relatively small, to have a low threshold and to fire continuously at a low frequency (e.g., 20 Hz), while those innervating fast fibers tend to be larger, to have a higher threshold, and to fire in brief high frequency (e.g., 100 Hz) bursts (Henneman et al., 1965; Hennig and Lømo, 1985). The ability of the nerve terminal to sustain ACh release is matched to these different intrinsic patterns.

2.1.1.3. The motor unit

To take advantage of the diverse functional properties of skeletal muscle fibers, it is essential that the nervous system can excite specific sets of muscle fibers with particular properties. Within its target muscle, each motor neuron innervates a number of muscle fibers. This number may be only a few, in small muscles of laboratory rodents, or more than 1000 in large muscles of humans (Cooper, 1966). All the muscle fibers innervated by a given motor neuron have very similar properties (Burke et al., 1973) which are well-matched to those of the motor neuron and NMJs, ensuring that each motor unit produces a contraction suited to a particular need. An important feature of this pattern of innervation is that every nerve impulse in the motor axon should reliably excite every muscle fiber in the motor unit.

2.1.2. The NMJ and the nature of the reliability of neuromuscular transmission

The normal reliability of neuromuscular transmission is the result of factors operating at many different levels of organization. These range from the detailed atomic structure of the proteins that make up the essential ion channels to the multimolecular complexes that mediate vesicle exocytosis and finally to the multicellular complex that is the NMJ itself. In any situation where impaired reliability is present, all these levels must be considered when trying to understand the basis of that impairment.

2.1.2.1. Structure of the NMJ

A detailed account of the structure and cell biology of the NMJ is given in Chapter 3. Here only certain key features will be reviewed to provide a basis for the following treatment of neuromuscular transmission. When the motor axon makes contact with its target muscle fibers, it loses its myelin sheath and branches repeatedly to form the presynaptic nerve terminals of the individual NMJs (Fig. 2.1A, B). These terminals are capped by processes of the several terminal Schwann cells associated with them (Fig. 2.1A, D, E). Instead of myelin, these terminal Schwann cells elaborate thin layers of cytoplasm that cover and insulate the nerve terminal.

The precise form of nerve terminal branching, and the sites of synaptic contact with the muscle formed by the branches, varies between species. In many cases, including humans, the terminal consists of numerous spot-like regions of synaptic contact, where the axon enlarges to a width of 3–5 μm, linked by lengths of axon with a finer caliber (Fig. 2.1B). In other cases the regions of synaptic contact are merged to varying degrees to make a more or less continuous band which, as in the frog, may extend several 100s of μm along the muscle fiber.

In all cases, transmitter release occurs at specialized "active zones" (AZs) in the presynaptic membrane. These consist of highly ordered arrays of protein molecules including both the structural molecules that promote exocytosis and the Ca^{++} channels that regulate it. Different forms of AZ occur in lower and higher vertebrates (see Section 2.6.1.2). In both groups, the AZs are located opposite the openings between the postsynaptic folds.

The postsynaptic membrane is distinguished by the presence of infoldings, which lie opposite the AZs (Fig. 2.1D). The AChR and $Na_V1.4$ proteins occupy separate postsynaptic domains (Fig. 2.1C, E). The AChRs are concentrated at the crest of the folds, near the nerve, while the $Na_V1.4$ channels are concentrated in the depths of the folds. A thin mesh of extracellular matrix, the basal lamina (BL), surrounds each muscle fiber and motor axon. A single common BL is present in the synaptic cleft between the nerve and the muscle. A number of molecules important for the short and long term activities of the NMJ are bound to this synaptic BL including acetylcholinesterase (AChE), which terminates ACh action, and agrin, which plays an essential role in the development and maintenance of postsynaptic differentiation.

2.1.2.2. Principles of neuromuscular transmission

In all vertebrates, neuromuscular transmission involves the release of ACh from the nerve terminal and its action on the muscle to trigger its excitation and contraction. The NMJ is highly specialized to ensure that the main events in this complex process take place within less than a millisecond. Within the cytoplasm

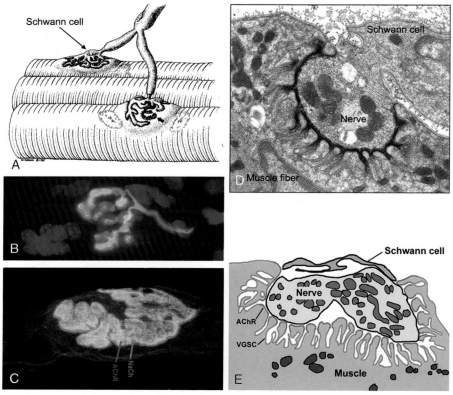

Fig. 2.1. Structure of the NMJ. (A) Diagram of mouse NMJ showing three muscle fibers, two of which are innervated by branches of a single motor axon. The highly branched nerve terminals are each capped by several Schwann cells. (From Salpeter, 1987, with permission.) (B) Human NMJ. The nerve terminal (green) branches extensively within the NMJ. The terminal boutons are aligned with regions of high AChR (red) density in the muscle fiber surface. Many nuclei (blue) from muscle and Schwann cells are seen. (C) Ion channels in the muscle fiber surface. AChR clusters (green) are surrounded by regions of high Na_V1 (red) density. Regions of optical overlap appear yellow. (D) Mouse NMJ showing nerve, muscle and Schwann cells. The AChRs have been labeled with an electron-dense conjugate of αBgTx and appear as a black labeling at the crests of the postsynaptic folds. (E) Diagram of ion channel domains at level of the electron microscope. The AChRs at the crests between the folds are shown in green and the Na_V1 channels in the depths of the folds in red.

of the presynaptic nerve terminal ACh is contained in membrane-bound vesicles. Each vesicle is believed to contain about 10 000 ACh molecules, which can be released within 100 µs or so following a nerve impulse. These multi-molecular packets, which are roughly uniform in size and effect at any given NMJ, are the elementary units of evoked ACh release. They are often referred to as "quanta" of ACh, by analogy with the elementary units of electromagnetic energy, and their release as "quantal" release. This release is normally triggered by an increase in the concentration of Ca^{++} in the nerve terminal, which results from the opening of voltage-gated Ca^{++} channels in the nerve terminal membrane by the nerve impulse. Normally a single nerve impulse causes 20–200 of these vesicles to release their contents, depending on the species and muscle.

The mechanism for ACh release from the nerve is complemented by a high density of AChRs in the postsynaptic membrane of the muscle fiber. These ligand-gated ion channels open briefly when ACh binds to them. This causes an influx of positive ions and a transient local depolarization of the muscle membrane. Since the NMJ is sometimes referred to as the endplate, the signals associated with this charge influx and subsequent depolarization are known as the endplate current (EPC), and the endplate potential (EPP), respectively (Fig. 2.2A). The analogous much smaller signals that result from the impact of spontaneously released single quanta of ACh are known as miniature EPCs and EPPs (Fig. 2.2). The EPP typically rises to a peak of some 25–45 mV (from the resting potential of about −75 mV) in about 1 ms. As it does so, it causes the opening of a second class of ion channels in the muscle fiber, the voltage-gated $Na_V1.4$ channels, thus initiating an action potential in the muscle fiber (Fig. 2.2B).

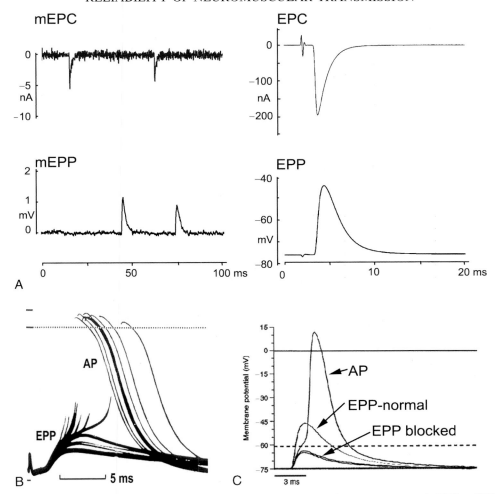

Fig. 2.2. Electrical events in neuromuscular transmission. (A) Events resulting from spontaneous (mEPC, mEPP) and evoked (EPC, EPP) release of ACh quanta. Note that the time course of the current transients (mEPC, EPC) is faster than the time course of the voltage transients (mEPP, EPP) that result from them. (B) EPPs and action potentials (AP) at an NMJ from a patient with myasthenia gravis. The EPP is much smaller than normal so it is often too small to evoke an AP. (From Elmqvist et al., 1964, with permission.) (C) Full-sized EPP from muscle in which the muscle AP has been blocked by μ-conotoxin ('normal') compared with EPP in muscle critically blocked by dTC ('blocked') so some EPPs are below the AP threshold (dashed horizontal line).

The action of the ACh is rapidly terminated by the action of the AChE associated with the synaptic BL, splitting ACh into acetate and choline. The choline is subsequently transported by a high affinity uptake system into the nerve terminal where it is eventually used to make more ACh.

2.1.2.3. The safety factor

The EPP that results from the summed effect of all the ACh released by a single motor nerve impulse normally depolarizes the muscle fiber more than is required to reach the electrical threshold for triggering an AP (Fig. 2.2C) (Wood and Slater, 2001). The significance of this safety factor is seen during intense activity when individual muscle fibers must be

activated repeatedly at high frequency. In these conditions, there is a temporary depletion of vesicles available for rapid release in the nerve terminal, resulting in a reduction of the amount of ACh release by individual nerve impulses. An adequate safety factor ensures that even in such circumstances, the EPP will still be able to activate the muscle fiber reliably.

2.1.3. Evidence for reliability at the human NMJ

Neuromuscular transmission is extremely reliable in healthy humans. It appears to be virtually impossible to bring about failure of transmission as a result of voluntary exertion (Bigland-Ritchie et al., 1978, 1982). Instead, normal fatigue during intense exertion seems to result primarily from reduced ability of the muscle fibers to contract, rather than from a failure of their excitation (Thomas and Zijdewind, 2006). In addition, "central fatigue", leading to a lowering of the frequency of nerve impulses in the motor neurons, may also occur during extreme fatigue (Bigland-Ritchie et al., 1978). It is important to appreciate that while the persistence of an undiminished EMG signal during extreme exertion may indicate that there has been no reduction in the number of active muscle fibers, the high safety factor may mask a substantial reduction in ACh release or EPP amplitude at many individual NMJs.

2.1.4. Effects of reduced reliability of neuromuscular transmission

In spite of the large reserve capacity of neuromuscular transmission, there are many important situations in which that reserve reaches its limit and transmission is significantly impaired. Among these the inherited and acquired myasthenias are of particular interest and the subject of this volume. In these conditions, the impairment of transmission is so severe that the EPP falls below the threshold for muscle activation, resulting in fatigue, weakness or paralysis. The process of neuromuscular transmission is a complex one, involving numerous specializations that all appear to be optimized to make the overall process as fast and reliable as possible. This means that there are many potential cellular and molecular targets for pathological processes that may lead to impaired transmission.

2.2. Presynaptic aspects of neuromuscular transmission

2.2.1. Introduction to the quantal release of ACh

ACh quanta are released from the motor nerve terminal within 100 µs or so of the arrival of the nerve impulse (Katz, 1969; Van der Kloot and Molgo, 1994). The events that allow the conversion of depolarization into secretion are complex. At the normal mammalian NMJ, they result in the release of more than enough ACh to ensure a postsynaptic depolarization that evokes an action potential in the muscle fiber (Wood and Slater, 2001). This section presents an account of the main events in the release process.

2.2.1.1. Early evidence for quantal release

Early studies of neuromuscular transmission using extracellular electrodes revealed that a motor nerve impulse is followed by a local depolarization of the muscle fiber, the EPP (Eccles et al., 1942). The introduction of intracellular recording techniques

allowed the true amplitude and time course of the EPP to be analyzed (Fatt and Katz, 1951). During this analysis much smaller events, with an amplitude of about 0.5–1 mV, were observed to occur spontaneously at a frequency of about 1 Hz (in the frog, Fig. 2.3A) (Fatt and Katz, 1952). These had a similar time course to EPPs and, like them, could only be recorded near the NMJ. Furthermore, like EPPs, they were blocked by the drug curare, which blocks the postsynaptic response to ACh. These similarities to EPPs led them to be called miniature EPPs (mEPPs).

A second key observation linked the spontaneous mEPPs to evoke release. In solutions containing low Ca^{++} (e.g., 0.2 mM instead of the usual 2 mM), and/or raised Mg^{++}, neuromuscular transmission was blocked because the EPP was too small to reach the action potential threshold. When the distribution of amplitudes of EPPs at a NMJ in low Ca^{++} was studied, it was found that some stimuli failed to evoke any response in the muscle. The responses that were observed had certain preferred amplitudes, which were integral multiples of a fundamental value (Fig. 2.3B, C) (del Castillo and Katz, 1954; Boyd and Martin, 1956). This fundamental value had the same mean as the amplitude of the mEPPs at the same NMJ.

The behavior of the NMJ in low Ca^{++} led to the hypothesis that EPPs result from the near simultaneous occurrence of a number of mEPPs. The mEPPs, in turn, were assumed to result from the action of a nearly constant number of prepackaged ACh molecules (see below). The analogy between fundamental units of chemical transmission and of electromagnetic energy led to the practice of referring to the ACh packets as "quanta". According to this view, each nerve-evoked EPP is caused by the release of an integral number of ACh quanta. This number is referred to as the "quantal content" of the EPP. In low Ca^{++}, fewer quanta are released (i.e., the quantal content is reduced) but the effect of the individual quanta is unchanged. It is important to realize that the term "quantal content" does *not* refer to the amount of ACh in a quantum, or to the number of quanta contained in a single nerve terminal.

Ultrastructural investigation of the NMJ soon suggested a likely structural basis of the ACh quanta. Membrane bound vesicles with a diameter of about 50 nm were seen in the motor nerve terminal (Reger, 1958; Birks et al., 1960) (see Chapter 3). It was suggested that each quantum represented the ACh molecules in a single such vesicle and that, somehow, the nerve impulse caused the near simultaneous fusion of a number of these vesicles with the nerve membrane, allowing them to discharge their contents into the synaptic cleft (del Castillo and Katz, 1956a). Although there is often a correlation between the frequency of

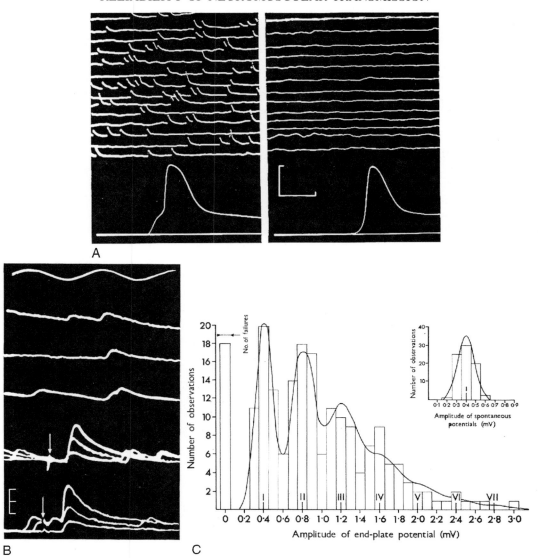

Fig. 2.3. Quantal release. (A) High and low gain recordings made close to a frog NMJ (left panel) and far from it (right panel). Note the randomly occurring mEPPs seen in the high gain recording and the 'kink' made by the EPP on the rising phase of the AP in recordings made near the NMJ. (B) Spontaneous (upper four traces) and evoked (lower two traces; arrows indicate stimulus) quantal events in low Ca^{++} medium at a frog NMJ. Note the similar degree of variation in both types of event. (C) Distribution of amplitudes of quantal events evoked at a rat NMJ in low Ca^{++} medium showing peaks at integral multiples of 0.4 mV, the mean of the sample of spontaneous mEPPs. (A, B from Fatt and Katz, 1952, with permission. C from Boyd and Martin, 1956, with permission.)

these spontaneous mEPPs and the quantal content of the evoked response, they respond quite differently to changes in the concentration of divalent cations. As a result, it is never safe to use mEPP frequency as a proxy measure of evoked release.

Numerous efforts have been made to establish the number of ACh molecules in a quantum. Probably the most accurate estimate was obtained by comparing the effect of nerve-derived ACh quanta on the frog NMJ with that of calibrated amounts of ACh ejected iontophretically from micropipettes onto the exposed

postsynaptic membrane in the same preparations (Kuffler and Yoshikami, 1975; Hartzell et al., 1976). This study found that fewer than 10 000 ACh molecules were required to mimic the effect of natural quanta. It is now generally accepted that a quantum usually contains 5000–10 000 ACh molecules.

2.2.1.2. Spatial aspects of quantal release

Subsequent experiments in the frog showed that ACh release occurred from many discrete sites located along the branches of the motor nerve terminals (del Castillo and Katz, 1956b). This conclusion was based on micro-electrode recordings of the currents flowing in the extracellular medium (Fig. 2.4A). These currents are highly localized and their site of origin can be determined to within 5–10 μm. In subsequent modifications of this approach, recordings were made simultaneously with 2 or 3 electrodes to provide even greater spatial resolution (Fig. 2.4B, C) (Benish et al., 1988; Zefirov and Cheranov, 1995). These showed that quanta are released from sites similar in size, shape and distribution to AZs (Fig. 2.4D). These electrophysiological findings were consistent with ultrastructural studies of frog NMJs frozen within a few milliseconds of nerve stimulation, which showed what were apparently the profiles of recently fused vesicles closely associated with the AZs (Heuser et al., 1979). These findings are described more fully in Chapter 3.

2.2.1.3. Temporal aspects of quantal release

The process of Ca^{++}-mediated exocytosis at the NMJ occupies less than a millisecond. Electrophysiological methods have been used to investigate the kinetics of quantal release. Initial studies were made in the frog, where individual branches of frog nerve terminals are up to 150 μm long. As a result, the action potential may reach the most distal end up to 0.3 ms after arising at the proximal end. This clearly complicates the investigation of the time course of release. To circumvent this problem, the method of extracellular recording was refined to restrict release to a small region of the frog nerve terminal (Katz and Miledi, 1965). This approach revealed that in the frog at 20°C, there was a period of about 0.5 ms between the peak active phase of the nerve action potential (indicated by the negative deflection of the extracellular record) and the earliest detectable release.

Analysis of a large sample of evoked uniquantal events, recorded in low Ca^{++}, showed that there is considerable variation in the time of their occurrence, relative to the peak of the action potential, even at a single site along the nerve terminal (Katz and Miledi, 1965). While most responses occurred about 1 ms after the peak of the nerve action potential, some occurred after only 0.5 ms and others as much as 2 ms later (Fig. 2.5). This temporal dispersion was interpreted as reflecting the time course of a transient increase in the probability of release of individual quanta of ACh, triggered by the increase in the concentration of free Ca^{++} in the cytoplasm.

When considering the entire NMJ, a further source of temporal dispersion in quantal release is introduced by the fact, referred to above, that the action potential invades the most distal part of the frog terminal as much as 0.3 ms later than the most proximal part. There is some evidence that this effect is partly compensated by a greater synchrony of quantal release in the most distal parts of the frog nerve terminal, though the basis of this is not yet clear (Bukharaeva et al., 2000). Because the linear extent of normal mammalian motor nerve terminals is much less than that of frogs, all regions of the nerve terminal probably become maximally depolarized by a nerve impulse within 100 μs. In some abnormal situations, in which the nerve terminal becomes elongated as a result of sprouting induced by inactivity, much longer distances and delays may be involved (see Section 2.7).

2.2.2. Depolarization of the nerve terminal by the action potential

It is now generally agreed that evoked quantal release is triggered by an increase in free Ca^{++} in the nerve terminal, which results from the opening of voltage-gated Ca^{++} channels in the nerve membrane when it is depolarized by an action potential.

The action potential in the motor axon travels to the NMJ by means of saltatory conduction. This mode of conduction results from the fact that the voltage-gated sodium channels responsible for the action potential are only present at the nodes of Ranvier, small (1 μm), widely separated (ca 1 mm) spots along the axon. These active regions are separated from each other by myelin, the insulating layers of plasma membrane of the Schwann cells associated with the axon. As a result, the active phase of the action potential "jumps" from one node to the next.

When the axon reaches the NMJ, both the highly restricted regions of excitability and the myelin sheath are lost. The motor nerve terminal contains many different classes of ion channel that may influence its excitability (Meir et al., 1999). Available evidence indicates that the excitability of the terminal axon differs between frogs, where the most detailed studies have been made, and mammals.

2.2.2.1. Frogs

The small diameter of the presynaptic axon terminals makes it difficult to make intracellular recordings of the action potential. However, important information can be gained by recording with extracellular electrodes, placed close to the nerve terminal (Fig. 2.5). In frogs, which have nerve terminals up to several 100 μm long, extracellular records indicate that the action potential propagates actively virtually to the end of the terminal. Further, blocking the invasion of the terminal by the action potential by local application of tetrodotoxin

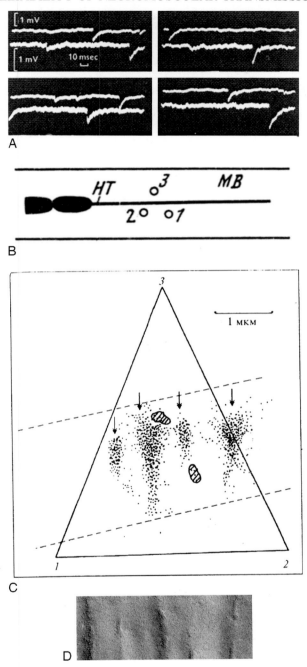

Fig. 2.4. Extracellular recording of quantal release. (A) Simultaneous extracellular recordings of spontaneous quantal events from two spots about 10 μm apart on a frog motor nerve terminal. Note that the events recorded by the two electrodes have very different amplitudes, indicating the very focal nature of the quantal currents. (B) Diagram of recording situation using three electrodes to determine the site of origin of individual quantal events by triangulation. A single muscle fiber with the last node of Ranvier (black) and a single branch of the nerve terminal, together with the numbered positions of the three electrodes. (C) Diagram showing outline of nerve terminal (parallel dashed lines) and positions of recorded quantal events determined by triangulation (dots). Note that these form four bands perpendicular to the nerve. (D) Electron micrograph of freeze fracture replica of frog nerve terminal showing positions of AZs. Magnification of C and D is the same. (A from del Castillo and Katz, 1956b, with permission. B from Benish et al., 1988, with permission. C from Zefirov and Cheranov, 1995, with permission. D from Heuser, 1976, with permission.)

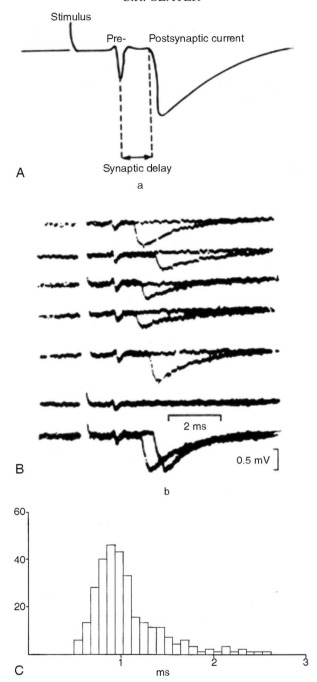

Fig. 2.5. Measurement of synaptic delay. Synaptic delay recorded at a frog NMJ. To prevent contraction and to restrict release to the recording site the preparation was bathed in a low Ca^{++} medium and Ca^{++} then restored locally at the recording site from a $CaCl_2$-filled micropipette. (A) Synaptic delay is defined as the elapsed time from the negative peak of the nerve AP, indicating the time of maximum inward current, to the onset of the evoked EPC in the muscle. (B) Records of several trials show variation in synaptic delay. (C) Distribution of delays recorded in many trials. The minimum is about 0.5 ms and the mode is about 0.9 ms. (From Katz and Miledi, 1965, with permission.)

(TTX) at the end of the last myelin segment completely abolishes the EPP (Katz and Miledi, 1967). Thus in frogs, active propagation of the action potential along the length of the nerve terminal is essential for normal neuromuscular transmission.

2.2.2.2. Mammals

Mammals have much smaller terminals than frogs. Initial studies concluded that the action potential does not invade the terminal actively (Brigant and Mallart, 1982) and that active Na^+ currents are present only in the most proximal part of the terminal axon. In contrast, repolarizing currents due to the efflux of K^+ are present throughout the terminal. While subsequent studies have found some evidence of active Na^+ currents in the distal terminal (Konishi and Sears, 1984; Konishi, 1985) these Na^+ currents are apparently not essential for normal quantal release. Thus it appears that in mammals quantal release is triggered largely by passive depolarization of the terminal by current drawn from the opening of Na^+ channels in the most distal nodes of Ranvier and the last "heminode".

2.2.2.3. Repolarization of the nerve terminal

The repolarization of the nerve terminal plays an important part in limiting the duration of Ca^{++} entry and thus preparing the NMJ for a further nerve impulse. This repolarization is primarily mediated by K^+ channels in the nerve. These include both voltage- and Ca^{++}-activated channels. The impact of these channels on quantal release is revealed when they are blocked by drugs such as 3,4-diamino pyridine (DAP) and its analogs (Katz and Miledi, 1979). These drugs can greatly increase the quantal content, making them useful both experimentally and clinically.

2.2.3. Ca^{++} entry

2.2.3.1. Calcium channels in the nerve terminal

Studies of the effect of Ca^{++} on quantal release imply that 3–5 Ca^{++} ions must bind to a target to trigger release (Dodge, Jr. and Rahamimoff, 1967). Observations of Ca^{++} concentration in the frog motor nerve terminal, using fluorescent indicator dyes, confirm that depolarization of the nerve terminal leads to the brief, highly localized, influx of Ca^{++} (Wachman et al., 2004). This influx is mediated by voltage-gated Ca^{++} channels present in the nerve terminal membrane (see Chapter 3).

While Ca^{++} channels of many different types are present at NMJs (Day et al., 1997) two of these, N and P/Q, predominate in vertebrate motor nerve terminals. Their activities can be distinguished by using highly specific natural toxins as selective blockers (Katz et al., 1995; Protti et al., 1996; Katz et al., 1997;

Urbano et al., 2002). In frogs and lizards, the main type is N, while in mammals it is P/Q. P/Q-type channels require less depolarization to open than N-type and less hyperpolarization to inactivate (Catterall et al., 2005). These functional differences may be related to the differences in active propagation of the action potential into the nerve terminal in frogs and mammals.

Fluorescent studies with a variety of specific labels have confirmed that Ca^{++} channels are concentrated in the motor nerve terminal (Robitaille et al., 1990; Sugiura et al., 1995; Day et al., 1997). In the frog, Ca^{++} channels are strategically placed immediately opposite the sites of highest AChR density in the postsynaptic membrane (Robitaille et al., 1990). Since this corresponds to the location of the AZs in the nerve terminal, it is generally assumed that the Ca^{++} channels are integral components of the AZs, and correspond to some or all of the intramembranous particles seen in freeze-fracture preparations. Detailed electrophysiological studies support this view (Yazejian et al., 2000).

2.2.3.2. Dynamics of calcium within the nerve terminal

The relationship between Ca^{++} entry into presynaptic terminals and quantal release is a topic of much current interest (Gentile and Stanley, 2005). Some studies of synapses in the CNS have suggested that many Ca^{++} channels must open, causing a generalized increase in Ca^{++} concentration in the presynaptic terminal, to bring about the release of an individual quantum. A different situation seems to apply at the frog NMJ. Following a single nerve impulse, Ca^{++} increases in the nerve terminal at a small number of discrete sites (Fig. 2.6A) (Wachman et al., 2004). The position of these sites changes from one response to the next. This suggests that only a small fraction of the Ca^{++} channels in the nerve terminal open in response to each action potential. As yet, comparable studies on mammalian NMJs have not been reported.

In order that neuromuscular transmission can operate reliably at high frequency, it is essential that the level of free Ca^{++} in the nerve terminal returns rapidly to its normally low level after each nerve impulse. A variety of mechanisms, including diffusion, binding to cytoplasmic proteins and uptake into intracellular organelles all appear to play a part in this process (Zucker and Regehr, 2002). During high frequency activation, there is often an increase in the quantal content. This is likely to result from the summed effect of the calcium that enters with each new impulse and residual calcium from previous stimuli that persists near the release sites (Katz and Miledi, 1968; Zucker and Regehr, 2002) (see Section 2.5.1).

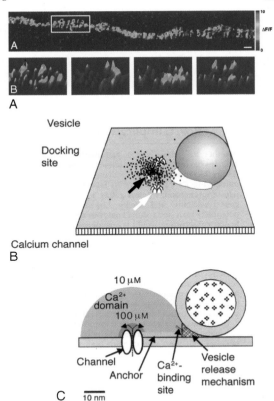

Fig. 2.6. Spatial dynamics of Ca^{++} entry. (A) Upper panel shows distribution of nerve-evoked Ca^{++} entry along a branch of a frog NMJ following a single stimulus. Lower panels show substantial trial-to-trial variation at a single site. Pseudocolor representation of Ca^{++} levels with low values shown in blue and high values in red. From Wachman et al. (2004) with permission. Copyright 2004 by The Society for Neuroscience. (B) Depiction of distribution of Ca^{++} (dots) entering through a single open channel (black arrow) next to a closed channel (white arrow) and close to a docked vesicle. (C) Spatial extent of regions where the Ca^{++} concentration reaches 100 μM and 10 μM, considered adequate to cause vesicle release. (B, C from Stanley, 1997, with permission.)

2.2.4. Exocytosis

2.2.4.1. Molecular basis of exocytosis at the NMJ

Much has been learned in recent years about the molecular events leading to exocytosis in general and at synapses in particular (Sudhof, 2004). It is now clear that the process of exocytosis involves interactions of one set of proteins in the membrane of the synaptic vesicles (V-SNARES including: synaptotagmin, and synaptobrevin) and another in the membrane of the nerve terminal (T-SNARES including syntaxins, and SNAP-25) (Fig. 2.7). An initial set of interactions leads to the "docking" of vesicles at the AZ as recognized by structural criteria, followed by an ATP-dependent step that leaves the vesicles in a

"primed" state, poised for release. The conversion of this "primed" state into full fusion is triggered when the concentration of free Ca^{++} in the cytoplasm reaches 10–20 μM (Stanley, 1997). This leads to Ca^{++} binding to the vesicle protein synaptotagmin, which saturates at a Ca^{++} concentration of about 10 μM (Hui et al., 2005). This, in turn, triggers a conformational change that results in further interactions between vesicle and terminal proteins that are believed to draw the vesicle toward the terminal membrane and cause fusion. Further details of the proteins involved in this process are described elsewhere in this volume (Chapter 3).

2.2.4.2. Calcium dynamics and exocytosis

Following the voltage-gated opening of Ca^{++} channels, the Ca^{++} ions that enter the nerve terminal must diffuse to their binding sites on synaptotagmin before release can occur. The earliest release events to occur after the nerve action potential therefore shed light on the distance between the sites of Ca^{++} entry and release. The probability of release begins to increase within 200 μs of the opening of these channels (Stanley, 1997; Gentile and Stanley, 2005). During this time, the region in which the Ca^{++} concentration reaches 10 μM extends about 25 nm from the opened channel. On the assumption that both the Ca^{++} channels and their targets are components of the AZ, this distance is so short as to indicate that the Ca^{++} entering the nerve terminal through a single opened Ca^{++} channel acts mainly on vesicles docked at the AZ of which the channel is a part.

It is generally thought that the intramembranous particles (IMPs) at AZs represent ion channels. At a mammalian AZ, there are usually about 20 IMPs in total (Fukunaga et al., 1983; Fukuoka et al., 1987), only some of which are likely to be Ca^{++} channels, the others are probably K^+ channels. Assuming that two vesicles are docked at each AZ, and the AZ is 50–100 nm long, only some of the Ca^{++} channels are likely to be close enough to each vesicle to play a part in its exocytosis. Thus fewer than 10 Ca^{++} channels, and possibly only one (Meriney et al., 1985; Stanley, 1997), may need to open to cause the release of a vesicle.

2.2.5. Determinants of quantal content

2.2.5.1. Number of release sites and efficiency of release

The local events described above, including Ca^{++} entry into the nerve terminal and the vesicle fusion events it triggers, form the basis of our understanding of the process of quantal release. However, to understand how it is that the nerve releases enough quanta to ensure reliable neuromuscular transmission, we

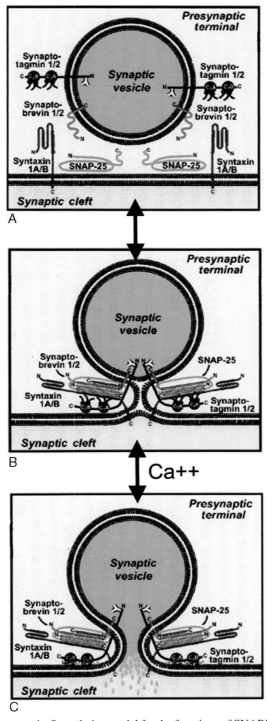

Fig. 2.7. Steps in synaptic vesicle exocytosis. Speculative model for the functions of SNARE proteins (synaptobrevin, SNAP-25, syntaxin 1/2) and synaptotagmins in exocytosis. In docked vesicles (A), SNAREs and synaptotagmins do not interact directly. During priming (B), SNARE complexes form, complexins (green) are bound to fully assembled complexes, and synaptotagmins constitutively associate with the assembled SNARE complexes. The synaptic vesicle membrane and plasma membranes are forced together by SNARE complex assembly, which results in an unstable intermediate. Ca^{++} influx (C) further destabilizes the fusion intermediate by triggering the C_2 domains of synaptotagmin to partially insert into the phospholipids. This action is proposed to cause a mechanical perturbation that opens the fusion pore. (From Sudhof, 2004, with permission.)

must consider the whole population of AZs in the nerve terminal and the efficiency of release from them.

Frog NMJs have been studied in the greatest detail. Their AZs occur at intervals of about 1 μm along the nerve terminal (Pawson et al., 1998). Since the average total length of the nerve terminal branches is about 1000 μm, there are about 1000 AZs per NMJ. Since the quantal content of the whole NMJ is about 100–200, this means that the probability of release from a single AZ is about 0.15, although estimates up to 0.75 have been suggested (Meriney et al., 1985). It is estimated that there are 20–30 docked vesicles at each AZ (Meriney et al., 1985), or about 25 000 per NMJ, implying that fewer than 1% of the docked vesicles are released per nerve action potential.

In mammals, the AZs are distributed apparently at random throughout the presynaptic membrane. Their density in mice and humans is 2.6 AZ/μm (Fukunaga et al., 1983; Fukuoka et al., 1987). At a typical rat or mouse NMJ, with an area of synaptic contact of about 400 μm^2 (Lyons and Slater, 1991; Wood and Slater, 1997), this implies that there are about 1000 AZs. Each AZ is believed to harbor no more than two docked vesicles (see Section 2.6.1.2, Fig. 2.22), making a maximum of 2000 per NMJ. The quantal content of EPPs in such a muscle is about 100, or about 0.1 per AZ. This means that about 5% of the docked vesicles are released by each nerve action potential. A similar conclusion applies to human NMJs. In each case, the number is substantially greater than in the frog. The explanation for this difference is not yet clear, but it is likely to be related to the different relationships between vesicles and AZ particles in frogs and mammals.

In spite of the differences in the "efficiency" of release of docked vesicles in different species, the number of quanta released per unit area of presynaptic membrane is roughly constant. Although there are clear exceptions, many NMJs release between 0.15–0.35 quanta/μm^2. This principle was first recognized in frogs, where a rough correlation between NMJ size and quantal content was found (Kuno et al., 1971). At NMJs such as those in humans where the nerve terminal is formed from many boutons about 3 μm in diameter, each bouton has about 50 AZs and 100 docked vesicles, of which 1–3 are typically released by a single nerve impulse.

At first, it seems strange that so reliable a process as neuromuscular transmission should be founded on such a low probability of release of individual docked vesicles. One possible explanation is related to the fact that muscle fiber activation, particularly of fast mammalian muscles (Hennig and Lømo, 1985) often consists of a burst of 5–10 nerve impulses at a frequency of around 100 Hz. If each impulse causes the release of a small fraction of docked vesicles "at random", this would ensure that there is always an adequate supply of vesicles ready to be released by following impulses. In any case, it is clear that an understanding of the reliability of release from the nerve terminal as a whole must take into account these spatial features of release.

2.2.5.2. Vesicle pools in the nerve terminal

The vesicles released by a single nerve impulse are a very small fraction of all the vesicles contained in the presynaptic terminal. In a variety of mammals, this total has been estimated at 100 000 to 300 000, e.g., Reid et al. (1999). Thus there is an enormous reserve capacity of vesicles potentially available for release. However, studies using repetitive nerve stimulation have shown that subpopulations, or "pools", of vesicles differ in their actual availability (Rizzoli and Betz, 2005). The docked and primed vesicles represent a "readily releasable" pool which can be replenished rapidly from a "recycling" pool. In addition, there is a much larger "reserve" pool in which vesicles are believed to be tethered to elements of the cytoskeleton. The properties of these pools, and how vesicles move from one pool to another, are topics of much current interest. This topic is discussed more fully in Section 2.5.

2.2.6. Statistical aspects of quantal release

An important aspect of the initial studies of quantal release was the effort to formulate statistical models that could describe the fluctuations in the quantal content (m) of the EPP in different situations (del Castillo and Katz, 1954; Katz, 1969). These models are relevant here because they have played an important part in many subsequent efforts to quantify quantal release in different situations (see Section 2.4.3.3). The general approach was to assume that within the nerve terminal there are a large number (n) of "units" (provisionally quanta) each with a finite probability (p) of being released by a given nerve impulse. Thus

$$m = np$$

For such a system, it should be possible to describe the distribution of quantal contents in a large series by a binomial distribution. Efforts to do this have been of limited value because it is unclear exactly what the variable n represents.

Many of the key observations on which the modeling was based were made in the presence of a low

Ca^{++} concentration in which the EPP was very small. Because the amplitude of the mEPPs was found not to be reduced, indicating that the size of the individual quanta did not change, it was assumed that the effect of reducing the concentration of Ca^{++} was to reduce m. In these experiments, there was either no response at all (a "failure"), or a response whose amplitude was approximately an integral multiple of the mEPP amplitude. Under these conditions the distribution of EPP amplitudes of a large number of events can be described by the Poisson distribution:

$$P_x = e^{-m} m^x / x!$$

where p is the probability of occurrence of a response resulting from x quanta and m is the mean number of quanta per response, or quantal content (del Castillo and Katz, 1954).

A useful feature of a Poisson distribution is that the entire distribution of responses can be predicted from a single variable. For example, if one determines the fraction of trials in which there is no response because zero quanta have been released, it is possible to determine the remaining fractions in which one, two or more quanta will be released, and therefore the value of m. This property is the basis for a widely used method for estimating m (the "failures" method). An alternative approach is based on the fact that the mean of a Poisson distribution (i.e., m) is inversely related to the variance. Thus, even in circumstances where individual quanta (mEPPs) cannot be recorded, m can be estimated from the variance of the response amplitudes (the "variance" method). An important limitation of the use of the Poisson distribution is that it is only valid when p, and hence m, are very small (<3). This makes it invalid to use the Poisson distribution as the basis for estimating m in conditions of normal release (discussed further in Section 2.4.3.3). A failure to recognize this limitation in some early studies of quantal release in mammals led to estimates of m that are now recognized as having been much too high.

2.2.7. Endocytosis and vesicle recycling

Following a nerve impulse, the membrane of the vesicles that fuse by exocytosis is added to the membrane of the nerve terminal, which therefore gets bigger. This process is balanced by recovery of the membrane by a process of endocytosis (see Chapter 3). The process of endocytosis, and the subsequent trafficking of the recovered vesicles, can be followed using fluorescent lipophilic dyes, most commonly FM1–43 (Cochilla et al., 1999), that become incorporated into the membranes of the endocytotic vesicles. Studies of

this sort have revealed much about the properties of the vesicle "pools" within the nerve terminal (Rizzoli and Betz, 2005). These pools play an important part in ensuring that the number of vesicles ready for release is normally adequate. This topic is discussed in more detail in Section 2.5.1 in the context of how the NMJ responds to repetitive activity such as occurs in vivo.

2.2.8. Conclusions

The number of vesicles released by a given nerve impulse is a very important determinant of the efficacy of transmission. It is clear that it depends on a large number of factors, reflecting the complexity of the release process (Atwood and Karunanithi, 2002). These factors may be classed into those that influence Ca^{++} entry into the terminal and those that influence how much ACh that Ca^{++} causes to be released. The former class includes: action potential amplitude and duration, determined by the number and types of Na^+ and K^+ channels in the membrane of the terminal, and the density, distribution and properties of the voltage-gated Ca^{++} channels. The latter class includes: synapse size, AZ density, the number of docked vesicles per AZ, and the fraction of docked vesicles that are primed for release. Additional factors probably include vesicle size and the concentration of ACh within them.

2.3. Postsynaptic aspects of neuromuscular transmission

2.3.1. Dynamics of ACh in the synaptic cleft

2.3.1.1. Diffusion of ACh in the cleft

The rising phase of the EPC lasts about 0.2 ms. During this time, ACh released from the nerve must diffuse across the synaptic cleft, bind to AChRs, which must then undergo a conformational change ("opening"), and Na^+ ions must diffuse into the muscle fiber to generate the EPC. The ACh released from a single vesicle diffuses rapidly in the synaptic cleft, with an estimated diffusion coefficient of 1.4×10^{-6} cm^{2}s^{-1} (Krnjević and Mitchell, 1960). In 0.2 ms, the mean diffusion distance of an ACh molecule from the site of release $= \sqrt{(2Dt)}$ (where D is the diffusion coefficient and t is the time) is about 0.25 μm. For a quantum of 10 000 molecules, in a synaptic cleft 50 nm wide, this would result in an average concentration of ACh of >0.5 mM, immediately adjacent to a region of postsynaptic membrane within 0.25 μm of the site of release.

2.3.1.2. Impact of the basal lamina and AChE on ACh dynamics

One may wonder whether all the ACh in a quantum would really reach the postsynaptic membrane, given the high concentration of AChE associated with the synaptic BL. The explanation lies in the fact that there are some 10 times fewer AChE molecules in the synaptic space encountered by a quantum of ACh than there are ACh molecules in a quantum (Anglister et al., 1994). As a result, something like 10% of the ACh rapidly occupies all the AChE molecules while 90% passes through the BL to reach the postsynaptic membrane. As the bound ACh molecules gradually dissociate from the AChRs during a period of a few ms, they are rapidly bound and hydrolyzed by the AChE, limiting both the temporal and spatial extent of action of each quantum of ACh (see Section 2.3.7).

2.3.2. Structure and function of the AChR

2.3.2.1. General structure of AChRs

The AChRs in the postsynaptic membrane of the vertebrate NMJ are of the class activated by nicotine, and are therefore referred to as nicotinic (e.g., nAChRs). Other AChRs activated by muscarine (mAChRs) are present on the presynaptic side of the NMJ and may act to modulate quantal release (see Section 2.5.4.1). Each postsynaptic AChR molecule is a cylindrical complex of 5 subunits (Fig. 2.8A). The long axis lies perpendicular to the plane of the membrane and both surrounds and gates a central cation-selective channel. At mature mammalian NMJs, the stoichiometry of the subunits is $\alpha_2,\beta,\delta,\varepsilon$. At immature or regenerating NMJs the ε-subunit is replaced by a γ-subunit, which is also commonly found in more primitive vertebrates. This replacement alters the kinetic properties of the cation channel (see below).

2.3.2.2. Properties of ACh-gated channels

Each AChR molecule has two ACh binding sites in the interfaces between the α/ε and α/δ subunits. At the concentration of ACh present in the synaptic cleft following a nerve impulse, binding to the AChRs occurs within microseconds. When both subunits are occupied the probability of the associated channel opening increases dramatically (Fig. 2.8B). The transition from closed to open occurs in less than 100 μs (Matsubara et al., 1992). The open channels are approximately equally permeable to Na^+ and K^+ (Takeuchi and Takeuchi, 1959) and are also slightly permeable to Ca^{++}. The flow of ions through an open channel is determined by the instantaneous value of the relevant electrochemical gradients.

At the normal resting potential the electrochemical driving force on Na^+ is much greater than that on K^+. The net result of opening AChR channels is to allow a positive charge in the form of Na^+ ions to enter the

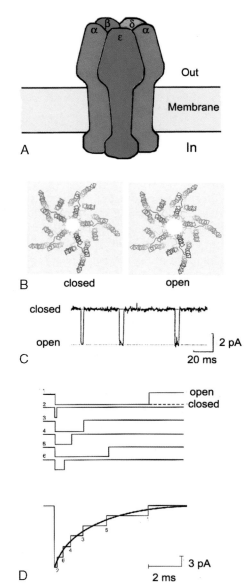

Fig. 2.8. From AChRs to mEPCs. (A) Schematic diagram of an AChR molecule in the membrane. The five subunits (2α, β, δ, ε) span the membrane and enclose the ion pore. (B) View along the axis of the pore of how the orientation and conformation of the subunits may change when the channel opens (kindly provided by Nigel Unwin). (C) Examples of current flowing through a single open channel during three opening events. (From Mishina et al., 1986, with permission.) (D) The mEPC results from the near simultaneous opening of a number of channels (only 6 of the 1000 or so that make up a mEPC are shown) followed by their gradual closure.

muscle fiber. The conductance of these channels when open is about 40–60 pS. At a normal resting potential of -90 to -70 mV, this corresponds to an inward current of some 4–5 pA. If the membrane potential is more positive than the resting potential, the driving force on Na^+ decreases and that on K^+ increases, causing the net current to decrease. At about 0 mV, the two currents balance each other and there is no net current through the open channels. If the membrane potential becomes more positive than this "reversal potential", the net current becomes outward, i.e., the efflux of K^+ is greater than the influx of Na^+.

2.3.2.3. Impact of subunit composition on channel properties

At immature NMJs, the AChRs present contain a γ-subunit in place of the ε-subunits present at NMJs in the adult (see Section 2.6). The presence of the γ-subunit reduces the conductance from 40–50 pS to about 30 pS but prolongs its mean open time from 1 to 4 ms. The net result is that more charge enters the muscle fiber per opening through a γ-subunit containing AChR, but it does so over a longer period of time, than for an ε-subunit containing AChR.

2.3.3. Generation of quantal currents

2.3.3.1. ACh binding to AChRs

The AChR density in the postsynaptic membrane is of the order of 10 000 per μm^2 (Matthews-Bellinger and Salpeter, 1983). Thus, within the region to which the 10 000 or so ACh molecules of a quantum diffuse in 0.2 ms, they would encounter about 2500 AChR molecules, each of which has two ACh binding sites. Because the concentration of ACh in the cleft (0.5 mM) is substantially higher than the K_D for the ACh–AChR interaction (3–8 $\times$ 10^{-5} M), ACh binds rapidly to the AChRs, saturating most of those present within the diffusion distance of about 0.25 μm (Land et al., 1981).

2.3.3.2. Time course of the EPC

The ACh molecules contained in a single quantum normally cause the opening of about 2000 AChR-associated channels (mouse) within less than 100 μs (see above). Following an opening event, each channel at a mature mammalian NMJ stays open for an average of 1 ms, excluding the very brief closures that characterize channel "bursting". Each channel has a conductance of about 60 pS. Initially, when all these channels are open, the total conductance increase is therefore about 100 nS. In physiological conditions, this gives rise to a peak mEPC of 3–5 nA (Fig. 2.2).

The individual channels opened by a single quantum close after a mean "open time" of about 1 ms. However, random variations in the open time mean that the number of channels still open at any time after the initial activation declines along an exponential time course. As it does so, the mEPC declines in parallel. These factors explain how the shape of the mEPC—a very rapid rise followed by a slower, exponential decline—arises from the summed effects of many "rectangular" single channel events (Fig. 2.8C).

2.3.4. From quantal currents to the EPC

Following a nerve impulse, each of the many separate quanta of ACh released acts on a small region of post-synaptic membrane. This region has a diameter of about 0.5 μm and contains about 2000 AChRs (see Section 2.3.1.1), or about 0.01% of all the AChRs at the NMJ (1–2 $\times$ 10^7). As a consequence of the fact that the probability of release of a vesicle at each AZ is low, the release sites are on average separated by about 2 μm. There is thus rarely any significant overlap of the "saturated disks" of AChRs associated with adjacent release events. As a result, each quantum acts independently on the postsynaptic membrane. For a quantal content of 50–100, the number of ACh-gated channels opened in response to a single nerve impulse is about 1% of those at the NMJ.

2.3.5. From the EPC to the EPP

2.3.5.1. Introduction to the cable properties of the muscle fiber

The effect of opening ACh-gated channels is to allow the entry of positive charge into the muscle fiber, giving rise to the EPC. The conversion of the EPC into the EPP is determined primarily by the passive cable properties of the muscle fiber, i.e., those that do not involve the voltage-gated Na^+ channel. These properties of the muscle fiber as a whole are determined by the electrical conductivity of the cytoplasm, the specific resistance and capacitance of the membrane (that is the resistance or capacitance per unit area), and by the diameter of the muscle fiber (Katz, 1966; Jack et al., 1975).

Current entering the fiber at a point, such as the NMJ, can flow both longitudinally in the cytoplasm and transversely across the membrane (Fig. 2.9A). However, only the latter pathway leads to a change in the membrane potential. The fraction of the current that takes each route depends on the relative resistance each pathway presents. When the diameter is relatively large, current can flow more easily along the interior of the fiber and is less likely to "leak" out across the membrane causing a change in membrane potential.

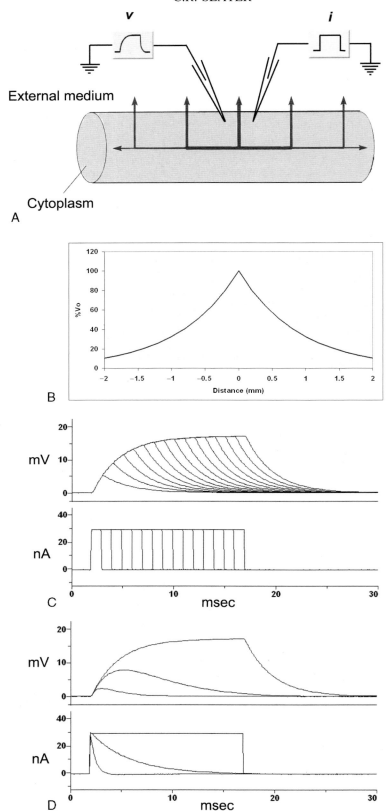

When the diameter is small, the opposite is true so the peak change in membrane potential caused by a given current is greater. For a cylindrical cell such as a muscle fiber, the peak voltage change caused by a continuous current entering the cell at a point is determined by the "input resistance" of the cell. Typical values for vertebrate muscle fibers are $0.2–1 \times 10^6$ Ohm. Other things being equal, the input resistance of a muscle fiber is inversely proportional to $(\text{diameter})^{3/2}$ (Katz, 1966).

2.3.5.2. Space constant

An important consequence of the "leakiness" of the muscle fiber membrane is that the change of membrane potential caused by current entering at a point decays with distance along the fiber away from that point. The decay of potential from a site of current injection, (e.g., the NMJ) can usually be approximately described by a single exponential (Fig. 2.9B). For many vertebrate muscle fibers the space constant of the decay, that is the distance required for the potential to drop to 37% $(1/e)$ of its value at the origin, is 0.5–2 mm. It is because of this that the ACh released from the nerve has little direct effect on the membrane potential more than a few mm away from the NMJ.

2.3.5.3. Effects of membrane capacitance

When current flows across a cell membrane, it causes the reorganization of charged molecules in the membrane. This takes time and energy. In response to an abrupt step change in current, the voltage changes to a new value along an approximately exponential time course. For a muscle fiber, the "charging time constant" is typically 2–5 ms (Fig. 2.9C). When a current transient such as an EPC occurs which is brief relative to the charging time constant of the muscle, the peak voltage change does not reach that predicted by Ohm's Law (Fig. 2.9C). Thus, for an EPC of 250 nA, and an input resistance of 0.4×10^6 Ohm, Ohm's Law predicts that the EPP should have an amplitude of 100 mV. In reality, the amplitude is usually only about half of that value.

2.3.5.4. Impact of cable properties on EPP

These biophysical factors have a major impact on the ability of ACh released from the nerve to trigger an action potential in the muscle fiber. The combined effect of the input resistance and capacitance of the muscle determines how big a mEPP will result from a quantum of ACh (Katz and Thesleff, 1957). Input resistance is particularly influenced by muscle fiber diameter. The effect of membrane capacitance is relatively constant in different muscles. Its importance as a determinant of synaptic efficacy is seen in situations in which the decay time constant of the mEPCs and EPCs vary, as during normal development or in a variety of pathological situations (see below). In such cases, the longer the decay time of the EPC, relative to that of the muscle fiber charging time constant, the greater the potential change caused by the EPC will be (Fig. 2.9D).

2.3.5.5. Non-linear summation of quanta

The amplitude of the EPP is also influenced by the value of the membrane potential. As the membrane potential approaches the reversal potential for the ACh-induced current (−10 to 0 mV), less current flows through the opened channels. As a result, when the quantal content increases, and with it the peak amplitude of the EPP, more quanta must be released to cause a further unit increase in EPP amplitude. This feature of the EPP is often referred to as "non-linear summation" of the effects of ACh quanta (McLachlan and Martin, 1981). Its importance relates to the relationship between the quantal content and the amplitude of the EPP and will be discussed in more detail in Section 2.4.3.3.

2.3.6. Initiation of the action potential

2.3.6.1. The threshold

In the great majority of mammalian muscles, the motor neurons activate the skeletal muscle fibers by generating an AP. As in all excitable cells, this requires reducing the internal negativity of the cell to the point where there are enough voltage-gated Na^+ channels

Fig. 2.9. Passive cable properties of muscle fibers. (A) The electrical properties of a muscle fiber are studied with two intracellular electrodes, one to pass current (I) and one to record the resulting changes in voltage (V). Current entering the muscle fiber at a point flows both internally along the fiber and transversely across the membrane. (B) The amplitude of the peak voltage change depends on the distance from the site of current entry. The voltage is shown as a fraction of that when the voltage and current electrodes are at the same position. (C) The time course of the voltage change is distorted by the membrane capacitance. The voltage changes shown were obtained by injecting rectangular current pulses of different lengths into a simple electrical model that approximates a muscle fiber. It takes about 10 ms for the voltage change to reach a plateau. When the current pulse is shorter than this, as is the case for the EPC, the voltage change does not reach the plateau. (D) For current transients that approximate EPCs, the peak voltage change depends on the decay time constant. Thus for a model EPC with a decay time constant of about 1 ms, as at adult mammalian NMJs, the peak voltage change is only about 40% of that when the time constant is 3–4 ms, as at immature mammalian NMJs.

open to cause a regenerative entry of positive charge into the cell (inward current). Subthreshold depolarizing currents have the effect of driving positive charge out of the cell (outward current). Only when the depolarization is great enough to cause the opening of voltage-gated Na^+ channels can it lead to the inward current that causes excitation.

A muscle fiber is normally excited by current flowing at a single site, the NMJ. A result of the cable properties of the muscle fiber (see above) is that when an EPC is just great enough to cause some Na^+ channels to open at the NMJ, the "active" region is surrounded by less depolarized membrane in which the induced current is still outward. At threshold, the net positive charge that is carried into the fiber by the inward current at the NMJ is equal to that carried out by the outward current in the surrounding membrane (Jack et al., 1975). When the depolarization is above threshold, the positive charge entering at the NMJ is greater than that leaving in the surrounding region. This excess of charge depolarizes the adjacent membrane to threshold, setting in train the regenerative process that underlies the action potential.

The depolarization required to reach threshold is usually determined experimentally by passing current into a muscle fiber from an intracellular microelectrode and measuring the resulting change in voltage with a second electrode placed nearby (cf. Fig. 2.9A). Conventionally this is done in a region of membrane away from the NMJ. For a typical mammalian muscle in experimental conditions, an action potential is generated when the membrane is depolarized from a resting level of about −80 mV to a new level of about −55 mV, i.e., a depolarization of 25 mV (Wood and Slater, 1994). In the muscles of laboratory rodents the EPP, measured after blocking the muscle action potential with the cone snail toxin μ-conotoxin GIIIB (μCTx, see below), is about 35 mV, clearly greater than needed to reach the action potential threshold (Wood and Slater, 1997).

2.3.6.2. Threshold at the NMJ

The postsynaptic region of vertebrate NMJs contains a much higher density of Na_V1 channels than is present away from the NMJ (Fig. 2.1C) (Haimovich et al., 1984; Flucher and Daniels, 1989; Ruff, 1992; Ruff and Whittlesey, 1992; Wood and Slater, 1998a). Analogy with the nodes of Ranvier in myelinated axons suggests that the threshold for action potential generation should be lower at the NMJ than in the non-junctional region, where threshold is conventionally measured. This prediction has been confirmed by determining the action potential threshold in response to

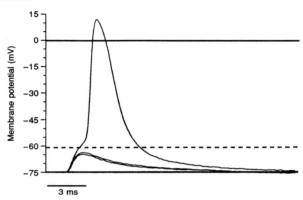

Fig. 2.10. Measuring AP threshold with EPPs. To determine the AP threshold using EPPs, the preparation (rat soleus muscle) was critically blocked with dTC (2×10^{-7} M) so that most EPPs were subthreshold but occasional ones were big enough to trigger an AP. The threshold was defined as the voltage at the inflection point on the rising phase of the response, and was about −60 mV, some 10 mV less positive than that obtained away from the NMJ. (From Wood and Slater, 1995, with permission.)

EPPs. To do this, rat muscles were exposed to a critical level of D-tubocurarine to create near-threshold EPPs (Wood and Slater, 1997). In this study, EPPs with a peak amplitude greater than about 10 mV triggered muscle action potentials (Fig. 2.10). Thus the depolarization of the immediate postsynaptic membrane required to trigger an action potential is less than half that required in the non-junctional region.

2.3.6.3. Folds and their electrical effects

An additional influence on the threshold at the NMJ is the geometry of the postsynaptic folds and the distribution of ion channels within them (Vautrin and Mambrini, 1989; Martin, 1994). The high concentration of AChRs at the crest of the folds (see Fig. 2.1D, E) means that during the EPC, positive charge enters the muscle fiber only at the crests of the folds (Fig. 2.11A). The onward "path of least resistance" for this current is through the cytoplasm of the junctional folds rather than across the folded membrane. However the sheet of cytoplasm within the folds, which may be as thin as 100 nm, offers a resistance some 10 times greater than the input resistance of the fiber as a whole (Fig. 2.11B) (Martin, 1994). During the flow of a single mEPC there is thus a potential gradient of about 10 mV between the tops of the folds and the bulk of the cytoplasm of the muscle fiber, where the voltage can be sampled by an intracellular electrode. Put another way, the amplitude of a typical mEPP, which is 0.5–1 mV when measured with a conventional electrode, would be about 10 mV if it could be measured at the tops of

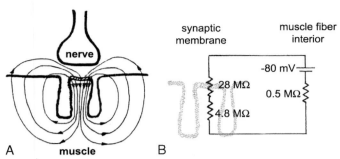

Fig. 2.11. Electrical effects of postsynaptic folds. (A) Current flow through a single junctional fold in response to ACh. Because the AChRs are concentrated at the crest of the folds, current enters the folds at that site. The path of least resistance is through the narrow sheet of cytoplasm within the junctional fold and then through the bulk cytoplasm and across the unfolded membrane. (B) Electrical model of a fold. The resistance of the intrafold cytoplasm (4.8 MΩ) is nearly ten times greater than the input resistance of the cell (0.5 MΩ). At mammalian NMJs, the current path created by the opened AChR channels has a very high resistance (28 MΩ).

the folds. The $Na_V1.4$ channels lining the lower portions of the junctional folds and the troughs of the synaptic clefts thus experience a greater depolarization from the EPC than if they were present on an unfolded membrane, as in the non-junctional region.

These two factors, the high local density of Na_V1 channels and the folding of the postsynaptic membrane, cooperate to lower the effective threshold at the NMJ. The observed magnitude of this effect is well-accounted for by the appropriate model of the postsynaptic region proposed by Martin (Martin, 1994). By lowering the effective threshold, the folds and the $Na_V1.4$ channels in them amplify the effects of the ACh released from the nerve. As a result, fewer ACh-gated ion channels need to be opened to generate an action potential than in the absence of these factors.

2.3.7. Termination of ACh action

The action of a quantum of ACh is terminated by a combination of diffusion of ACh molecules within the synaptic cleft and their enzymatic destruction by the AChE associated with the synaptic BL. If ACh were cleared from the cleft solely by diffusion, it would take many milliseconds for an average ACh molecule to diffuse out of reach of any AChRs. During this time, the molecules would be free to bind to further AChRs and thus prolong the EPC well after the initial muscle fiber action potential has terminated.

The AChE in the synaptic cleft greatly speeds up the process of ACh clearance. As described above, most of the ACh molecules released from the nerve bind rapidly to underlying AChRs, where they remain bound for about 1 ms. During this time, the ACh molecules that bind initially to AChE are cleaved and the AChE becomes available. As ACh molecules unbind from the AChRs, they quickly encounter and bind to

AChE and are cleaved. The net effect of the AChE is to limit both the lateral spread of ACh molecules in a quantum and the duration of their action (Fig. 2.12) (Hartzell et al., 1975). In physiological conditions, it is believed that as a result, most AChRs open only a single time in response to a quantum of ACh. If AChE is absent, or its effectiveness is impaired, both the duration and magnitude of the effect of a quantum are increased.

2.3.8. Conclusions

Each quantum of ACh released from the nerve acts on a discrete "response domain" in the muscle fiber surface. This consists of the AChR molecules at the crests of the 1–2 folds adjacent to the site of release, the high resistance sheets of cytoplasm within the junctional folds, and the $Na_V1.4$ channels contained in the membrane of the folds themselves. Each response domain occupies an area of about 0.2 μm^2 of the postsynaptic surface in contact with the nerve, or about 0.05% of the total synaptic surface at a typical mammalian NMJ. As a result, even when the quantal content is as much as 100, there is little probability that the ACh molecules from one released quantum will compete for AChRs with those from an adjacent quantum.

An important concept developed in recent years concerns the role of the postsynaptic folds. These previously enigmatic structures are now believed to act as amplifiers of ACh action. As such, they play an important role in ensuring the reliability of neuromuscular transmission.

2.4. Safety factor of neuromuscular transmission: definition and measurement

The previous sections have described the two core aspects of neuromuscular transmission: the quantal

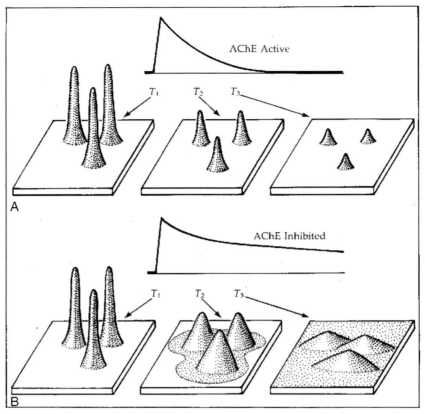

Fig. 2.12. Effect of AChE activity on synaptic events. A representation of the impact of AChE activity at the NMJ on the change in concentration in space and time of ACh released from the nerve. In the presence of normal AChE activity (upper part) the ACh released as a quantum from a given site on the nerve terminal is cleaved before it has spread into the 'territory' of another quantum. When the AChE is blocked, ACh spreads away from the release site and into the territories of adjacent quanta, thus activating additional AChRs with increasing time and prolonging the falling phase of the EPC. (From Hartzell et al., 1975, with permission.)

release of ACh by the nerve impulse and the action of that ACh on the muscle fiber to initiate an action potential. In practice, it is the balance between these two processes that determines whether the neural activation of muscle is successful. Many studies have shown that in a wide variety of conditions more ACh is released by each nerve impulse than is required to excite the muscle fiber. The terms "safety factor" or "safety margin" of neuromuscular transmission are used, more or less interchangeably, to describe this excess. For the clinician, an important implication of this safety factor is that by the time clinical weakness becomes apparent, considerable impairment of neuromuscular transmission may already have occurred.

This section addresses the questions of how the safety factor has been experimentally defined and its size estimated. Consideration of these topics is important because it gives insight into the various methods that have been used and the particular limitations they bring to the estimates of safety factor derived from them. It also provides a quantitative basis for understanding the normal reliability of neuromuscular transmission and how that may be altered in disease. This material has been reviewed in detail elsewhere (Wood and Slater, 2001).

2.4.1. Origin of the concept of a safety factor in excitable cells

The concept of a safety factor for cell excitation was initially developed in the context of AP propagation in unmyelinated axons (Rushton, 1937). Subsequent studies of myelinated axons suggested that the longitudinal current flowing within an axon from an active to an inactive node of Ranvier was 5–10 times greater than that required to initiate an AP (Hodgkin and Rushton, 1946). Further studies pointed out that the critical factor for the initiation of an AP is that the charge transferred, and the membrane depolarization it causes, should be distributed in such a way that enough sodium channels are opened to allow a net influx of positive charge (Jack et al., 1975), thus setting in train the regenerative events that constitute the AP (see Section 2.3.6.1).

Studies of isolated nerve-muscle preparations have established that during normal neuromuscular transmission more ACh is released from the nerve, causing more positive charge to enter the muscle at the NMJ, than is required to depolarize the muscle fiber to the threshold for AP generation (Wood and Slater, 1997). The safety factor of neuromuscular transmission is thus an expression of how much greater an effect the nerve has on the muscle fiber than is required to generate an AP (reviewed in Wood and Slater, 2001).

2.4.2. Definitions of the safety factor for neuromuscular transmission

A number of different working definitions of the safety of neuromuscular transmission have been proposed. The differences between them generally reflect the type of experiment carried out. In pharmacological studies, the safety factor was defined as the fraction of AChRs that could be blocked before AP generation was prevented (Paton and Waud, 1962; Chang et al., 1975). In electrophysiological studies, the safety factor has often been defined as the ratio of the estimated peak amplitude of the EPP to the threshold depolarization required to generate an AP (Harris and Ribchester, 1979a; Kelly and Robbins, 1983; Engel, 2004). Another approach has been to estimate the magnitude of the postsynaptic current flowing in response to a nerve impulse (Magleby, 1994), defining the safety factor as the excess current generated in response to a nerve impulse over that required to reach the AP threshold. Since the quantal content of the EPP is the feature of neuromuscular transmission that varies most during normal neuromuscular activity (see Section 2.5.1), still another approach is to define the safety factor as the ratio of the number of transmitter quanta released to the number required to excite the muscle fiber (Wood and Slater, 1997). This is the approach which will be emphasized in this section.

2.4.3. Estimating safety factor at the NMJ

To estimate the safety factor in terms of the number of quanta, it is necessary to estimate both the number of quanta released per nerve impulse and the number required to initiate an AP. In general this requires using intracellular microelectrodes to record both quantal and nerve-evoked synaptic events. To make

this possible, it is first necessary to block the generation of muscle fiber APs, both to allow the effect of the transmitter to be measured in the absence of the AP and to prevent the mechanical disturbance resulting from contraction. This leads to a fundamental difficulty in determining the safety factor; it is inherently impossible to determine both the amount of transmitter normally released by a nerve impulse and the amount required to trigger an AP in the same experimental conditions. Many different approaches have been taken to resolve this problem, each with its own limitations. A number of these are considered below. Further details can be found elsewhere (Prior et al., 1993; Isaacson and Walmsley, 1995).

2.4.3.1. Blocking action potential generation

Numerous methods have been used to block AP generation. Reducing the ratio of Ca^{++} to Mg^{++} concentrations in the bathing solution reduces transmitter release to levels that are too low to generate an AP (del Castillo and Katz, 1954). This method has the obvious limitation that it does not allow the full quantal content to be measured. Nonetheless, its simplicity makes it potentially useful for assessing the relative values of quantal content in different situations (Alshuaib and Fahim, 1990; Lyons and Slater, 1991). However, it must be borne in mind that even this use depends on the assumption that the sensitivity to Ca^{++} is constant in the situations being compared, and this may not be so.

An alternative that was used in many early studies was to partially block the response of the muscle to ACh with D-tubocurarine to reduce the amplitude of the EPP to a sub-threshold level (Fatt and Katz, 1951). Using this approach in mammals, 80% or more of the AChRs must be blocked to ensure that contraction is fully abolished and intracellular recordings can be made (Paton and Waud, 1962; Chang et al., 1975). As a result the mEPPs are usually too small to measure. Therefore, when a measure of the quantal content is required, indirect estimates based on the analysis of variation of EPP amplitudes must be used. These are inherently inaccurate in any situation that allows normal release (see Section 2.2.6) (Martin, 1955; Slater et al., 1992). A further limitation is that D-tubocurarine may also reduce the amount of transmitter released by interacting with presynaptic nicotinic autoreceptors (see Section 2.5.4.1) (Glavinović, 1979b; Magleby et al., 1981; Bowman et al., 1988; Ferry and Kelly, 1988).

An approach used successfully in a number of studies is to damage the muscle fibers, usually by cutting them some distance from the NMJ (Barstad and Lilleheil, 1968; Glavinović, 1979c; Maselli et al., 1991; Slater et al., 1992). This causes depolarization of the membrane, usually to a resting potential of about −40 mV. This, in turn, leads to inactivation of the voltage-gated sodium channels, thereby blocking AP generation in the muscle. This has the advantage that no drugs are required. However there are several disadvantages. The low resting membrane potential and reduced input resistance of the muscle fibers caused by the damage means that both EPPs and mEPPs are small and therefore difficult to record. This effect can be partially overcome by injecting a steady current into the muscle through a second intracellular electrode to restore the resting potential locally to a more negative value. A further complication is that extensive damage to the muscle results in the leakage of K^+ into the extracellular space. Unless care is taken to wash the muscle thoroughly, this may depolarize the intramuscular nerve branches, leading to a failure of propagation of the nerve impulse into the presynaptic terminal. In spite of these limitations, this approach has provided much useful information.

Recently, a natural toxin has become available which, in appropriate circumstances, blocks APs in the muscle but not in the nerve. In principle, this is currently the best available approach to the study of evoked release. μ-conotoxin GIIIB (μCTX) is a component of the venom of the cone snail *Conus geographus*. In initial studies, it was found that μCTX blocks rat muscle fiber sodium channels while having no effect on those from nerve or brain (Cruz et al., 1985; Moczydlowski et al., 1986). In subsequent studies, concentrations of μCTX were found which blocked action potentials in muscles of guinea pig (Muraki et al., 1991), mouse (Gonoi et al., 1989), rat (Plomp et al., 1992) and frog (Sosa and Zengel, 1993) but not in their nerves. However, it was subsequently shown that at high concentrations, μCTX blocks sodium currents in mouse nerves (Braga et al., 1992). While it is generally believed that the relative specificity for $Na_V1.4$ channels allows the use of μCTX to block all vertebrate NMJs, this is unfortunately not the case. In some human and chicken tissues, μCTX blocks the nerve impulse at concentrations lower than that required to block muscle APs (Plomp et al., 1995; Wood and Slater, 1998b). This raises the possibility that in some circumstances, the use of μCTX may lead to partial block of the nerve impulse and the reduction of transmitter release.

2.4.3.2. Estimating transmitter release using electrophysiology

The effect of the released transmitter on the muscle can be measured and expressed in several ways. The most straightforward is to record and measure the peak amplitude of full-sized EPPs in a situation in which the muscle fiber action potential has been blocked.

To make accurate recordings of synaptic events with intracellular electrodes, it is important to place the electrodes close (<100 μm) to the NMJ. Otherwise, the passive cable properties of the muscle membrane result in the amplitude of the EPP declining as the recording electrode is placed increasingly far from the NMJ (Fatt and Katz, 1951; Betz et al., 1984). This effect is best overcome by making recordings in a situation where the NMJ can be directly visualized. The can be done most directly by using fluorescent dyes such as 4-di-2-asp (a mitochondrial dye; (Magrassi et al., 1987)) or FM1–43 (see Section 2.2.7). In favorable conditions, it may also be possible to visualize the NMJ without fluorescent dyes, simply using bright field or Nomarski interference contrast optics. As an alternative, recordings may be limited to those where the rise time of the EPP is faster than some preset value (e.g., 1 ms), since EPP rise time is a function of distance from the NMJ (Fatt and Katz, 1951; Betz et al., 1984).

While the amplitude of the EPP provides a measure of transmitter effect, it is not an accurate reflection of the amount of transmitter released from the nerve. This is because of the non-linear relationship between the amount of transmitter released and the resulting depolarization of the muscle fiber membrane (see Section 2.3.5.5). As a result, the amplitude of the EPP generally underestimates the number of quanta that give rise to it (McLachlan, 1978; Slater et al., 1992). This confounding factor becomes greater as the quantal content increases.

Various formulas for adjusting the EPP amplitude to take account of this "non-linear summation" have been devised (Martin, 1976; Stevens, 1976; McLachlan and Martin, 1981), such as;

$$v' = v/(1 - v/E)$$

where v' is the adjusted EPP amplitude, v is the recorded EPP amplitude and E is the difference between the resting potential and the reversal potential for transmitter action, usually between 0 and −10 mV. In practise there are considerable uncertainties involved in using these corrections. This is because, in addition to the effect of non-linear summation, the magnitude of the peak depolarization of the recorded EPP is also influenced by the capacitative properties of the muscle fiber membrane (see Section 2.3.5.3). Efforts have been made to account for this, for example by introducing an additional variable (f) into some of the equations (Martin, 1976) as follows;

$$v' = v/(1 - fv/E)$$

Unfortunately, the value of f can only be determined empirically, greatly reducing the usefulness of the whole approach.

A better way around the difficulties raised by non-linear summation is to make recordings of synaptic currents rather than potentials. To do this, two micro-electrodes need to be inserted within 100 µm of the NMJ and used to "voltage-clamp" the muscle fiber. EPCs can then be recorded over a range of membrane potentials (Takeuchi and Takeuchi, 1959; Magleby and Stevens, 1972; Glavinović, 1979c; Slater et al., 1992). This method provides a more direct estimate of transmitter release since the amplitudes of the recorded currents are linearly related to the number of ion channels opened by the released ACh and hence to the amount of ACh released (McLachlan, 1978).

2.4.3.3. Estimating quantal content

To estimate the safety factor in terms of the number of quanta normally released by a nerve impulse, it is necessary to determine the quantal content. The most direct way to do this is to determine the ratio between the peak amplitude of the EPCs and the mEPCs. Since there is statistical variation in both the effect of individual quanta and of the number of quanta released, even at the same NMJ in the same experiment, mean amplitudes of a suitable number of events must always be used in these calculations. Another important consideration is that the quantal content varies depending on the pattern and frequency of activity (see Section 2.5.1). In isolated nerve-muscle preparations from frogs and mammals, stimulation at frequencies greater than about 0.2–1 Hz results in a frequency dependent reduction in quantal release (see below). In what follows, values for quantal content have been derived from studies in which the frequency of stimulation was not greater than 1Hz. It must be emphasized that while this approach allows comparison of quantal content in differing situations, it does not represent the values expected to apply during natural patterns of activity.

The amplitude of synaptic events depends on the membrane potential at which they are recorded. It is therefore important either to record both spontaneous and evoked events at the same membrane potential, or to make some correction for differences in membrane potential. One approach is to use two intracellular electrodes in a "current clamp" configuration to maintain a constant membrane potential that is sufficiently negative to allow mEPPs to be recorded even from cut fiber preparations (Slater et al., 1992). In many species, spontaneous quantal events occur at a frequency of about 1 Hz and 50–100 events can be recorded with no difficulty. In some cases, such as normal humans or immature rodents, the frequency is much lower—of the order of a few per minute. One way around this, which is effective in human nerve-muscle preparations, is to stimulate the nerve at high frequency (50 Hz) for up to 10 s. This results in a great increase in the frequency of quantal events, which lasts from 10–20 s (Magleby, 1994). In our experience, the mean amplitude of mEPPs recorded this way does not differ significantly from those recorded without stimulation, though this may not be true for more exhaustive stimulation (Van der, 1991; Glavinović, 1995).

Once the mean amplitudes of mEPCs and EPCs have been determined the quantal content (m) can be calculated as:

$$m = \text{EPC amplitude}/m\text{EPC amplitude}$$

This "direct" method can also be used with EPPs and mEPPs but then corrections must be made for both variations of resting membrane potential and non-linear summation (see Section 2.3.5.5) and these are likely to lead to inaccuracies in the final value:

$$m = \text{NLS}_{\text{corr}}\text{EPP amplitude}/m\text{EPP amplitude}$$

where "NLS$_{\text{corr}}$EPP amplitude" is the amplitude of the EPP corrected for non-linear summation. Reported values of quantal content obtained in comparable conditions using the "direct" method, with either potential or current recording, are generally from 20–200.

Many early estimates of quantal content were made in situations where quantal events could not be resolved so direct estimates of quantal content were not possible. In the absence of a measured value of quantum size, the assumption was made that the responses could be described by the Poisson distribution. On this basis, the mean quantal content could be estimated from a measure of the variance of the amplitude of the EPP (see Section 2.2.6). While this seems an attractive method to be used in preparations blocked by D-tubocurarine, it overlooks the fact that the Poisson approximation is only justified in situations where the probability of release from the nerve terminal, and hence the quantal content, is very low. When, as in solutions of normal Ca^{++} concentration, this is not true, the "variance" method significantly overestimates the quantal content (Fig. 2.13) (Martin, 1965; McLachlan, 1978; Slater et al., 1992).

For a long time, the use of the "variance" method to estimate quantal content led to the belief that the quantal content at mammalian, including human, NMJs was around 200, similar to that in frogs (Ginsborg and Jenkinson, 1976). Figures such as this may still be found in common text books. It is now clear, however, that at a stimulus frequency of 1 Hz, the true value at rat NMJs is between 50–100 (Glavinović, 1979a; Catterall and Coppersmith, 1981; Plomp et al., 1992; Wood and Slater, 1995) while in humans it is lower still, 20–50 (Fig. 2.21, Section 2.6.1.1) (Cull-Candy et al., 1980; Engel et al., 1990; Slater et al., 1992; Plomp et al., 1995).

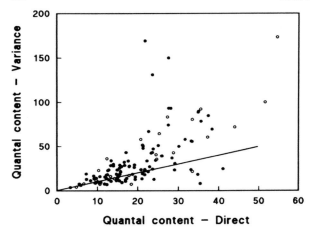

Fig. 2.13. Comparison of direct and variance estimates of quantal content. Data from human NMJs, in a solution allowing normal ACh release, show that use of the "variance method" substantially overestimates the value of the quantal content. (From Slater et al., 1992, with permission.)

In summary, the most accurate way to estimate quantal release is to record EPCs and mEPCs from muscle in which action potentials have been blocked and to use the direct method to calculate quantal content. In species where μCTX cannot be used, or when quantal events cannot be resolved, it may be necessary to resort to other less direct approaches as described above.

2.4.3.4. Measuring the "threshold quantal content"

Having obtained a measure of transmitter release per nerve impulse, it is then necessary to estimate how much transmitter is "required" to generate an action potential. This involves first determining the threshold at the NMJ, as described in Section 2.3.6.2 , and then estimating the number of quanta that must be released to reach that threshold. The number of quanta that would have to act to reach threshold can be estimated from the mean amplitude of threshold EPCs recorded during partial block by D-tubocurarine (Wood and Slater, 1997). This amplitude must then be divided by the mean amplitude of mEPCs recorded in the absence of D-tubocurarine to arrive at an estimate of the threshold quantal content. For both the "fast" EDL and the "slow" soleus muscles of the rat, the value of threshold quantal content is about 13. This is about 25% of the normal quantal content at these NMJs.

2.4.3.5. Comparison of reported values of safety factor at rat NMJs

The concept of a safety factor for neuromuscular transmission was first discussed in detail nearly 40 years ago (Paton and Waud, 1967). Since then there have

been remarkably few efforts to assess it quantitatively and those that have been made have used a variety of methods and preparations and are not, therefore, strictly comparable. Nonetheless, they provide a general consensus that at NMJs in most mammalian limb muscles, studied in vitro, the safety factor is between 2 and 10 (Table 2.1).

Some of the highest estimates of safety factor come from pharmacological experiments at mammalian NMJs (Paton and Waud, 1962; Chang et al., 1975). By blocking increasing fractions of AChRs with D-tubocurarine, it was found that 80–90% of the receptors could be blocked before there was any failure of indirectly evoked contraction. These studies suggest that, at low frequencies, 5–10 times more ACh-gated channels are normally opened than is required to generate an action potential. Such experiments also established that there is a substantial excess of AChRs at the NMJ (Ginsborg and Jenkinson, 1976). However, the distributed nature of transmitter release and the short distance over which the ACh in a single quantum acts (see Section 2.3.8) means that in spite of this nominal excess, most of the AChRs are out of range of the ACh released by any given nerve impulse.

Many studies have used intracellular recording techniques to estimate the safety factor. In their classic study of the EPP in mammalian muscle, Boyd and Martin (1956) estimated that the EPP, in the absence of an action potential, would be about 35–40 mV while a depolarization of only 10–20 mV would be required to generate an action potential. Thus, a safety factor of 2–4 can be derived from their data. In other studies, the amplitude of the full-sized EPP was estimated from the product of the quantal content and the mEPP amplitude and then "corrected" for non-linear summation (Kelly, 1978; Harris and Ribchester, 1979b). In these studies, the quantal content was estimated from the variance of EPPs recorded at NMJs blocked with D-tubocurarine. Since the variance method substantially overestimates the quantal content (Section 2.4.3.3) this approach is likely to overestimate the EPP amplitude. In the same studies, the action potential threshold was measured by passing rectangular current pulses through the membrane some distance from the NMJ. This is likely to overestimate the threshold (Section 2.3.6.2). Since both components of the safety factor ratio are overestimated, the errors generated tend by chance to cancel each other out.

A value for safety factor has been defined based on how many more quanta are released per nerve impulse than are required to trigger an action potential. Using the methods described in Section 2.4.3, values within the range observed by others were obtained (Wood and Slater, 1997). In rat soleus and EDL, the normal

Table 2.1

The range of reported safety factors for neuromuscular transmission in different muscles. In some cases the values are derived from data presented in the paper referred to. These values are not directly comparable with one another since different methods have been used to estimate the safety factor (see Section 2.4) and different experimental conditions such as temperature, pattern of activity and age of animals may influence the reported value (see Section 2.6).

Species	Muscle	Safety factor	Source
Rat	Soleus	1.8	Gertler and Robbins (1978)
		3.5	Wood and Slater (1997)
	EDL	2.0	Gertler and Robbins (1978)
		5.0	Wood and Slater (1997)
	Diaphragm	3.0–5.0	Chang et al. (1975)
		2.0–3.6	Kelly (1978)
		1.7–2.8	Wareham et al. (1994)
Mouse	Soleus	4.6–5.8	Banker et al. (1983)
	EDL	2.4–2.8	Harris and Ribchester (1979b)
		3.2–5.8	Banker et al. (1983)
Human	Intercostal	2.0	Elmqvist et al. (1964)
Cat	Tennuissimus	2.0–4.0	Boyd and Martin (1956)
	Tibialis	4.0–12.0	Paton and Waud (1967)
	Sartorius	4.0–12.0	Paton and Waud (1967)
Frog	Cutaneous pectoris	4.0	Grinnell and Herrerra (1980)
	Sartorius	1.0	Grinnell and Herrerra (1980)
		3.1–5.5	Adams (1989)

quantal content is 46.3 and 65.1, respectively, while the corresponding threshold quantal contents are 13.3 and 13.0. Thus, the calculated safety factors are 3.5 for soleus and 5.0 for EDL.

2.4.4. Conclusions

Whatever methodological approach has been used, studies of the safety factor at normal mammalian NMJs stimulated in vitro at or near 1 Hz suggest a typical value of about 4 (Table 2.1). While some estimates appear to be based on more firm methodological foundations than others, it is important to reiterate that all must be considered imperfect estimates of the true value *in vivo*, where varying patterns of activity and the actions of many modulating factors may play an important part in determining the safety factor at any moment. The most important of these modulating factors are considered in the following section.

2.5. Modulation of safety factor during normal use

Why is the safety factor for neuromuscular transmission so high? During natural use of the neuromuscular system, the pattern and amount of activity change over a wide range. The ability of the nerve to release transmitter varies significantly as the frequency of activation changes. In particular, during high frequency activity, the quantal content declines significantly. Most published estimates of quantal content that have been used to estimate safety factor (Table 2.1) were determined at low frequencies (0.1–1 Hz) and are assumed to represent close to the maximum release of which the NMJ is capable in physiological conditions. During normal usage, the quantal content is almost certainly lower.

There are many factors in the nerve terminal that influence its response to different activity patterns (Van der Kloot and Molgo, 1994; Atwood and Karunanithi, 2002). Most important are the dynamics of Ca^{++} concentration and the synaptic vesicle "pools" in the nerve terminal, and the action of chemical modulators on the nerve terminal and the Schwann cells associated with it. Although our understanding of these factors, and the interactions between them, is still very incomplete, it is likely that they play an important part in regulating the efficacy of neuromuscular transmission.

2.5.1. The effects of repetitive activity on release

When isolated nerve-muscle preparations are stimulated repetitively at frequencies much above 0.1 Hz,

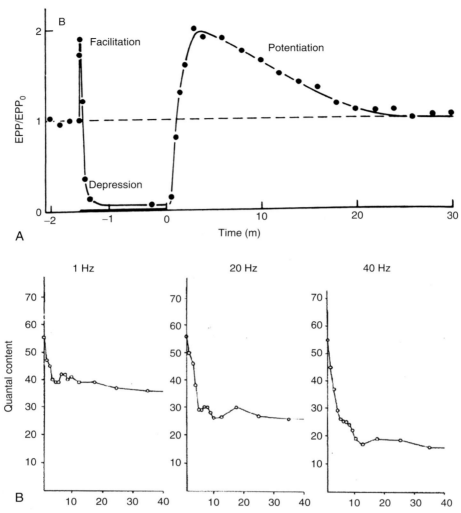

Fig. 2.14. Changes in neuromuscular transmission during repetitive activation. (A) The effect of 90 s stimulation at 100 Hz on the amplitude of the EPP, relative to that during an initial period of stimulation at 0.1 Hz, at a partially curarized (dTC, 3 μM) frog NMJ. An initial increase due to facilitation of ACh release is followed by a decline due to depression of release. When the 100 Hz stimulation stops, there is a further phase of increased EPP amplitude reflecting post-activation potentiation of ACh release. (From Magleby, 1994, with permission. (B) The quantal content at NMJs in human intercostal muscle declines during repetitive activation. (From Kamenskaya et al., 1975, with permission.) Note that there is little evidence of facilitation at mammalian NMJs when the quantal content is normal, in contrast to frog NMJs.

the quantal content varies in ways that depend both on the frequency, duration of stimulation, and the species and type of muscle. These changes in release involve both increases and decreases, each of which may occur on several different time scales (Fig. 2.14A) (Magleby, 1994; Zucker and Regehr, 2002).

2.5.1.1. Decreases in quantal content

With mammalian nerve-muscle preparations in physiological concentrations of Ca^{++} (e.g., 2mM), the predominant effect of repetitive stimulation at 1–100 Hz

is a progressive reduction in quantal content that often has several components that vary in time course and magnitude (Liley and North, 1953; Elmqvist and Quastel, 1965; Kamenskaya et al., 1975). The fastest component of depression generally lasts for 10–20 stimuli so that at 50–100 Hz, this phase thus lasts <0.5 s (Fig. 2.14B). During this time the quantal content typically falls to 30–80% of its value at 1 Hz, depending on the frequency.

It is generally believed that the decline in quantal content during high frequency stimulation reflects the depletion of the population of vesicles docked at the AZs (Rizzoli and Betz, 2005). It is likely that the docked vesicles exist in different states of readiness for release. In particular they may be in various stages of "priming", in the sense that they have undergone ATP-dependent associations with the release proteins of the nerve membrane that represent the first steps in exocytosis (Fig. 2.7). The process of priming is complex and involves members of the Munc and Rab protein families (Sudhof, 2004). Current estimates of the priming process suggest that it takes place on a timescale of a few seconds (Rettig and Neher, 2002). These primed vesicles are considered to form a "readily releasable pool" (RRP, see Section 2.5.2).

Only a small fraction of the vesicles in the terminal are docked at AZs at any time. For a typical mammalian NMJ, the total number of vesicles is about 250 000–350 000. Of these, no more than about 1000–2000 can be docked (2/AZ, 2.6 AZ/μm^2, synaptic area 200–400 μm^2). The probability of any one docked vesicle being released by a given nerve impulse is about 0.05–0.1 at rest, giving a quantal content of about 50–100. In the frog, if the RRP is rapidly depleted, it refills within a few seconds (Kalkstein and Magleby, 2004). In any physiological situation, the instantaneous quantal content is therefore likely to reflect a balance between the rates of depletion and refilling of the RRP. The higher the frequency of simulation, the more fully the RRP is depleted and the lower the instantaneous quantal content.

Prolonged stimulation causes further, slower, components of reduced quantal content on timescales of seconds and minutes (Magleby, 1994). The first of these ($\sim$5 s) is believed to reflect the "priming" of vesicles already close to the AZ into a releasable state. The slowest component of depression is believed to reflect the movement of vesicles from a reserve pool held at some distance from the AZs to the vicinity of the AZs (see below) (Rizzoli and Betz, 2005).

2.5.1.2. Increases in quantal release

In addition to processes that lead to decreases in quantal content, others do the opposite. At least three distinct phases of increasing quantal content have been defined: facilitation (<1 s), augmentation (5–10 s) and potentiation (10 s of seconds to minutes) (Kamenskaya et al., 1975; Magleby, 1979). Facilitation has long been believed to result from the persistence of "residual Ca^{++}" in the nerve terminal after an initial nerve impulse (Katz and Miledi, 1968). If a second impulse arrives before the effect of the Ca^{++} that entered during the first has fully subsided, then the residual Ca^{++} is expected to sum with that entering during the second impulse and "facilitate" quantal release (Zucker and Regehr, 2002).

In bathing solutions with normal Ca^{++} concentration (2 mM), facilitation is not a marked feature of the response at normal mammalian NMJs. This is because the amount of Ca^{++} entering the opened Ca^{++} channels is already enough to cause a near maximal effect. However, as the external Ca^{++} is lowered, or Ca^{++} entry is reduced by a pathological process, the response falls below the maximal and the facilitating effect of any residual Ca^{++} becomes obvious. Thus there is often an inverse relationship between the low frequency quantal content and the amount of facilitation. An important clinical example of this is seen in the Lambert–Eaton Myasthenic Syndrome (see Section 2.8).

The factors accounting for augmentation and potentiation are less clear. All phases of enhanced quantal release are associated in time with the accumulation of Ca^{++} in the nerve terminal (Zucker and Regehr, 2002). One likely source of the prolonged increase in Ca^{++} associated with potentiation is the slow release from mitochondria of Ca^{++} taken up during intense activity (David and Barrett, 2003) (see below).

2.5.1.3. Relationship to clinical EMG protocols

How do the many components of frequency-dependent modulation of quantal release, described above, interact to determine the real instantaneous quantal content and safety factor *in vivo*? This question is of great importance to the clinical neurophysiologist who needs to devise tests that can reveal the functional state of the nerve terminals in patients. One of the most common tests uses the response of the compound muscle action potential (CMAP) to nerve stimulation at 3–5 Hz to test for the efficacy of neuromuscular transmission. At this frequency, facilitation is low so depression can be readily detected.

2.5.2. Vesicle pools and their dynamics

Underlying much of our understanding of the modulation of quantal release by activity is the notion that synaptic vesicles exist in different states within the nerve terminal. These are defined both by the location of the vesicles, in particular their proximity to the AZs, and by their functional state. Studies of the various temporal phases of depression and enhancement of release during repetitive stimulation have led to the notion that vesicles exist in distinct "pools", and that they can move from one pool to another with definable kinetics (Fig. 2.15) (Rizzoli and Betz, 2005). Recent investigation of the dynamics of these pools has utilized the activity-dependent labeling of vesicles with fluorescent dyes, most notably steryl dyes including FM1-43 and analogs of it (Cochilla et al., 1999).

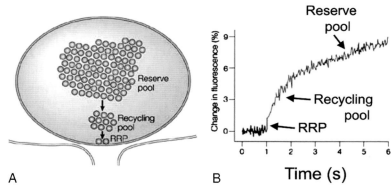

Fig. 2.15. Vesicle pools at the NMJ. (A) Schematic representation of the three physiologically distinct pools of vesicles in a nerve terminal: the reserve pool, the recycling pool and the readily releasable pool (RRP). See text for further details. In reality, the vesicles of the recycling and reserve pools are intermingled and not topographically separate. (B) During depolarization of retinal bipolar cells, fluorescent dye contained in the vesicles is released revealing the kinetic relationships between the pools. The RRP is released virtually instantaneously, the recycling pool is emptied within a few seconds, and the reserve pool is released more gradually over a period of minutes. Similar kinetic relationships characterize the vesicle pools at NMJs. (From Rizzoli and Betz, 2005, with permission.)

The vesicles of the RRP represent only a small fraction (<1%) of all the vesicles in a motor nerve terminal. It is depleted within less than 1 s by stimulation at 10–100 Hz. Most vesicles (80–90%) are located some distance from the AZs and are believed to be tethered to the actin cytoskeleton by phosphorylation-dependent bonds with synapsin 1 (Rizzoli and Betz, 2005). Periods of stimulation lasting minutes are required to release vesicles from this "reserve pool". Between the reserve pool and the RRP are vesicles that are available for rapid docking, the so-called "recycling pool". This pool typically contains 10–20% of the vesicles in the terminal and vesicles from it are released by stimulation lasting more than a few seconds. While it is clear that movement of vesicles between these pools can occur in experimental conditions, little is known about their dynamics in vivo.

2.5.3. Mitochondria as modulators of quantal release

As mentioned above, many of the short-term changes in quantal content induced by repetitive activity appear to reflect changes in the concentration of free Ca^{++} in the nerve terminal. A number of factors influence how, and at what rate, the increase in Ca^{++} concentration in the nerve associated with a single nerve impulse is restored to the resting level. The mitochondria, which are prominent components of the presynaptic cytoplasm (Fig. 2.1D), are one of these factors.

The most familiar role of mitochondria is to provide ATP to power a wide variety of cellular activities, such as the complex and demanding processes of exocytosis and ionic regulation during intense activity. However,

mitochondria also act to sequester Ca^{++}, and are therefore well placed to play a key role in Ca^{++} homeostasis in the nerve terminal (Alnaes and Rahamimoff, 1975; David et al., 1998). Depolarization of mitochondria by drugs such as CCCP (*m*-chlorophenyl-hydrazone) blocks Ca^{++} uptake into the mitochondria and thus allows a build up of Ca^{++} in the nerve terminal during intense activity. This, in turn, increases the rate of spontaneous mEPPs that is very pronounced during and after high frequency stimulation (David and Barrett, 2003).

When NMJs poisoned by CCCP are studied at normal Ca^{++} concentration, intense stimulation (50 Hz for 10 s) leads to a much greater decline in quantal release than in normal medium (Fig. 2.16A, C). This effect is paradoxical in that an increase in Ca^{++} within the nerve terminal would be expected to increase evoked release, as during facilitation (see above). The explanation seems to lie in a great increase in the frequency of spontaneous quantal release (Fig. 2.16B). This increase in "asynchronous" release is so great that it rapidly depletes the RRP, thus reducing evoked release.

It is possible to visualize and measure the levels of Ca^{++} in the nerve terminal using Ca^{++}-sensitive fluorescent dyes, injected into the terminal (David et al., 1997). During bursts of high frequency stimulation, the level of Ca^{++} increases first in the cytoplasm and then in the mitochondria. After such a burst, the elevated Ca^{++} persists in the mitochondria after it has declined in the cytoplasm. If mitochondrial function is blocked, using drugs that abolish the mitochondrial proton gradient, the increase in Ca^{++} in the cytoplasm is greatly exaggerated (David and Barrett, 2003). Thus, the observed changes in release all have parallels in the levels of cytoplasmic Ca^{++} and these

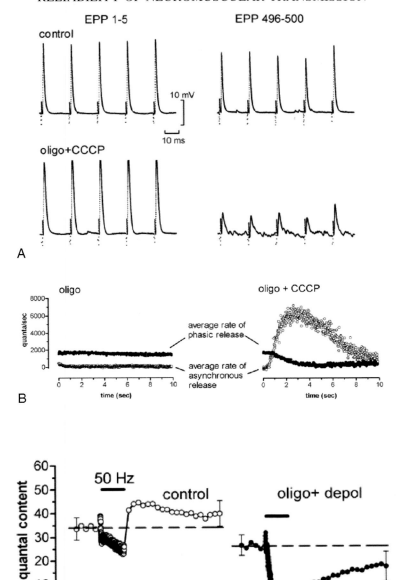

Fig. 2.16. Role of mitochondrial function in maintaining quantal release. Mouse NMJs were stimulated at 50 Hz for 10 s. (A) EPPs recorded at the beginning (EPP 1–5) and end (EPP 496–500) of the train of stimuli. The lower traces show the much greater decline of EPP amplitude when mitochondria are depolarized by CCCP than in the control solution. Note also the great increase in mEPP frequency at the CCCP treated NMJ. (B) Changes in quantal release per second due to evoked ("phasic") release and spontaneous ('asynchronous') release during the train. Note that in CCCP blocked preparations, asynchronous release rapidly outstrips evoked release. (C) Changes in quantal content during and after the train. Note the greater and more prolonged reduction at NMJs when the mitochondria had been blocked. (From David and Barrett, 2003, with permission.)

appear to be closely regulated by the mitochondria. The effects of specific mitochondrial blockers show that these relatively short-term effects of the mitochondria are dependent on the state of the proton gradient rather than on the ability of the mitochondria to supply ATP (David and Barrett, 2003).

It is clear from these studies that mitochondria can exert a modulatory influence on quantal release at the NMJ. While it is difficult to assess the significance of this effect in vivo, it seems possible that the general metabolic state of an animal could have a real impact on the efficacy and reliability of neuromuscular transmission.

2.5.4. Effects of chemical modulators on release

There is extensive evidence that quantal release of ACh at the NMJ is subject to modulation by a variety of naturally occurring chemical mediators (Van der Kloot and Molgo, 1994). The history of this field is complex, partly because many of the effects are on a modest scale, partly because it is difficult to establish the site of action of bath applied drugs, and partly because of real differences in the properties of NMJs in frogs on the one hand and the mammals that have been studied. Nonetheless, there is now extensive evidence of negative modulation of quantal release both by ACh itself and by ATP (or its metabolite adenosine) released along with ACh, and of positive modulation by noradrenaline. In principle, these modulatory effects could reduce the safety factor during normal activity or enhance it in times of stress ("fight or flight").

2.5.4.1. Autocrine effects on release: cholinergic

For many years there has been evidence that ACh acts presynaptically as well as postsynaptically at the NMJ. Early pharmacological studies suggested that ACh exerted a direct depolarizing effect on the nerve terminals that acted to decrease quantal content (Hubbard and Wilson, 1970; Ferry and Kelly, 1988). This effect was believed to be blocked by both D-tubocurarine and atropine, leaving doubts about the nature of the cholinergic receptors involved. Subsequent studies have provided clear evidence that muscarinic AChRs (mAChRs) are present at mammalian NMJs and that bath-applied muscarine reduces quantal content at mouse NMJs maintained in a physiological concentration of Ca^{++} (Fig. 2.17) (Minic et al., 2002). This suggests that a mechanism exists whereby ACh can limit its own release.

The mechanism of mAChR regulation of quantal release is complicated. In mice with active AChE, muscarine activates M_2 mAChRs to cause a pertussis toxin-dependent reduction in quantal content. However,

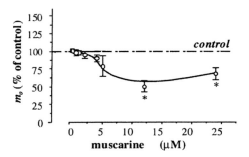

Fig. 2.17. Muscarinic effects on quantal release of ACh. Muscarine causes a dose-dependent reduction in the quantal content at NMJs in the mouse diaphragm. Muscles were studied in low Ca^{++} (0.4 mM) and high Mg^{++} (6–8 mM) to reduce the EPP amplitude and thus abolish contraction and stimulated at 0.3 Hz. (From Minic et al., 2002, with permission.)

when AChE is absent or its activity is blocked, muscarine causes an enhancement of quantal content that is not blocked by pertussis toxin and is therefore likely to be due to activations of M_1 mAChRs (Minic et al., 2002; Santafe et al., 2003; Slutsky et al., 2003).

Similar biphasic effects have been described at frog NMJs, where it has also been shown that the enhancement of release caused by activation of M_2 mAChRs is associated with an increase in the amplitude of the presynaptic Ca^{++} current (Slutsky et al., 1999, 2001). No change in Ca^{++} current was observed following activation of M_1 mAChRs. Since M1 and M2 mAChRs act via different G-protein coupled pathways, it is clear that the balance between the effects of these two mAChR types is likely to be influenced by many aspects of the physiology of the nerve terminal.

2.5.4.2. Autocrine effects on release: purinergic

Synaptic vesicles contain and release ATP as well as ACh (Silinsky and Hubbard, 1973; Silinsky, 1975). Once in the synaptic cleft, ATP is broken down by ectonucleotidases, releasing adenosine. There is evidence that both exogenous ATP and adenosine can depress quantal release and that purinergic receptors for both compounds are present at the NMJ (Deuchars et al., 2001; Moores et al., 2005). As with cholinergic modulation of release, the effects of activation of these receptors are complex. Exposure of isolated nerve-muscle preparations to ATP reduces quantal release. It seems likely that this is due in part to direct effects of ATP on P_2 receptors (Hong and Chang, 1998; Sokolova et al., 2003) and in part to the effects of adenosine released following ATP breakdown.

In physiological conditions, exogenous adenosine inhibits quantal release (Ginsborg and Hirst, 1972),

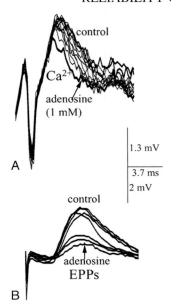

Fig. 2.18. Adenosine reduces quantal release. Exogenous adenosine (1 mM) reduces both the Ca^{++} current in the nerve terminal at mouse NMJs (A) and the amplitude of the EPP (B). (From Silinsky, 2004, with permission.)

an effect mediated by P_1A_1 purinergic receptors (Silinsky, 1980). At mouse NMJs, this effect is accompanied by a reduction in the presynaptic Ca^{++} current (Fig. 2.18A, B) (Silinsky, 2004). However, activation of P_1A_2 receptors, detected after inhibiting the downstream effects of P_1A_1 receptors, increased ACh release (Silinsky et al., 1989). To add further to the complexity of purinergic modulation of quantal release at the NMJ, there is also evidence of cross-talk between the muscarinic and purinergic systems (Oliveira et al., 2002).

2.5.4.3. Effects of reactive oxygen species

The events associated with neuromuscular transmission and muscle contraction require a constant and immediate supply of ATP. Reactive oxygen species (ROS) such as superoxide, H_2O_2 and the hydroxyl radical are generated as consequences of ATP synthesis by mitochondria. Recent studies have provided evidence that ROS exert a negative effect on quantal release (Giniatullin and Giniatullin, 2003; Kovyazina et al., 2003). This may serve to limit ACh output during intense activity.

2.5.4.4. Schwann cells and modulation of quantal release

While it is clear that multiple effects of ACh and ATP/ adenosine can be demonstrated at mammalian and frog NMJs, it is difficult to know where the receptors mediating these effects are located. Although it is

often assumed that these "presynaptic" receptors are on the nerve terminals, they could also be on the terminal Schwann cells (Minic et al., 2002). There is considerable evidence from the frog NMJ that Schwann cells play an active role in the regulation of quantal release (Auld et al., 2003). The terminal Schwann cells express functional muscarinic and P_2X and P_2Y purinergic receptors. Activation of these receptors leads to an increase in cytoplasmic Ca^{++}, probably as a result of release of Ca^{++} from intracellular stores (Jahromi et al., 1992; Robitaille, 1995; Robitaille et al., 1997). This increase in Schwann cell Ca^{++} is associated with a parallel increase in quantal release from the nerve. However, the link between these events is unclear.

Both mAChRs and P_2Y purinergic receptors act via G-protein coupled pathways. The effects on quantal release of direct injections of non-hydrolysable GTP and GDP analogues into the Schwann cells, designed to mimic receptor activation and inhibition respectively, have therefore been investigated (Robitaille, 1998). Injection of GTPγS, a non-hydrolyzable analog of GTP, which activates G-proteins, led to a significant reduction in quantal release in response to high frequency stimulation (Fig. 2.19). By contrast, injection of GDPβS, which antagonizes G proteins, had no such effect. It thus seems that in the frog, the terminal Schwann cells may play an active part in regulating quantal release from the motor nerve terminal. While it is less clear that the same effects occur at mammalian NMJs, it has been shown that activation of mAChRs leads to increases in cytoplasmic Ca^{++} in mammalian Schwann cells (Rochon et al., 2001).

It is thus clear that there is a rich network of potential autoregulatory presynaptic effects at the NMJ. These bear similarities to regulatory pathways at CNS synapses, and to the involvement of astrocytes as modulators of synaptic strength. What remains unclear is how important these effects are at normal NMJs in vivo. Many of them are most prominent at high frequencies of stimulation, and may serve to protect against the deleterious effects of excessive ACh action on the postsynaptic region (see below).

2.5.4.5. NO as a modulator of release

Nitric oxide synthase (NOS) is concentrated at NMJs in frogs and mammals (Kusner and Kaminski, 1996; Descarries et al., 1998) although its cellular distribution remains controversial (Rothe et al., 2005). There is considerable evidence that its product, NO, inhibits quantal release at frog NMJs (Lindgren and Laird, 1994; Thomas and Robitaille, 2001; Etherington and Everett, 2004). The mechanism of the effects of NO appears to depend on the frequency of stimulation.

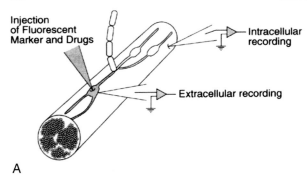

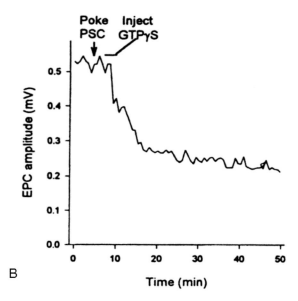

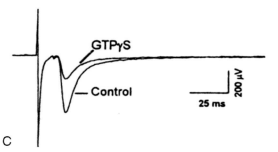

Fig. 2.19. Schwann cells influence ACh release from the nerve. (A) Injection of a stable analog of ATP (GTPγS) into terminal Schwann cells at frog NMJs. (B) Time course of reduction of EPC amplitude during stimulation at 10 Hz. (C) Sample EPCs before (control) and 30 min after injection of GTPγS. (From Auld et al., 2003, with permission.)

Thus at low frequency they are cGMP-dependent but at high frequency they are not (Thomas and Robitaille, 2001; Etherington and Everett, 2004). While the presence of NOS at mammalian NMJs suggests that NO may be a modulator of transmission in mammals, this has not been directly demonstrated.

2.5.4.6. Adrenergic modulation of quantal release

In addition to the potential modulatory effects mediated by ACh and ATP released at the NMJ, there are other effects mediated by circulating factors. The best known of these is the action of noradrenaline. It has long been recognized that stimulation of the sympathetic nerve supply can potentiate neuromuscular transmission in fatigued frog muscles (Orbeli, 1923). Modern microelectrode studies agree that this effect involves an increase in the amplitude of the EPP, but there has been little consensus about its origin. Thus increases in both mEPP size (Van der and van der Kloot, 1986) and quantal content (Hutter and Loewenstein, 1955; Krnjević and Miledi, 1958; Jenkinson et al., 1968; Vizi, 1991) have been suggested. Recently, a further effect of noradrenaline on frog NMJs has been reported (Bukchareva et al., 1999). Using focal extracellular recording (see Fig. 2.4 above), it has been found that bath applied noradrenaline increases the synchrony of quantal release (Fig. 2.20). This allows more effective summation of the effects of the individual quanta and results in a larger EPP. This effect is mediated by a signaling pathway involving activation of protein kinase A and an increase in cAMP concentration (Bukharaeva et al., 2002).

The potential biological significance of an enhancement of quantal release mediated by activation of adrenergic receptors presumably lies in its ability to ensure effective muscle activation in times of stress. Since most of the experimental evidence for such a modulatory pathway comes from work on frogs, its significance to mammalian and human physiology is unclear. Ephedrine, a sympathomimetic, has been used to treat patients with impaired neuromuscular transmission due to myasthenia gravis (MG) and several congenital myasthenic syndromes (see Section 2.8.7.1). When tested on canine NMJs in vitro, ephedrine has mixed effects, involving both enhanced quantal release and block of ACh-gated ion channels (Shinnick-Gallagher and Gallagher, 1979; Sieb and Engel, 1993; Milone and Engel, 1996). At concentrations associated with clinically beneficial effects in humans, it had little effect in vitro. One possible explanation of these findings is that ephedrine has some central effects in humans (Molenaar et al., 1993).

2.5.4.7. Modulation of quantal release by peptides and proteins

An influence of peptides on neuromuscular transmission activity is common in invertebrates and in the enteric nervous system of vertebrates (Shaw, 1996). At the vertebrate NMJ, there is some evidence that a variety of proteins or peptides may also exert a modulating effect. Many of these studies have been made on cultured nerve and muscle cells in vitro and have concentrated on the

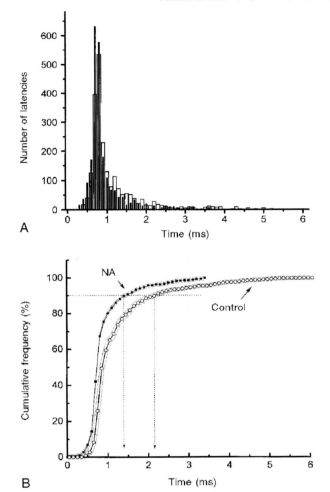

Fig. 2.20. Effect of noradrenaline on synchrony of release. Both the mean and the variance of the latency of EPCs recorded with extracellular electrodes from frog NMJs, bathed in low Ca^{++} (0.2 mM) medium to reduce ACh release and block contraction (see Fig. 2.5), are reduced by addition of noradrenaline (NA, 1×10^{-5} M). (A) Distribution of latencies in the control solution (open bars) and in NA (solid bars). (B) Cumulative histogram of latencies showing that 90% of latencies are less than 1.5 ms in NA compared to 90% in less than 2.2 ms in the control. (From Bukchareva et al., 1999, with permission.)

possible effects of neurotrophins (Poo, 2001; Lu and Je, 2003). Studies on nerve-muscle co-cultures from *Xenopus laevis* have shown enhancing effects of BDNF and NT-3 on both spontaneous (mEPPs) and evoked quantal release (Lohof et al., 1993). BDNF induces potentiation of quantal release associated with an increase in the cytosolic Ca^{++} in the nerve terminal (Stoop and Poo, 1996). By contrast, in the same system, CNTF potentiates quantal release in the absence of an effect on cytosolic Ca^{++} (Stoop and Poo, 1996).

Effects of neurotrophins have also been shown to influence quantal release in mammalian nerve-muscle preparations. BDNF and NT-4 both increase neuromuscular transmission in the rat diaphragm (Mantilla et al., 2004). A number of neurotrophins and related compounds were tested on nerve-muscle preparations from neonatal mice (Ribchester et al., 1998). While GDNF increased mEPP frequency, none of the other seven compounds tested had any effect. The significance of peptidergic modulation of neuromuscular transmission in adult mammals thus remains unclear.

Other peptides or proteins are released from motor nerve terminals along with ACh (Van der Kloot and Molgo, 1994). These include CGRP and agrin. Both these substances have effects on NMJ development and/or maintenance. However, there is no convincing evidence that they, or any other proteins released from the nerve have direct effects on quantal release.

2.5.5. Effects of muscle length on transmission

Contracting muscles generally change their length. Motor nerve terminals are mechanically coupled to the muscle fiber through adhesive interactions of both cells with the basal lamina. As a result, changes in muscle length have an impact on the length of the nerve terminal. In the frog, muscle stretch causes a significant increase in both spontaneous and evoked quantal release (Grinnell et al., 2003). Because frog terminals consist of straight branches running along the long axis of the muscle fiber, they are likely to experience a fractional change in length similar to that of the muscle fiber. The sensitivity of quantal release to muscle length is mediated by integrins present at the surface of both pre- and postsynaptic elements of the NMJ.

There is little evidence for sensitivity of mammalian neuromuscular transmission to muscle length. Although integrins are present at mammalian NMJs (Martin et al., 1996), studies of the rat diaphragm revealed no obvious sensitivity of quantal release to stretching (Grinnell et al., 2003). Whether this is due to the relatively compact and symmetric mechanical arrangement of mammalian NMJs or to the lack of the molecular components that transduce length changes is not known.

2.5.6. Conclusions

It is clear that many factors can influence the short-term efficacy of neuromuscular transmission at mammalian NMJs. Those that have been investigated most extensively are the pattern of activity, Ca^{++} sequestration by mitochondria and the effects of a wide variety of possible chemical modulators. Nearly all of these factors exert their effects on quantal release from the nerve. There are very few well-documented examples of short-term changes that influence the postsynaptic effect of ACh once it has been released.

Each of these many factors may be viewed as influencing the safety factor of neuromuscular transmission. Thus, each has an impact on the likelihood that a given nerve impulse in a motor neuron will cause contraction of the muscle fibers it innervates. However, with the exception of those activity-related effects, which appear to have their origins in the inherent properties of the release mechanism, the real physiological significance of many of the potential modulating factors that have been detected in vitro remains unclear.

2.6. Biological aspects of safety factor

The description presented so far of the factors that determine the reliability of neuromuscular transmission has been concerned almost entirely with the mature NMJs of normal adult animals. Further, although some mention has been made of differences between the NMJs of frogs and mammals, little attention has been paid to how NMJs in different species, or even within the same species, might differ. The first part of Section 2.6 will consider how NMJs vary between and within species. While a comparative approach may at first seem inappropriate or redundant to some clinical readers, it will become apparent that an appreciation of how different species achieve reliability has provided valuable insight into the way human NMJs achieve the same end.

The second part will consider how the factors that determine reliability in the adult come about, and how those factors change as individuals age. It will focus almost entirely on NMJs in mammals, including humans.

2.6.1. Variation between vertebrate species

There are substantial differences in the NMJs in different vertebrate species. At the level of the whole NMJ, some are much bigger than others and have different "shapes". Within the NMJ, there are also important variations in the details of both the pre- and postsynaptic specializations. These variations all have an impact on the efficacy of neuromuscular transmission.

2.6.1.1. NMJ size and shape
The NMJ of the frog is often presented as the "typical" NMJ. Yet it differs in important ways from those in

many other vertebrates in its conformation, overall size, and detailed structure. The frog motor nerve terminal consists of 5–10 elongate branches that run along the length of the muscle fiber. The overall length is typically 300 μm but the summed length of all the branches is typically about 1000 μm (Nudell and Grinnell, 1982). The axonal branches are overlaid by terminal Schwann cells. At intervals of about 1 μm, small finger-like projections of the Schwann cells wrap around the axon, intruding into the synaptic cleft. These effectively divide the axon into functional units about 1 μm long.

In mammals, including humans, a similar subdivision of the nerve terminal exists. As mentioned above (Section 2.1.2.1), mammalian terminals often consist of a series of roughly circular spot-like boutons, interconnected by fine axon branches (Fig. 2.1A, B). The area and volume of these boutons are roughly similar to the longitudinal units of the frog NMJ. In rats and mice, the boutons are sometimes fused, forming elongate terminal segments that are nonetheless much shorter than the major branches in the frog. The overall area of the NMJ in rats and mice is typically less than 25% of that in frogs. In humans, the NMJs are usually made up of clearly separated spot contacts and are even smaller than in rats and mice.

The functional significance of the natural variation in NMJ size is revealed when one compares the quantal content in the different species (Fig. 2.21). In frogs, the quantal content is typically 100–200 while in humans it is only 20–50, with rats and mice somewhere in between. When one compares the quantal content/unit area, however, all species are much more similar. Thus, there appears to be a relatively fixed "intrinsic release density" of about 0.2 quanta/μm^2 (Wood and Slater, 2001). At the same time, there is real variation around this basic value even in the same species and when NMJs on muscle fibers of similar size, and input resistance, are compared. This is likely to reflect adaptation of the release system to the specific functions of different motor units.

2.6.1.2. Release mechanism
In addition to the differences in the overall conformation or shape of the NMJs in different species, there are also differences on a smaller scale that influence quantal release. Of particular importance is the difference in AZ structure. In frogs, where the first detailed structural analysis of AZs was made (Hirokawa and Heuser, 1982; Harlow et al., 2001), the AZ consists of two parallel linear arrays of membrane proteins about 1 μm long and separated by about 50 nm. About 30 docked vesicles are normally associated with each AZ, lying on either

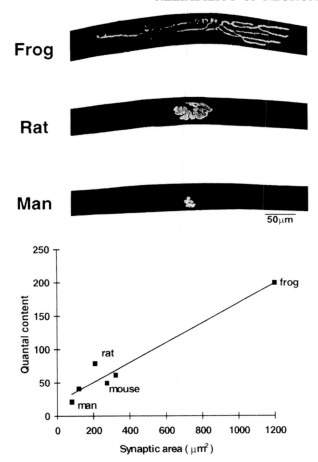

Fig. 2.21. Quantal content is related to NMJ size in different species. Typical NMJs of frog, rat and man are shown in the top part, all at the same magnification. The NMJs are shown in white and the muscle fibers in black. Note the small size of human NMJs. There is a roughly linear relationship between quantal content and synaptic area (bottom part).

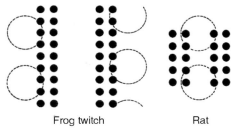

Frog twitch   Rat

Fig. 2.22. Active zone structure in frogs and rats. Scale drawing of active zones at frog and rat NMJs. Only a small part of a frog AZ is shown. Vesicles (dotted circles) are 50 nm in diameter. Note that in mammals each vesicle is in contact with intramembrane particles (dots), probably representing Ca^{++} and K^+ channels as well as attachment sites to exocytosis proteins, on two sides. In frogs, this contact is only on one side. (From Walrond and Reese, 1985, with permission. Copyright 1985 The Society for Neuroscience.)

is not yet certain, it seems likely to be related to the greater number of contacts between each vesicle and AZ particles seen in mammals.

Like the AZs as a whole, the Ca^{++} channels within them also differ between frogs and mammals. In lower vertebrates, including fish, amphibia and reptiles, activity-dependent release is regulated by N-type Ca^{++} channels whereas in mammals it is P/Q channels (see Section 2.2.3.1). Differences in the number and properties of the Ca^{++} channels may contribute to the greater efficiency of release at mammalian NMJs.

In summary, mammalian NMJs appear to be designed to allow more efficient quantal release than those of frogs. When release/area is compared, mammals release 0.2–0.4 quanta/μm^2/nerve impulse, while for frogs the comparable number is 0.1–0.2. This helps mammals to achieve reliable transmission with smaller NMJs than frogs.

2.6.1.3. Postsynaptic specializations

The quantal content at human NMJs is so low that at first it is hard to understand how the safety factor can be large enough to ensure reliable transmission. Comparison with different species suggests that there must be compensating factors that ensure adequate transmission in humans. Insight into the nature of such factors has come from examination of electron micrographs (Fig. 2.23). These reveal significant differences in the extent of postsynaptic folding (Wood and Slater, 2001). In frogs, the folds are not very extensive and increase the postsynaptic surface area about 2-fold. In rats and mice, the folds are more extensive, and in humans they increase the area about 8-fold (Slater et al., 1992). Thus in these species, there is an inverse relationship between quantal content and folding.

side of the paired array (Fig. 2.22). Each docked vesicle is contacted on one side by 2–4 lateral "ribs" that extend from the particle arrays (Harlow et al., 2001). By contrast, in mammals, the AZs are much smaller, consisting of a total of about 20 particles in two parallel arrays about 0.1 μm long (see Chapter 3). Each mammalian AZ can accommodate no more than two docked vesicles that lie between the paired arrays.

The possible functional significance of these differences in AZ structure is seen when the probability of release of individual docked vesicles in frogs and mammals is compared. In frogs, less than 1% of the 30 000 or so docked vesicles at each NMJ are released by a single action potential, whereas in mammals, about 5% are released. While the explanation for this

The functional significance of these anatomical relationships appears to be related to the amplifying effect of the folds, described above (Section 2.3.6.3). At human NMJs, the very extensive folds would provide greater amplification than the shallower folds of frogs and might thus compensate for the relatively low quantal content and size of the EPP. The inverse relationship between quantal content and folding (Fig. 2.23) implies that different species achieve an adequate safety factor in different ways, depending on different balances between presynaptic and postsynaptic factors. Frogs have large nerve terminals that release many quanta and need little postsynaptic amplification. For humans the reverse is true.

What might account for the particular balance between pre- and postsynaptic factors that has evolved in each species? There is at present no definitive answer. One possibility is related to the fact that in mammals, and possibly other groups, when large and small species are compared the number of muscle fibers increases with body size much more than the number of motor neurons (Cooper, 1966). Thus each motor neuron innervates more muscle fibers in larger animals. Considerations of cellular economy may demand that as the number of NMJs per motor neuron increases, the volume of each nerve terminal is kept small. According to this view, human NMJs are small because humans are relatively large. Unfortunately, there is little appropriate information about the NMJ in other large species to allow a good test of this hypothesis. Nonetheless, it forms a useful starting point for the interpretation of the functional implications of some examples of NMJ pathology (see Section 2.8 below).

2.6.2. Variation between NMJs in the adult

There is considerable variation of NMJ properties within the same species, and even within the same muscle in the same individual. These differences are related to the range of tasks that muscles must perform, from maintaining posture, to allowing delicate manipulations of individual digits, to rapid forceful movements of the whole body. As motor units range from slow, low threshold units with relatively small caliber muscle fibers that develop relatively little force to fast units with large caliber fibers that develop much force, the properties of the NMJs vary in parallel with the muscle fibers.

2.6.2.1. Matching NMJ size to muscle fiber size

It has long been clear that NMJs on small muscle fibers are themselves smaller than those on large fibers

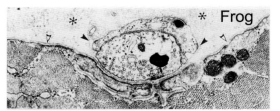
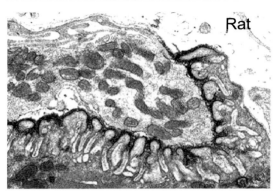
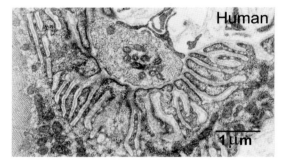
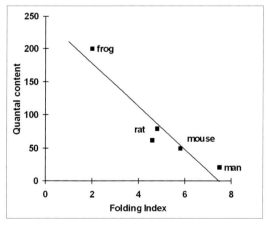

Fig. 2.23. The extent of folding is inversely related to quantal content. Electron micrographs of normal NMJs from frog, rat and human. Note the greater extent of postsynaptic folding in mammals. There is an inverse relationship between the extent of folding ("Folding Index", the factor by which the folding increases the postsynaptic area) and quantal content in these species.

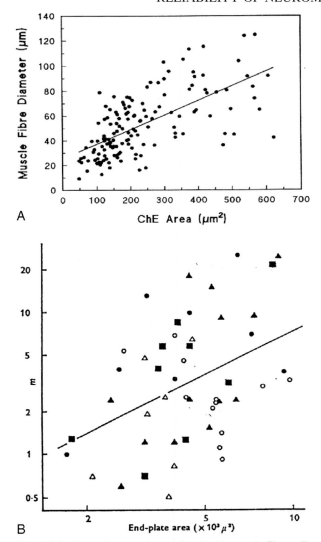

A

B

Fig. 2.24. Quantal content is correlated with muscle fiber caliber. (A) There is a significant correlation between muscle fiber diameter and NMJ size (ChE area, the area of high AChE activity), here shown for human muscles. (B) There is also a significant correlation between quantal content (*m*) and NMJ area (end-plate area), here shown for frogs. Taken together these imply that quantal content is correlated with muscle fiber caliber. (From Kuno et al., 1971; Slater et al., 1992, with permission.)

(Fig. 2.24) (Kuno et al., 1971; Harris and Ribchester, 1979b). As the quantal content/area is relatively constant, large NMJs release more quanta than small ones. This results in a matching of the quantal content to the input resistance of the muscle fiber. Large fibers have relatively low input resistance and so need more ACh-induced current to reach the threshold potential for action potential generation. The matching of NMJ size to muscle fiber diameter helps to ensure that the EPP

is large enough in big fibers, and not bigger than necessary in small ones.

The factors that regulate NMJ size are poorly understood. It has recently been found that mutations in the human gene encoding the protein Dok-7 result in NMJs that are about 50% of the normal size (Beeson et al., 2006). This appears to be responsible for a similar reduction in quantal content in many patients with limb-girdle myasthenia (LGM). It is likely that many other factors also influence NMJ size.

2.6.2.2. Matching of functional properties of NMJs to activity patterns

Motor units in mammalian muscles differ not only in the properties of the muscle fibers they contain, but also in their patterns of activity. In rats, where such patterns have been most carefully studied (Hennig and Lømo, 1985), motor neurons innervating slow, low threshold units tend to fire in long trains at about 10–20 Hz that last many seconds. By contrast, motor neurons innervating fast, high threshold units tend to fire in short bursts of 5–10 impulses with a mean frequency of about 100 Hz.

The release properties of the NMJs innervating these two types of motor unit are adapted to the appropriate pattern of activity (Fig. 2.25) (Reid et al., 1999). Thus, NMJs in the predominantly slow soleus muscle of rats are better at maintaining quantal content during prolonged stimulation than are those of the predominantly fast EDL. At the NMJs of the fast EDL, where the quantal content "runs down" relatively rapidly, a larger fraction of docked vesicles is released per impulse than in the slow soleus (Reid et al., 1999). This suggests that fast NMJs are specialized to release more quanta per impulse, thus ensuring adequate activation of the muscle during short high frequency trains of impulses. It may be this very specialization that prevents fast NMJs from maintaining high quantal output during prolonged stimulation in an experimental situation.

In addition to the differences in release properties, NMJs in fast and slow rat muscles differ in some postsynaptic features. In fast muscle fibers of the diaphragm, the folds are deeper and more numerous than in the slow fibers (Padykula and Gauthier, 1970). Although it is not clear that this difference is a feature of fast and slow NMJs in all rat muscles (Wood and Slater, 1997), it suggests that the extent of postsynaptic amplification may be matched to the activity pattern.

The result of the distinct features of fast and slow NMJs in rats is a high safety factor in both types of motor unit (Wood and Slater, 1997). By achieving this reliability in slightly different ways, the properties of

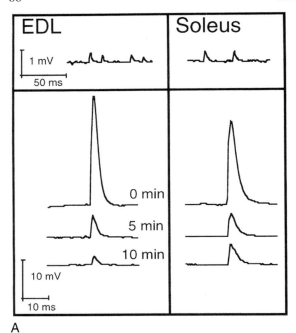

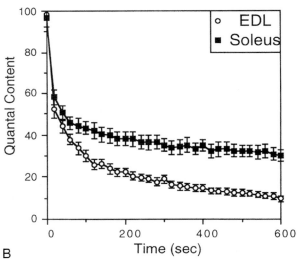

B

Fig. 2.25. Rundown of quantal content in fast and slow rat muscles. (A) Examples of spontaneous mEPPs and evoked EPPs at NMJs in rat EDL and soleus muscles. EPPs were recorded at different times after starting stimulation at 20 Hz. (B) Decline of quantal content during repetitive stimulation at 20 Hz in EDL and soleus. Note that NMJs in soleus, which is normally activated by long trains at about 20 Hz, declines less than in EDL, which is normally activated in short, high-frequency bursts. (From Reid et al., 1999, with permission. Copyright 1999 The Society for Neuroscience.)

transmission are effectively matched to the patterns of activity different motor units usually experience. This presumably helps to strike a balance between reliability and economy.

2.6.2.3. Activity-dependent plasticity of the NMJ

How is the matching of NMJ properties to functional demand achieved? One possibility is that the NMJ responds to different patterns of activity by adjusting its own properties so as to be able to support the prevailing pattern. An experimental approach to this question has been to subject NMJs to imposed patterns of activity by means of stimulating electrodes implanted close to the peripheral nerves (Reid et al., 2003). When rat EDL nerves were stimulated with a pattern of activity characteristic of the slow soleus muscle for several weeks, their release properties became much more like those of the soleus (Fig. 2.26). Conversely, when the soleus nerve was stimulated with a "fast" pattern quantal release from the soleus NMJs became more like that from the normal EDL. Activity-dependent changes in NMJ structure also take place that are consistent with transformation from fast to slow and vice versa (Waerhaug and Lømo, 1994). While the mechanisms of these changes are not known, it is clear that adult mammalian NMJs can undergo long-term changes that adapt them to the pattern of imposed activity.

2.6.3. Development of the mammalian NMJ

The distinctive features of the adult mammalian NMJ arise during a series of developmental stages that lasts several weeks (Sanes and Lichtman, 1999). At each of these stages, even when the NMJs are still structurally and functionally very immature, they function in a way that is appropriate for the degree of maturity of the animal. The products of this developmental process are NMJs that are not only reliable in a general sense, but are well matched to the functional requirements of the motor units of which they are a part. The following account of NMJ development is based on studies of rats and mice.

2.6.3.1. Development of the motor neuron

Motor neurons are among the earliest nerve cells to be "born", i.e., undergo their final round of DNA synthesis and begin to extend an axon and dendrites (Jacobson, 1970). In mammals, the motor neurons that innervate an individual muscle are usually grouped into a longitudinally oriented "column" that occupies 2–3 spinal segments. Their axons grow out of the spinal cord or brain stem even before muscles have formed. As they grow, they select paths that lead to the muscles they are destined to innervate. This selection involves decisions that are based on local cues. The ability of an immature motor neuron to make such decisions indicates that it has some "knowledge" of its identity, and

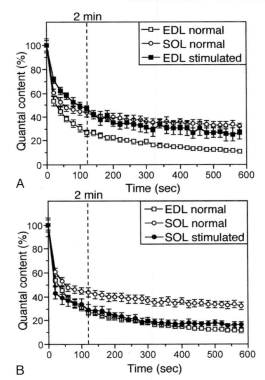

Fig. 2.26. Chronic effects of activity on quantal rundown at rat NMJs. Activity pattern-dependent plasticity at stimulated fast (EDL) and slow (SOL) NMJs in the rat. Graphs show decline of quantal content, normalized to the initial value, during 10 min stimulation at 20 Hz. (A) Quantal content rundown at NMJs in fast EDL muscles that had been chronically stimulated below a TTX block of the nerve in vivo with a "slow" stimulus pattern (200 pulses at 20 Hz every 30 s) for 3–4 weeks. Note that the chronically stimulated EDL NMJs resemble normal SOL NMJs in their ability to maintain their response to intense stimulation. (B) Quantal content rundown at NMJs in slow SOL muscles chronically stimulated with fast pattern (150 pulses at 150 Hz every 60 s). Note that the NMJs in the chronically stimulated SOL come to resemble those in the normal EDL. (From Reid et al., 2003, with permission. Copyright 1999 The Society for Neuroscience.)

that different motor neurons have different identities. Once contact with the appropriate pre-muscle mass has been established, but not before, the axons branch extensively. In rats and mice, functional contacts with newly formed muscle are first present around E14 (embryonic day 14), a week before birth. A similar stage occurs in humans at week 9 of gestation (Hesselmans et al., 1993).

Motor neurons in neonatal rats and mice fire at a uniformly low frequency. The first evidence of faster, more adult-like firing patterns, and of differences between the firing patterns of different motor neurons, is seen about 2 weeks after birth (Vrbova et al., 1985;

Personius and Balice-Gordon, 2001). The onset of these more adult-like firing properties of motor neurons coincides with the time of myelination of the most distal intramuscular nerve branches (Slater, 1982). It is likely that before this happens, the small caliber unmyelinated branches would be unable to fire at high frequencies and would therefore filter out any high frequency activity.

2.6.3.2. Development of the muscle

Mammalian skeletal muscle fibers arise during development from the fusion of many mononucleated myogenic cells (often called myoblasts). Fusion is just one stage of a process that involves withdrawal of proliferating myoblasts from DNA synthesis, alignment of the spindle shaped myoblasts into "strings" of cells in the premuscle masses and then their fusion to form the myotubes. The myotubes incorporate further myoblasts, as they grow into mature muscle fibers. In adult muscle fibers, there is typically 1 nucleus for every 10 μm of length. Thus a single fiber in a large human muscle, such as vastus lateralis, which has fibers up to 20 cm long, has up to 20 000 nuclei.

The distinctive properties of muscle fibers of different functional types are determined by the pattern of gene expression. Since the nuclei away from the NMJ all express the same set of genes, an important developmental question concerns how that homogeneity of nuclear gene expression within a given fiber comes about. There is evidence for two very different, though not at all mutually exclusive, mechanisms. On the one hand, there is evidence that myoblasts differ in their properties from a very early stage in development. Thus, there may be "fast" and "slow" myoblasts before myotube formation occurs (Nikovits Jr et al., 2001), and these may fuse more or less selectively to make myotubes containing nuclei with intrinsically similar properties. On the other hand, there is very strong evidence, particularly in mammals, that the properties of adult muscle fibers can be fundamentally changed by imposing on it different patterns of activity (Lømo, 1989). This indicates that the properties of a muscle fiber may be modified after innervation by the activity pattern of the particular motor neuron that innervates it. Both schemes lead to important questions about how the innervation of muscle fibers arises so as to result in motor units in which all the muscle fibers have the same properties.

2.6.3.3. Synapse formation and elimination

Muscle fibers become innervated very soon after they first form. In rats and mice signs of innervation can already be detected within a day or two of myotube formation. At about this time, clusters of AChRs form in the muscle fiber membrane at the sites of nerve contact, followed a few days later by the appearance of AChE in the basal lamina (Sanes and Lichtman, 1999).

An important feature of the early motor innervation of vertebrates is that several motor neurons initially innervate each muscle fiber (Jansen and Fladby, 1990). This innervation occurs at a single postsynaptic site that is contacted by the terminal axons of several motor neurons (Fig. 2.27A). Over a period of several weeks (rats, mice), a process of local competition between these branches results in the contacts with all but one motor neuron being eliminated (Fig. 2.27B). Although the nature of this process of synapse elimination has been extensively investigated, its details remain largely obscure. There is evidence that each branch of a motor axon competes locally at a given NMJ (Kasthuri and Lichtman, 2003) and that axons with the strongest input to a given NMJ are more likely to survive the competitive process than weaker ones (Buffelli et al., 2003). However neither of these findings fully explains the final outcome of the competition in which a single

motor axon, with appropriately matched properties, innervates each muscle fiber.

Neuromuscular transmission is effective throughout the processes of synapse elimination and NMJ maturation. In the early stages, when polyneuronal innervation is present, quantal content and mEPP frequency are both very low (Diamond and Miledi, 1962). However, because the muscle fibers have a small caliber at this time, their input resistance is very high. As a result, very little current is required to bring the membrane potential to the action potential threshold. Thus, even spontaneous mEPPs may sometimes trigger muscle fiber action potentials (Jaramillo et al., 1988). As a result, at the peak of polyneuronal innervation, each of the several motor neurons innervating a muscle fiber is able to trigger its contraction (Jansen and Fladby, 1990).

An important consequence of the process of synapse elimination is that each motor neuron ends up innervating muscle fibers with similar properties. Clear signs of functional homogeneity of the muscle fibers within

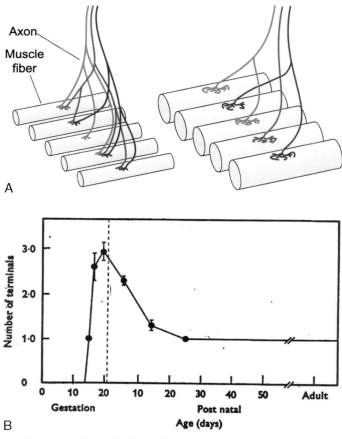

Fig. 2.27. Development of muscle innervation. (A) Comparison of polyneuronal innervation of muscles in newborn rats or mice (left) with the adult state (right). (B) Changes in the number of axon terminals innervating NMJs in rat diaphragm with age. (From Bennett and Pettigrew, 1974, with permission.)

motor units are seen in mice 2 weeks after birth, as synapse elimination nears completion but before the distinctive patterns of activity of different motor units are clearly developed (Fladby and Jansen, 1988). It therefore seems unlikely that differences in activity patterns between motor neurons play a decisive role in either survival selection or in matching the properties of motor neurons to the muscle fibers they innervate. A possible alternative is that the initial matching of nerve and muscle cells is achieved by a molecular recognition system that involves activity-dependent expression of surface and/or diffusible molecules that interact to promote survival of the most compatible pairs at each developing NMJ. Such a mechanism could depend on activity as a driving force, without the pattern of activity determining the specific outcome of the competition.

2.6.3.4. Structural maturation of the developing NMJ

As NMJ maturation progresses, and the elimination of supernumerary synapses comes to completion, a number of structural and molecular changes take place that have the combined effect of enhancing the speed of neuromuscular transmission and matching its efficacy to the enlarging muscle fibers. Soon after synapse elimination is complete, the terminals of the sole surviving axon begin to enlarge (Fig. 2.28) (Slater, 1982; Marques et al., 2000) and the quantal content increases. The postsynaptic specializations, most notably the accumulation of AChRs and AChE, become restricted to the region of the muscle fiber in immediate contact with the expanding nerve terminals.

The postsynaptic folds begin to develop soon after birth (Fig. 2.29) (Kelly and Zacks, 1969; Matthews-Bellinger and Salpeter, 1983; Bewick et al., 1996). It appears likely that the folds form by the addition of a new membrane to their depths. However the factors that control the distribution and growth of the folds are poorly understood. It has been suggested that the opening of the fold represents a site of reduced nerve–muscle adhesion, possibly related to the presence of the AZs in the nerve (Marques et al., 2000). The structural maturation of the NMJ is largely complete 3–4 weeks after birth (Slater, 1982).

2.6.3.5. Molecular maturation of the developing NMJ

As these structural changes take place, immature forms of three key classes of ion channel, Ca_V1, AChRs and Na_V1, are replaced by adult ones. The Ca_V1 channels that control evoked quantal release from motor nerve terminals in rat embryos are mostly of the N-type. During the first week after birth, these are replaced by the P/Q-type (Rosato and Uchitel, 1999). Since the P/Q-type channels require less depolarization to open (see Section 2.2.3.1) this apparent "recapitulation of phylogeny" (see Section 2.6.1.2) may help to ensure that passive depolarization of the enlarging nerve terminal causes adequate numbers of channels to open in response to each nerve impulse.

Two distinct forms of the AChR protein are expressed by mammalian muscles. The form that predominates at immature NMJs has $\alpha(2)$, β, γ, and δ subunits. In the adult form, the γ subunit is replaced by an ϵ subunit. The two forms differ in their channel properties: in humans, the immature form has a mean open time of about 7–8 ms and a conductance of 44 pS while the adult form has a mean open burst time of 1–2 ms and a conductance of 60 pS (Sine et al., 2002). As a result, a single opening of average duration of an immature AChR channel allows 3–4 times as much charge to enter the cell as an adult channel. This makes the immature channels more efficient at converting bound ACh to charge entry.

Immature muscle fibers usually have a small diameter and therefore a high input resistance. This results in a greater depolarization per unit charge. However, the increase in input resistance leads to an increase in the passive charging time constant of the fiber (see Section 2.3.5.5) which tends to reduce the depolarization due to a brief inflow of current (see Fig. 2.9C, D). The slower kinetics of the currents mediated by AChRs with a γ-subunit are thus better matched to the passive cable properties of the immature fibers than those in the adult. On the other hand, because of their slower kinetics, they are less well adapted to transmit the high frequency repetitive activity that occurs in the mature animal. It is thus relevant that the change in AChR properties occurs at about the same time that the adult firing patterns of the motor neuron, and the myelination of the most distal axons which allows those patterns to reach the NMJ, appear.

Conversion between the two AChR forms occurs during the period when synapse elimination is nearing completion. In rats and mice the conversion begins about the time of birth and is complete at the end of the second week after birth. Studies in adult animals show that expression of the immature form is suppressed by the normal activity of the muscle (Lømo and Rosenthal, 1972; Goldman et al., 1988). In contrast, expression of the ϵ-subunit that characterizes the adult form is insensitive to muscle or nerve activity, as it must be to persist at the adult NMJ. Even when the nerve is cut at birth, expression of ϵ-AChR mRNA is initiated in the first week after birth as usual (Brenner et al., 1990).

A similar isoform switch of Na_V1 also occurs during NMJ maturation (Lupa et al., 1993; Stocksley et al., 2005). The immature $Na_V1.5$ form differs from

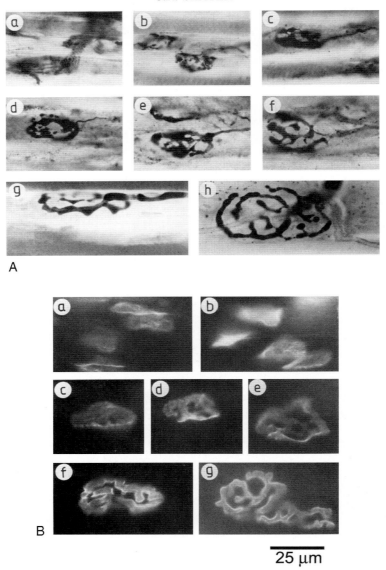

Fig. 2.28. Structural maturation of mouse NMJs. Changes in overall structure of NMJs in postnatal mouse EDL muscles. (A) Nerve terminals, labeled with ZIO. a. newborn, b. 1 week. c–f. 2 weeks. g. 3 weeks. h. adult. (B) AChRs labeled with R-α-bungarotoxin. a. newborn. b. 1 week. c–e. 2 weeks. f. 3 weeks. g. adult. Note loss of polyaxonal innervation, enlargement of surviving nerve terminal and increasing segregation of AChR cluster. (From Slater, 1982, with permission.)

the adult $Na_V1.4$ form in that it is opened at more negative membrane potentials. As a result, less depolarization is required to trigger an action potential in an immature than a mature muscle. Although the initial accumulation of Na_V1 channels at developing NMJs occurs later than that of AChRs, the isoform switch occurs during the same period of 2–3 weeks postnatal. Thus newborn rats have nearly all $Na_V1.5$ channels, while by 1 month most channels are $Na_V1.4$ (Lupa et al., 1993; Stocksley et al., 2005).

The regulation of expression of the two isoforms of Na_V1 has close similarities to that of AChRs. Thus expression of $Na_V1.5$ is repressed by imposed activity (Awad et al., 2001) whereas that of $Na_V1.4$ is insensitive to activity. The insensitivity of the expression of the adult forms of AChR and Na_V1 to activity ensures that they persist in adequate numbers on active muscle fibers. However it leaves open the question of the nature of the developmental switch that initiates their expression.

A likely candidate for a factor regulating the expression of adult channels at mammalian NMJs is agrin (McMahan, 1990). Agrin is synthesized by motor neurons and released from their terminals, after which it

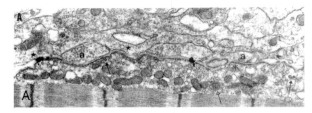

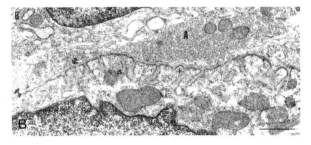

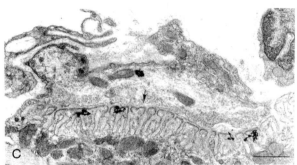

Fig. 2.29. Ultrastructural maturation of mouse NMJs. Development of postsynaptic folds at NMJs in postnatal mouse EDL muscles. (A) Newborn, few folds are present. (B) 2 weeks, folds are present but less well-developed than in adult. (C) Adult, folds are well formed and closely packed. Scale bars = 1 μm. (From Matthews-Bellinger and Salpeter, 1983, with permission. Copyright 1983 The Society for Neuroscience.)

binds to the synaptic BL. From there, it can interact with a muscle specific receptor kinase (MuSK) in the muscle membrane (Glass et al., 1996). Activation of MuSK promotes many aspects of the differentiation of the postsynaptic membrane. These include the accumulation of AChR, AChE and Na_V1 molecules at the NMJ and expression of the genes that encode their mature forms by the 5–10 myonuclei closest to the junction (Cohen et al., 1997; Meier et al., 1997).

The switch to expression of adult $Na_V1.4$ channels occurs at the same time as the development of the postsynaptic folds, during the first 2–3 weeks after birth. It is likely that the folds form by the incorporation of new membrane into the depths of the folds. At the time that this is happening, the mRNA encoding the $Na_V1.4$ is concentrated in the postjunctional region (Stocksley et al., 2005). It is therefore likely that the

membrane being added to the folds already bears a high concentration of $Na_V1.4$.

There is some evidence that as the density of Na_V1 channels at the NMJ begins to increase, those channels are at least partially excluded from the crest of the folds where the concentration of AChRs is already very high (Bailey et al., 2003). It may be that the complex of molecules that supports the junctional AChR cluster forms a barrier to Na_V1 channel entry. Such a barrier might thus account for the sharp boundary between the main postsynaptic ion channel domains (Winckler et al., 1999).

2.6.3.6. Functional consequences of NMJ maturation

The many changes in the structural and molecular properties of the NMJ that occur during its maturation adapt it for reliable high-frequency activation of mature muscle fibers. These changes are matched to complementary changes in the nerve and the muscle. Their overall effect is the conversion of an immature system that is good at generating slow muscle contractions in response to low frequency activity in the nerve to a much faster system, adapted to the needs of a freely moving and increasingly independent animal. For example, in the hind limb muscles of rats and mice, the timing of these changes corresponds to the time when the animal can first support its hind quarters against gravity and begin to walk. While the factors influencing the reliability of neuromuscular transmission change during development, at all stages, the process remains well-suited to the tasks it needs to perform.

The events that give rise to the mature NMJ are part of a coherent developmental program that defines the patterns of expression of a number of proteins, such as ion channels, that play central roles in neuromuscular transmission. In addition it determines the size and conformation of the NMJ. Both aspects of the program have important consequences for the efficacy and reliability of the mature NMJ. This program can be reactivated in the adult in circumstances where neuromuscular transmission is impaired, as during normal aging (see below) or in response to cellular damage or chemical intoxication of the NMJ (see Section 2.7).

2.6.4. Changes in the NMJ affecting safety factor during normal aging

It is well-known that muscle power is reduced in humans during old age. Changes in muscle innervation make an important contribution to this phenomenon. There is good evidence from clinical neurophysiological studies of a decrease in the number of motor units, particularly in distal muscles, after the age of 60 (Campbell et al., 1973; Sica et al., 1974; Galea, 1996) and for some deterioration in the efficacy of neuromuscular transmission (Larsson and Ansved, 1995; Galea, 1996). Anatomical studies show that the number of large cell bodies in the ventral horn is reduced (Kawamura et al., 1977; Tomlinson and Irving, 1977), while electrophysiological estimates of motor unit numbers (Galea, 1996) also point to a loss of motor neurons. Thus single fiber EMG (SFEMG) studies show an increase in fiber density and MACRO EMG studies show an increase in amplitude of motor unit potentials (Stalberg and Trontelj, 1979; Stalberg and Fawcett, 1982). These findings are all consistent with the death of some motor neurons during old age and a compensating reinnervation of the denervated muscle fibers by newly formed branches of the surviving axons. More direct evidence for such a phenomenon is presented below.

Anatomical studies in animals and humans suggest that the structure of NMJs changes with age (Fig. 2.30) (Barker and Ip, 1966; Tuffery, 1971; Bennett and Stenbuck, 1980; Bennett and Davis, 1982; Arizono et al., 1984; Oda, 1984; Cardasis and LaFontaine, 1987; Diaz et al., 1989; Wokke et al., 1990; Rich et al., 1998). In most cases, these changes involve increased local complexity of axonal branching within individual NMJs (Oda, 1984; Andonian and Fahim, 1989; Prakash and Sieck, 1998), which may (Waerhaug, 1992), or may not (Fahim and Robbins, 1982; Fahim et al., 1983), be associated with an overall change in the total area of the NMJ. Some studies have also found an increase in preterminal branching (Barker and Ip, 1966; Tuffery, 1971; Arizono et al., 1984; Oda, 1984; Wokke et al., 1990), though this has not been seen in all such studies (Wokke et al., 1990). On the postsynaptic side, a number of studies have reported an increase in the complexity and branching of the regions of specialized postsynaptic membrane, which parallels the presynaptic changes. In addition, there is an increasing amount of specialized postsynaptic membrane that is not in contact with the nerve terminal, suggesting a partial withdrawal of the nerve (Arizono et al., 1984; Cardasis and LaFontaine, 1987). These changes all suggest that there is considerable structural remodeling of mature NMJs, particularly in association with senescence.

In light of the general impact of NMJ structure on its function, it seems likely that changes in neuromuscular transmission would accompany the remodeling seen in old age. While this is suggested by the SFEMG data referred to above, there is little information about the detailed functional properties of the NMJ in elderly humans. From animal studies, mostly in rats and mice, it seems that an adequate safety factor of

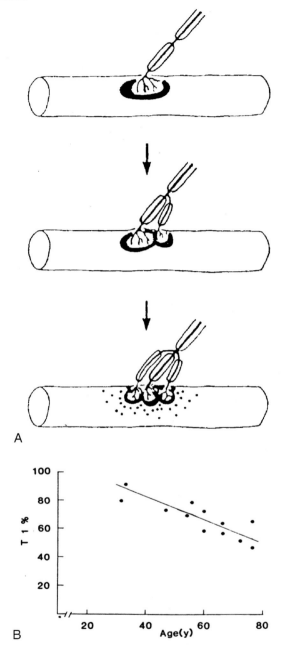

Fig. 2.30. Changes in preterminal branching patterns of human NMJs with age. (A) Drawing at top shows "normal" state with a single unbranched preterminal axon, referred to as T_1 innervation. Lower drawings show gradual increase in branching with age. (B) Graph shows that the fraction of simple T_1 NMJs declines with age. (From Oda, 1984, with permission.)

transmission is generally maintained in spite of the structural changes that accompany old age. In rat diaphragm, the safety factor was reported to increase steadily from about 4 to 10 during the first 9 months of life and then to decline (Kelly, 1978; Kelly and

Robbins, 1983). The reported changes in safety factor were accompanied by similar changes in quantal content (though the values given are very high due to the use of the "variance" method (Section 2.4.3.3) to determine them). On the basis of existing evidence, it seems likely that the changes in quantal content are a major determinant of the changes in the safety factor during aging.

All these observations suggest that a gradual process of NMJ remodeling becomes much more intense during old age as a fraction of motor neurons die. Recent studies have shown that the terminal Schwann cells play an important part in the induction of nerve terminal sprouting following partial denervation (Son et al., 1996) and it is likely that they also influence the remodeling of the presynaptic terminal nerve during aging. So long as this process maintains the total extent of the nerve terminals and synaptic contact, it is likely that the safety factor would be maintained. Eventually, however, the presence of "unoccupied" postsynaptic membrane suggests that this endeavor fails. While the increasing complexity of the postsynaptic surface may represent an effort to enhance the effect of a reduction of quantal content, the overall effect may be a decline of safety factor in old age.

2.6.5. Conclusions

Patterns of muscle use vary widely between species and muscle types, and at different stages in an animal's life. The properties of NMJs are adapted to these patterns in order to ensure reliable activation of muscle throughout life. These adaptations occur at every level of organization, from molecular (e.g., Ca_V1, AChR and Na_V1 isoforms) to "system" (e.g., poly- to mononeuronal innervation). An important focus of current investigation is the effort to understand how this adaptation is controlled at a molecular level. Experimental studies of how NMJs respond to, and recover from, traumatic injury and toxic assault have done much to reveal the main processes that underlie this ability of the NMJ to adapt to changing circumstances so as to maintain reliable muscle activation.

2.7. Response of the neuromuscular junction to trauma or intoxication

The vertebrate neuromuscular system, including the NMJ, is extremely good at repairing itself and restoring function after many sorts of damage. Several different types of cellular mechanism contribute to this ability and help to ensure that effective and reliable activation of muscle is maintained or re-established. Thus motor axons regenerate well and can form new presynaptic terminals in a few days. For their part, muscle fibers can regenerate after complete destruction and accept and respond to new innervation on a similar time scale. This Section reviews some of the key experiments that have revealed the processes that underlie this important ability of the NMJ.

2.7.1. Nerve transection and regeneration

2.7.1.1. Degeneration of severed axons

Damage to peripheral nerves is a common occurrence and may result from sports activities, domestic, motor or industrial accidents or a wide variety of other causes. Whatever be the nature of the damage, the distal segments of any severed axons degenerate. Paradoxically, the first part of the isolated axon segment to degenerate is that furthest from the site of injury, the presynaptic nerve terminal (Slater, 1966; Miledi and Slater, 1970). This is followed by degeneration of the remainder of the axon by a complex process known as Wallerian degeneration (Coleman, 2005).

2.7.1.2. Axon regeneration

Peripheral nerves are capable of extensive regeneration. The success of this regeneration, in terms of the restoration of effective muscle control, depends on whether continuity of the BL and connective tissue sheaths surrounding the nerve and its axons are left intact. If they are, the axons can regenerate within them and make their way back to their original target muscle fibers and reinnervate them at the site of the original NMJ. Under these circumstances, regeneration occurs in mammals at a rate of 2–5 mm/day (Hoffman and Lasek, 1980). If the sheath is cut through, although regenerating axons may eventually return to the denervated muscles, they are unlikely to return to the muscle of origin, much less to the same muscle fibers and synaptic sites (Bennett et al., 1973). As a result, even if new synaptic contacts are made, they may be of little use. Thus the connective tissue sheath, which appears to play only a passive "supporting" role, is, in fact a key factor in ensuring re-establishment of effective motor innervation.

2.7.1.3. Structural reinnervation of the muscle

Once an axon regenerates to the site of an original NMJ, differentiated presynaptic terminals form rapidly and effective synaptic contact is re-established within a few days (Bennett et al., 1973). This appears to be due in part to the presence of molecules associated with the synaptic basal lamina, which survive axon degeneration and act as "stop signals", arresting growth of the regenerating axon and triggering presynaptic differentiation (Glicksman and Sanes, 1983).

These are likely to include agrin (see Section 2.6.3.5) (Sanes, 1989; McMahan, 1990; Campagna et al., 1995; Ruegg and Bixby, 1998). If a regenerating motor axon makes contact with a muscle fiber away from the region of normal innervation, there is a strong tendency for it to grow along the muscle until it makes contact with the site of the original NMJ and re-establish synaptic contact there (Bennett et al., 1973).

In some circumstances, most notably after denervation of the "slow" soleus muscle of rats and mice, implanted "foreign" nerves can make new NMJs at ectopic sites on the muscle fiber away from the original NMJs. Most of the experiments on ectopic innervation have been made on the rat soleus muscle, normally innervated by the tibial nerve, by implanting a branch of the peroneal nerve away from the original NMJ. If the normal innervation is then cut or blocked, the foreign nerve makes new functional NMJs within 1–2 weeks (Fex and Thesleff, 1967; Jansen et al., 1973; Lømo and Slater, 1978). The ability of the foreign axons to make such ectopic NMJs is triggered by inactivity: if the denervated muscle is kept active by direct stimulation, then ectopic NMJs fail to form (Jansen et al., 1973; Lømo and Slater, 1978). One mediator of this effect may be the nerve–cell adhesion molecule (NCAM). NCAM is normally present in a higher concentration at the NMJ than elsewhere. Following denervation its expression away from the NMJ is greatly increased (Covault and Sanes, 1985). NCAM may help to bring nerve and muscle close together and thus facilitate subsequent interactions in synaptogenesis (Walsh et al., 2000).

2.7.1.4. Response of the muscle to denervation

Acquiring an increased responsiveness to innervation is one of a number of changes in the muscle that are triggered by inactivity and promote the restoration of effective innervation. One of the best studied of these is the expression of AChRs. Functional AChRs are normally expressed primarily in the region of the NMJ, with lower levels also present at the myotendinous junctions (Miledi and Zelena, 1966). Elsewhere, that expression is largely inhibited by muscle activity (Lømo and Rosenthal, 1972). Within a few days of denervation, AChRs appear all along the muscle fiber (Lømo and Slater, 1978). These new AChRs resemble those at developing NMJs in having slow kinetics, characteristic of those containing a γ- rather than an ε-subunit (Brenner and Sakmann, 1978). Although their density ($500/\mu m^2$) is much less than at the normal NMJ ($10\,000/\mu m^2$), it is much higher than in normally active muscles. The presence of AChRs away from the original NMJ allows growing motor axons to depolarize the muscle fiber membrane, and this may help to initiate the events leading to new NMJ formation.

At the original NMJ, the density of AChRs remains much higher than in the extrajunctional region even after denervation or paralysis. However, activity of AChE, particularly of the asymmetric form most specifically associated with the mammalian NMJ, declines significantly (Hall, 1973). This has the effect of enhancing the activity of any ACh released from immature regenerating nerve terminals.

Several other changes in the muscle fiber induced by inactivity have the effect of increasing muscle excitability. These include a reduction of membrane potential, typically from -80 mV to -60 mV, which brings the resting potential close to the AP threshold. This probably occurs as a result of decreased permeability to K^+ (Nicholls, 1956). In addition, $Na_V 1.5$ channels, which open at a less depolarized membrane potential than the $Na_V 1.4$ channels of active muscle, are expressed both at the NMJ and in the extrajunctional region (Caldwell and Milton, 1988; Kallen et al., 1990; Catterall, 1995; Awad et al., 2001). Finally, inactivity generally causes muscle fiber atrophy. The reduction of fiber caliber, together with that of K^+ permeability, gives rise to an increase in input resistance (see Section 2.3.5.2). As a result, less synaptic current is required to achieve a given change in membrane potential. All these factors cooperate to increase the excitability of the muscle fiber, so less charge needs to enter the fiber to initiate contraction. Thus loss of normal activity as a result of nerve transection triggers a constellation of changes in the muscle that promote restoration of effective innervation.

2.7.1.5. Functional reinnervation of the muscle

The functional properties of reinnervated mammalian NMJs often return to near normal values (Bennett et al., 1973; McArdle and Albuquerque, 1973; Tonge, 1974b; Slack and Hopkins, 1982; Katz et al., 1996). During the first few weeks after damage by nerve crush, which leaves the nerve sheath intact to promote reinnervation, the quantal content increases progressively from an initially low value to near normal (Fig. 2.31). In the early stages, when quantal content is low, evoked release is sensitive to blockers of both P-type Ca^{++} channels, as normal, and to L-type channels (Katz et al., 1996). With time the contribution of the L-type channels is lost. N-type channels, which contribute to evoked release at NMJs in early development, do not appear to be re-expressed during nerve regeneration.

2.7.2. Partial denervation

2.7.2.1. Axon sprouting and muscle fiber type conversion

There are many situations in which only a fraction of fibers in a muscle lose their innervation. Such "partial

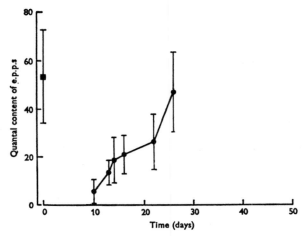

Fig. 2.31. Recovery of neuromuscular transmission during reinnervation of mouse muscle. Mouse soleus muscles show the first signs of functional reinnervation 10 days after nerve crush in the thigh. The efficacy of innervation increases to normal over the next 2–3 weeks. (From Tonge, 1974b, with permission.)

denervation" may result from trauma, normal aging, or a variety of diseases including most notably amyotrophic lateral sclerosis (ALS). In these cases, new intramuscular sprouts grow out from the surviving motor axons and often reinnervate the NMJs on the denervated muscle fibers (Brown et al., 1981; Gordon et al., 2004). This may lead to a local increase in the number of fibers innervated by individual motor axons that can be detected as an increase in fiber density during SFEMG investigation in a clinical setting. It is often the case that the sprouting axon is from a motor unit whose properties are different from those of the muscle fiber it comes to innervate. In such cases, the nerve may impose its "type" on the muscle fiber, leading to the phenomenon of "fiber type grouping" (Banker and Engel, 2004).

The influence of the nerve on the "type" of adult muscle fiber is mediated by the pattern of activity (Salmons and Vrbova, 1969; Windisch et al., 1998). If a denervated muscle is stimulated directly with implanted electrodes its type, based largely on the pattern of expression of the genes encoding myosin heavy chains, is determined by the pattern of imposed activity (Windisch et al., 1998). The fact that new patterns of innervation resulting from axonal sprouting lead to new patterns of muscle fiber type indicates that the new synaptic connections are sufficiently effective to stimulate muscle activity. In most cases, it seems that these new connections are established at the sites of the original NMJ. This raises the question of how axonal sprouts "find" those sites.

2.7.2.2. Schwann cells promote axon sprouting

A key factor in the guidance of axonal sprouts to denervated NMJs is the Schwann cell. When muscle fibers are denervated by a nerve crush, the terminal Schwann cells extend long sprouts along the muscle fibers, similar in appearance to those that grow out from axons in partially denervated muscles (Reynolds and Woolf, 1992). The Schwann cells guide regenerating axons back to the original NMJs. In some cases the axons "overshoot" the NMJs and grow along the Schwann cell sprouts, occasionally innervating other muscle fibers (Fig. 2.32).

In a partially denervated muscle, Schwann cell sprouts grow out only from the denervated muscle fibers (Fig. 2.33). These sprouts then appear to guide axonal sprouts from intact motor neurons to the denervated NMJs (Son et al., 1996). The signaling pathways that trigger Schwann cell sprouting are unclear. If a muscle is completely denervated, there is extensive Schwann cell sprouting from all NMJs, suggesting that inactive muscle fibers may release molecules that promote Schwann cell growth. On the other hand, in partially denervated muscles, Schwann cell sprouts appear to make "bridges" preferentially with NMJs that are still innervated and active (Love and Thompson, 1999). One possibility is that Schwann cell sprouts grow out initially at random and are then withdrawn (Reynolds and Woolf, 1992) unless they make contact with an innervated NMJ (Love and Thompson, 1999).

2.7.3. Muscle damage

The integrity of the NMJ may also be disrupted by damage to the muscle. This may happen as a result of traumatic injury or the action of natural myotoxins, or occur as a feature of inherited muscle diseases such as muscular dystrophies. In one frequently used experimental model intramuscular injection of notexin, one active component of the venom of the snake *Notechis scutatus scutatus*, into the rat soleus muscle causes destruction of the muscle fibers but leaves intact the population of myogenic satellite cells (Harris and Johnson, 1978). These cells proliferate rapidly following muscle damage. Within 2 days of the complete destruction of the rat soleus muscle, each satellite cell divides about three times and these myoblasts fuse to make new myotubes, one in each original BL sheath (Fig. 2.34A). If the nerve is undamaged, or only its terminals are damaged, the nerve reoccupies the original postsynaptic sites within a few days (Jirmanova and Thesleff, 1972; Grubb et al., 1991). The first signs of neuromuscular transmission appear within less than a week of the return of the nerve (Fig. 2.34B)

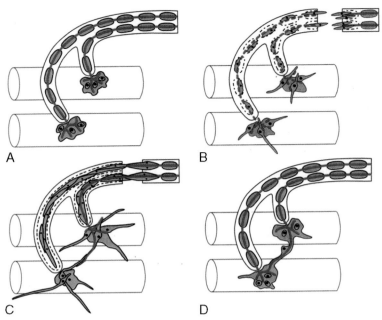

Fig. 2.32. Schwann cells guide reinnervation of muscle after a nerve crush. (A) Normal NMJs showing two muscle fibers with the associated nerve terminals (red) and Schwann cells (blue). (B) After cutting the nerve, the nerve terminals degenerate and processes of the Schwann cells grow away from the NMJ. C. Regenerating axons follow the Schwann cell processes to the original, and sometimes to other, NMJs. D. Following functional reinnervation, the processes of the Schwann cells retract. (From Son et al., 1996, with permission.)

and quantal content returns to normal within 3 weeks (Fig. 2.34C) (Grubb et al., 1991).

The rapid functional reinnervation of damaged muscle implies that both the pre- and postsynaptic components of the NMJ can be reassembled within a few days. A number of studies indicate that this process is facilitated by the presence of molecular signals associated with synaptic basal lamina. The best studied of these is agrin (see Section 2.6.3.5). Indeed, much of the early evidence indicating the presence of persistent signals at the NMJ that might direct its own regeneration were made on regenerating muscles (Burden et al., 1979; McMahan and Slater, 1984; Brenner et al., 1992; Jo and Burden, 1992). These studies show that such signals direct both the structural and molecular differentiation of the postsynaptic membrane and the expression of synapse specific genes in the newly formed myonuclei that accumulate at the regenerating NMJ.

Particularly striking demonstrations of these properties of the synaptic BL come from experiments in which all the cellular constituents of the NMJ were destroyed and then selected cells (e.g., nerve or muscle) were allowed to regenerate (Sanes et al., 1978; Burden et al., 1979; Glicksman and Sanes, 1983; McMahan and Slater, 1984). In each case, local differentiation of the regenerated cell occurred in the absence of its normal synaptic partner, presumably as a result of the signals persisting in the synaptic BL.

Although agrin remains fixed to the BL after muscle damage, the NMJs that form on regenerating muscle fibers often differ structurally from the original NMJs at the same site. For example, after damage induced in mouse muscle by the myotoxin from *Dendroaspis jamesoni* (Duchen et al., 1974) or that occurring in *mdx* mice, which have an inherited form of muscular dystrophy (Nagel et al., 1990; Lyons and Slater, 1991; Personius and Sawyer, 2005), the reformed NMJs consist of a collection of distinct spot contacts rather than the normal bands of synaptic contact (Fig. 2.35). This suggests that the nerve is able to lay down agrin at new sites, and that agrin at sites unapposed by a nerve may break down.

2.7.4. Toxins and the NMJ

2.7.4.1. Introduction to the toxins

There are many natural toxins that attack the nervous system in general and the NMJ in particular. In addition to their clinical significance, a number of these toxins have been used extensively in an experimental context to explore the covert plasticity of the mature NMJ. In contrast to the CNS, where the blood–brain barrier protects synapses from many foreign molecules, the NMJ is much more easily accessible to molecular attack. Bacteria, plants and both invertebrate and vertebrate animals all produce neurotoxins that act on the NMJ. These toxins can be classified

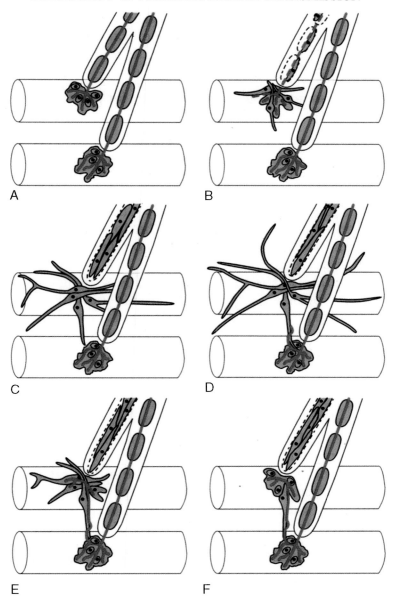

Fig. 2.33. Reinnervation of muscle after partial denervation. (A) Normal NMJs, showing nerves (red) and Schwann cells (blue). (B, C) Following partial denervation Schwann cell sprouts grow out from the denervated NMJs. (D, E) If Schwann cell sprouts make contact with an innervated NMJ, they may induce sprouting of the intact axons, causing them to grow back to the denervated NMJ. (F) These axonal sprouts may make effective synaptic contacts with the originally denervated muscle fiber. If so, the Schwann cell sprouts retract. (From Son et al., 1996, with permission.)

according to their site and mode of action. Thus, toxins may act preferentially on the presynaptic nerve terminal or postsynaptically on the muscle fiber, and they may act to block ion channels, to disrupt critical cellular processes such as exocytosis, or to cause cell damage. In addition to these natural toxins, there is a wide variety of man-made "environmental" toxins that have a deleterious effect on the NMJ.

The great diversity of natural toxins, both in terms of their origins and their modes of action, make the toxicology of the NMJ a rich field in its own right, that goes well beyond what is appropriate for this Chapter. The reader is referred to more specialized articles (e.g., Van der Kloot and Molgo, 1994; Schiavo et al., 2000; Harris et al., 2003) and texts on neurotoxicology. Here the responses of the NMJ to several toxins that have been extensively investigated, and which exemplify different modes of action, are described. They are of particular interest because of what they reveal about the regenerative capacity of the NMJ.

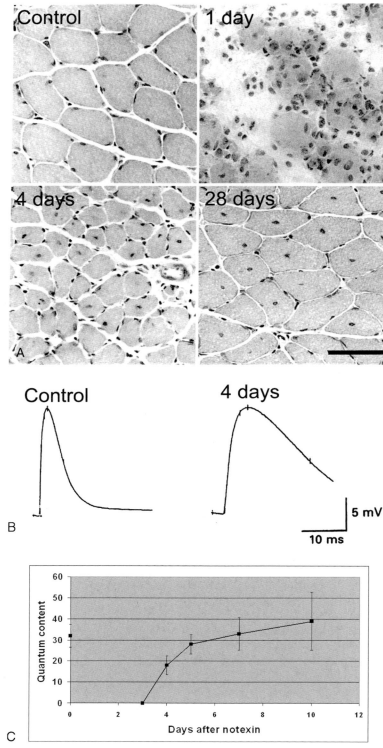

Fig. 2.34. Innervation of regenerating muscles. The response of rat soleus muscles to a single perimuscular injection of notexin (2 µg). (A) Histological preparations (H&E) show that the muscle fibers undergo breakdown within 1 day and that new fibers are present 2–3 days later. By 28 days, the fibers have reached normal size but retain centrally located nuclei. (B) Typical EPPs recorded from normal muscles (control) and at an early stage of innervation of the regenerating muscle fibers (4 days). Note that the EPP is much slower at the reinnervated NMJ, both because γ-AChRs are present and because AChE activity is reduced. (C) Mean quantal content at NMJs on regenerating muscles. The earliest EPPs are seen 4 days after intoxication and the normal level of release is reached a week later. (From Grubb et al., 1991, with permission.)

Control   *mdx*

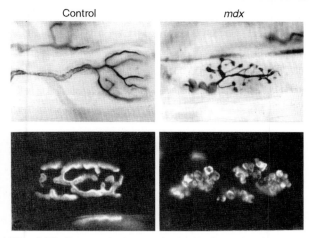

Fig. 2.35. Structural changes in NMJs in *mdx* mice. The NMJs on regenerated muscle fibers in *mdx* mice consist of a set of discrete boutons with associated postsynaptic specializations. Upper panels show nerve terminals (silver impregnation), lower panels show AChRs (R-α-bungarotoxin). (From Lyons and Slater, 1991, with permission.)

2.7.4.2. Presynaptic toxins that block release

Numerous toxins block the activation of voltage-gated Na^+ and Ca^{++} channels. The best known of these is the puffer fish toxin, tetrodotoxin, which blocks Na_V1 channels and thus prevents action potentials from depolarizing the nerve terminal. A variety of toxins derived from invertebrates exist that block Ca^{++} channels in the nerve terminal. Among these are ones that specifically block the various different types of Ca^{++} channel that may be present at mammalian NMJs, e.g., N-, P/Q- and L- (Uchitel, 1997). The effect of these toxins on release depends on which Ca^{++} channels are present and in what relative abundance. This, in turn, depends on the biological state of the NMJ (see Section 2.6).

Perhaps the best known, and most clinically relevant, presynaptic toxins are those produced by the anaerobic bacterium *Clostridium botulinum*. These toxins bind to specific polysaccharide groups on the motor nerve terminal (Jahn, 2006) by their heavy chains and are taken into the cytoplasm where their light chains catalyze the cleavage of one or more SNARE proteins involved in quantal release from the nerve terminal (see Section 2.2.4.1) (Schiavo et al., 2000; Montecucco and Molgo, 2005). This leads to profound blocking of quantal ACh release and the paralysis that characterizes clinical botulism. There are seven different serotypes of botulinum neurotoxin (BoNT/A–G), which differ in the particular SNARE proteins they cleave.

These toxins, in particular BoNT/A, are of considerable therapeutic importance because they can be used to effect partial paralysis of selected muscles in the treatment of a variety of dystonias and spasticity. In addition, BoNT/A is used by large numbers of people as a cosmetic agent that reduces myogenic facial wrinkling. In many situations the NMJ is eventually able to recover, at least partially, from BoNT/A on a timescale of several months. This necessitates multiple treatments to maintain a useful effect. Understanding how the NMJ regains reliable function is thus of interest both because of what it reveals about the mechanisms for maintaining reliable neuromuscular transmission, and for what it may reveal about the effects of repeated exposure to BoNT/A in a clinical setting.

Recovery from botulism occurs at a rate that depends on the particular serotype involved. It seems that the duration of action depends, at least in part, on the particular SNARE protein cleaved, and even on the site of cleavage within that protein. For example, BoNT/A and BoNT/E both cleave SNAP-25, though at different sites (Fig. 2.7). However, recovery from BoNT/E is much faster than from BoNT/A. Following BoNT/A intoxication of rat or mouse muscles, neuromuscular transmission recovers on a timescale of weeks. Functional recovery from BoNT/A is associated with the outgrowth of axonal sprouts from the motor nerve terminal which occurs as early as a week after exposure to BoNT/A (Fig. 2.36A) (Duchen, 1970; Tonge, 1974a; Juzans et al., 1996; de Paiva et al., 1999; Santafe et al., 2000). Some of these sprouts make new synaptic contacts with the muscle fiber, complete with high concentrations of AChRs and AChE, at varying distances from the original NMJ. This recovery is associated with a steady increase of quantal content back to its normal value (Fig. 2.36B) (Tonge, 1974a; de Paiva et al., 1999; Santafe et al., 2000). This is a dramatic example of the rerunning of the developmental program that brings about postsynaptic differentiation in response to the inductive influence of the nerve.

There are varying accounts in the literature of the natural history of the sprouts and new synaptic contacts induced by BoNT/A. Some authors have reported that the ectopic contacts persist and the original nerve terminals eventually withdraw, leaving a highly abnormal innervation pattern (Duchen, 1970). Other accounts describe the eventual withdrawal of the ectopic contacts and the simultaneous recovery of quantal release at the original NMJs (de Paiva et al., 1999; Meunier et al., 2002). Still in doubt is how much the new contacts contribute to the overall functional recovery of the NMJ and the question of whether the NMJs that eventually result from the recovery process are fully normal.

A different pattern of recovery is seen when BoNT serotypes with a shorter duration of action are used

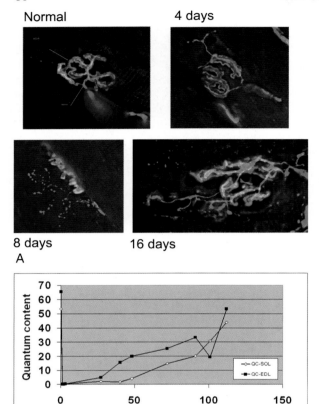

Fig. 2.36. Recovery of mouse muscles from BoNT/A intoxication. (A) Following a single injection of BoNT/A axonal sprouts (green, neurofilament immunolabeling) grow away from the NMJ and make new synaptic contacts with associated postsynaptic specializations (AChRs, red, R-α-bungarotoxin). Times shown are days after BoNT/A injection. (C.R. Slater and L. Gurney, unpublished images). (B) Quantal content recovers on a timescale of several months, sooner in fast muscles (EDL) than slow (SOL). (From Tonge, 1974a, with permission.)

(Meunier et al., 2003). Following the shortest acting form, BoNT/E, recovery occurs in a few days and does not involve the formation of axonal sprouts. With BoNT/F, functional recovery takes about 3 weeks and is accompanied by a brief period of sprout formation. Thus, it seems that paralysis lasting more than 1–2 weeks elicits a process of sprouting from the nerve that appears to be aimed at bringing about functional recovery by the formation of new synaptic contacts which may, or may not, persist long after BoNT administration.

The signaling pathways that trigger axonal sprouting after BoNT are not known. Early studies showed that imposing activity on muscle paralyzed by BoNT/A reduced the extent of sprouting (Brown et al.,

1977). This suggests axonal sprouting is suppressed by normal activity. A number of studies have tried to identify molecules whose expression by the muscle is activity-dependent and which suppress axonal sprouting. Although some candidates, such as IGF1 (Caroni and Schneider, 1994), have been implicated it is not clear that any single signaling pathway can account for the wide range of events that occur after BoNT intoxication.

What is clear from studying both recovery from BoNT, and the response to partial denervation, is that the NMJ is capable of a high degree of "adaptive plasticity", which allows it to recover useful function after long term block. Nonetheless, a number of important questions about that recovery remain unanswered. One such question is: how complete is recovery? In a clinical setting, movement of a small fraction of all muscle fibers may lead to recovery of useful function. Further, at the level of the individual NMJ, a quantal content several-fold lower than normal may be adequate to elicit some contraction. Thus assessment of clinically detectable recovery of function may not be a good indicator of recovery at the level of the NMJ. A second important question is: what is the effect of repeatedly blocking the NMJ? There have been few detailed studies of the recovery after repeated BoNT/A injections, and none of these have been done in situations where the structural and functional properties of the NMJ could be adequately assessed. When these two issues are taken together, considerable uncertainty remains about the possible cumulative effects of repeated BoNT/A injections.

2.7.4.3. Presynaptic toxins that damage the nerve

A second class of presynaptic toxins are those that damage the nerve terminal. These toxins are exemplified by β-bungarotoxin (β-BgTx), a phospholipase A_2 component of the venom of kraits of the genus *Bungarus sp.* (Prasarnpun et al., 2005). Both in vivo and in vitro, β-BgTx causes acute (<1 h) block of neuromuscular transmission. This results from impaired release of ACh and is associated with a profound reduction in the number of synaptic vesicles in the nerve terminal. When the damage to the nerve is local, the terminal can begin to regenerate within a few days and functional innervation is restored within a week.

A second class of presynaptic toxin is exemplified by the α-latrotoxin (αLTX) from the black widow spider *Latrodectus mactans* (Ushkaryov et al., 2004). This toxin has a complex mode of action, but its most dramatic effect is a great increase in the rate of spontaneous release of ACh quanta from the nerve. This is a result of binding of the toxin to neurexins in the motor nerve terminal and then forming tetrameric Ca^{++} permeable pores in the membrane. It is the flow of Ca^{++} into the nerve through these pores that enhances spontaneous release. In addition, αLTX binds to latrophilins in the nerve terminal. This leads to activation of a G-protein mediated cascade that also promotes spontaneous quantal release. During the action of αLTX, evoked release of ACh quanta is impaired. Ultimately, the action of αLTX leads to destruction of the nerve terminal, but this damage may be quite local. As with β-BgTx, regeneration of the terminal can occur starting a few days after intoxication, and substantially full recovery is possible (Robbins et al., 1990).

2.7.4.4. Postsynaptic toxins that block AChRs

Much of what is known about the action of ACh at the NMJ is owed to the existence of natural compounds that interfere with AChR function. The first of these to be discovered was curare, a concoction of substances extracted from plants such as *Strychnos toxifera,* used in the production of poisoned darts by various South American indigenous peoples. The principal active component, the alkaloid D-tubocurarine (dTC), is a reversible competitive blocker of AChRs at the NMJ and is now used clinically as a muscle relaxant. When dTC binds to the AChRs it prevents their activation by ACh and thus reduces the sensitivity of the postsynaptic membrane to released ACh. This reduces the amplitude of the mEPPs and EPPs. In sufficient doses it reduces the EPP to below the threshold for activation of the muscle, causing paralysis. At a critical dose, transmission may be effective at low frequencies of stimulation but fail at higher frequencies when the quantal content is depressed (see Section 2.5.1.1).

A second AChR blocker of great historical importance is α-bungarotoxin (αBgTx). This small (MW 8000 Daltons), highly stable protein is a component of the venom of the banded krait *Bungarus multicinctus* and is an example of the postsynaptically active toxins of elapid and hydrophiid snakes. It is an irreversible blocker of the ACh binding site of the AChRs at the NMJ. It is easily conjugated to fluorescent or electron-dense groups or made radioactive through conjugation to [125]I. The irreversible nature of its binding has made αBgTx extremely useful in a wide variety of experimental situations, not least in the purification and visualization of the AChRs. Its effect on neuromuscular transmission is similar to that of dTC with the notable exception that it is virtually irreversible.

2.7.4.5. Postsynaptic toxins that damage the muscle
Numerous myotoxins are known that cause catastrophic breakdown of muscle fibers, usually as a result of phospholipase activity. Mention has already been made of notexin and how the muscle and NMJ respond to it (see Section 2.7.3).

2.7.4.6. Environmental toxins

The toxicity of man-made compounds may be intentional, as in insecticides, or incidental. Of the intentionally toxic compounds, some of the best known are the compounds that act by blocking the AChE at the NMJ (Blain, 1999). Examples are sarin and the organophosphate pesticides. Since these compounds block AChE activity, they allow ACh released from the nerve to persist in the synaptic cleft longer than usual. This leads to repeated opening of the AChRs and a prolongation of the decay of the EPC. In the short term, this potentiates neuromuscular transmission but soon the high concentration of ACh in the cleft leads to depolarization of the postsynaptic membrane, which inactivates the Na_V1 channels responsible for the action potential. Further, desensitization of the AChRs may occur as a result of persistent binding of ACh. In addition, the entry of Ca^{++} into the muscle fiber through the open AChRs may cause local activation of lytic processes in the cell that lead to breakdown of the postsynaptic apparatus (Leonard and Salpeter, 1979).

2.7.5. Conclusions

The ability of the NMJ to recover from a wide variety of mechanical and chemical assaults indicates the evolutionary importance of effective and reliable neuromuscular transmission. The BL, and the presence in it of molecules that can direct the rapid reconstruction of the NMJ after its constituent cells have been damaged, play an important part in this recovery. In many circumstances, the reconstruction of the NMJ in an adult mammal occurs more rapidly than its original development. Finally, it is increasingly clear that the Schwann cells play an important part in facilitating the adaptive plasticity of the nerve terminal.

2.8. The impact of disease on safety factor

2.8.1. Overview

The efficacy and reliability of neuromuscular transmission depend on many factors operating at numerous levels of functional organization. As a result many molecules could be targets of pathogenic processes that might interfere with the reliability of neuromuscular transmission. It is perhaps surprising, therefore, that diseases in the NMJ are rare. For example, myasthenia gravis (MG), the most common disease affecting the

NMJ directly, has a prevalence in Western countries of only 10–20/100 000 (Flachenecker, 2006). Since the NMJ is so important for survival, it is likely that many such conditions would be lethal if expressed during early development, and this is the case for many engineered mutations of key NMJ molecules in mice. On the other hand, the remarkable ability of the NMJ to respond adaptively to interference may result in adequate functional compensation so that some conditions remain unrecognized. However rare, conditions leading to impaired neuromuscular transmission are highly debilitating and represent a significant clinical problem. Other chapters in this Handbook deal with these individual diseases in detail. Here, the aim is to consider more generally the ways in which the main functional components of the NMJ are influenced by disease processes.

Two broad classes of disease, distinguished by their etiology, account for most of the recognized conditions affecting neuromuscular transmission. The first class to be recognized contains the acquired autoimmune disorders, including MG, the Lambert–Eaton Myasthenic syndrome (LEMS), neuromyotonia (NMT) and the Miller–Fisher variant of the Guillain–Barré syndrome (MFS). The second class contains the inherited conditions known collectively as Congenital Myasthenic Syndromes (CMS) (Beeson et al., 2005). Many of these conditions involve attack on, or abnormalities of, molecules that play a central role in the immediate events of neuromuscular transmission, such as voltage-gated ion channels, AChE and the AChR. However it has become clear in recent years that a number of other conditions result from direct structural damage to the NMJ (e.g., MFS, Overell and Willison, 2005) or abnormalities of the events that account for the development and maintenance of the normal structure of the NMJ (e.g., Chevessier et al., 2004; Slater et al., 2006). It is thus important, when trying to understand the basis of impaired neuromuscular transmission in any particular case, to keep in mind the broad aspects of the cell biology of the NMJ as well as the immediate events and molecules that mediate transmission.

Regardless of their etiology, diseases affecting neuromuscular transmission may be distinguished by whether the initial effect on transmission is positive or negative. In some cases, such as MG or the congenital AChR deficiencies, the primary effects are to impair transmission. In others, such as neuromyotonia, the slow channel syndrome or AChE deficiency, the initial effects are to exaggerate transmission. In the longer term, the increased transmitter effect associated with these conditions may lead to structural damage to the NMJ that contributes to symptoms (see Section 2.7.4.6).

2.8.2. Conditions influencing transmitter release

A number of conditions are known in which the amount of ACh released from the nerve terminal is less than normal. This can be either because the amount of ACh per vesicle is reduced, or because the number of vesicles released by a nerve impulse is low.

2.8.2.1. Impaired ACh synthesis
The events leading to quantal release of ACh begin with ACh synthesis from acetylCoA and choline. This is mediated by the enzyme choline acetyltransferase (ChAT), which is present in the cytoplasm of the nerve terminal. When the gene encoding ChAT is completely inactivated in mice, the result is lethal at birth and there is no evidence of ACh synthesis, indicating that there is no effective alternative pathway for ACh synthesis (Misgeld et al., 2002).

Pathogenic mutations of the gene encoding this enzyme have been found to be the basis of a form of CMS known as CMS with episodic apnea (CMS-EA, formerly referred to as Familial Infantile Myasthenia) (Ohno et al., 2001). In this condition, neuromuscular transmission is close to normal at rest. However, abnormal fatigue is apparent during sustained exertion. When NMJs from these patients are studied in vitro, a decline in EPP amplitude is seen only after repetitive stimulation (10 Hz) for 5 min. This decline is a result of decreasing mEPP amplitude and is not accompanied by any change in quantal content. It is, however, associated with a reduction in size of the vesicles, consistent with the view that the amount of ACh/vesicle is lower than normal in these patients (Mora et al., 1987). Thus it appears that the safety factor of transmission is reduced in CMS-EA because the abnormally low rate of ACh synthesis is not able to keep up with intense demand.

Once synthesized, ACh must be taken up into synaptic vesicles before it can be released. So far, there are no reported conditions in which this uptake process is impaired.

2.8.2.2. Reduced quantal content of the EPP
Quantal content can be reduced for a number of reasons. For example, failure of the nerve impulse to depolarize the nerve terminal leads to greatly reduced release. An example of this is seen in the naturally occurring mouse mutant motor endplate disease (*med*) (Harris and Pollard, 1986). In this mouse, a profound impairment of quantal ACh release results from a mutation in the gene encoding the voltage-gated sodium channel in the nerve (SCN8a) (Burgess et al., 1995; Kohrman et al., 1996). No similar condition has yet been described in humans.

However, at least four conditions are known in humans in which the safety factor is reduced because the number of quanta released is too small. These are LEMS, "limb-girdle myasthenia" (LGM), congenital endplate AChE deficiency (Engel et al., 1977) and botulism. In LEMS, autoantibodies are present that react with the voltage-gated Ca^{++} channels in the nerve terminal (Vincent et al., 1989). Binding of these antibodies at the extracellular face of the channels leads to a decrease in the number of Ca^{++} channels in the nerve terminal, presumably as a result of cross-linking and subsequent endocytosis, and disruption of the AZs (Fukuoka et al., 1987). As a result, the amount of Ca^{++} entering the nerve in response to a nerve impulse is less than normal. This, in turn, results in fewer quanta being released than normal. This effect is typically great enough so that transmission fails at many NMJs and the CMAP at rest is much smaller than normal. During exercise, however, the weakness associated with LEMS may be reduced. This is assumed to be a result of the build-up of residual Ca^{++} in the nerve terminal, leading to enhanced quantal release (see Section 2.5.1.2) and a marked increase in the amplitude of the CMAP. However, this does not last long after exercise stops. This effect forms the basis for a clinical test for LEMS.

LGM is a condition characterized by weakness primarily of the proximal muscles with little involvement of facial or eye muscles (see below). The reduction of quantal content in LGM has a completely different basis from that in LEMS, and therefore provides an interesting comparison. In LGM, the average quantal content is about 50% of normal but the size of the mEPPs is only slightly reduced. The average size of the NMJ is also about 50% of normal. Thus, the quantal release per unit area is normal, indicating that the reduction in ACh output is not primarily a result of an impairment of the release mechanism per se, but rather a "secondary" consequence of the reduction in NMJ size (Slater et al., 2006).

In congenital endplate cholinesterase deficiency the amount of AChE at the NMJ is severely reduced (Section 2.8.3.4). The quantal release from the nerve is also reduced, and this is associated with a reduction in size of the nerve terminals, many of which are completely or partially encased by Schwann cells. In botulism, as described above (Section 2.7.4.2), one or more proteins that play a key role in the process of exocytosis are cleaved by the toxin and thus inactivated. As a result the quantal content is dramatically reduced.

The comparison of the first three conditions points out the important influence of structural factors as determinants of the reliability of neuromuscular transmission.

2.8.2.3. Prolonged release due to impaired repolarization

In addition to conditions in which quantal release is impaired, there is at least one condition in which the opposite is true. In neuromyotonia (NMT), as in myogenic myotonia, muscle relaxation is slowed after contraction. In NMT this results from slowed repolarization of the nerve terminal membrane after a nerve impulse rather than from a similar effect in the muscle cell. Repolarization is normally mediated by the opening of voltage-gated K^+ channels (see Section 2.2.2). In at least some forms of NMT, autoantibodies are present (Shillito et al., 1995; Newsom-Davis, 1997) that recognize the K^+ channels in the nerve terminal, presumably causing them to be removed by endocytosis. As a result, the density of K^+ channels is less than normal, the repolarizing current is reduced and the period of repolarization extended. This, in turn, extends the period of Ca^{++} entry into the nerve terminal and with it, the release and action of ACh. The resulting prolonged EPP causes the generation of multiple action potentials in the muscle fiber and persisting contraction after individual motor nerve impulses.

2.8.2.4. Lytic damage to nerve terminals by autoantibodies

Destruction of the nerve terminal is the most extreme way of impairing ACh release. In the Miller–Fisher variant of the Guillain–Barré Syndrome (MFS), autoantibodies are elaborated, often in response to bacterial infections, which are specific for polysaccharides of the GQ1b class. These groups are present on motor nerve terminals, and are bound by the circulating antibodies. This, in turn, leads to local recruitment of the complement system, and lysis of the nerve terminal (O'Hanlon et al., 2002). In this sense, their action resembles that of certain presynaptically active natural toxins, e.g., β-bungarotoxin (see Section 2.7.4.3). In both cases, the ready access of substances in the blood to the NMJ is an important aspect of the pathogenic process.

Following acute lytic attack on the nerve terminal, axonal sprouting and the reinnervation of the original NMJ normally lead to recovery on a timescale of weeks to months. Indeed, it is in recovery from diseases of this kind that the real value of the adaptive plasticity of the NMJ is seen. During this recovery phase, it is likely that the reliability of neuromuscular transmission is reduced, as during reinnervation following mechanical or toxic injury.

2.8.3. Conditions influencing transmitter action

Once ACh is released from the nerve, it must bind to the AChRs and cause their channels to open before there is any excitatory effect on the muscle. Two important classes of NMJ disorders are associated with changes in the number or properties of the AChRs in the postsynaptic membrane.

2.8.3.1. Abnormal ACh-gated channel function

Mutations of the genes encoding the subunits of the AChR can influence either the abundance or the functional properties of the AChR, or both. An important group of CMSs are those associated with abnormal function of the AChRs.

A number of mutations in different AChR subunits, and different domains of the individual subunits, result in changes in the rate of closing of the opened AChR ion channel (Engel and Sine, 2005). When the channel closes too rapidly, the amount of positive charge entering the muscle fiber per nerve impulse is reduced and with it, the amount of depolarization associated with the action of each quantum of transmitter. As a result, the EPP is smaller than normal and the safety factor correspondingly reduced. There is evidence in some of these diseases of increased expression of AChRs containing a γ-subunit (Milone et al., 1998). These may act to compensate for the loss of normal ε-subunit function, and may thus represent an important compensatory strategy that allows toleration of some mutations in the ε-subunit. This strategy is not available for compensation from mutations in the other AChR subunits, and this probably accounts for the relative predominance of ε-AChR mutations in patients with CMS caused by mutations in AChR genes.

A second group of AChR mutations, resulting in slowing of closure of the ion channel, underlie the "slow-channel syndromes" (SCS). Initially such mutations would be expected to increase the safety factor since more positive charge than normal would enter the muscle fiber following each channel opening event. However, the weakness seen in these patients results from a paradoxical impairment of transmission. This is associated with focal degeneration of junctional folds and loss of acetylcholine receptors in the membrane (Engel et al., 1982) as well as a depolarization block developing in the course of physiologic activity. Degeneration of the junctional folds is attributed to excessive Ca^{++} entry during the prolonged synaptic response; the Ca^{++} conductance of the mutant slow-channels is not increased (Fucile et al., 2006). Degeneration of the junctional folds is also associated with block of AChE activity by chemical toxins (e.g., sarin, organophosphates, see Section 2.7.4.6) or inherited deficiency of AChE.

2.8.3.2. Inherited AChR deficiency

A reduction in the local density of AChRs in the postsynaptic membrane most often occurs either as a result

Control

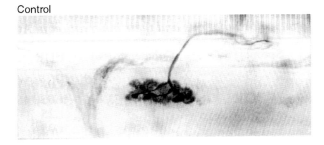

AChR deficiency

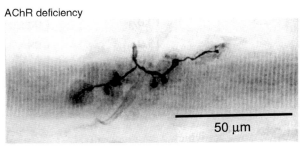

50 μm

Fig. 2.37. Elongated NMJs in AChR deficiency. NMJs from human *vastus lateralis* visualized after silver impregnation and histochemical demonstration of AChE activity. Control shows normal compact form. In the patient with AChR deficiency the NMJ is elongated in a manner suggestive of induced axonal sprouting. (From Slater et al., 1997, with permission.)

of a mutation in one of the AChR subunit genes in various forms of CMS (usually the ε-subunit), or as a result of the action of autoantibodies specific for the AChR, as in MG (see below). Mutations in the AChR genes that affect the promoter or disrupt the reading frame can result in severe inherited deficiencies in expression of the subunit in question. Most such mutations have been found in the gene encoding the ε-subunit, since this is the only subunit that can be replaced by an analogous subunit (γ-AChR) (Engel and Sine, 2005).

A frequent feature of inherited AChR deficiencies is an abnormally elongated NMJ (Fig. 2.37) (Vincent et al., 1981; Slater et al., 1997). This appearance suggests that in these cases, the nerve terminal has undergone a phase of sprouting and formation of new synaptic contacts. As in the response to partial denervation or BoNT/A (see Sections 2.7.2.1 and 2.7.4.2), this remodeling is presumably induced by some consequence of the reduced muscle activity. It is noteworthy, however, that in these cases of AChR deficiency, this adaptive plasticity is inadequate to reestablish the normal level of reliability of the NMJ. The explanation for this is unknown.

The accumulation of AChRs in the postsynaptic membrane depends on a complex set of interactions involving numerous proteins in addition to the AChRs themselves (see Section 2.6.3.5). Of particular importance is rapsyn, a 43 kD protein, which is essential for AChR clustering (Gautam et al., 1995). A number of patients with a severe form of CMS have recently been found to harbor mutations in the gene encoding rapsyn (Ohno et al., 2002; Engel and Sine, 2005). In these patients, both the density of AChRs and the intensity of postsynaptic folding at the NMJ are greatly reduced. In addition, the NMJs have a strikingly elongate conformation. Thus, the NMJs in these patients are similar to those in patients with mutations of the AChR itself. In both cases, it is obvious that the reliability of neuromuscular transmission is profoundly compromised by the reduction in AChR density.

MuSK is a key component of the signaling cascade by which neurally-derived agrin induces a high density of AChRs in the postsynaptic membrane (see Section 2.6.3.5) (Strochlic et al., 2005). As with rapsyn, which must be phosphorylated by MuSK to cause AChR clustering, mice in which the gene for MuSK has been knocked-out are unable to form functional NMJs and therefore die at birth (DeChiara et al., 1996). A number of patients with CMS have now been found with mutations in the gene encoding MuSK (Chevessier et al., 2004). Although little is known about the functional properties of the NMJs in these patients, their conformation is abnormal, with some similarities to that in other cases of AChR deficiency.

These patients with defects of rapsyn and MuSK exemplify the point that due to the highly interactive nature of the processes that ensure the normal reliability of the NMJ, there are many molecular targets for pathogenic attack.

2.8.3.3. Acquired AChR deficiency

The most familiar disease that has its primary impact on the reliability of neuromuscular transmission is MG. In most patients with this condition, the pathogenic agents are autoantibodies to the AChR. The majority of these do not act as functional blockers of the AChR or its channel. Rather, they bind to and cross-link the AChRs causing them to be internalized and degraded. The result is a profound reduction in the density of AChRs in the postsynaptic membrane, a reduction in the amplitude of mEPPs and EPPs (Elmqvist et al., 1964; Cull-Candy et al., 1980) and an attendant loss of efficacy and reliability of neuromuscular transmission. In addition to the downregulation of AChRs, there is also a disorganization of the postsynaptic apparatus, with a widening of the folds (Engel and Santa, 1971). This is presumably caused by the lytic process associated with complement binding to the AChRs in the postsynaptic

membrane. In light of the current view of the function of the folds (see Section 2.3.6.3), it is likely that their disruption exacerbates the effects of the primary deficiency of AChRs on transmission.

Axonal sprouting can also occur in autoimmune MG. This is associated with a second form of adaptive plasticity, an increase in the output of quanta per unit area of synaptic contact (Plomp et al., 1995). The magnitude of this increase is inversely correlated with the amplitude of the mEPPs at individual NMJs. The basis of this effect is not known. Possible explanations include a change in the type or density of Ca^{++} channels or in their modulation by G-protein coupled mediators, or an alteration in the duration of the nerve action potential, possibly by changes in the properties or number of K^+ channels in the nerve terminal. As with those examples of inherited AChR deficiency cited above, the adaptive response of the nerve in MG is clearly inadequate to normalize the reliability of transmission.

A significant fraction of patients with MG do not have detectable serum antibodies to AChRs. Some of these "seronegative" patients have antibodies to MuSK in their serum (Hoch et al., 2001; McConville et al., 2004), although there is doubt about whether these antibodies account for the functional defect in any or all of these patients (Selcen et al., 2004).

2.8.3.4. Prolonged ACh action due to AChE deficiency

The action of ACh on the postsynaptic membrane is normally terminated by hydrolysis catalyzed by the AChE associated with the synaptic basal lamina (see Section 2.3.4). A number of patients have been identified in whom the duration of the synaptic potentials is greatly prolonged and virtually all AChE activity is absent (Engel et al., 1977). It has recently been found that these patients have mutations in the gene encoding the AChE molecule, most commonly in the region encoding the collagenous tail (COL Q), which is involved in binding the enzyme to the basal lamina (Ohno et al., 1998). In the absence of normal AChE activity, ACh molecules that unbind from AChR after the initial activation are free to rebind to AChRs and thus to trigger repeated openings. In these circumstances, the termination of ACh action after the release of a quantum of transmitter is determined by the rate at which it diffuses away from the release site, resulting in a decreased local concentration.

The consequences for the NMJ of a profound deficiency of AChE are similar to those of the prolongation of the AChR open time in the SCS. In NMJ AChE deficiency, however, the opening events of the AChR channel are normal but the individual channels open repeatedly owing to the prolonged lifetime of ACh in the synaptic space. In both cases, excessive entry of Ca^{++} occurs, resulting in local degeneration of the postsynaptic apparatus. In NMJ AChE deficiency, neuromuscular transmission is compromised by the combination of decreased quantal release by nerve impulses from small nerve terminals, many of which are encased by Schwann cells, a depolarization block during physiologic activity, and structural changes in the junctional folds that alter the geometry of the NMJ. The two conditions can be distinguished by the absence of any beneficial response in cases of AChE deficiency. Although anticholinesterase treatment may in principle alleviate the symptoms of SCS, it is obvious that, in the long term, this approach would only intensify the pathogenic process.

2.8.4. Conditions influencing muscle excitation

Muscle contraction is normally activated by an action potential that propagates along the full length of the fiber. Unless the muscle fiber action potential occurs, the depolarization of the EPP causes at most a local graded contraction that is of no functional significance. Two classes of disease are known in which the triggering of muscle fiber action potentials at the NMJ is impaired.

2.8.4.1. Abnormal $Na_V1.4$ properties

One patient has been described in whom mutations of the gene encoding $Na_V1.4$ results in abnormally rapid inactivation of the channels (Tsujino et al., 2003). As a result, the number of $Na_V1.4$ channels that are opened by a full-sized EPP is reduced and action potential generation is impaired. In this patient, all aspects of ACh release and action appear to be normal. It is important to realize that $Na_V1.4$ is normally expressed only in skeletal muscle. As a result, these mutations do not directly influence the function of nerve or cardiac muscle. Other mutations affecting the structure of $Na_V1.4$ have been described and are the basis of the periodic paralyses and myotonias (Jurkat-Rott and Lehmann-Horn, 2005). These mutations generally result in a gain of function, in the sense that the activated channels remain open longer than normal, leading to the generation of multiple action potentials that is the defining feature of myotonias. The rarity of this form of CMS, in which there is a loss of function of $Na_V1.4$, presumably reflects the lethality of many other mutations affecting this essential channel.

2.8.4.2. Disturbances of folding

The second class of conditions affecting the generation of muscle fiber action potentials is less well defined, but probably much more common. In these conditions, the characteristic folding of the postsynaptic membrane is disrupted and/or reduced. This may occur as a result of mutations affecting postsynaptic proteins, of attack by autoantibodies as in MG (Engel et al., 1976), or as a result of local degeneration induced by excess Ca^{++} entry through opened AChR channels in SCS or AChE deficiency. Current views about the significance of the folds as amplifiers of ACh action are described above (Section 2.3.6.3).

The cellular processes that account for the formation and maintenance of the folds are poorly understood. It is noteworthy that mutations affecting many postsynaptic proteins, both integral membrane proteins and components of the cytoskeleton, lead to reduced folding (De Kerchove et al., 2002). These proteins include AChR (Engel et al., 1982), rapsyn (Ohno et al., 2002), utrophin (Deconinck et al., 1997; Grady et al., 1997), dystrophin (Torres and Duchen, 1987; Lyons and Slater, 1991), and syntrophin (Adams et al., 2004). A similar reduction in folding has also been seen in cases of limb-girdle myasthenia (Slater et al., 2006). It thus seems likely that the very extensive folding, which is a feature of human NMJs, is sensitive to subtle mechanical properties of the postsynaptic membrane that are influenced by many proteins.

Folding may also be disrupted as a result of antibody-dependent degeneration of the postsynaptic apparatus. In MG, this results from a complement-mediated attack on the postsynaptic membrane (Engel et al., 1976). Associated with this effect on the folds, in both MG and an animal model of it, is a reduction in the number of $Na_V1.4$ channels and an increase in action potential threshold (Ruff and Lennon, 1998). Similar effects are likely to be associated with local postsynaptic degeneration in CMS and AChE deficiency, although this has not been directly established in these conditions.

It is thus clear that a wide variety of circumstances give rise to reduced or disorganized folding. In few of these situations has the impact of this effect on muscle fiber action potential generation been quantified. Nonetheless, it seems clear that what may often be "secondary" effects of a pathological process at the NMJ may have significant functional consequences.

2.8.5. Conditions influencing NMJ size

Many of the well-defined pathological conditions that lead to impaired neuromuscular transmission have their primary effect on either the pre- or the postsynaptic component of the NMJ. In some conditions, however, both components are clearly affected. An example of this is limb-girdle myasthenia (LGM) (Slater et al., 2006). In LGM patients, the effects of individual quanta on the muscle fiber are substantially normal, indicating that the function and local density of AChRs is normal (Fig. 2.38). However there is a reduction in quantal content to about 50% of its normal value. This is associated with, and probably caused by, a reduction in the overall size of the NMJs. At the same time, the extent of postsynaptic folding is also reduced to about 50% of its normal value. It is likely that the reduction in folding raises the effective threshold for action potential initiation in the muscle (see Section 2.3.6.3), thus exacerbating the effect of the reduced quantal content.

It has recently been found that many cases of LGM, including those described immediately above, result from mutations in the gene encoding Dok-7, a protein that modulates the activity of MuSK (Beeson et al., 2006). This is the first gene to be identified that influences the efficacy of neuromuscular transmission primarily by an effect on NMJ size and conformation ("synaptopathy"), rather than on the properties or density of one of the molecules that mediate the immediate events of neuromuscular transmission. Further investigation of the normal action of Dok-7 may shed light on the question of how one of the most distinctive and functionally important features of the NMJ, its size, is determined.

2.8.6. Impaired transmission associated with diseases of the motor neuron

In a number of conditions, the reliability of neuromuscular transmission is compromised as part of a broad decline in the state of health of the motor neuron. A comprehensive review of these conditions would go beyond the remit of this chapter. Nonetheless, it is worth mentioning two examples of this group which, though still poorly described or understood, are of considerable clinical importance. These are the early stages of ALS and the so-called post-polio syndrome. In both these conditions, loss of reliability of neuromuscular transmission occurs before, or in the absence of, overt necrosis of the motor neuron.

2.8.6.1. Early stages of ALS

Several reports document decreased reliability of neuromuscular transmission during the early stages of ALS (e.g., Stalberg et al., 1975; Denys and Norris, Jr, 1979). This reduced efficacy of transmission is associated with the expansion of motor units that survive the motor neuron death that defines this condition. In the early stages of the disease, when relatively few motor neurons have died, there are still many surviving motor neurons available to provide innervation for the muscle fibers that have become denervated.

It is likely that transmission at the earliest of these re-established NMJs is fully effective. However, as the extent of motor neuron death increases, the surviving motor neurons become increasingly extended. At this stage it is likely that the general level of reliability of transmission declines, leading to clinically significant weakness.

The one detailed study of transmission at NMJs in 10 patients with ALS found a decline in quantal content to about 50% of normal values (Maselli et al., 1993). Whether this was a loss of release efficacy, or a result of a reduction in the size of individual NMJs, was not determined. The decline in quantal content was associated with a decline in mEPP amplitude to about 67% of normal. In that study, it was not possible to determine whether the NMJs from which recordings were made were original or newly formed, or how much the axons in question had sprouted. It is therefore unclear whether the observations represent a decline in function of origin NMJs, or a failure of newly formed innervation to reach a normal level of reliability, or a mixture of both.

Some animal studies suggest that changes at the NMJ are among the earliest signs of motor neuron degeneration in some forms of inherited motor neuron disease (Frey et al., 2000). In three stains of mutant mice with motor neuron loss, structural degeneration of some motor nerve terminals was observed before signs of clinical weakness were apparent or there was detectable motor neuron loss. The first nerve terminals to be lost were those of fast motor units. While no functional studies were made, it seems that events leading to overt degeneration of the nerve terminal may occur at an early stage in these conditions. Whether this is also true of the more common sporadic forms of ALS in man is unclear.

2.8.6.2. Post-polio syndrome

A second condition in which decreased reliability of neuromuscular transmission is associated with motor neuron pathology is the post-polio syndrome (PPS) (Trojan and Cashman, 2005). In this condition, patients who have had polio as children experience a new phase of increased weakness typically 35–40 years later. This new weakness appears to be due in large part to impaired neuromuscular transmission. SFEMG studies reveal that the extent of the observed increase in "jitter", an indication of a decline in the safety factor of neuromuscular transmission, is correlated with the enlargement of the motor unit as indicated by increased fiber density (Maselli et al., 1992). Detailed studies of neuromuscular transmission in isolated biopsy samples have found varying degrees of impairment involving decreases in

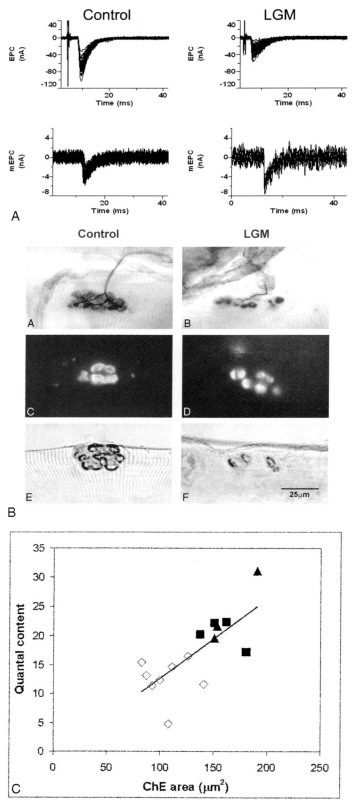

Fig. 2.38. Abnormalities of the NMJ in LGM. (A) The evoked EPC is reduced in amplitude at LGM NMJs but the amplitude of mEPCs is normal, indicating reduced quantal release from the nerve. (B) The NMJs are abnormally small in LGM patients. Top row, nerve terminal visualized after silver impregnation and histochemical demonstration of AChE activity. Middle row, AChRs labeled with R-α-bungarotoxin. Bottom row, histochemical demonstration of AChE activity. (C) Both quantal release and NMJ size are reduced in LGM patients (open symbols) compared to controls (filled symbols). (From Slater et al., 2006, with permission.)

both quantal content and mEPP amplitude (Maselli et al., 1995). In the absence of appropriate morphological studies, the basis of these changes is unclear.

The most generally accepted hypothesis concerning the basis of PPS is that motor nerve terminals that have undergone an expansion of their territory experience a time-dependent decline in function that eventually leads to the observed clinical weakness (Wiechers, 1988). The typical age of onset of the renewed phase of weakness in PPS is about 50 years of age, a decade or so earlier than the onset of motor neuron death that occurs in the normal population (see Section 2.6.4).

The biological bases of these aspects of age-dependent decline in motor neuron function are not understood. Nor is it clear how they are related to the normal processes of motor neuron aging and degeneration.

2.8.7. Treatments and their basis

Given the wide variety of conditions that alter the normal reliability of neuromuscular transmission, there are very few drugs available to treat their symptoms. These drugs can be divided broadly into those that alter quantal ACh release, and those that alter ACh action. Practical experience with different treatments is described in the chapters of this Handbook dealing with specific diseases. Here, only some brief general comments about the available drugs and their action will be made. Treatments of the autoimmune basis of the acquired diseases of the NMJ will not be covered.

2.8.7.1. Drugs that alter ACh release

The drug most commonly used to enhance evoked ACh release is 3,4-diaminopyridine (DAP). This drug blocks voltage-gated K^+ channels in muscle and nerve (see Section 2.2.2.3). Its most relevant action at the NMJ is to prolong the nerve terminal action potential and thus increase the entry of Ca^{++}. This in turn increases the number of quanta released. This drug has been particularly effective in the treatment of LEMS but is also useful in other conditions.

Sympathomimetic drugs have an enhancing effect on neuromuscular transmission (see Section 2.5.4.6), which may be related to their ability to synchronize quantal release. Ephedrine, a plant alkaloid, has sympathomimetic effects but has little effect in vitro on neuromuscular transmission in therapeutically achievable concentrations. It has nonetheless proven useful in some patients with limb-girdle myasthenia (Slater et al., 2006) and with AChE deficiency (Bestue-Cardiel et al., 2005). In the latter case the beneficial effect may be related to ephedrine's action as an open channel blocker with an associated speeding up of AChR channel closure (Milone and Engel, 1996).

2.8.7.2. Drugs that alter ACh action

The drugs used most commonly to treat impaired reliability of neuromuscular transmission are the anticholinesterases. Blocking the activity of the AChE in the synaptic cleft prolongs the period of action of the ACh released from the nerve, allowing it to remain active until diffusion away from the site of release lowers the local concentration to an inactive level. This allows AChR channels to remain open longer than normal and more positive charge to enter the muscle for every nerve impulse, thus enhancing the chance of generating an action potential in the muscle fiber. In many conditions of impaired transmission, regardless of whether they are pre- or postsynaptic in origin, this type of treatment is potentially effective. Obvious exceptions are AChE deficiencies and SCS, where even if there is a potential short term benefit, the long term effect is absent or negative (see Section 2.8.3).

Blockers of ACh action have potential use in conditions where overactivation of AChRs occurs. Quinidine and related compounds are open channel blockers that hasten the closure of open AChR channels (Sieb et al., 1996). This results in reduced amplitude and rapid decay of the mEPCs and EPPs. Quinidine has been used effectively in cases of SCS (Fukudome et al., 1998). Some patients treated with quinidine develop an allergy to it. In these patients fluoxetine (Prozac), also an open channel blocker (Garcia-Colunga et al., 1997), has been useful (Harper et al., 2003).

2.8.8. Conclusions

There have been enormous advances during the last 50 years in understanding the basic mechanisms that account for the process of neuromuscular transmission and for its great reliability in mammals. This knowledge has provided the essential foundation for efforts to understand the basis of impaired transmission in the many different human diseases in which the NMJ is the primary target. In many cases, it has also allowed the development of effective therapies to treat those conditions. Several important conclusions for the future can be drawn from these efforts.

2.8.8.1. Many levels of organization contribute to the reliability of neuromuscular transmission

The process of fast chemical transmission of signals at synapses is one of the most remarkable products of evolution. The specific form of this process found at mammalian NMJs is one of many, and represents a particular specialization for very fast and reliable transmission. Many different levels of organization contribute to this reliability. At one end of the spectrum are the individual molecules involved in transmission such as the key ion channels and the proteins that mediate exocytosis. Many of these molecules are present in multimolecular complexes, such as those regulating exocytosis and the distribution of ion channels in the postsynaptic apparatus. These molecular complexes are strategically located in subcellular units subserving the essential functions of transmission. Thus the AZs and the vesicles immediately associated with them are exactly positioned opposite the opening of the postsynaptic folds and the distinct ion channel domains associated with them, forming what may be thought of as a "unit of transmission". In many species, these units are in turn associated with distinct regions of the NMJ based on the boutons of the nerve terminal. In humans, there are typically 50 or so such units associated with each bouton. The NMJ as a whole is composed of a number of boutons, or analogous regions.

An important consequence of this hierarchical organization of the NMJ is that the great reliability of neuromuscular transmission can arise from events that individually have low probability. These include the opening of individual Ca^{++} channels in the nerve, the release of individual docked vesicles, and the activation of individual AChRs in the muscle fiber membrane. As a result of the way the NMJ is organized, the transmission of a single nerve impulse uses only a small fraction of the molecular components present. During repetitive activation each unit of transmission is only used in response to approximately every tenth nerve impulse. This allows time between periods of activity for local recovery processes such as restoration of ion concentrations and uptake of choline into the nerve terminal.

2.8.8.2. Many factors may modulate the efficacy of neuromuscular transmission

The mammalian NMJ has evolved to be able to operate with great reliability in a wide variety of circumstances. The basic structure and molecular organization of the NMJ play the major part in delivering that reliability. At the same time, there is much evidence for an extensive and highly interactive network of influences that can modulate the efficacy of transmission on a time-scale of seconds and minutes. The various autocrine and endocrine effects described in Section 2.6 all seem to be capable of influencing the reliability of transmission, mainly by regulating quantal release from the nerve. These effects appear to be exerted both directly on the nerve terminal and indirectly via the Schwann cells. What remains to be established in the future is how significant these effects are in the intact individual.

2.8.8.3. Different factors may determine reliability in different species and different stages of development

It is clear that different species achieve reliability of neuromuscular transmission in somewhat different ways. This makes it important to be cautious when interpreting observations in one species, e.g., humans, on the basis of findings made in a different species, e.g., frog. One example of this is provided by the differences in the quantal release mechanisms in frogs and mammals. The substantially greater probability of an individual docked vesicle being released at mammalian versus frog NMJs is very likely due to the differences in both the structural features of the AZs and the type of Ca^{++} channels present. While a detailed explanation of these differences is not yet available, it seems likely that more detailed knowledge of how release occurs at mammalian NMJs will be an important basis for understanding the defects of human transmission.

Another example is provided by the differing balance between pre- and postsynaptic factors in achieving reliability in different species. In frogs the emphasis is on the release of many quanta, with relatively little postsynaptic amplification. In humans, the opposite is true, with small nerve terminals releasing relatively few quanta and extensive postsynaptic folds providing more substantial amplification. The biological factors that account for the particular strategy used in a given species are unknown. Nonetheless it is important, when considering defects at human NMJs, to be aware of the important contribution to reliability of transmission likely to be made by the folds and the numerous molecular disturbances that seem to lead to reduced folding.

Major gaps exist in our understanding of the events leading to the development of the mature transmission mechanism in any species and in mammals in particular. It is clear that the key ion channels supporting transmission all undergo changes in type during NMJ maturation. Less is known about the structural changes at the developing NMJ and the molecular basis for them. For example, little is known about the sequence of events leading to the formation of mature AZs, or when that process occurs in development relative to other recognized milestones. The presence of N-type Ca^{++} channels at immature mammalian NMJs suggests an example of "ontogeny recapitulating phylogeny", since N-type channels predominate in frogs and possibly other lower vertebrates. It remains unclear whether these N-type channels at the immature NMJ function in the context of AZs whose structure is characteristically mammalian.

It is tempting to look for common principles of function and organization of the NMJ across many species. While it is true that the most basic principles of quantal release and ligand-mediated activation of postsynaptic receptors are common to NMJs from nematodes to man, there are also many very important differences. Attention to the origins and significance of these differences is likely to continue to provide important insights into the properties of human NMJs.

2.8.8.4. The potential for adaptive plasticity of the NMJ has limits that are poorly understood

The NMJ has a remarkable ability to respond to conditions that impair transmission so as to compensate for the functional loss. This adaptive plasticity includes both structural plasticity of the nerve and the ability to rerun programs of coordinated molecular expression that operate in the immature animal to promote effective transmission at structurally immature NMJs. It is clear that changes in activity exert a powerful regulatory influence over the adaptive process. Considerable insight has been gained recently into the molecular mechanisms underlying the links between activity and patterns of gene expression, particularly in muscle. However there is still little detailed knowledge about how the key process of axonal growth and sprouting is regulated, either during development or during adaptive responses in the adult.

Given the striking potential for responding in an adaptive way to impaired transmission, it seems odd that in many diseases this response has obviously been inadequate. In some cases, it may be that the adaptive response is so good that the effects of impaired transmission are rendered undetectable. In many other cases, where weakness is all too obvious an outcome, the question arises whether the response mechanism has reached some inherent limits, or is itself defective. In either case, better knowledge of the factors regulating the adaptive plasticity of the NMJ might lead to ways of enhancing the restoration of more normal function.

References

Adams BA (1989). Temperature and synaptic efficacy in frog skeletal muscle. J Physiol (Lond) 408: 443–455.

Adams ME, Kramarcy N, Fukuda T, et al. (2004). Structural abnormalities at neuromuscular synapses lacking multiple syntrophin isoforms. J Neurosci 24: 10302–10309.

Alnaes E, Rahamimoff R (1975). On the role of mitochondria in transmitter release from motor nerve terminals. J Physiol 248: 285–306.

Alshuaib WB, Fahim MA (1990). Effect of exercise on physiological age-related change at mouse neuromuscular junctions. Neurobiol Aging 11: 555–561.

Andonian MH, Fahim MA (1989). Nerve terminal morphology in C57BL/6nnia mice at different ages. J Gerontol 44: B43–B51.

Anglister L, Stiles JR, Salpeter MM (1994). Acetylcholinesterase density and turnover number at frog neuromuscular junctions, with modeling of their role in synaptic function. Neuron 12: 783–794.

Arizono N, Koreto O, Iwai Y, et al. (1984). Morphometric analysis of human neuromuscular junction in different ages. Acta Pathol Jpn 34: 1243–1249.

Atwood HL, Karunanithi S (2002). Diversification of synaptic strength: presynaptic elements. Nat Rev Neurosci 3: 497–516.

Auld DS, Colomar A, Belair EL, et al. (2003). Modulation of neurotransmission by reciprocal synapse–glial interactions at the neuromuscular junction. J Neurocytol 32: 1003–1015.

Awad SS, Lightowlers RN, Young C, et al. (2001). Sodium channel mrnas at the neuromuscular junction: distinct patterns of accumulation and effects of muscle activity. J Neurosci 21: 8456–8463.

Bailey SJ, Stocksley MA, Buckel A, et al. (2003). Nav1 channels and ankyrin G occupy a different postsynaptic domain from achrs from an early stage of neuromuscular junction formation in rats. J Neurosci 23: 2102–2111.

Banker BQ, Engel AG (2004). Basic Reactions of Muscle. In: AG Engel, C Franzini-Armstrong (Ed.), Myology. McGraw-Hill, Inc., New York, pp. 691–747.

Banker BQ, Kelly SS, Robbins N (1983). Neuromuscular transmission and correlative morphology in young and old mice. J Physiol 339: 355–377.

Barker D, Ip MC (1966). Sprouting and degeneration of mammalian motor axons in normal and de-afferentated skeletal muscle. Proc R Soc Lond B Biol Sci 163: 538–554.

Barstad JAB, Lilleheil G (1968). Transversely cut diaphragm preparations from rat. Archives internationales de pharmacodynamie et thérapie 175: 373–390.

Beeson D, Hantai D, Lochmuller H, et al. (2005). 126th International Workshop: Congenital Myasthenic Syndromes, 24–26 September 2004, Naarden, the Netherlands. Neuromuscul Disord 15: 498–512.

Beeson D, Higuchi O, Palace J, et al. (2006). Dok-7 mutations underlie a neuromuscular junction synaptopathy. Science 313: 1975–1978.

Benish TV, Zefirov AL, Fatkullin NF (1988). [Identification of the site of mediator release in the frog motor nerve ending using 3 extracellular microelectrodes]. Dokl Akad Nauk SSSR 302: 477–480.

Bennett MR, Pettigrew AG (1974). The formation of synapses in striated muscle during development. J Physiol 241: 515–545.

Bennett MR, McLachlan EM, Taylor RS (1973). The formation of synapses in reinnervated mammalian striated muscle. J Physiol 233: 481–500.

Bennett V, Davis J (1982). Immunoreactive forms of human erythrocyte ankyrin are localized in mitotic structures in cultured cells and are associated with microtubules in brain. Cold Spring Harb Symp Quant Biol 46(Pt 2): 647–657.

Bennett V, Stenbuck PJ (1980). Human erythrocyte ankyrin. Purification and properties. J Biol Chem 255: 2540–2548.

Bestue-Cardiel M, Saenz DC-A, Capablo-Liesa JL, et al. (2005). Congenital endplate acetylcholinesterase deficiency responsive to ephedrine. Neurology 65: 144–146.

Betz WJ, Caldwell JH, Kinnamon SC (1984). Increased sodium conductance in the synaptic region of rat skeletal muscle fibres. J Physiol 352: 189–202.

Bewick GS, Young C, Slater CR (1996). Spatial relationships of utrophin, dystrophin, beta-dystroglycan and beta-spectrin to acetylcholine receptor clusters during postnatal maturation of the rat neuromuscular junction. J Neurocytol 25: 367–379.

Bigland-Ritchie B, Jones DA, Hosking GP, et al. (1978). Central and peripheral fatigue in sustained maximum voluntary contractions of human quadriceps muscle. Clin Sci Mol Med 54: 609–614.

Bigland-Ritchie B, Kukulka CG, Lippold OC, et al. (1982). The absence of neuromuscular transmission failure in sustained maximal voluntary contractions. J Physiol 330: 265–278.

Birks RI, Huxley H, Katz B (1960). The fine structure of the neuromuscular junction of the frog. J Physiol 150: 134–144.

Blain PG (1999). Neurotoxicology of organophosphates, with special regard for chemical warfare agents. In: PG Blain, JB Harris (Eds.), Medical Neurotoxicology. Arnold, London, pp. 237–253.

Bowman WC, Marshall IG, Gibb AJ, et al. (1988). Feedback control of transmitter release at the neuromuscular junction. Trends Pharmacol Sci 9: 16–20.

Boyd IA, Martin AR (1956). The end-plate potential in mammalian muscle. J Physiol 132: 74–91.

Braga MF, Anderson AJ, Harvey AL, et al. (1992). Apparent block of K^+ currents in mouse motor nerve terminals by tetrodotoxin, mu-conotoxin and reduced external sodium. Br J Pharmacol 106: 91–94.

Brenner HR, Sakmann B (1978). Gating properties of acetylcholine receptor in newly formed neuromuscular synapses. Nature 271: 366–368.

Brenner HR, Witzemann V, Sakmann B (1990). Imprinting of acetylcholine receptor messenger RNA accumulation in mammalian neuromuscular synapses. Nature 344: 544–547.

Brenner HR, Herczeg A, Slater CR (1992). Synapse-specific expression of acetylcholine receptor genes and their products at original synaptic sites in rat soleus muscle fibres regenerating in the absence of innervation. Development 116: 41–53.

Brigant JL, Mallart A (1982). Presynaptic currents in mouse motor endings. J Physiol 333: 619–636.

Brown MC, Goodwin S, Ironton R (1977). Prevention of motor nerve sprouting in botulinum toxin poisoned mouse soleus muscles by direct stimulation of the muscle. J Physiol 248: 44P–45P.

Brown MC, Holland RL, Hopkins WG (1981). Motor nerve sprouting. Annu Rev Neurosci 4: 17–42.

Buffelli M, Burgess RW, Feng G, et al. (2003). Genetic evidence that relative synaptic efficacy biases the outcome of synaptic competition. Nature 424: 430–434.

Bukchareva EA, Kim KC, Moravec J, et al. (1999). Noradrenaline synchronizes evoked quantal release at frog neuromuscular junctions. J Physiol 517: 879–888.

Bukharaeva EA, Kim KK, Nikol'skii EE, et al. (2000). Synchronization of evoked secretion of quanta of mediator as a mechanism facilitating the action of sympathomimetics. Neurosci Behav Physiol 30: 139–146.

Bukharaeva EA, Samigullin D, Nikolsky E, et al. (2002). Protein kinase A cascade regulates quantal release dispersion at frog muscle endplate. J Physiol 538: 837–848.

Burden SJ, Sargent PB, McMahan UJ (1979). Acetylcholine receptors in regenerating muscle accumulate at original synaptic sites in the absence of the nerve. J Cell Biol 82: 412–425.

Burgess DL, Kohrman DC, Galt J, et al. (1995). Mutation of a new sodium channel gene, Scn8a, in the mouse mutant "motor endplate disease". Nat Genet 10: 461–465.

Burke RE, Levine DN, Tsairis P, et al. (1973). Physiological types and histochemical profiles in motor units of the cat gastrocnemius. J Physiol 234: 723–748.

Caldwell JH, Milton RL (1988). Sodium channel distribution in normal and denervated rodent and snake skeletal muscle. J Physiol 401: 145–161.

Campagna JA, Ruegg MA, Bixby JL (1995). Agrin is a differentiation-inducing "stop signal" for motoneurons in vitro. Neuron 15: 1365–1374.

Campbell MJ, McComas AJ, Petito F (1973). Physiological changes in ageing muscles. J Neurol Neurosurg Psychiatry 36: 174–182.

Cardasis CA, LaFontaine DM (1987). Aging rat neuromuscular junctions: a morphometric study of cholinesterase-stained whole mounts and ultrastructure. Muscle Nerve 10: 200–213.

Caroni P, Schneider C (1994). Signaling by insulin-like growth factors in paralyzed skeletal muscle: rapid induction of IGF1 expression in muscle fibers and prevention of interstitial cell proliferation by IGF-BP5 and IGF-BP4. J Neurosci 14: 3378–3388.

Catterall WA (1995). Structure and function of voltage-gated ion channels. Annu Rev Biochem 64: 493–531.

Catterall WA, Coppersmith J (1981). High-affinity saxitoxin receptor sites in vertebrate heart. Evidence for sites associated with autonomic nerve endings. Mol Pharmacol 20: 526–532.

Catterall WA, Perez-Reyes E, Snutch TP, et al. (2005). International Union of Pharmacology. XLVIII. nomenclature and structure-function relationships of voltage-gated calcium channels. Pharmacol Rev 57: 411–425.

Chang CC, Chuang S-T, Huang MC (1975). Effects of chronic treatment with various neuromuscular blocking agents on the number and distribution of acetylcholine receptors in the rat diaphragm. J Physiol 250: 161–173.

Chevessier F, Faraut B, Ravel-Chapuis A, et al. (2004). MUSK, a new target for mutations causing congenital myasthenic syndrome. Hum Mol Genet 13: 3229–3240.

Cochilla AJ, Angleson JK, Betz WJ (1999). Monitoring secretory membrane with FM1–43 fluorescence. Annu Rev Neurosci 22: 1–10.

Cohen I, Rimer M, Lømo T, et al. (1997). Agrin-induced postsynaptic-like apparatus in skeletal muscle fibers in vivo. Mol Cell Neurosci 9: 237–253.

Coleman M (2005). Axon degeneration mechanisms: commonality amid diversity. Nat Rev Neurosci 6: 889–898.

Cooper S (1966). Muscle spindles and motor units. In: BL Andrew, (Ed.), Control and Innervation of Skeletal Muscle. University of St, Andrews, Dundee, pp. 9–16.

Covault J, Sanes JR (1985). Neural cell adhesion molecule (N-CAM) accumulates in denervated and paralyzed skeletal muscles. Proc Natl Acad Sci U S A 82: 4544–4548.

Cruz LJ, Gray WR, Olivera BM, et al. (1985). Conus geographus toxins that discriminate between neuronal and muscle sodium channels. J Biol Chem 260: 9280–9288.

Cull-Candy SG, Miledi R, Trautmann A, et al. (1980). On the release of transmitter at normal, myasthenia gravis and myasthenic syndrome affected human end-plates. J Physiol 299: 621–638.

David G, Barrett EF (2003). Mitochondrial Ca2+ uptake prevents desynchronization of quantal release and minimizes depletion during repetitive stimulation of mouse motor nerve terminals. J Physiol 548: 425–438.

David G, Barrett JN, Barrett EF (1997). Stimulation-induced changes in [Ca2+] in lizard motor nerve terminals. J Physiol 504(Pt 1): 83–96.

David G, Barrett JN, Barrett EF (1998). Evidence that mitochondria buffer physiological Ca2+ loads in lizard motor nerve terminals. J Physiol 509: 59–65.

Day NC, Wood SJ, Ince PG, et al. (1997). Differential localization of voltage-dependent calcium channel alpha1 subunits at the human and rat neuromuscular junction. J Neurosci 17: 6226–6235.

DeChiara TM, Bowen DC, Valenzuela DM, et al. (1996). The receptor tyrosine kinase musk is required for neuromuscular junction formation in vivo. Cell 85: 501–512.

Deconinck AE, Potter AC, Tinsley JM, et al. (1997). Postsynaptic abnormalities at the neuromuscular junctions of utrophin-deficient mice. J Cell Biol 136: 883–894.

De Kerchove D'E, Cartaud J, et al. (2002). Expression of mutant Ets protein at the neuromuscular synapse causes alterations in morphology and gene expression. EMBO Rep 3: 1075–1081.

del Castillo J, Katz B (1954). Quantal components of the end-plate potential. J Physiol 124: 560–573.

del Castillo J, Katz B (1956a). Biophysical aspects of neuromuscular transmission. Prog Biophys Biophys Chem 6: 121–170.

del Castillo J, Katz B (1956b). Localization of active spots within the neuromuscular junction of the frog. J Physiol 132: 630–649.

Denys EH, Norris FH Jr (1979). Amyotrophic lateral sclerosis. Impairment of neuromuscular transmission. Arch Neurol 36: 202–205.

de Paiva A, Meunier FA, Molgo J, et al. (1999). Functional repair of motor endplates after botulinum neurotoxin type A poisoning: biphasic switch of synaptic activity between nerve sprouts and their parent terminals. Proc Natl Acad Sci U S A 96: 3200–3205.

Descarries LM, Cai S, Robitaille R, et al. (1998). Localization and characterization of nitric oxide synthase at the frog neuromuscular junction. J Neurocytol 27: 829–840.

Deuchars SA, Atkinson L, Brooke RE, et al. (2001). Neuronal P2X7 receptors are targeted to presynaptic terminals in the central and peripheral nervous systems. J Neurosci 21: 7143–7152.

Diamond J, Miledi R (1962). A study of foetal and new-born rat muscle fibres. J Physiol 162: 393–408.

Diaz J, Molgo J, Pecot-Dechavassine M (1989). Sprouting of frog motor nerve terminals after long-term paralysis by botulinum type A toxin. Neurosci Lett 96: 127–132.

Dodge FA Jr, Rahamimoff R (1967). Co-operative action of calcium ions in transmitter release at the neuromuscular junction. J Physiol 193: 419–432.

Duchen LW (1970). Changes in motor innervation and cholinesterase localization induced by botulinum toxin in skeletal muscle of the mouse: differences between fast and slow muscles. J Neurol Neurosurg Psychiatry 33: 40–54.

Duchen LW, Excell BJ, Patel R, et al. (1974). Changes in motor end-plates resulting from muscle fibre necrosis and regeneration. A light and electron microscopic study of the effects of the depolarizing fraction (cardiotoxin) of Dendroaspis jamesoni venom. J Neurol Sci 21: 391–417.

Eccles JC, Katz B, Kuffler SW (1942). Effects of eserine on neuromuscular transmission. J Neurophysiol 5: 211–230.

Elmqvist D, Quastel DM (1965). A quantitative study of end-plate potentials in isolated human muscle. J Physiol 178: 505–529.

Elmqvist D, Hofmann WW, Kugelberg J, et al. (1964). An electrophysiological investigation of neuromuscular transmission in myasthenia gravis. J Physiol 174: 417–434.

Engel AG (2004). The neuromuscular junction. In: AG Engel, C Franzini-Armstrong (Eds.), Myology. McGraw-Hill, New York, pp. 325–372.

Engel AG, Santa T (1971). Histometric analysis of the ultrastructure of the neuromuscular junction in myasthenia gravis and in the myasthenic syndrome. Ann N Y Acad Sci 183: 46–63.

Engel AG, Sine SM (2005). Current understanding of congenital myasthenic syndromes. Curr Opin Pharmacol 5: 308–321.

Engel AG, Tsujihata M, Lindstrom JM, et al. (1976). The motor end plate in myasthenia gravis and in experimental autoimmune myasthenia gravis. A quantitative ultrastructural study. Ann N Y Acad Sci 274: 60–79.

Engel AG, Lambert EH, Gomez MR (1977). A new myasthenic syndrome with end-plate acetylcholinesterase deficiency, small nerve terminals, and reduced acetylcholine release. Ann Neurol 1: 315–330.

Engel AG, Lambert EH, Mulder DM, et al. (1982). A newly recognized congenital myasthenic syndrome attributed to a prolonged open time of the acetylcholine-induced ion channel. Ann Neurol 11: 553–569.

Engel AG, Walls TJ, Nagel A, et al. (1990). Newly recognized congenital myasthenic syndromes: i. Congenital paucity of synaptic vesicles and reduced quantal release. ii. High-conductance fast-channel syndrome. iii. Abnormal acetylcholine receptor (achr) interaction with acetylcholine. iv. Achr deficiency and short channel-open time. Prog Brain Res 84: 125–137.

Etherington SJ, Everett AW (2004). Postsynaptic production of nitric oxide implicated in long-term depression at the mature amphibian (Bufo marinus) neuromuscular junction. J Physiol 559: 507–517.

Fahim MA, Robbins N (1982). Ultrastructural studies of young and old mouse neuromuscular junctions. J Neurocytol 11: 641–656.

Fahim MA, Holley JA, Robbins N (1983). Scanning and light microscopic study of age changes at a neuromuscular junction in the mouse. J Neurocytol 12: 13–25.

Fatt P, Katz B (1951). An analysis of the end-plate potential recorded with an intra-cellular electrode. J Physiol 115: 320–370.

Fatt P, Katz B (1952). Spontaneous subthreshold activity at motor nerve endings. J Physiol 117: 109–128.

Ferry CB, Kelly SS (1988). The nature of the presynaptic effect of (+)-tubocurarine at the mouse neuromuscular junction. J Physiol 403: 425–437.

Fex S, Thesleff S (1967). The time required for innervation of denervated muscles by nerve implants. Life Sci 6: 635–639.

Flachenecker P (2006). Epidemiology of neuroimmunological diseases. J Neurol 253: v2–v8.

Fladby T, Jansen JK (1988). Selective innervation of neonatal fast and slow muscle fibres before net loss of synaptic terminals in the mouse soleus muscle. Acta Physiol Scand 134: 561–562.

Flucher BE, Daniels MP (1989). Distribution of Na+ channels and ankyrin in neuromuscular junctions is complementary to that of acetylcholine receptors and the 43 kd protein. Neuron 3: 163–175.

Frey D, Schneider C, Xu L, et al. (2000). Early and selective loss of neuromuscular synapse subtypes with low sprouting competence in motoneuron diseases. J Neurosci 20: 2534–2542.

Fucile S, Sucapane A, Grassi F, et al. (2006). The human adult subtype ach receptor channel has high Ca2+ permeability and predisposes to endplate Ca2+ overloading. J Physiol 573: 35–43.

Fukudome T, Ohno K, Brengman JM, et al. (1998). Quinidine normalizes the open duration of slow-channel mutants of the acetylcholine receptor. Neuroreport 9: 1907–1911.

Fukunaga H, Engel AG, Lang B, et al. (1983). Passive transfer of Lambert–Eaton myasthenic syndrome with igg from man to mouse depletes the presynaptic membrane active zones. Proc Natl Acad Sci U S A 80: 7636–7640.

Fukuoka T, Engel AG, Lang B, et al. (1987). Lambert–Eaton myasthenic syndrome: I. Early morphological effects of igg on the presynaptic membrane active zones. Ann Neurol 22: 193–199.

Galea V (1996). Changes in motor unit estimates with aging. J Clin Neurophysiol 13: 253–260.

Garcia-Colunga J, Awad JN, Miledi R (1997). Blockage of muscle and neuronal nicotinic acetylcholine receptors by fluoxetine (Prozac). Proc Natl Acad Sci U S A 94: 2041–2044.

Gardiner PF, Kernell D (1990). The "fastness" of rat motoneurones: time-course of afterhyperpolarization in relation to axonal conduction velocity and muscle unit contractile speed. Pflugers Arch 415: 762–766.

Gautam M, Noakes PG, Mudd J, et al. (1995). Failure of postsynaptic specialization to develop at neuromuscular junctions of rapsyn-deficient mice. Nature 377: 232–236.

Gentile L, Stanley EF (2005). A unified model of presynaptic release site gating by calcium channel domains. Eur J Neurosci 21: 278–282.

Gertler RA, Robbins N (1978). Differences in neuromuscular transmission in red and white muscles. Brain Res 142: 160–164.

Giniatullin AR, Giniatullin RA (2003). Dual action of hydrogen peroxide on synaptic transmission at the frog neuromuscular junction. J Physiol 552: 283–293.

Ginsborg BL, Hirst GDS (1972). The effect of adenosine on the release of the transmitter from the phrenic nerve of the rat. J Physiol 224: 629–645.

Ginsborg BL, Jenkinson DH (1976). Transmission of impulses from nerve to muscle. In: E Zaimis (Ed.), Neuromuscular Junction, Handbook of Experimental Pharmacology. Vol. 42. Springer-Verlag, Berlin, pp. 229–364.

Glass DJ, Bowen DC, Stitt TN, et al. (1996). Agrin acts via a musk receptor complex. Cell 85: 513–523.

Glavinović MI (1979a). Change of statistical parameters of transmitter release during various kinetic tests in unparalysed voltage-clamped rat diaphragm. J Physiol 290: 481–497.

Glavinović MI (1979b). Presynaptic action of curare. J Physiol 290: 499–506.

Glavinović MI (1979c). Voltage clamping of unparalysed cut rat diaphragm for study of transmitter release. J Physiol 290: 467–480.

Glavinović MI (1995). Decrease of quantal size and quantal content during tetanic stimulation detected by focal recording. Neuroscience 69: 271–281.

Glicksman MA, Sanes JR (1983). Differentiation of motor nerve terminals formed in the absence of muscle fibres. J Neurocytol 12: 661–671.

Goldin AL, Barchi RL, Caldwell JH, et al. (2000). Nomenclature of voltage-gated sodium channels. Neuron 28: 365–368.

Goldman D, Brenner HR, Heinemann S (1988). Acetylcholine receptor alpha-, beta-, gamma-, and delta-subunit mrna levels are regulated by muscle activity. Neuron 1: 329–333.

Gonoi T, Hagihara Y, Kobayashi J, et al. (1989). Geographutoxin-sensitive and insensitive sodium currents in mouse skeletal muscle developing in situ. J Physiol 414: 159–177.

Gordon T, Hegedus J, Tam SL (2004). Adaptive and maladaptive motor axonal sprouting in aging and motoneuron disease. Neurol Res 26: 174–185.

Grady RM, Merlie JP, Sanes JR (1997). Subtle neuromuscular defects in utrophin-deficient mice. J Cell Biol 136: 871–882.

Grinnell AD, Chen BM, Kashani A, et al. (2003). The role of integrins in the modulation of neurotransmitter release from motor nerve terminals by stretch and hypertonicity. J Neurocytol 32: 489–503.

Grinnell AD, Herrera AA (1980). Physiological regulation of synaptic effectiveness at frog neuromuscular junctions. J Physiol 307: 301–317.

Grubb BD, Harris JB, Schofield IS (1991). Neuromuscular transmission at newly formed neuromuscular junctions in the regenerating soleus muscle of the rat. J Physiol 441: 405–421.

Haimovich B, Bonilla E, Casadei J, et al. (1984). Immunocytochemical localization of the mammalian voltage-dependent sodium channel using polyclonal antibodies against the purified protein. J Neurosci 4: 2259–2268.

Hall ZW (1973). Multiple forms of acetylcholinesterase and their distribution in endplate and non-endplate regions of rat diaphragm muscle. J Neurobiol 4: 343–361.

Harlow ML, Ress D, Stoschek A, et al. (2001). The architecture of active zone material at the frog's neuromuscular junction. Nature 409: 479–484.

Harper CM, Fukodome T, Engel AG (2003). Treatment of slow-channel congenital myasthenic syndrome with fluoxetine. Neurology 60: 1710–1713.

Harris JB, Johnson MA (1978). Further observations on the pathological responses of rat skeletal muscle to toxins isolated from the venom of the Australian tiger snake, Notechis scutatus scutatus. Clin Exp Pharmacol Physiol 5: 587–600.

Harris JB, Pollard SL (1986). Neuromuscular transmission in the murine mutants "motor end-plate disease" and "jolting." J Neurol Sci 76: 239–253.

Harris JB, Ribchester RR (1979a). Muscular dystrophy in the mouse: neuromuscular transmission and the concept of functional denervation. Ann N Y Acad Sci 317: 152–170.

Harris JB, Ribchester RR (1979b). The relationship between end-plate size and transmitter release in normal and dystrophic muscles of the mouse. J Physiol 296: 245–265.

Harris JB, Vater R, Wilson M, et al. (2003). Muscle fibre breakdown in venom-induced muscle degeneration. J Anat 202: 363–372.

Hartzell HC, Kuffler SW, Yoshikami D (1975). Postsynaptic potentiation: interaction between quanta of acetylcholine at the skeletal neuromuscular synapse. J Physiol 251: 427–463.

Hartzell HC, Kuffler SW, Yoshikami D (1976). The number of acetylcholine molecules in a quantum and the interaction between quanta at the subsynaptic membrane of the skeletal neuromuscular synapse. Cold Spring Harb Symp Quant Biol 40: 175–186.

Henneman E, Somjen G, Carpenter DO (1965). Excitability and inhibitability of motoneurons of different sizes. J Neurophysiol 28: 599–620.

Hennig R, Lømo T (1985). Firing patterns of motor units in normal rats. Nature 314: 164–166.

Hesselmans LF, Jennekens FG, Van den Oord CJ, et al. (1993). Development of innervation of skeletal muscle fibers in man: relation to acetylcholine receptors. Anat Rec 236: 553–562.

Heuser JE (1976). Morphology of synaptic vesicle discharge and reformation at the frog neuromuscular junction. In: S Thesleff (Ed.), Motor Innervation of Muscle. Academic Press, London, pp. 51–115.

Heuser JE, Reese TS, Dennis MJ, et al. (1979). Synaptic vesicle exocytosis captured by quick freezing and correlated with quantal transmitter release. J Cell Biol 81: 275–300.

Hirokawa N, Heuser JE (1982). Internal and external differentiations of the postsynaptic membrane at the neuromuscular junction. J Neurocytol 11: 487–510.

Hoch W, McConville J, Helms S, et al. (2001). Auto-antibodies to the receptor tyrosine kinase musk in patients with myasthenia gravis without acetylcholine receptor antibodies. Nat Med 7: 365–368.

Hodgkin AL, Rushton WAH (1946). The electrical constants of a crustacean nerve fibre. Proc R Soc Lond B Biol Sci 133: 444–479.

Hoffman PN, Lasek RJ (1980). Axonal transport of the cytoskeleton in regenerating motor neurons: constancy and change. Brain Res 202: 317–333.

Hong SJ, Chang CC (1998). Evaluation of intrinsic modulation of synaptic transmission by ATP in mouse fast twitch muscle. J Neurophysiol 80: 2550–2558.

Hubbard JI, Wilson DF (1970). Reduction of the quantum content of endplate potentials by atropine. Experientia 26: 1234–1235.

Hui E, Bai J, Wang P, et al. (2005). Three distinct kinetic groupings of the synaptotagmin family: candidate sensors for rapid and delayed exocytosis. Proc Natl Acad Sci U S A 102: 5210–5214.

Hutter OF, Loewenstein WR (1955). Nature of neuromuscular facilitation by sympathetic stimulation in the frog. J Physiol 130: 559–571.

Isaacson JS, Walmsley B (1995). Counting quanta: direct measurements of transmitter release at a central synapse. Neuron 15: 875–884.

Jack JJB, Noble D, Tsien RW (1975). Electric Current Flow in Excitable Cells. Oxford University Press, Oxford.

Jacobson M (1970). Developmental Neurobiology. Holt, Reinhart and Winston, Inc., New York.

Jahn R (2006). Neuroscience. A neuronal receptor for botulinum toxin. Science 312: 540–541.

Jahromi BS, Robitaille R, Charlton MP (1992). Transmitter release increases intracellular calcium in perisynaptic Schwann cells in situ. Neuron 8: 1069–1077.

Jansen JKS, Fladby T (1990). The perinatal reorganization of the innervation of skeletal muscle in mammals. Prog Neurobiol 34: 39–90.

Jansen JK, Lømo T, Nicolaysen K, et al. (1973). Hyperinnervation of skeletal muscle fibers: dependence on muscle activity. Science 181: 559–561.

Jaramillo F, Vicini S, Schuetze SM (1988). Embryonic acetylcholine receptors guarantee spontaneous contractions in rat developing muscle. Nature 335: 66–68.

Jenkinson DH, Stamenovic BA, Whitaker BD (1968). The effect of noradrenaline on the end-plate potential in twitch fibres of the frog. J Physiol 195: 743–754.

Jirmanova I, Thesleff S (1972). Ultrastructural study of experimental muscle degeneration and regeneration in the adult rat. Z Zellforsch Mikrosk Anat 131: 77–97.

Jo SA, Burden SJ (1992). Synaptic basal lamina contains a signal for synapse-specific transcription. Development 115: 673–680.

Jurkat-Rott K, Lehmann-Horn F (2005). Muscle channelopathies and critical points in functional and genetic studies. J Clin Invest 115: 2000–2009.

Juzans P, Comella JX, Molgo J, et al. (1996). Nerve terminal sprouting in botulinum type-A treated mouse levator auris longus muscle. Neuromuscul Disord 6: 177–185.

Kalkstein JM, Magleby KL (2004). Augmentation increases vesicular release probability in the presence of masking depression at the frog neuromuscular junction. J Neurosci 24: 11391–11403.

Kallen RG, Sheng ZH, Yang J, et al. (1990). Primary structure and expression of a sodium channel characteristic of denervated and immature rat skeletal muscle. Neuron 4: 233–242.

Kamenskaya MA, Elmqvist D, Thesleff S (1975). Guanidine and neuromuscular transmission. II. Effect on transmitter release in response to repetitive nerve stimulation. Arch Neurol 32: 510–518.

Kasthuri N, Lichtman JW (2003). The role of neuronal identity in synaptic competition. Nature 424: 426–430.

Katz B (1966). Nerve, Muscle and Synapse. McGraw-Hill, New York.

Katz B (1969). The Release of Neural Transmitter Substances. Liverpool University Press, Liverpool.

Katz B, Miledi R (1965). The measurement of synaptic delay, and the time course of acetylcholine release at the neuromuscular junction. Proc R Soc Lond B Biol Sci 161: 483–495.

Katz B, Miledi R (1967). Tetrodotoxin and neuromuscular transmission. Proc R Soc Lond B Biol Sci 167: 8–22.

Katz B, Miledi R (1968). The role of calcium in neuromuscular facilitation. J Physiol 195: 481–492.

Katz B, Miledi R (1979). Estimates of quantal content during "chemical potentiation" of transmitter release. Proc R Soc Lond B Biol Sci 205: 369–378.

Katz B, Thesleff S (1957). On the factors which determine the amplitude of the "miniature end-plate potential". J Physiol 137: 267–278.

Katz E, Ferro PA, Cherksey BD, et al. (1995). Effects of Ca2+ channel blockers on transmitter release and presynaptic currents at the frog neuromuscular junction. J Physiol 486: 695–706.

Katz E, Ferro PA, Weisz G, et al. (1996). Calcium channels involved in synaptic transmission at the mature and regenerating mouse neuromuscular junction. J Physiol 497: 687–697.

Katz E, Protti DA, Ferro PA, et al. (1997). Effects of Ca2+ channel blocker neurotoxins on transmitter release and presynaptic currents at the mouse neuromuscular junction. Br J Pharmacol 121: 1531–1540.

Kawamura Y, O'Brien P, Okazaki H, et al. (1977). Lumbar motoneurons of man II: the number and diameter distribution of large- and intermediate-diameter cytons in "motoneuron columns" of spinal cord of man. J Neuropathol Exp Neurol 36: 861–870.

Kelly SS (1978). The effect of age on neuromuscular transmission. J Physiol 274: 51–62.

Kelly SS, Robbins N (1983). Progression of age changes in synaptic transmission at mouse neuromuscular junctions. J Physiol 343: 375–383.

Kelly AM, Zacks SI (1969). The fine structure of motor endplate morphogenesis. J Cell Biol 42: 154–169.

Kernell D (2006). The Motoneurone and its Muscle Fibres. Oxford University Press, Oxford.

Kohrman DC, Harris JB, Meisler MH (1996). Mutation detection in the med and medj alleles of the sodium channel Scn8a. Unusual splicing due to a minor class AT-AC intron. J Biol Chem 271: 17576–17581.

Konishi T (1985). Electrical excitability of motor nerve terminals in the mouse. J Physiol 366: 411–421.

Konishi T, Sears TA (1984). Electrical activity of mouse motor nerve terminals. Proc R Soc Lond B Biol Sci 222: 115–120.

Kovyazina IV, Nikolsky EE, Giniatullin RA, et al. (2003). Dependence of miniature endplate current on kinetic parameters of acetylcholine receptors activation: a model study. Neurochem Res 28: 443–448.

Krnjević K, Miledi R (1958). Some effects produced by adrenaline upon neuromuscular propagation in rats. J Physiol 141: 291–304.

Krnjević K, Mitchell JF (1960). Diffusion of acetylcholine in agar gels and in the isolated rat diaphragm. J Physiol 153: 562–572.

Kuffler SW, Yoshikami D (1975). The number of transmitter molecules in a quantum: an estimate from iontophoretic application of acetylcholine at the neuromuscular synapse. J Physiol 251: 465–482.

Kuno M, Turkanis SA, Weakly JN (1971). Correlation between nerve terminal size and transmitter release at the neuromuscular junction of the frog. J Physiol 213: 545–556.

Kusner LL, Kaminski HJ (1996). Nitric oxide synthase is concentrated at the skeletal muscle endplate. Brain Res 730: 238–242.

Land BR, Salpeter EE, Salpeter MM (1981). Kinetic parameters for acetylcholine interaction in intact neuromuscular junction. Proc Natl Acad Sci U S A 78: 7200–7204.

Larsson L, Ansved T (1995). Effects of ageing on the motor unit. Prog Neurobiol 45: 397–458.

Leonard JP, Salpeter MM (1979). Agonist-induced myopathy at the neuromuscular junction is mediated by calcium. J Cell Biol 82: 811–819.

Liley AW, North KA (1953). An electrical investigation of effects of repetitive stimulation on mammalian neuromuscular junction. J Neurophysiol 16: 509–527.

Lindgren CA, Laird MV (1994). Nitroprusside inhibits neurotransmitter release at the frog neuromuscular junction. Neuroreport 5: 2205–2208.

Lohof AM, Ip NY, Poo MM (1993). Potentiation of developing neuromuscular synapses by the neurotrophins NT-3 and BDNF. Nature 363: 350–353.

Lømo T (1989). Long-term effects of altered activity on skeletal muscle. Biomed Biochim Acta 48: S432–S444.

Lømo T, Rosenthal J (1972). Control of ach sensitivity by muscle activity in the rat. J Physiol 221: 493–513.

Lømo T, Slater CR (1978). Control of acetylcholine sensitivity and synapse formation by muscle activity. J Physiol 275: 391–402.

Love FM, Thompson WJ (1999). Glial cells promote muscle reinnervation by responding to activity-dependent postsynaptic signals. J Neurosci 19: 10390–10396.

Lu B, Je HS (2003). Neurotrophic regulation of the development and function of the neuromuscular synapses. J Neurocytol 32: 931–941.

Lupa MT, Krzemien DM, Schaller KL, et al. (1993). Aggregation of sodium channels during development and maturation of the neuromuscular junction. J Neurosci 13: 1326–1336.

Lyons PR, Slater CR (1991). Structure and function of the neuromuscular junction in young adult mdx mice. J Neurocytol 20: 969–981.

Magleby KL (1979). Facilitation, augmentation, and potentiation of transmitter release. Prog Brain Res 49: 175–182.

Magleby K (1994). Neuromuscular transmission. In: AG Engel, C Franzini-Armstrong (Eds.), Myology, McGraw-Hill, New York, pp. 442–463.

Magleby K, Stevens CF (1972). The effect of voltage on the time course of end-plate currents. J Physiol 223: 151–171.

Magleby KL, Palotta BS, Terrar DA (1981). The effect of (+)-tubocuarine on neuromuscular transmission during repetitive stimulation in the rat, mouse and frog. J Physiol 312: 97–113.

Magrassi L, Purves D, Lichtman JW (1987). Fluorescent probes that stain living nerve terminals. J Neurosci 7: 1207–1214.

Mantilla CB, Zhan WZ, Sieck GC (2004). Neurotrophins improve neuromuscular transmission in the adult rat diaphragm. Muscle Nerve 29: 381–386.

Marques MJ, Conchello JA, Lichtman JW (2000). From plaque to pretzel: fold formation and acetylcholine receptor loss at the developing neuromuscular junction. J Neurosci 20: 3663–3675.

Martin AR (1955). A further study of the statistical composition of the end-plate potential. J Physiol 130: 114–122.

Martin AR (1965). Quantal nature of synaptic transmission. Physiol Rev 46: 51–66.

Martin AR (1976). The effect of membrane capacitance on non-linear summation of synaptic potentials. J Theoret Biol 59: 179–187.

Martin AR (1994). Amplification of neuromuscular transmission by postjunctional folds. Proc R Soc Lond B Biol Sci 258: 179–187.

Martin PT, Kaufman SJ, Kramer RH, et al. (1996). Synaptic integrins in developing, adult, and mutant muscle: selective association of alpha1, alpha7a, and alpha7b integrins with the neuromuscular junction. Dev Biol 174: 125–139.

Maselli RA, Mass DP, Distad BJ, et al. (1991). Anconeus muscle: a human muscle preparation suitable for in-vitro microelectrode studies. Muscle & Nerve 14: 1189–1192.

Maselli RA, Cashman NR, Wollman RL, et al. (1992). Neuromuscular transmission as a function of motor unit size in patients with prior poliomyelitis. Muscle Nerve 15: 648–655.

Maselli RA, Wollman RL, Leung C, et al. (1993). Neuromuscular transmission in amyotrophic lateral sclerosis. Muscle Nerve 16: 1193–1203.

Maselli RA, Wollman RL, Roos R (1995). Function and ultrastructure of the neuromuscular junction in post-polio syndrome. Ann N Y Acad Sci 753: 129–137.

Matsubara N, Billington AP, Hess GP (1992). How fast does an acetylcholine receptor channel open? Laser-pulse photolysis of an inactive precursor of carbamoylcholine in the microsecond time region with BC3H1 cells. Biochemistry 31: 5507–5514.

Matthews-Bellinger JA, Salpeter MM (1983). Fine structural distribution of acetylcholine receptors at developing mouse neuromuscular junctions. J Neurosci 3: 644–657.

McArdle JJ, Albuquerque EX (1973). A study of the reinnervation of fast and slow mammalian muscles. J Gen Physiol 61: 1–23.

McConville J, Farrugia ME, Beeson D, et al. (2004). Detection and characterization of musk antibodies in seronegative myasthenia gravis. Ann Neurol 55: 580–584.

McLachlan EM (1978). The statistics of transmitter release at chemical synapses. Int Rev Physiol 17: 49–117.

McLachlan EM, Martin AR (1981). Non-linear summation of end-plate potentials in the frog and mouse. J Physiol 311: 307–324.

McMahan UJ (1990). The agrin hypothesis. Cold Spring Harb Symp Quant Biol 55: 407–418.

McMahan UJ, Slater CR (1984). The influence of basal lamina on the accumulation of acetylcholine receptors at synaptic sites in regenerating muscle. J Cell Biol 98: 1453–1473.

Meier T, Hauser DM, Chiquet M, et al. (1997). Neural agrin induces ectopic postsynaptic specializations in innervated muscle fibers. J Neurosci 17: 6534–6544.

Meir A, Ginsburg S, Butkevich A, et al. (1999). Ion channels in presynaptic nerve terminals and control of transmitter release. Physiol Rev 79: 1019–1088.

Meriney SD, Gray DB, Pilar G (1985). Morphine-induced delay of normal cell death in the avian ciliary ganglion. Science 228: 1451–1453.

Meunier FA, Schiavo G, Molgo J (2002). Botulinum neurotoxins: from paralysis to recovery of functional neuromuscular transmission. J Physiol Paris 96: 105–113.

Meunier FA, Lisk G, Sesardic D, et al. (2003). Dynamics of motor nerve terminal remodeling unveiled using SNARE-cleaving botulinum toxins: the extent and duration are dictated by the sites of SNAP-25 truncation. Mol Cell Neurosci 22: 454–466.

Miledi R, Slater CR (1970). On the degeneration of rat neuromuscular junctions after nerve section. J Physiol 207: 507–528.

Miledi R, Zelena J (1966). Sensitivity to acetylcholine in rat slow muscle. Nature 210: 855–856.

Milone M, Engel AG (1996). Block of the endplate acetylcholine receptor channel by the sympathomimetic agents ephedrine, pseudoephedrine, and albuterol. Brain Res 740: 346–352.

Milone M, Wang HL, Ohno K, et al. (1998). Mode switching kinetics produced by a naturally occurring mutation in the cytoplasmic loop of the human acetylcholine receptor epsilon subunit. Neuron 20: 575–588.

Minic J, Molgo J, Karlsson E, et al. (2002). Regulation of acetylcholine release by muscarinic receptors at the mouse neuromuscular junction depends on the activity of acetylcholinesterase. Eur J Neurosci 15: 439–448.

Misgeld T, Burgess RW, Lewis RM, et al. (2002). Roles of neurotransmitter in synapse formation: development of neuromuscular junctions lacking choline acetyltransferase. Neuron 36: 635–648.

Mishina M, Takai T, Imoto K, et al. (1986). Molecular distinction between fetal and adult forms of muscle acetylcholine receptor. Nature 321: 406–411.

Moczydlowski E, Olivera BM, Gray WR, et al. (1986). Discrimination of muscle and neuronal Na-channel subtypes by binding competition between [3H]saxitoxin and mu-conotoxins. Proc Natl Acad Sci U S A 83: 5321–5325.

Molenaar PC, Biewenga JE, van Kempen GT, et al. (1993). Effect of ephedrine on muscle weakness in a model of myasthenia gravis in rats. Neuropharmacology 32: 373–376.

Montecucco C, Molgo J (2005). Botulinal neurotoxins: revival of an old killer. Curr Opin Pharmacol 5: 274–279.

Moores TS, Hasdemir B, Vega-Riveroll L, et al. (2005). Properties of presynaptic P2X7-like receptors at the neuromuscular junction. Brain Res 1034: 40–50.

Mora M, Lambert EH, Engel AG (1987). Synaptic vesicle abnormality in familial infantile myasthenia. Neurology 37: 206–214.

Muraki K, Imaizumi Y, Watanabe M (1991). Sodium currents in smooth muscle cells freshly isolated from stomach fundus of the rat and ureter of the guinea-pig. J Physiol 442: 351–375.

Nagel A, Lehmann-Horn F, Engel AG (1990). Neuromuscular transmission in the mdx mouse. Muscle Nerve 13: 742–749.

Newsom-Davis J (1997). Autoimmune neuromyotonia (Isaacs' syndrome): an antibody-mediated potassium channelopathy. Ann N Y Acad Sci 835: 111–119.

Nicholls JG (1956). The electrical properties of denervated skeletal muscle. J Physiol 131: 1–12.

Nikovits W Jr, Cann GM, Huang R, et al. (2001). Patterning of fast and slow fibers within embryonic muscles is established independently of signals from the surrounding mesenchyme. Development 128: 2537–2544.

Nudell BM, Grinnell AD (1982). Inverse relationship between transmitter release and terminal length in synapses on frog muscle fibers of uniform input resistance. J Neurosci 2: 216–224.

Oda K (1984). Age changes of motor innervation and acetylcholine receptor distribution on human skeletal muscle fibres. J Neurol Sci 66: 327–338.

O'Hanlon GM, Bullens RW, Plomp JJ, et al. (2002). Complex gangliosides as autoantibody targets at the neuromuscular junction in Miller Fisher syndrome: a current perspective. Neurochem Res 27: 697–709.

Ohno K, Brengman J, Tsujino A, et al. (1998). Human endplate acetylcholinesterase deficiency caused by mutations in the collagen-like tail subunit (colq) of the asymmetric enzyme. Proc Natl Acad Sci U S A 95: 9654–9659.

Ohno K, Tsujino A, Brengman JM, et al. (2001). Choline acetyltransferase mutations cause myasthenic syndrome associated with episodic apnea in humans. Proc Natl Acad Sci U S A 98: 2017–2022.

Ohno K, Engel AG, Shen XM, et al. (2002). Rapsyn mutations in humans cause endplate acetylcholine-receptor deficiency and myasthenic syndrome. Am J Hum Genet 70: 875–885.

Oliveira L, Timoteo MA, Correia-de-Sa P (2002). Modulation by adenosine of both muscarinic M1-facilitation and M2-inhibition of [3H]-acetylcholine release from the rat motor nerve terminals. Eur J Neurosci 15: 1728–1736.

Orbeli LA (1923). Die sympatetische Innervation der Skelletmuskeln. Bull Inst Sci St Petersb 6: 194–197.

Overell JR, Willison HJ (2005). Recent developments in Miller Fisher syndrome and related disorders. Curr Opin Neurol 18: 562–566.

Padykula HA, Gauthier GF (1970). The ultrastructure of the neuromuscular junctions of mammalian red, white, and intermediate skeletal muscle fibers. J Cell Biol 46: 27–41.

Paton WDM, Waud DR (1962). Neuromuscular blocking agents. Br J Anaesth 34: 251–259.

Paton WD, Waud DR (1967). The margin of safety of neuromuscular transmission. J Physiol 191: 59–90.

Pawson PA, Grinnell AD, Wolowske B (1998). Quantitative freeze-fracture analysis of the frog neuromuscular junction synapse—I. Naturally occurring variability in active zone structure. J Neurocytol 27: 361–377.

Personius KE, Balice-Gordon RJ (2001). Loss of correlated motor neuron activity during synaptic competition at developing neuromuscular synapses. Neuron 31: 395–408.

Personius KE, Sawyer RP (2005). Terminal Schwann cell structure is altered in diaphragm of mdx mice. Muscle Nerve 32: 656–663.

Plomp JJ, van Kempen GT, Molenaar PC (1992). Adaptation of quantal content to decreased postsynaptic sensitivity at single endplates in alpha-bungarotoxin-treated rats. J Physiol 458: 487–499.

Plomp JJ, van Kempen GT, De Baets MB, et al. (1995). Acetylcholine release in myasthenia gravis: regulation at single end-plate level. Ann Neurol 37: 627–636.

Poo MM (2001). Neurotrophins as synaptic modulators. Nat Rev Neurosci 2: 24–32.

Prakash YS, Sieck GC (1998). Age-related remodeling of neuromuscular junctions on type-identified diaphragm fibers. Muscle & Nerve 21: 887–895.

Prasarnpun S, Walsh J, Awad SS, et al. (2005). Envenoming bites by kraits: the biological basis of treatment-resistant neuromuscular paralysis. Brain 128: 2987–2996.

Prior C, Dempster J, Marshall IG (1993). Electrophysiological analysis of transmission at the skeletal neuromuscular junction. J Pharmacol Toxicol Methods 30: 1–17.

Protti DA, Reisin R, Mackinley TA, et al. (1996). Calcium channel blockers and transmitter release at the normal human neuromuscular junction. Neurology 46: 1391–1396.

Reger JF (1958). The fine structure of neuromuscular synapses of gastrocnemii from mouse and frog. Anat Rec 130: 7–23.

Reid B, Slater CR, Bewick GS (1999). Synaptic vesicle dynamics in rat fast and slow motor nerve terminals. J Neurosci 19: 2511–2521.

Reid B, Martinov VN, Nja A, et al. (2003). Activity-dependent plasticity of transmitter release from nerve terminals in rat fast and slow muscles. J Neurosci 23: 9340–9348.

Rettig J, Neher E (2002). Emerging roles of presynaptic proteins in Ca++-triggered exocytosis. Science 298: 781–785.

Reynolds ML, Woolf CJ (1992). Terminal Schwann cells elaborate extensive processes following denervation of the motor endplate. J Neurocytol 21: 50–66.

Ribchester RR, Thomson D, Haddow LJ, et al. (1998). Enhancement of spontaneous transmitter release at neonatal mouse neuromuscular junctions by the glial cell line-derived neurotrophic factor (GDNF). J Physiol 512(Pt 3): 635–641.

Rich MM, Pinter MJ, Kraner SD, et al. (1998). Loss of electrical excitability in an animal model of acute quadriplegic myopathy. Ann Neurol 43: 171–179.

Rizzoli SO, Betz WJ (2005). Synaptic vesicle pools. Nat Rev Neurosci 6: 57–69.

Robbins N, Kuchynski M, Polak J, et al. (1990). Motor nerve terminal restoration after focal destruction in young and old mice. Int J Dev Neurosci 8: 667–678.

Robitaille R (1995). Purinergic receptors and their activation by endogenous purines at perisynaptic glial cells of the frog neuromuscular junction. J Neurosci 15: 7121–7131.

Robitaille R (1998). Modulation of synaptic efficacy and synaptic depression by glial cells at the frog neuromuscular junction. Neuron 21: 847–855.

Robitaille R, Adler EM, Charlton MP (1990). Strategic location of calcium channels at transmitter release sites of frog neuromuscular synapses. Neuron 5: 773–779.

Robitaille R, Jahromi BS, Charlton MP (1997). Muscarinic Ca2+ responses resistant to muscarinic antagonists at perisynaptic Schwann cells of the frog neuromuscular junction. J Physiol 504: 337–347.

Rochon D, Rousse I, Robitaille R (2001). Synapse–glia interactions at the mammalian neuromuscular junction. J Neurosci 21: 3819–3829.

Rosato S, Uchitel OD (1999). Calcium channels coupled to neurotransmitter release at neonatal rat neuromuscular junctions. J Physiol 514(Pt 2): 533–540.

Rothe F, Langnaese K, Wolf G (2005). New aspects of the location of neuronal nitric oxide synthase in the skeletal muscle: a light and electron microscopic study. Nitric Oxide 13: 21–35.

Ruegg MA, Bixby JL (1998). Agrin orchestrates synaptic differentiation at the vertebrate neuromuscular junction. Trends Neurosci 21: 22–27.

Ruff RL (1992). Na current density at and away from end plates on rat fast- and slow-twitch skeletal muscle fibers. Am J Physiol 262: C229–C234.

Ruff RL, Lennon VA (1998). End-plate voltage-gated sodium channels are lost in clinical and experimental myasthenia gravis. Ann Neurol 43: 370–379.

Ruff RL, Whittlesey D (1992). Na+ current densities and voltage dependence in human intercostal muscle fibres. J Physiol 458: 85–97.

Rushton WAH (1937). Initiation of the propagated disturbance. Proc R Soc B 124: 210–243.

Salmons S, Vrbova G (1969). The influence of activity on some contractile characteristics of mammalian fast and slow muscles. J Physiol 201: 535–549.

Salpeter MM (1987). Vertebrate neuromuscular junctions: general morphology, molecular organization, and functional consequences. In: MM Salpeter (Ed.), The Vertebrate Neuromuscular Junction, Alan R. Liss, Inc., New York, pp. 1–54.

Sanes JR (1989). Extracellular matrix molecules that influence neural development. Annu Rev Neurosci 12: 491–516.

Sanes JR, Lichtman JW (1999). Development of the vertebrate neuromuscular junction. Annu Rev Neurosci 22: 389–442.

Sanes JR, Marshall LM, McMahan UJ (1978). Reinnervation of muscle fiber basal lamina after removal of myofibers. Differentiation of regenerating axons at original synaptic sites. J Cell Biol 78: 176–198.

Santafe MM, Urbano FJ, Lanuza MA, et al. (2000). Multiple types of calcium channels mediate transmitter release during functional recovery of botulinum toxin type A-poisoned mouse motor nerve terminals. Neuroscience 95: 227–234.

Santafe MM, Salon I, Garcia N, et al. (2003). Modulation of ach release by presynaptic muscarinic autoreceptors in the neuromuscular junction of the newborn and adult rat. Eur J Neurosci 17: 119–127.

Schiavo G, Matteoli M, Montecucco C (2000). Neurotoxins affecting neuroexocytosis. Physiol Rev 80: 717–766.

Selcen D, Fukuda T, Shen XM, et al. (2004). Are musk antibodies the primary cause of myasthenic symptoms? Neurology 62: 1945–1950.

Shaw C (1996). Neuropeptides and their evolution. Parasitology 113: S35–S45.

Shillito P, Molenaar PC, Vincent A, et al. (1995). Acquired neuromyotonia: evidence for autoantibodies directed against K+ channels of peripheral nerves. Ann Neurol 38: 714–722.

Shinnick-Gallagher P, Gallagher JP (1979). Ephedrine: a postsynaptic depressant drug at the mammalian neuromuscular junction. Neuropharmacology 18: 755–761.

Sica RE, McComas AJ, Upton AR, et al. (1974). Motor unit estimations in small muscles of the hand. J Neurol Neurosurg Psychiatry 37: 55–67.

Sieb JP, Engel AG (1993). Ephedrine: effects on neuromuscular transmission. Brain Res 623: 167–171.

Sieb JP, Milone M, Engel AG (1996). Effects of the quinoline derivatives quinine, quinidine, and chloroquine on neuromuscular transmission. Brain Res 712: 179–189.

Silinsky EM (1975). On the association between transmitter secretion and the release of adenine nucleotides from mammalian motor nerve terminals. J Physiol 247: 145–162.

Silinsky EM (1980). Evidence for specific adenosine receptors at cholinergic nerve endings. Br J Pharmacol 71: 191–194.

Silinsky EM (2004). Adenosine decreases both presynaptic calcium currents and neurotransmitter release at the mouse neuromuscular junction. J Physiol 558: 389–401.

Silinsky EM, Hubbard JI (1973). Release of ATP from rat motor nerve terminals. Nature 243: 404–405.

Silinsky EM, Solsona C, Hirsh JK (1989). Pertussis toxin prevents the inhibitory effect of adenosine and unmasks adenosine-induced excitation of mammalian motor nerve endings. Br J Pharmacol 97: 16–18.

Sine SM, Shen XM, Wang HL, et al. (2002). Naturally occurring mutations at the acetylcholine receptor binding site independently alter ach binding and channel gating. J Gen Physiol 120: 483–496.

Slack JR, Hopkins WG (1982). Neuromuscular transmission at terminals of sprouted mammalian motor neurones. Brain Res 237: 121–135.

Slater CR (1966). Time course of failure of neuromuscular transmission after motor nerve section. Nature 209: 305–306.

Slater CR (1982). Postnatal maturation of nerve–muscle junctions in hindlimb muscles of the mouse. Dev Biol 94: 11–22.

Slater CR, Lyons PR, Walls TJ, et al. (1992). Structure and function of neuromuscular junctions in the vastus lateralis of man. A motor point biopsy study of two groups of patients. Brain 115: 451–478.

Slater CR, Young C, Wood SJ, et al. (1997). Utrophin abundance is reduced at neuromuscular junctions of patients with both inherited and acquired acetylcholine receptor deficiencies. Brain 120: 1513–1531.

Slater CR, Fawcett PR, Walls TJ, et al. (2006). Pre- and postsynaptic abnormalities associated with impaired neuromuscular transmission in a group of patients with "limb-girdle myasthenia". Brain 129: 2061–2076.

Slutsky I, Parnas H, Parnas I (1999). Presynaptic effects of muscarine on ach release at the frog neuromuscular junction. J Physiol 514: 769–782.

Slutsky I, Silman I, Parnas I, et al. (2001). Presynaptic M(2) muscarinic receptors are involved in controlling the kinetics of ach release at the frog neuromuscular junction. J Physiol 536: 717–725.

Slutsky I, Wess J, Gomeza J, et al. (2003). Use of knockout mice reveals involvement of M2-muscarinic receptors in control of the kinetics of acetylcholine release. J Neurophysiol 89: 1954–1967.

Sokolova E, Grishin S, Shakirzyanova A, et al. (2003). Distinct receptors and different transduction mechanisms for ATP and adenosine at the frog motor nerve endings. Eur J Neurosci 18: 1254–1264.

Son YJ, Trachtenberg JT, Thompson WJ (1996). Schwann cells induce and guide sprouting and reinnervation of neuromuscular junctions. Trends Neurosci 19: 280–285.

Sosa MA, Zengel JE (1993). Use of mu-conotoxin GIIIA for the study of synaptic transmission at the frog neuromuscular junction. Neurosci Letts 157: 235–238.

Stalberg E, Fawcett PR (1982). Macro EMG in healthy subjects of different ages. J Neurol Neurosurg Psychiatry 45: 870–878.

Stalberg E, Trontelj JV (1979). Single Fiber Electropmyography The Miravalle Press Ltd, Old Woking, Surrey.

Stalberg E, Schwartz MS, Trontelj JV (1975). Single fibre electromyography in various processes affecting the anterior horn cell. J Neurol Sci 24: 403–415.

Stanley EF (1997). The calcium channel and the organization of the presynaptic transmitter release face. Trends Neurosci 20: 404–409.

Stevens CF (1976). A comment on Martin's relation. Biophys J 16: 891–895.

Stocksley MA, Awad SS, Young C, et al. (2005). Accumulation of Na(V)1 mrnas at differentiating postsynaptic sites in rat soleus muscles. Mol Cell Neurosci 28: 694–702.

Stoop R, Poo MM (1996). Synaptic modulation by neurotrophic factors: differential and synergistic effects of brain-derived neurotrophic factor and ciliary neurotrophic factor. J Neurosci 16: 3256–3264.

Strochlic L, Cartaud A, Cartaud J (2005). The synaptic muscle-specific kinase (musk) complex: new partners, new functions. Bioessays 27: 1129–1135.

Sudhof TC (2004). The synaptic vesicle cycle. Annu Rev Neurosci 27: 509–547.

Sugiura Y, Woppmann A, Miljanich GP, et al. (1995). A novel omega-conopeptide for the presynaptic localization of calcium channels at the mammalian neuromuscular junction. J Neurocytol 24: 15–27.

Takeuchi A, Takeuchi N (1959). Active phase of frog's end-plate potential. J Neurophysiol 22: 395–411.

Thomas S, Robitaille R (2001). Differential frequency-dependent regulation of transmitter release by endogenous nitric oxide at the amphibian neuromuscular synapse. J Neurosci 21: 1087–1095.

Thomas CK, Zijdewind I (2006). Fatigue of muscles weakened by death of motoneurons. Muscle Nerve 33: 21–41.

Tomlinson BE, Irving D (1977). The numbers of limb motor neurons in the human lumbosacral cord throughout life. J Neurol Sci 34: 213–219.

Tonge DA (1974a). Chronic effects of botulinum toxin on neuromuscular transmission and sensitivity to acetylcholine in slow and fast skeletal muscle of the mouse. J Physiol 241: 127–139.

Tonge DA (1974b). Physiological characteristics of reinnervation of skeletal muscle in the mouse. J Physiol 241: 141–153.

Torres LF, Duchen LW (1987). The mutant mdx: inherited myopathy in the mouse. Morphological studies of nerves, muscles and end-plates. Brain 110: 269–299.

Trojan DA, Cashman NR (2005). Post-poliomyelitis syndrome. Muscle Nerve 31: 6–19.

Tsujino A, Maertens C, Ohno K, et al. (2003). Myasthenic syndrome caused by mutation of the SCN4A sodium channel. Proc Natl Acad Sci U S A 100: 7377–7382.

Tuffery AR (1971). Growth and degeneration of motor end-plates in normal cat hind limb muscles. J Anat 110: 221–247.

Uchitel OD (1997). Toxins affecting calcium channels in neurons. Toxicon 35: 1161–1191.

Urbano FJ, Rosato-Siri MD, Uchitel OD (2002). Calcium channels involved in neurotransmitter release at adult, neonatal and P/Q-type deficient neuromuscular junctions (Review). Mol Membr Biol 19: 293–300.

Ushkaryov YA, Volynski KE, Ashton AC (2004). The multiple actions of black widow spider toxins and their selective use in neurosecretion studies. Toxicon 43: 527–542.

Van der Kloot W (1991). The regulation of quantal size. Prog Neurobiol 36: 93–130.

Van der Kloot W, van der Kloot TE (1986). Catecholamines, insulin and ACTH increase quantal size at the frog neuromuscular junction. Brain Res 376: 378–381.

Van der Kloot WG, Molgo J (1994). Quantal acetylcholine release at the vertebrate neuromuscular junction. Physiol Rev 74: 899–991.

Vautrin J, Mambrini J (1989). Synaptic current between neuromuscular junction folds. J Theoret Biol 140: 479–498.

Vincent A, Cull-Candy SG, Newsom-Davis J, et al. (1981). Congenital myasthenia: end-plate acetylcholine receptors and electrophysiology in five cases. Muscle Nerve 4: 306–318.

Vincent A, Lang B, Newsom-Davis J (1989). Autoimmunity to the voltage-gated calcium channel underlies the Lambert-Eaton myasthenic syndrome, a paraneoplastic disorder. Trends Neurosci 12: 496–502.

Vizi S (1991). Evidence that catecholamines increase acetylcholine release from neuromuscular junctions through stimulation of α-1 adrenoceptors. Naunyn-Schmiedebergs Arch Pharmacol 343: 435–438.

Vrbova G, Navarrete R, Lowrie M (1985). Matching of muscle properties and motoneurone firing patterns during early stages of development. J Exp Biol 115: 113–123.

Wachman ES, Poage RE, Stiles JR, et al. (2004). Spatial distribution of calcium entry evoked by single action potentials within the presynaptic active zone. J Neurosci 24: 2877–2885.

Waerhaug O (1992). Postnatal development of rat motor nerve terminals. Anat Embryol (Berl) 185: 115–123.

Waerhaug O, Lømo T (1994). Factors causing different properties at neuromuscular junctions in fast and slow rat skeletal muscles. Anat Embryol (Berl) 190: 113–125.

Walrond JP, Reese TS (1985). Structure of axon terminals and active zones at synapses on lizard twitch and tonic muscle fibers. J Neurosci 5: 1118–1131.

Walsh FS, Hobbs C, Wells DJ, et al. (2000). Ectopic expression of NCAM in skeletal muscle of transgenic mice results in terminal sprouting at the neuromuscular junction and altered structure but not function. Mol Cell Neurosci 15: 244–261.

Wareham AC, Morton RH, Meakin GH (1994). Low quantal content of the endplate potential reduces safety factor for neuromuscular transmission in the diaphragm of the newborn rat. Br J Anaesth 72: 205–209.

Wiechers DO (1988). New concepts of the reinnervated motor unit revealed by vaccine-associated poliomyelitis. Muscle Nerve 11: 356–364.

Winckler B, Forscher P, Mellman I (1999). A diffusion barrier maintains distribution of membrane proteins in polarized neurons. Nature 397: 698–701.

Windisch A, Gundersen K, Szabolcs MJ, et al. (1998). Fast to slow transformation of denervated and electrically stimulated rat muscle. J Physiol 510: 623–632.

Wokke JH, Jennekens FG, Van den Oord CJ, et al. (1990). Morphological changes in the human end plate with age. J Neurol Sci 95: 291–310.

Wood SJ, Slater CR (1994). Action potential generation in the isolated rat soleus muscle. J Physiol 480: 125P.

Wood SJ, Slater CR (1995). Action potential generation in rat slow- and fast-twitch muscles. J Physiol 486: 401–410.

Wood SJ, Slater CR (1997). The contribution of postsynaptic folds to the safety factor for neuromuscular transmission in rat fast- and slow-twitch muscles. J Physiol 500: 165–176.

Wood SJ, Slater CR (1998a). Beta-Spectrin is colocalized with both voltage-gated sodium channels and ankyring at the adult rat neuromuscular junction. J Cell Biol 140: 675–684.

Wood SJ, Slater CR (1998b). Quantal content at neuromuscular junctions that lack postsynaptic folds. J Physiol 511: 142P.

Wood SJ, Slater CR (2001). Safety factor at the neuromuscular junction. Prog Neurobiol 64: 393–429.

Yazejian B, Sun XP, Grinnell AD (2000). Tracking presynaptic Ca2+ dynamics during neurotransmitter release with Ca2+-activated K+ channels. Nat Neurosci 3: 566–571.

Zefirov AL, Cheranov SI (1995). [Localization of origination sites of anomalous end-plate miniature currents in the neuromuscular synapse]. Biull Eksp Biol Med 120: 235–238.

Zucker RS, Regehr WG (2002). Short-term synaptic plasticity. Annu Rev Physiol 64: 355–405.

Handbook of Clinical Neurology, Vol. 91 (3rd series)
Neuromuscular junction disorders
A.G. Engel, Editor

Chapter 3

The neuromuscular junction

ANDREW G. ENGEL*

*3M McKnight Professor of Neuroscience, Mayo Clinic College of Medicine, Consultant,
Department of Neurology, Mayo Clinic, Rochester, MN, USA*

3.1. Basic definitions

The neuromuscular junction (NMJ) is a chemical synapse that is anatomically and functionally differentiated for the transmission of a signal from the motor nerve terminal to a circumscribed postsynaptic region on the muscle fiber. The position of NMJs on the muscle fiber, the configuration of the nerve terminals within the NMJ, and the extent of development of the postsynaptic region can vary according to phylum and species, between different muscles in a given species, and between different fibers in a given muscle. Despite these differences, all NMJs have five principal components: 1. A Schwann cell process that forms a cap above that portion of the nerve terminal that does not face the postsynaptic region. 2. A nerve terminal that contains the neurotransmitter. 3. A synaptic space lined with a basement membrane. 4. A postsynaptic membrane that contains the receptor for the neurotransmitter. 5. Junctional sarcoplasm that provides structural and metabolic support for the postsynaptic region (Fig. 3.1). In vertebrate voluntary muscle the neurotransmitter is acetylcholine (ACh), the receptor is the nicotinic ACh receptor (AChR), and the synaptic space contains ACh esterase (AChE).

3.2. Patterns of motor innervation

Mature muscle receives a topographic projection of nerve fibers from its motor neuron pool (Bennett, 1983). The rostrocaudal axis of the motor pool is systematically mapped onto the rostrocaudal axis of the muscle. This is associated with segmental ordering of axons in the nerve and may be aided by axonal guidance at branch points in the nerve and by positional labels within the muscle (Laskowski and Sanes, 1987).

The nerve trunks that enter muscle carry both motor and sensory fibers. The motor nerve fibers terminate on extrafusal muscle fibers; β motor nerve fibers terminate on both extra- and intrafusal muscle fibers; and γ motor nerve fibers terminate on intrafusal muscle fibers. The sensory nerves are destined to reach intrafusal and Golgi tendon end-organs. In normal mature muscle a single extrafusal muscle fiber receives its innervation from a single motor neuron, but each motor neuron supplies more than one muscle fiber. The motor neuron and the muscle fibers innervated by it constitute the motor unit. A nerve fiber from a given motor neuron divides into its terminal branches close to the muscle fibers it innervates, but not all fibers in a motor unit are immediately adjacent to each other. In focally innervated muscles preterminal axons tend to course perpendicularly to the long axis of the muscle fibers (Letinsky and Morrison-Graham, 1980); in muscles with distributed innervation, preterminal axons run parallel to the direction of the muscle fibers (Bennett and Pettigrew, 1974c).

3.2.1. Focal, distributed and myoseptal innervation

Focally innervated muscle fibers have single NMJs near their center. This, however, does not imply that all NMJs in a focally innervated muscle are in the central, or equatorial, region of the muscle. There are two reasons for this: not all muscle fibers in a given muscle extend through the entire length of the muscle; and muscle fibers may run parallel (e.g., biceps) or obliquely (e.g., rectus femoris) to the long axis of the muscle (Fig. 3.2C). Focally innervated muscle fibers are fast phasic fibers: the end-plate potential triggers an all-or-none muscle fiber action potential.

*Correspondence to: Dr Andrew G. Engel, MD, Department of Neurology, Mayo Clinic, Rochester, MN 55905, USA.
E-mail: age@mayo.edu, Tel: 1-507-284-5102, Fax: 1-507-284-5831.

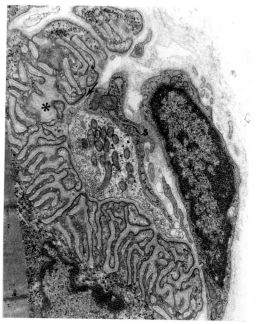

Fig. 3.1. Electron micrograph of normal human NMJ. The nerve terminal is covered by Schwann cells (S) on the right and faces the synaptic space on the left. The junctional sarcoplasm (X) contains glycogen granules, ribosomes, small tubular profiles, and nucleus. Arrow and asterisk mark primary and secondary synaptic clefts, respectively. Original magnification ×30 600. (From Engel, 2004, with permission.)

A muscle fiber that receives a distributed innervation has multiple NMJs positioned on its surface at regular intervals. The number of junctions per fiber may be as small as 2 to 5, as in the slow fibers of the frog cruralis muscle (Verma and Reese, 1984), or considerably higher, as in the avian anterior latissimus dorsi muscle.

Muscle fibers receiving distributed innervation are either slow tonic fibers whose end-plate potential propagates electrotonically without triggering an all-or-none action potential, as in avian anterior latissimus dorsi fibers, or in fast phasic fibers, as in frog sartorius fibers (Katz and Kuffler, 1941). Cross-reinnervation studies during development indicate that the pattern of synaptic sites on muscle fibers is determined by the nerve fibers (Bennett and Pettigrew, 1974b; Bennett, 1983).

In most mammalian muscles all extrafusal fibers are focally innervated. Distributed innervation in mammalian muscles occurs in intrafusal fibers (Bennett and Pettigrew, 1974a), and a small proportion of extrafusal fibers in extraocular (Peachey et al., 1974; Fraterman et al., 2006), facial, laryngeal and lingual (Hines, 1932; Cöers, 1967) muscles.

Myoseptal innervation, most frequently observed in myotomes of the lowest vertebrates (e.g., *Cyclotomes*), consists of basket-like nerve endings applied close to the origin and insertion of muscle fibers. This innervation becomes less important in higher vertebrates but still persists in some of the myotomal tail muscles of tadpoles and reptiles. Myoseptal innervation was first illustrated by Retzius (1892) and initially was thought to be associated with stretch receptors until Cöers (1967) demonstrated its motor character. This type of innervation has not been investigated in recent years.

3.2.2. Types of nerve ending

Plate-like (*en plaque*) nerve endings form round or elliptical loops on the muscle fiber surface (Fig. 3.2A, B). On mature muscle fibers the diameter of the innervated zone ranges from 10 to 80 μm with an average of 33 μm, and is proportionate to the muscle fiber diameter (Cöers, 1967). Plate-like endings occur with focal or distributed innervation and generate a propagated action potential. Plate-like terminals are the most common moiety in mammals and reptiles, but also occur in birds and lower vertebrates (Kühne, 1887).

Grape-like (*en grappe*) nerve endings consist of a spray of fine varicose filaments that end in minute expansions (Tschiriew, 1879; McMahan et al., 1972). They are typically found in birds and reptiles on "slow tonic fibers" with distributed innervation that cannot propagate an action potential, but may also occur on focally innervated fibers. Not all muscle fibers with distributed innervation have grape-like terminals (Hess, 1970; McMahan et al., 1972). Cöers (1967) emphasized that the distinction between grape- and plate-like terminals was originally based on gold or silver impregnation methods and that the configuration of the nerve endings cannot be used to identify mammalian muscle fibers that do not propagate action potentials. This argument is supported by methylene blue studies of rat diaphragm end-plates: white (type 2B) fibers have grape-like terminals, red (type 1) fibers have plate-like terminals, and intermediate (type 2A) fibers have intermediate-type terminals (Korneliussen and Waerhaug, 1973). Thus, grape-like endings can be found on mammalian fibers with the shortest contraction times, and all fibers in the rat diaphragm propagate an action potential.

Grape-like nerve endings are also present in multiple-innervated slow-twitch external ocular muscles that do not propagate an action potential. Interestingly, the AChRs of slow-twitch external ocular muscles harbor the fetal γ subunit whereas the fast-twitch

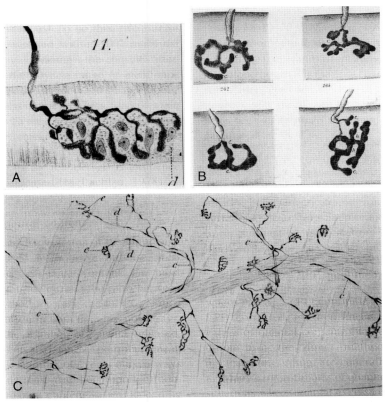

Fig. 3.2. Early accurate camera lucida drawings of intramuscular nerve endings. (A) Plate-like nerve terminal on a lizard muscle fiber, supravital staining. (B) Plate-like nerve endings on guinea pig muscle fibers visualized by a gold impregnation technique. (C) Intramuscular nerve branches and terminals in salamander muscle visualized by supravital staining. An intramuscular nerve coursing from lower left to upper right gives off small branches (c) that divide into single nerve fibers (d) that form terminals (e) on individual muscle fibers. The muscle fibers course vertically. The fine horizontal lines on the fibers represent cross striations. (A and B are from Dogiel, 1890; C is from Kühne, 1887).

external ocular muscles harbor the adult AChR that contains the ε-subunit (Fraterman et al., 2006).

End-brush (*Endbüschel*) nerve endings consist of long, slender, branches, most of which course parallel to the long axis of the muscle fiber for several hundred micrometers. They are commonly observed in frogs and turtles, and generate propagated muscle fiber action potentials. At these junctions the active zones and junctional folds course perpendicularly to the long axis of the nerve terminals. This highly oriented arrangement is particularly favorable for anatomic and physiologic studies.

Basket nerve endings are associated with myoseptal innervation, as described above. The comparative anatomy of the myoseptal nerve endings in different species has not been adequately investigated to date.

Trail nerve endings are found in the juxtaequatorial region of intrafusal fibers on multiply innervated bag$_2$- and chain-type fibers innervated by γ-motor neurons.

The terminal axons consist of fine branches bearing varicose dilations.

3.3. The presynaptic region

The preterminal myelinated nerve fiber is surrounded by a sheath of perineural epithelial cells (Henle's sheath), which is partially surrounded by fibroblasts and other connective tissue elements. The myelinated nerve fibers and Henle's sheath are covered by basement membrane, but the fibroblasts are not. Sparse collagen fibrils traverse the spaces between the myelinated nerve fiber and Henle's sheath, and between Henle's sheath and the fibroblasts. Within a few micrometers of the NMJ the myelin sheath ends abruptly at the last node of Ranvier. Between the last node of Ranvier and the NMJ the terminal axon is enveloped by the Schwann cell which is surrounded by Henle's sheath (Fig. 3.3). A 10–30-nm gap intervenes

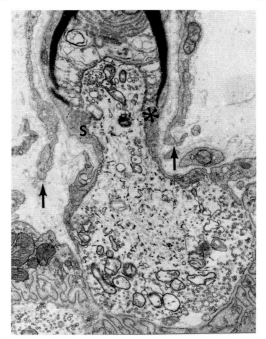

Fig. 3.3. Approach of a preterminal nerve fiber to the NMJ. The myelin sheath ends abruptly at the last node of Ranvier (asterisk). The rest of the preterminal nerve fiber (p) is surrounded by Schwann cell processes (S). Henle's sheath terminates shortly beyond the last node of Ranvier (arrows). The preterminal axon contains mitochondria, neurofilaments, and sparse synaptic vesicles. The basal lamina covers Schwann cells and Henle's sheath, and extends into the synaptic space. Original magnification ×11 900. (From Engel, 2004, with permission.)

between the axolemma and the Schwann cell plasma membrane, and a distance of 0.1 μm to about 1.0 μm separates the outer Schwann cell surface from Henle's sheath. Henle's sheath ends abruptly a short distance above the NMJ (Saito and Zacks, 1969) (Fig. 3.3), but the Schwann cell extends to cover that aspect of the nerve terminal that does not face the postsynaptic region (Fig. 3.3). At some nerve terminals the Schwann cell also sends finger-like extensions into the synaptic space extensions at regular intervals at frog but not at mammalian NMJs. The basement membrane overlying the Schwann cell laterally becomes continuous with the extrasynaptic basement membrane of the muscle fiber; medially it merges with the synaptic basement membrane (Figs. 3.1 and 3.3). Therefore, at the lateral borders of the NMJ basement membrane only separates the synaptic from the extracellular space.

The Schwann cell process overlying the terminal axon and nerve terminal contains numerous microfilaments, smooth and rough endoplasmic reticulum, mitochondria and, depending on the plane of the section, the cell's nucleus (Fig. 3.1). The terminal axon

contains neurofilaments, microtubules, smooth endoplasmic reticulum, a variable number of mitochondria, and a few synaptic vesicles.

3.3.1. The nerve terminal

The nerve terminal contains abundant small synaptic vesicles with clear contents, fewer giant synaptic vesicles with clear contents, coated vesicles, dense-core vesicles, mitochondria, and a varying complement of neurofilaments, microtubules, smooth endoplasmic reticulum, glycogen granules, lysosomal structures, and larger canaliculi and cisternae (Figs. 3.1 and 3.4–3.6). The relative abundance of the subcellular components in nerve terminals can vary within a given NMJ and from junction to junction; and with stage of development, aging, and neural activity. Morphometric studies of human and rat NMJs in the resting state indicate that

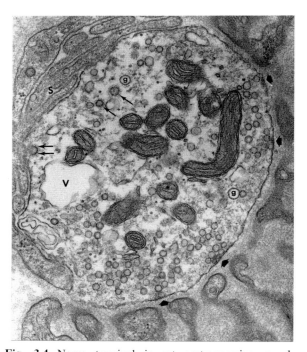

Fig. 3.4. Nerve terminal in rat gastrocnemius muscle. Synaptic vesicles are concentrated near the presynaptic membrane; mitochondria cluster near the center of the terminal. A few giant vesicles (g) and coated vesicles (arrows) are present. A coated pit (double arrows) is budding from the axolemma-covered Schwann cell (S). The nerve terminal also contains glycogen granules, a small vacuole (V), and an amorphous finely granular matrix. Solid arrows indicate four active zones that consist of dense spots on the inner surface of the presynaptic membrane and associated synaptic vesicles. The active zones are in register with the secondary synaptic clefts. Note dense membrane specializations on the terminal expansions of the junctional folds. Original magnification ×63 000. (From Engel, 2004, with permission.)

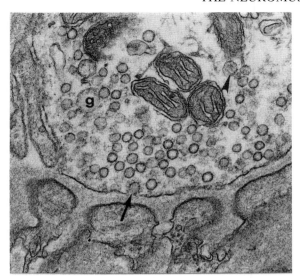

Fig. 3.5. Part of a nerve terminal and underlying postsynaptic region. Note coated vesicle budding from the presynaptic membrane (arrow) and giant synaptic vesicle (g). The synaptic space is filled with basal lamina. Original magnification ×51 800. (From Engel, 2004, with permission.)

mitochondria account for approximately 15% of the nerve terminal volume, and there are 50–70 synaptic vesicles per μm^2 of the nerve terminal area.

3.3.1.1. Giant synaptic vesicles

In the rested nerve terminal a small proportion of the synaptic vesicles are two to three times larger than the average synaptic vesicle (Figs. 3.4–3.6). These giant vesicles increase in number during recovery from tetanic stimulation (Heuser, 1974), or after exposure to lanthanum when most synaptic vesicles have been replaced by cisternae (Heuser and Miledi, 1971). Similar vesicles also appear in frog nerve terminals treated with vinblastine (Pécot-Dechavassine and Couteaux,

1975). The giant vesicles could arise from coalescence of smaller vesicles (Pécot-Dechavassine and Couteaux, 1975), or may represent intermediates of membrane recycling (Heuser, 1974). The appearance of giant vesicles after prolonged transmitter release has been correlated with that of giant miniature end-plate potentials (MEPPs) (Heuser, 1974). This suggests that each giant vesicle contains multiple ACh quanta, and that either the giant vesicle or its parent structure can concentrate ACh from the cytosol.

3.3.1.2. Coated vesicles

Few vesicles in the rested nerve terminal are coated by fuzzy material (Düring, 1967; Nickel et al., 1967; Zacks and Saito, 1969) (Figs. 3.4–3.6). In quick-freeze, deep-etch, rotary-shadow preparations the coat consists of a polyhedral surface lattice (Heuser, 1980b). The coated vesicles arise from endocytotic pits in the axolemma (Figs. 3.4 and 3.5) and pinch off from even those regions of the axolemma covered by Schwann cell processes (Heuser and Reese, 1973) (Fig. 3.4). The coated vesicles are also the first ones to pinch off from the axolemma and take up an extracellular marker when the nerve is tetanically stimulated in tracer-containing media (Heuser and Reese, 1973; Heuser, 1978), and they proliferate in the terminal when ACh secretion is accelerated (Heuser and Miledi, 1971; Heuser and Reese, 1973). Under these conditions they merge with, or bud from, cisternae and canaliculi within the nerve terminal (Heuser, 1978).

The polygonal network of the coated vesicles is made up of clathrin heavy and light chains (Ungewickell, 1984). These chains are present in the three-legged building blocks (triskelions) of the polygons. Within the network the centers and legs of triskelions become the corners and edges of the polygons, respectively

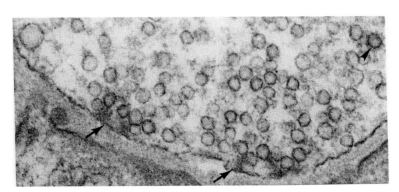

Fig. 3.6. Nerve terminal with two active zones (arrows). The dense material on the cytoplasmic surface of the active zone surrounds the associated synaptic vesicles. The synaptic space contains strands of basal lamina. The crests of two junctional folds face the active zone. Arrowhead points to a coated vesicle. Original magnification ×114 000. (From Engel, 2004, with permission.)

(Schmidt et al., 1984). Disassembly of the triskelions and denuding of the vesicles is induced by a cytosolic uncoating enzyme. This enzyme is an ATPase that interacts with clathrin light chains (Schmidt et al., 1984). Immunocytochemical (Cheng et al., 1980) and biochemical (Cheng and Wood, 1982) studies localize clathrin in the nerve terminal in the lattice of the coated vesicles, and in a "soluble" form in the axoplasmic matrix.

3.3.1.3. Dense-core vesicles

Normal nerve terminals contain sparse, randomly distributed vesicles with dense cores in their confines whose diameters are 1.5- to 2-fold larger than the diameters of the small clear synaptic vesicles (Fig. 3.5). These vesicles are morphologically and biochemically related to the secretory granules of endocrine cells. Dense-core vesicles are relatively abundant in nerve growth cones and sprouts, and in regenerating nerve terminals (De Iraldi and De Robertis, 1968). In different parts of the nervous system the dense-core vesicles contain neuropeptides, condensed proteins, and small nonprotein molecules. The presence of dense-core vesicles in adrenergic nerve terminals has been correlated with catecholamine associated fluorescence (De Iraldi and De Robertis, 1968; Heuser and Reese, 1977). At the NMJ the dense-core vesicles may contain agrin, calcitonin gene-related peptide (CGRP) (Matteoli et al., 1988; Hall and Sanes, 1993) and probably other neuroactive substances that can modify synaptic structure and function. Dense-core vesicles possess a vacuolar proton pump but lack synaptotagmin, synaptobrevin and synapsin. Their release from the nerve terminal is regulated by calcium and Munc18-1 (Voets et al., 2001), modulated by synaptotagmin (Wang et al., 2001), and, in *Drosophila*, by a calcium activated protein for secretion (Renden et al., 2001). The release mechanism differs from that for the small synaptic vesicles in several respects: the release is not preferentially at the active zones (Pow and Morris, 1989); the rate of release is not enhanced by α-latrotoxin (Matteoli et al., 1988; De Camilli and Jahn, 1990); and the release mechanism is relatively slow, occurring after about 50 ms of high-frequency stimulation, which results in a gradual increase of calcium concentration in the depth of the nerve terminal (Smith and Augustine, 1988; De Camilli and Jahn, 1990). Following exocytosis, the dense-core vesicles are recycled but their refilling requires a passage through the Golgi system (Jessell and Kandel, 1993).

3.3.1.4. Small clear synaptic vesicles

The smooth-surfaced clear synaptic vesicles with a mean diameter of 50–60 nm represent the predominant vesicle species in the nerve terminal (Engel and Santa, 1971; Engel et al., 1976), and from here on will be referred to simply as *synaptic vesicles*. The lumen of the synaptic vesicles contains ACh, ATP, GTP, a relatively high concentration of calcium and magnesium ions, and a vesicle-specific proteoglycan (Wagner et al., 1978; Whittaker, 1984; Volnandt and Zimmermann, 1986; Stadler and Kiene, 1987). The vesicles are more abundant near the presynaptic membrane than elsewhere in the terminal, whereas mitochondria and other organelles are concentrated in the center and upper part of the terminal (Anderson-Cedergren, 1959; Birks et al., 1960; Düring, 1967) (Figs. 3.1 and 3.4). The synaptic vesicles tend to be focused over dense spots on the presynaptic membrane (Figs. 3.4 and 3.6) that are part of the active zones and from where the vesicles exocytose their contents into the synaptic space (De Robertis and Bennett, 1955; Birks et al., 1960; Couteaux and Pécot-Dechavassine, 1970; Dreyer et al., 1973; Couteaux and Pécot-Dechavassine, 1974).

Synaptic vesicle precursors, associated with different sets of synaptic vesicle proteins, are produced in the body of the anterior horn cell and then are carried to nerve terminals by kinesin-like motors via fast axonal transport (Bööj et al., 1986; Kiene and Stadler, 1987; Llinás et al., 1989; Okada et al., 1995) by means of tubulovesicular organelles (Nakata et al., 1998). Further maturation of the vesicle precursors and their packaging with ACh occurs within the nerve terminal. A reduced number of synaptic vesicles, associated with a decrease in the number of readily releasable quanta, occurs in a congenital myasthenic syndrome. The putative cause of the syndrome is impaired axonal transport of synaptic vesicle components to the nerve terminal (see Chapter 10).

A current atomic model of the synaptic vesicle indicates that ~20% of the vesicle membrane is occupied by transmembrane regions of vesicle-associated proteins. Because each transmembrane region is surrounded by a ring of fixed phospholipids, the vesicle membrane is likely rigid (Sudhof, 2006; Takamori et al., 2006). Individual vesicles are associated with more than 400 different proteins but not all these copurify with the vesicles. Some vesicular proteins are more abundant than others: there are 70 copies of synaptobrevin, 30 of synaptophysin-1, and 15 of synaptotagmin-1 per vesicle, but there is only 1 copy of the vesicular proton pump, though this large molecule accounts for 20% of the membrane occupied by transmembrane regions (Sudhof, 2006; Takamori et al., 2006). Functions of these proteins will be discussed in subsequent sections of this chapter.

The functions and activities of the synaptic vesicles include: 1. the concentrative uptake and storage of

ACh; 2. movement to and docking at the active zones; 3. fusion with the presynaptic membrane to release ACh by exocytosis; and 4. recycling (Südhof and Jahn, 1991; Greengard et al., 1993; Jessell and Kandel, 1993; Kelly, 1993). During recycling, the vesicles are retrieved from the presynaptic membrane, and then recharged with ACh. Performance of these tasks requires the interaction of highly specialized vesicular, cytosolic, and target membrane proteins.

3.3.1.5. Vesicular ACh uptake

The synthesis of ACh from choline and acetate takes place in the cytoplasm of the nerve terminal in a reaction catalyzed by choline acetyltransferase (ChAT). Uptake of the newly formed ACh into the synaptic vesicles is mediated by a vacuolar proton-pump ATPase, which lowers the intravesicular pH and drives ACh uptake through the vesicular ACh transporter (VAChT) (Anderson et al., 1982; Parsons et al., 1982; McMahon and Nicholls, 1991). The same VAChT transiently exports ACh from the nerve terminal when, due to exocytosis, the inner surface of the vesicular membrane is exposed to the synaptic space.

The entire coding region of the *VAChT* gene is contained in the first intron of the *ChAT* gene, and the two genes share common regulatory elements for transcription (Eiden, 1998). The structural information that specifically targets VAChT to the synaptic vesicles resides within the cytoplasmic C-terminal domain of VAChT. An isoform of VAChT, VMAT2, is targeted to the large, dense-core synaptic vesicles, where it subserves the concentrative uptake of neuroactive substances other than ACh (Varochi and Eriksson, 1998). Recessive mutations in ChAT reduce the expression or catalytic activity of CHAT causing a highly disabling congenital myasthenic syndrome associated with abrupt episodes of apnea (Ohno et al., 2001) (see Chapter 10).

3.3.2. Synaptic vesicle pools

Electron microscopy studies, observations by fluorescence microscopy of the position and movement of synaptic vesicles labeled with styryl dyes, and electrophysiology recordings of capacitance changes when synaptic vesicles fuse with the presynaptic membrane as well as the postsynaptic response to released transmitter quanta define three functionally distinct synaptic vesicle pools at the frog NMJ and in other synaptic systems (Rizzoli and Betz, 2005).

A readily releasable pool comprises synaptic vesicles primed for release and in physical contact with the presynaptic membrane where it traverses the active zone. However, not all vesicles docked at the active zones are primed for release. This pool accounts for ~1–2% of all synaptic vesicles in the nerve terminal. Vesicles from this pool exocytose at the onset of physiologic stimulation, are recycled within a few seconds, and then rapidly mix with a recycling pool.

The recycling pool accounts for ~10–20% of all synaptic vesicles in the nerve terminal. Vesicles from this pool exocytose within a few seconds after the start of stimulation, are recycled within a few seconds, and then rapidly replete the readily releasable pool and slowly mingle with a reserve pool of vesicles.

The reserve pool comprises ~80–90% of all synaptic vesicles in the nerve terminal. Vesicles from this pool exocytose only after stimulation lasting tens of seconds or minutes, are recycled slowly over minutes, and mix slowly with other vesicle pools. Although the three vesicle pools are functionally distinct, only the readily releasable vesicles have a distinct anatomic locus at the active zones; vesicles in the recycling and reserve pools are intermingled above the active zones and in deeper parts of the nerve terminal and cannot be identified by simple inspection of electron micrographs (Rizzoli and Betz, 2005).

3.3.2.1. Movement of synaptic vesicles

Vesicles in the recycling pool likely move to the active zones by simple diffusion (Gaffield et al., 2006). Movement of the synaptic vesicles from the reserve pool involves several proteins.

Synapsin I, a vesicle specific phosphoprotein, links synaptic vesicles to the cytoskeleton in the reserve pool of vesicles. Synapsins II and III subserve similar roles in different sets of neurons (Valtorta et al., 1988b; Hirokawa et al., 1989; Südhof and Jahn, 1991; Valtorta et al., 1992; Hosaka and Südhof, 1998; Hilfiker et al., 1999). Although partly homologous, the three synapsins are encoded by three distinct genes, and the *a* and *b* isoforms of each synapsin arise from differential splicing of their primary transcripts. Vesicle binding proteins for synapsin include Ca^{2+}-calmodulin-dependent protein kinase II (CaM kinase II), c-src, and possibly other proteins. Synapsin I also binds to cytoskeletal actin, spectrin, and tubulin and thus anchors the vesicles to the cytoskeleton. In addition, synapsin I promotes the polymerization of actin monomers into actin filaments and the formation of thick bundles of actin filaments.

Four sites on synapsin I are substrates for phosphorylation by different protein kinases. Phosphorylation by a cAMP-dependent protein kinase A of a conserved serine in the N-terminal domain of all synapsins promotes neurite growth in the developing nervous system (Kao et al., 2002).

Phosphorylation of synapsin I by synaptic vesicle-associated CaM kinase II has at least three effects: (i) it reduces the affinity of synapsin I for the subunit of

CaM kinase II and causes synapsin to dissociate from the vesicles (Tarelli et al., 1992); (ii) it inhibits the effect of synapsin I on the polymerization of monomeric actin; and (iii) it abrogates the ability of synapsin I to bundle actin filaments (Benfenati et al., 1992). Other studies, however, have questioned that synapsin I restrains synaptic vesicles from movement because F-actin is concentrated in nonrelease domains of the frog nerve terminal (Dunaevsky and Connor, 2006).

Once freed from cytoskeletal constraints, the synaptic vesicles in the reserve pool can move closer to the active zone. Filamentous actin and myosin likely play a role in this movement because (i) blocking actomyosin-dependent movements by inhibiting myosin light-chain kinase restricts vesicle release in hippocampal synapses (Ryan, 2001), (ii) Staurosporine, an inhibitor of a wide spectrum of protein kinases, impairs vesicle movement from the reserve pool to the active zones (Becherer et al., 2001), and (iii) disruption of actin restricts movement of vesicles from the reserve pool at the *Drosophila* NMJ (Bi et al., 1997; Kuromi and Kidokoro, 2000; Nunes et al., 2006). Additional proof for the role of myosin in mobilizing vesicles from the reserve pool has come from mice deficient in NCAM (Polo-Parada et al., 2001; Polo-Parada et al., 2004, 2005). Mice lacking the 140 kDa or 180 kDa NCAM isoform show a cyclic failure of neuromuscular transmission on high-frequency stimulation. Seven C-terminal NCAM residues (KENESCA) are involved in NCAM-mediated signaling, which activates myosin light-chain kinase and hence myosin II. Introduction of KENESCA heptapeptide into wild-type NMJs results in cyclic failure of neuromuscular transmission as observed in NCAM-180 null mice (Polo-Parada et al., 2005). From the above observations, one may infer that actin filaments serve as tracks for movements of the vesicles by myosin motors.

3.3.2.2. Docking of synaptic vesicles at the active zones

Following mobilization, the synaptic vesicles must be docked and then primed for release at the active zones. It was previously thought that docking was due to the formation of a complex between vesicular synaptobrevin and syntaxin and SNAP-25 on the presynaptic membrane. However, cleavage of these three proteins by clostridial neurotoxins or deletion of syntaxin in *Drosophila* does not prevent vesicle docking (Robinson and Martin, 1998). More recent studies implicate interaction of vesicular synaptotagmin with presynaptic membrane neurexin and the voltage-gated Ca^{2+} channel in vesicle docking (see Section 3.3.7).

3.3.3. The exocytotic machinery

Ca^{2+}-regulated exocytosis of the synaptic vesicles involves the coordinated interaction of highly conserved proteins located on the synaptic vesicle, in the cytosol, and on the presynaptic membrane. The key proteins are 1. synaptobrevin and synaptotagmin associated with the synaptic vesicles; 2. NSF (N-ethylamide-sensitive ATPase) and α-SNAP (soluble NSF attachment protein) in the cytosol; and 3. syntaxin, SNAP-25 (synaptic vesicle associated 25 kDa protein), and voltage-gated Ca^{2+} channels associated with the presynaptic membrane. Because isoforms of several of the above proteins and of other exocytosis-related proteins play a universal role on vesicle–target membrane fusion, the specificity of the docking and fusion process at different vesicle–target membrane sites in different cells must depend on specificity of the receptors on the vesicular or target membranes and presence of other accessory molecules (Jahn and Scheller, 2006). In addition to these key proteins, numerous other proteins have been implicated in synaptic vesicle exocytosis in model systems that include hippocampal neurons in culture and *Drosophila*, *C. elegans* and frog NMJs. However, some proteins that participate in the exocytotic machinery in model systems may not be expressed or play a significant role at the mammalian NMJ.

3.3.3.1. The SNARE complex

Vesicular synaptobrevin, together with presynaptic membrane syntaxin and SNAP-25, serve as a receptor for α-SNAP. Therefore, synaptobrevin is referred to as a v-SNARE (vesicular SNAP receptor), and syntaxin and SNAP-25 are called t-SNAREs (target membrane SNAP receptors) (Robinson and Martin, 1998). The requirement of t- and v-SNAREs for exocytosis is revealed by the effects of clostridial neurotoxins. Botulinum toxins B, D, F and G, and tetanus toxin, cleave synaptobrevin; botulinum toxins A and E cleave SNAP-25; and botulinum toxin C cleaves syntaxin (Jahn et al., 1995; Südhof, 1995). In each case, the result is an arrest of exocytosis.

Biophysical (Lin and Scheller, 1997; Fasshauer et al., 1997a, b, c), quick-freeze/deep-etch electron microscopy (Hanson et al., 1997), and crystallography (Sutton et al., 1998) studies have elucidated the structure and function of the SNARE complexes (Götte and von Mollard, 1998; Jahn and Hanson, 1998; Weis and Scheller, 1998; Giraudo et al., 2006; Jahn and Scheller, 2006; Pobbati et al., 2006). The cytoplasmic portion of each SNARE protein contains repeats of

7 amino acids that can assume an α-helical conformation. Monomeric SNAREs are largely unstructured; after combining with each other, they become highly α-helical, assume a coiled coil configuration, and acquire enhanced thermodynamic stability.

Assembly of the t- and v-SNARES occurs in three steps. First, monomeric SNAP-25, anchored to the presynaptic membrane by palmitoyl side chains, binds two molecules of syntaxin and the complex assumes a coiled-coil configuration. Second, the v-SNARE synaptobrevin binds to the preassembled t-SNARES by displacing one of the two syntaxin molecules bound to SNAP-25. The entire complex is now a coiled-coil in which α-helices are strongly held together by hydrophobic interactions. The complex, also referred to as the SNAREpin, is a 12- to 14-nm-long and ~2-nm-wide cylindrical bundle, with the N termini of each component at one end and the C termini at the membrane anchor end. Third, the complex is stabilized by complexin, a small soluble neuronal protein that binds to the complex in an antiparallel α-helical conformation to seal the groove between synaptobrevin and syntaxin (Chen et al., 2002b) (see Fig. 3.7). Complexin has now been shown to act as a reversible clamping protein that can freeze the SNAREpin as an assembled intermediate en-route to fusion. When calcium binds to the calcium sensor synaptotagmin, the complexin clamp is released (Giraudo et al., 2006) (also see Section 3.3.3.3). Because the v-SNAREs and t-SNAREs are anchored in two different membranes facing each other, the formation of SNAREpins brings vesicle and target membranes into very close proximity. This, together with a strong basic charge at the C-terminal end of the SNAREpins, may provide the driving force behind membrane fusion (Sutton et al., 1998). Multiple SNAREpins are probably needed to trigger fusion of a single synaptic vesicle, and the pins are likely arranged in a ring-like structure at the contact point (Weber et al., 1998). When v- and t-SNAREs are reconstituted into separate liposomal vesicles they assemble to form SNAREpins that link adjacent vesicles (Weber et al., 1998); this process is inefficient but is dramatically accelerated when a stabilized syntaxin/SNAP-25 acceptor complex is used (Pobbati et al., 2006).

3.3.3.2. Priming of the docked synaptic vesicles

A proportion of the synaptic vesicles in the nerve terminal are recruited and docked on the plasma membrane of the nerve terminal. However, only a fraction of these vesicles are in a primed state capable of calcium-evoked fusion, i.e., in a readily releasable state. Munc13 (Unc13 in *C. elegans*) is required for vesicle priming. Munc13 stabilizes the open conformation of syntaxin that was forced into a closed conformation by Munc18; this drives syntaxin to interact with SNAP25 and synaptobrevin and thus to form a SNAREpin. Tomosyn, on the other hand, inhibits this interaction (Becherer and Rettig, 2006). Thus, priming is modulated by the balance between tomosyn and

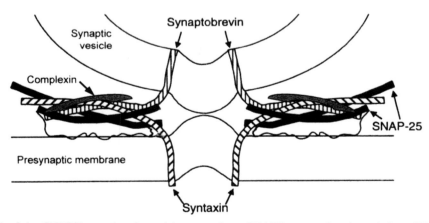

Fig. 3.7. A model of the SNARE complex formed between the v-SNARE synaptobrevin and the t-SNAREs syntaxin and SNAP-25. Two complexes are imaged. Synaptobrevin and syntaxin are anchored by transmembrane regions in the lipid bilayer of the synaptic vesicle (above) and presynaptic membrane (below), respectively. SNAP-25 is linked to the presynaptic membrane by a polypeptide chain (indicated by a thin undulating line). The complex is stabilized by complexin which binds in an α-helical conformation to seal the groove between synaptobrevin and syntaxin. The cytoplasmic domains of the v- and t-SNARES form a coil that pulls the synaptic vesicle and the presynaptic membrane into close proximity. Impending fusion is suggested by bulging regions of the vesicular and presynaptic membranes. This diagram is based on models proposed by Sutton et al. (1998), Weber et al. (1998) and Chen et al. (2002b).

Munc13, which probably regulates the availability of open-syntaxin (Rettig and Neher, 2002; Martin, 2003; McEwen et al., 2006).

3.3.3.3. Synaptotagmin-1

Synaptotagmin-1, a 65 kDa molecule, belongs to a large family of membrane proteins involved in membrane fusion in brain and other organs (Südhof and Rizo, 1996). Synaptotagmin-1 has a short, glycosylated intravesicular N-terminal domain, a transmembrane domain, and a cytoplasmic domain that harbors two Ca^{2+} regulatory C2 domains (C2A and C2B) connected by a short linker and separated from the transmembrane domain by a highly charged sequence.

The C2A domain binds phospholipids and two Ca^{2+} ions held in position by five negatively charged aspartate residues on two peptide loops (Shao et al., 1996). Fast vesicle exocytosis is driven by Ca^{2+}-dependent binding of syntagmin to the SNARE complex and to membrane phospholipids (Pang et al., 2006).

The Ca^{2+} concentration for half-maximal binding (EC50) is 200 μM, and is attained only in close proximity to the active zones. When the C2A domain binds Ca^{2+}, it acquires a large positive electrostatic potential and then binds syntaxin (Shao et al., 1997). Both syntaxin and synaptotagmin are highly associated with the presynaptic voltage-gated Ca^{2+} channels (Sheng et al., 1998).

The C2B domain of synaptotagmin binds to β-SNAP, which like α-SNAP binds to NSF, polyinositol phosphates, and the vesicular protein SV2A (Schivell et al., 1996; Südhof and Rizo, 1996). Ca^{2+} inhibits the interaction between SV2A and synaptotagmin, with an EC50 of 10 μM. The C-terminus of synaptotagmin binds neurexin, the presynaptic membrane receptor for α-latrotoxin (the active component of black-widow spider venom that causes massive exocytosis). The C2B domain also participates in endocytosis (see Section 3.3.9). Finally, an unknown region of synaptotagmin binds Munc13 (Südhof and Rizo, 1996). In mutant mice deficient in synaptotagmin, the Ca^{2+}-dependent evoked synaptic response is severely depressed. Consequently, the animals die shortly after birth (Geppert et al., 1994).

Synaptotagmin also binds to the voltage-gated Ca^{2+} channel as well as to syntaxin and neurexin which, in turn, are attached to the presynaptic Ca^{2+} channel (Rettig et al., 1997; Sheng et al., 1998). Hence, synaptotagmin could also participate in docking. Activation of synaptotagmin by Ca^{2+} is a likely trigger for exocytosis (Söllner et al., 1993; Südhof and Rizo, 1996). Recent studies have shed further light on the manner in which synaptotagmin regulates synaptic vesicle exocytosis by interaction with complexin. In a model system, SNARE proteins were flipped, so that instead

of being expressed on intracellular membranes they were exposed on the cell surface. Cells expressing such flipped SNAREs fused spontaneously. The introduction of complexin clamped the SNARE pins after they began to assemble but before they were fully zippered, and thereby prevented cell–cell fusion. Adding synaptotagmin and then calcium to the SNARE-complexin intermediate again allowed cell–cell fusion. According to this attractive model, synaptotagmin couples the calcium signal to SNAREs in a mechanism that requires complexin (Giraudo et al., 2006).

3.3.3.4. Steps in exocytosis

On the basis of recent studies, vesicle exocytosis can be postulated to involve the following major steps:

1. Partial and reversible assembly of the SNARE complex primes docked synaptic vesicles for exocytosis prior to the arrival of the Ca^{2+} trigger (Chen et al., 2001).
2. Following Ca^{2+} ingress into the nerve terminal, Ca^{2+} binds to synaptotagmin, enabling it to interact with syntaxin and SNAP-25 (Desai et al., 2000; Yoshihara and Littleton, 2002; Zhang et al., 2002), and to inhibit the clamping effect of complexin on SNAREpin assembly (Giraudo et al., 2006).
3. Syntaxin and SNAP-25 now firmly engage synaptobrevin to complete formation of the SNAREpins.
4. Full assembly of the SNAREpins brings vesicular and target membranes into close proximity, which initiates membrane fusion in a probabilistic manner (Hu et al., 2000).

3.3.4. Other proteins modulating exocytosis

3.3.4.1. Rab3a, rabphilin-3a, and RIM

Rab3a, a small GTP-binding protein, is also implicated in synaptic vesicle docking and fusion (Monck and Fernandez, 1992). The rab proteins belong to the p21ras superfamily, whose members regulate membrane fusion-fission events by cycling between membrane-bound and membrane-free states. When attached to a synaptic vesicle, rab3a binds GTP. Rab3a-GTP binds rabphilin-3a, a cytosolic protein with zinc-finger and C2 domains, and RIM (Wang et al., 1997). Both rabphilin-3a and RIM bind to rab3a through sequences contained in their zinc-finger domains.

At the time of exocytosis, activation of a GTPase converts rab3a-GTP to rab3a-GDP, whereupon both rab3a-GDP and rabphilin-3a dissociate from the synaptic vesicle (von Mollard et al., 1991; Bean and Scheller, 1997; Wang et al., 1997). Subsequently, rab3a-GDP becomes attached to another synaptic vesicle and recaptures GTP by nucleotide exchange. Evidence to date suggests that rab3a decreases the probability of quantal release (Geppert et al., 1997), RIM promotes transmitter release (Wang et al., 1997), and rabphilin-3a plays a regulatory role in both exocytosis and endocytosis (Burns et al., 1998). Recently it was shown that binding of rabphilin to SNAP-25 regulates exocytosis after the readily releasable pool of synaptic vesicles has been exhausted (Deák et al., 2006).

3.3.4.2. Rab5

This protein is involved in endosomal fusion events in different tissues and is present on the synaptic vesicles in high concentrations. It likely plays a part in interaction between the vesicles and endosomes during the vesicle cycle. Mutations in rab5 in *Drosophila* impair evoked transmitter release (Wucherpfennig et al., 2003).

3.3.4.3. SV2

This protein is found in synaptic vesicles and endocrine-cells. It is present in two major (SV2A and SV2B) and one minor isoforms (SV2C), which are highly homologous. The molecular structure of SV2 suggests that it functions as an ion channel transporter but this remains to be established. As noted above, SV2A interacts with the C2B domain of synaptotagmin in the absence of Ca^{2+}. The major phosphorylation site of SV2 is at its cytoplasmic amino terminus, and phosphorylation increases its affinity for synaptotagmin (Pyle et al., 2000). Neurons lacking both SV2 isoforms show increased Ca^{2+}-dependent transmitter release (Janz et al., 1999). Some evidence suggests that SV2 modulates the formation of protein complexes required for fusion and therefore the progression of vesicles to a fusion competent state (Xu and Bajjalieh, 2001).

3.3.4.4. Synaptophysin

Synaptophysin, a 38 kDa glycoprotein, is an abundant integral membrane protein of the synaptic vesicles (Wiedenmann and Franke, 1985). It has properties of a cation selective channel, with higher selectivity for K^+ than other cations, but is impermeable to Ca^{2+} (Ginzel and Shoshan-Barmatz, 2002). It is phosphorylated by a tyrosine kinase (Jena et al., 1997), interacts with a subunit of the vacuolar proton pump (Siebert et al., 1994), and may interact with synaptobrevin during exocytosis (Washbourne et al., 1995). When overexpressed at the *Xenopus* NMJ, synaptophysin increases the frequency of spontaneous quantal release and augments the number of quanta released by nerve impulse (Alder et al., 1995). In the yeast two-hybrid system, synapto-

physin interacts with the AP1-adaptor protein, γ-adaptin, and may thus play a role in endocytosis. However, synaptophysin null mice show no functional or morphologic abnormality (Eshkind and Leube, 1995).

3.3.4.5. Cysteine string protein (CSP), heat shock protein 70 (Hsc70), and SGT chaperone complex

These three proteins interact with each other to form a stable trimeric complex located on the surface of the synaptic vesicles. The complex functions as an ATP-dependent chaperone reactivating denatured substrates (Tobaben et al., 2001).

CSP itself is a 34 kDa protein anchored via palmitoyl groups to the synaptic vesicle so that its C- and N-termini are cytoplasmic (Calakos and Scheller, 1996; Buchner and Gundersen, 1997). CSP harbors an N-terminal J domain, characteristic of heat-shock proteins, and a central multiply palmitoylated string of cysteine residues. By increasing the ATPase activity of Hsc70, CSP co-chaperones with Hsc70 to promote the formation or dissociation of protein complexes and to regulate conformational changes in proteins (Braun et al., 1996; Chamberlain and Burgoyne, 1997). CSP also binds to the P/Q type Ca^{2+} channel with high affinity (Leveque et al., 1998) and interacts with synaptotagmin (Evans and Morgan, 2002). In *Drosophila* mutants lacking CSP, the exocytotic machinery is preserved but calcium entry into the nerve terminal and calcium activation of exocytosis, or both, are impaired (Ranjan et al., 1998). Injection of CSP into the chick ciliary neuron increases the Ca^{2+} current due to recruitment of dormant Ca^{2+} channels (Chen et al., 2002a). In mice deficient in the CSPa isoform, the NMJ degenerates, synaptic transmission is impaired, and the mice die at ~2 months of age (Fernandez-Chacon et al., 2004).

3.3.5. Presynaptic cytoskeletal components

Quick-freeze, deep-etch electron microscopy shows that the main cytoskeletal elements in the nerve terminal consist of actin filaments and microtubules (Heuser, 1980a; Hirokawa and Heuser, 1982; Landis and Reese, 1983; Hirokawa et al., 1989). The actin filaments honeycomb the nerve terminal. They are most closely packed adjacent to the synaptic membrane, and become more sparse with distance from the membrane. Those filaments terminating against the active zone tend to be perpendicularly oriented to the presynaptic membrane. The filaments are straight, often intersect, and extend from vesicle to vesicle, and from vesicle to presynaptic membrane. The actin filaments are linked to the synaptic vesicles by approximately 30-nm-long filaments that represent single synapsin I molecules. Synapsin I molecules also link microtubules to the synaptic vesicles and crosslink the microtubules (Hirokawa et al., 1989). A similar cytoskeletal network exists in Purkinje cell dendrites (Landis and Reese, 1983).

3.3.6. The active zone

The active zone is an anatomically differentiated region of the presynaptic membrane that defines the site of synaptic vesicle docking and fusion. That transmitter release occurs near active zones has been proposed by early studies of both central (Palay, 1958) and neuromuscular (De Robertis and Bennett, 1955; Birks et al., 1960) synapses. The position of the active zone in the nerve terminal is marked by a dense spot above which synaptic vesicles appear in clusters (Fig. 3.6). The dense spot contains a matrix of interconnected fibrils and particles that participate in vesicle exocytosis and membrane retrieval (Phillips et al., 2001). Proteins within the matrix of the active zone include RIM1, CAST, Bassoon, and Munc13-1. CAST binds directly to Bassoon and to RIM1 (rab interacting molecule 1) and indirectly to Munc13-1. RIM1 and Munc13-1 bind to each other. RIM1 binds to the C-terminus and Bassoon binds to the central region of CAST. RIM1 and Munc13-1 are implicated in synaptic vesicle priming. RIM null animals show a severe defect in spontaneous or evoked vesicle release but can dock vesicles at the active zone. Other proteins present in the active zones are considered in Section 3.3.7. Thus, the active zone matrix is a network of protein–protein, important for regulating synaptic vesicle exocytosis and organization of the active zone (Ohtsuka et al., 2002; Takao-Rikitsu et al., 2004; Schoch and Gundelfinger, 2006).

At the NMJ of fast-twitch frog muscle fibers the active zones recur at regular intervals, so that in longitudinal sections each zone is positioned above a secondary synaptic cleft that is flanked by two junctional folds. The long axis of each active zone is perpendicular to the long axis of the nerve terminal (Birks et al., 1960; Couteaux and Pécot-Dechavassine, 1970; Heuser and Reese, 1973; Couteaux and Pécot-Dechavassine, 1974; Heuser et al., 1974; Heuser and Reese, 1977). These features are clearly shown by freeze-fracture studies (Fig. 3.8). The precise alignment of the active zones with the crests of the junctional folds is also shown by dual immunofluorescence localization of the active zones with ω-conotoxin and of AChR with α-bungarotoxin (Robitaille et al., 1990; Tarelli et al., 1991). Treatment with proteolytic enzymes displaces and disorganizes

the active zones and clusters the active zone particles (Nystrom and Ko, 1988). Therefore precise alignment of the active zones on the presynaptic membrane depends, at least in part, on a factor in the basal lamina.

Freeze-fracture studies of the presynaptic membrane show additional features in the active zone. These are best observed on the protoplasmic (P) face of the fractured membrane. In the fast twitch frog muscle fiber the presynaptic membrane P face displays a ribbon-like convexity corresponding to the dense bar seen within the terminal by conventional transmission electron microscopy. The convexity is flanked on each side by a double parallel row of large (10–12 nm) intramembrane particles that represent voltage-gated Ca^{2+} channels (Dreyer et al., 1973; Heuser et al., 1974; Ceccarelli and Hurlbut, 1980) (Fig. 3.8). A remarkable electron microscope tomography study by McMahan and coworkers of the active zone of the frog cutaneous pectoris muscle reveals the spatial relationships and structural linkages between the docked synaptic vesicles, the presynaptic Ca^{2+} channels, and the related macromolecules (Harlow et al., 2001). According to this study, individual active zones are flanked on each side by a row of docked vesicles that flank the Ca^{2+} channels, which flank the ribbon-like convexity of the presynaptic membrane. Running in the center of the convexity are a series of ~75-nm-long "beams" whose orthogonal lateral extensions, or "ribs," associate with docked vesicles, about three ribs reaching each vesicle. The individual ribs are separated from the presynaptic membrane by a <7-nm gap, which is bridged at intervals by "pegs," with one or two pegs connecting each rib to regions of the membrane containing macromolecules that include the Ca^{2+} channel. While the molecular identity of the components of active zone scaffold are not yet known, the Ca^{2+} channels could be components of the pegs, and the ribs may contain proteins, such as syntaxin and synaptotagmin, which mediate the effects of Ca^{2+} on vesicle fusion.

The mammalian NMJ is less elongated and more convoluted than the linear NMJ on the fast-twitch frog muscle fiber. At the mammalian NMJ, the active zones retain the relationship to the underlying junctional folds but are shorter and less regularly disposed and the convexity between the double parallel rows of particles is usually absent (Rash and Ellisman, 1974; Fukunaga et al., 1982; Rash, 1983) (Fig. 3.9). The presynaptic membrane curves more steeply and irregularly at the mammalian than frog NMJ. However, the area of the mammalian membrane can still be determined by stereometric analysis (Engel et al., 1982). Using this approach, Fukunaga et al. (1982) found that

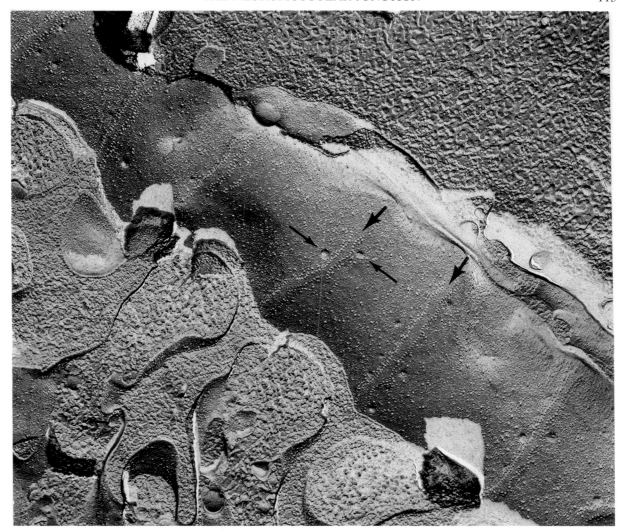

Fig. 3.8. Freeze-fractured frog NMJ stimulated during fixation in dilute aldehyde fixative. The fracture lane exposes a large expanse of the presynaptic membrane P face. The active zones are represented by a convex ridge flanked on each side by a double parallel row of large intramembrane particles (heavy arrows). The active zones run perpendicular to the long axis of the nerve terminal and are in register with the secondary synaptic clefts. Dimples adjacent to the active zones (light arrows) indicate exocytotic events that occurred during stimulation. Original magnification ×55 000. This micrograph was prepared by Dr. John Heuser. (From Heuser et al., 1974, with permission.)

in presynaptic membranes in human intercostal muscle the average density of active zones was $2.6/\mu m^2$, the density of active zone particles was $51/\mu m^2$, the average active zone had 5 particles per row and, on average, there were 19 particles per active zone. The same investigators obtained essentially identical values in freeze-fractured presynaptic membranes of the mouse diaphragm (Fukunaga et al., 1983). At the frog NMJ, the number of quanta released per nerve impulse varies with the total active zone length and total number of active zone particles per junction with quantal release from the same junctions (Propst and Ko, 1987).

3.3.7. The voltage-gated Ca^{2+} channels

The voltage-gated Ca^{2+} channels open when the presynaptic membrane is depolarized by the nerve action potential. The resultant Ca^{2+} entry peaks within 200 μs and lasts ∼800 μs (Llinas et al., 1995). During this time, the docked vesicles are engulfed in microdomains in which the Ca^{2+} concentration reaches ∼200–300 μM (Sheng et al., 1998). A synaptic vesicle within 20-nm from a Ca^{2+} channel can exocytose with high probability within a few hundred microseconds if the local Ca^{2+} concentration rises above 100 μM. It is

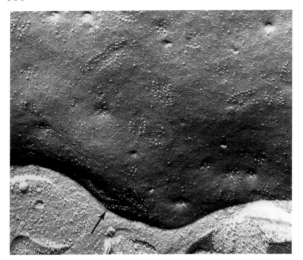

Fig. 3.9. Freeze-fracture electron microscopy reveals the voltage-sensitive Ca^{2+} channels of the presynaptic membrane as large membrane particles arrayed in double parallel rows. The fracture plane also traverses the synaptic space. Dimples on the presynaptic membrane represent exocytotic or endocytotic events occurring during fixation. Several dimples abut on, or are very close to, the active zones. Original magnification ×120 000. (From Engel, 2004, with permission.)

estimated that exocytosis of a single vesicle requires the opening of >60 Ca^{2+} channels and the entry of ~13 000 Ca^{2+} ions into the nerve terminal (Borst and Sakmann, 1996).

The voltage-gated Ca^{2+} channels at mammalian NMJs are predominantly of the P/Q type; a lesser number of L-type channels are also present at the mouse NMJ (Urbano and Uchitel, 1999), and N-type Ca^{2+} channels are transiently expressed at the neonatal rat NMJ (Siri and Uchitel, 1999). The P/Q channels consist of a pore-forming α_{1A} subunit, a partly extracellular $\alpha_2\delta$ subunit, a transmembrane γ subunit, and an intracellular β subunit. P/Q channels differ from N-type channels, which contain an α_{1B} subunit, and from L-type channels, which contain α_{1C} or α_{1D} subunits. Unlike the N- and L-type channels, the P/Q channels are selectively sensitive to ω-agatoxin IVA (<10 nM for the P-type channel and >10 nM for the Q-type channel) but are insensitive to dihydropyridines (Birnbaumer et al., 1994). All types of α_1 subunits are composed of four conserved and homologous transmembrane domains (I–IV) linked by nonconserved intracellular hydrophilic loops. The cytoplasmic loop ($L_{II–III}$) between homologous domains II and III of the α_{1A} subunit of the P/Q channel interacts in a Ca^{2+}-dependent manner with t-SNAREs syntaxin and SNAP-25 (Rettig et al., 1996), with vesicular synaptotagmin (Charvin et al., 1997), and CSP (Leveque et al., 1998). Each molecule binds to a specific "synprint" (an acronym for synaptic protein interaction) sequence on

the $L_{II–III}$ loop. The sequential and Ca^{2+}-dependent interactions of the t-SNAREs and synaptotagmin with Ca^{2+}-synprints may play a role in the cascade of reactions leading to vesicle docking and fusion (Sheng et al., 1998).

An immune-mediated downregulation of the number of presynaptic voltage-gated Ca^{2+} channels results in the Lambert–Eaton myasthenic syndrome (see Chapter 9). An electrophysiologically similar syndrome also occurs in a congenital setting. Here the defect could reside in the presynaptic voltage-gated Ca^{2+} channels, any of the SNARE components, or in other molecules that regulate exocytosis (see Chapter 10).

3.3.7.1. Voltage-gated K^+ channels of the presynaptic membrane

At mammalian motor nerve endings, the voltage-gated Na^+ channels disappear between the last node of Ranvier and the point where the terminal axon becomes associated with the NMJ (see Fig. 3.3). Therefore, the presynaptic membrane harbors K^+ and Ca^{2+} channels, but not Na^+ channels (Brigant and Mallart, 1982; Boudier et al., 1988), and the depolarizing current that reaches the presynaptic membrane originates from a preterminal nerve branch. The voltage-gated K^+ channels of the presynaptic membrane are rapidly acting delayed rectifiers that close the voltage-gated Ca^{2+} channels by restoring the resting membrane potential. Consequently, a deficiency of the presynaptic K^+ channels, as in patients with neuromyotonia (see Chapter 14), or their blockage by 3,4-diaminopyridine, prolong Ca^{2+} influx into the depolarized nerve terminal and enhance quantal release (see Chapters 9 and 10).

3.3.8. Morphologic correlates of quantal transmitter release

Depolarization of the nerve terminal by lanthanum (Heuser and Miledi, 1971) or facilitation of quantal release by black widow spider venom (Clark et al., 1972) markedly accelerate quantal ACh release as shown by a marked increase of the MEPP frequency. After a prolonged period of increased quantal release, the nerve terminal increases in size, the synaptic vesicles become depleted, and the MEPPs become less frequent and then disappear. After a long period of exposure to lanthanum many cisternae and small vacuoles, and numerous coated vesicles, appear in the nerve terminal (Heuser and Miledi, 1971).

Electric stimulation of the frog nerve terminal at 10 Hz for 1 min causes a 30% decrease in synaptic vesicle density, which is balanced by a corresponding increase in presynaptic membrane length. If stimulation is continued for 15 min, synaptic vesicle density decreases by 60% and numerous membrane bound cisternae appear within the nerve terminal (Heuser and Reese, 1973). After rest for 15 min the synaptic vesicles reappear and the cisternae become less numerous. If stimulation is in the presence of peroxidase, the marker appears in coated vesicles, larger cisternae, and in synaptic vesicles in this sequence (Heuser and Reese, 1973). Finally, evidence for synaptic vesicle exocytosis and endocytosis has been obtained by the stimulation of nerve terminals containing synaptic vesicles labeled with a fluorescent, lipid-soluble dye (Betz and Bewick, 1992, 1993; Betz et al., 1992). These experiments are consistent with the notion that ACh quanta reside in synaptic vesicles; that quantal release is by vesicle exocytosis; that membrane added to the axolemma during exocytosis is retrieved by endocytosis; and that cisternae and vacuoles in the nerve terminal represent transient sites of membrane storage.

In another study, stimulation of the frog nerve terminal for 3–4.5 h at 2 Hz significantly decreased the MEPP amplitude and quantal release without depleting the synaptic vesicles. Stimulation for 20 min at 10 Hz reduced not only the MEPP amplitude, but also depleted the synaptic vesicles (Ceccarelli et al., 1973). These findings are still consistent with the vesicle hypothesis but indicate that during prolonged low-frequency stimulation the resynthesis or packaging of ACh diminishes before the formation of new synaptic vesicles is affected. This can also be inferred from the lack of synaptic vesicle depletion when vesicular ACh stores are reduced by stimulation in the presence of hemicholinium-3 (Gorio et al., 1978).

Further evidence that synaptic vesicle exocytosis accompanies quantal release has come from capturing synaptic vesicle openings during stimulated transmitter release by 1. immersion of the NMJ in a dilute aldehyde fixative during electric stimulation (Heuser et al., 1974) (Fig. 3.8); 2. immersion of the NMJ in cool, dilute fixative containing sucrose or 20 mM KCl (Pécot-Dechavassine, 1982); 3. pretreatment of the NMJ with 4-aminopyridine (an agent that augments quantal release by nerve impulse), followed by a single electric shock, followed by ultra-rapid freezing of the NMJ within a few ms, followed either by freeze-fracture or by freeze-substitution fixation and thin sectioning (Heuser, 1977; Heuser, 1978; Heuser et al., 1979; Heuser and Reese, 1981). Under these conditions, exocytotic figures appear immediately adjacent to the active zones. These images are omega-shaped in thin sections and appear as dimples in the freeze-fractured presynaptic membrane P-face (Fig. 3.8).

In the presence of 4-aminopyridine a single electric shock discharges 3000–6000 synaptic vesicles from each nerve terminal. Exocytosis begins as soon as 2.5 ms after the stimulus, the vesicles fuse with the axolemma at the same time as the quanta are released, and the number of exocytotic figures corresponds to the estimated number of quanta released (Heuser et al., 1979; Torri-Tarrelli et al., 1985). Membrane sites where exocytosis had occurred are marked by clusters of two to four large intramembrane particles that derive from the concave cytoplasmic fracture face of the original synaptic vesicle (Heuser et al., 1979; Heuser and Reese, 1981). This is excellent evidence that the synaptic vesicles collapse into the presynaptic membrane rather than open and close at the same site (Heuser et al., 1979). Finally, there is convincing immunocytochemical evidence that synaptic vesicle membrane-specific antigens become incorporated into the presynaptic membrane during stimulated vesicle exocytosis (von Wedel et al., 1981; Valtorta et al., 1988a, b).

3.3.9. Endocytotic events and the formation of new synaptic vesicles

Following the exocytotic release of ACh, the membrane of the synaptic vesicle is retrieved from the presynaptic membrane. Paradoxically, the rate of endocytosis is reduced by the increased cytosolic Ca^{2+} concentration that occurs immediately after prolonged or repetitive stimulation (Matthews, 1996). Two major mechanisms of vesicle retrieval have been proposed. The first model postulates clathrin-mediated endocytotic uptake of the vesicular membrane either directly from the presynaptic membrane or from endosomal intermediates and away from the sites into which the vesicles collapsed during exocytosis (Heuser and Reese, 1973; Heuser, 1980b). Consistent with this is the increase in coated vesicles in the nerve terminal after increased transmitter release. A second clathrin-independent, or "kiss-and-run," model postulated rapid closure of a transient exocytotic fusion pore and ultra-fast retrieval of the synaptic vesicle. This model allows the vesicle to retain its identity, and remain in the pool of vesicles near the active zone (von Wedel et al., 1981; Valtorta et al., 1988a). So far, there is no convincing evidence for kiss-and-run endocytosis at the frog or mammalian NMJ. At the frog NMJ vesicles released from the recycling pool are endocytosed directly from the presynaptic membrane and rejoin the recycling pool; vesicles released from the reserve pool are recaptured by slow endocytosis that proceeds through formation of infoldings of the presynaptic membrane and formation of endosomal vacuoles from which vesicles are pinched off to join the reserve pool (Wilkinson and Cole, 2001; Richards et al., 2002,

2003; Rizzoli and Betz, 2004). Both mechanisms are clathrin dependent (Voglmaier et al., 2006). Clathrin-mediated endocytosis is also the dominant mechanism at hippocampal synapses (Granseth et al., 2006).

The major steps in the clathrin-mediated endocytosis at the NMJ are now well understood (De Camilli and Takei, 1996; Brodin et al., 1997; Murthy and De Camilli, 2003). First, the adaptor protein AP2 is recruited to the synaptic vesicle-derived patch of the presynaptic membrane; this results from the binding of AP2 to the C2B domain of vesicular synaptotagmin. Different residues in the C2B domain of synaptotagmin affect the rate of endocytosis and control the size of the synaptic vesicles (Poskanzer et al., 2006). Next, AP2 molecules form a lattice over the patch and recruit three-legged clathrin building blocks (triskelions) (Schmidt et al., 1984; Ungewickell, 1984). Another adaptor protein, AP180, also promotes clathrin cage formation and, in addition, affects the size of the synaptic vesicle by defining the amount of presynaptic membrane retrieved into clathrin cages during endocytosis (Zhang et al., 1998). In a process that requires ATP hydrolysis and GTP, the triskelions assemble into a polygonal network that invaginates a membrane patch that becomes a coated pit (De Camilli and Takei, 1996; Brodin et al., 1997). Complete separation of the coated pit from the presynaptic membrane begins with the amphiphysin-assisted assembly of dynamin molecules at the neck of the coated pit (David et al., 1996; Wigge et al., 1997). The dynamin molecules first form a choke ring, and then effect fission of the coated pit in a GTP-dependent way. In the last step, an uncoating ATPase denudes the internalized vesicle by dismantling its clathrin coat (Schmidt et al., 1984).

3.4. The synaptic space

The synaptic space is situated between the presynaptic and postsynaptic membranes. The space is somewhat arbitrarily divided into a primary and a number of secondary clefts. The primary cleft is limited by the presynaptic membrane on one side and, on the opposite side, by an imaginary plane tangential to the terminal expansions of the junctional folds (Figs. 3.4, 3.5 and 3.10). It is approximately 70 nm wide and its length is coextensive with that of the presynaptic membrane. The primary cleft lacks lateral boundaries except basement membrane and, therefore, communicates with the extracellular space. The secondary clefts are spaces between the junctional folds, and each secondary cleft communicates with the primary cleft (Figs. 3.1, 3.4, 3.8 and 3.9). At the frog NMJ, secondary cleft openings are in register with the overlying presynaptic active zones (Fig. 3.8). A similar arrangement also

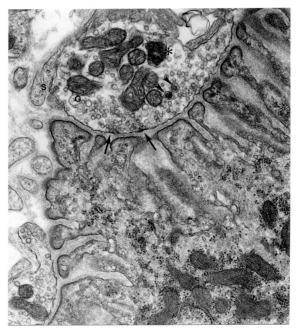

Fig. 3.10. Electron micrograph of a normal neuromuscular junction. The nerve terminal contains mitochondria, small clear synaptic vesicles, giant synaptic vesicles (G), dense-core vesicles (arrowheads), agglutinated vesicles surrounded by membrane (asterisk) and active zones (arrows) in register with the secondary synaptic clefts. The terminal expansions of the junctional folds are covered by dense postsynaptic specializations. Numerous microtubules, other tubular and vesicular structures, ribosomes, and pinocytotic vesicles can be observed in the junctional folds. The junctional sarcoplasm contains abundant mitochondria, rough and smooth-surfaced endoplasmic reticulum, microtubules, and abundant microfilaments. S, Schwann cell process. Original magnification ×40 400. (From Engel, 2004, with permission.)

exists at the mammalian NMJ (Fukunaga et al., 1982) (Fig. 3.9). Finger-like extensions of Schwann cell cytoplasm cover small segments of the presynaptic membrane, isolating it from the synaptic space. These extensions appear at varying intervals between the active zones and are more frequent and regularly spaced at the frog than at the mammalian NMJ. The transverse tubules of the muscle fiber extend to, and open into, the secondary synaptic clefts (Zacks and Saito, 1970).

The synaptic space is occupied by the synaptic basal lamina, which harbor numerous molecular components that regulate the formation and maintenance of the NMJ as described below.

3.5. The synaptic basal lamina

In conventionally fixed and embedded NMJs a layer of basement membrane covers both the pre- and postsynaptic membranes (Figs. 3.1 and 3.4). A different image appears with quick freezing followed either by freeze-substitution fixation and thin sectioning, or by freeze-fracture, deep-etching and rotary shadowing. The center of the synaptic cleft is occupied by a feathery 10–15 nm lamina from which wisps of material extend laterally toward both the pre- and postsynaptic membranes. In the primary synaptic cleft these extensions form bridges between the two opposed membranes (Heuser, 1980a).

The synaptic basal lamina plays an important role in NMJ development and regeneration, and in specifying the molecular architecture and physiologic properties of the pre- and postsynaptic membranes. Thus, the synaptic basal lamina contains factors that guide regenerating nerve terminals to previously denervated NMJs, induce physiologic and morphologic maturation of the nerve terminal even in the absence of the muscle fiber, and induce regeneration of the junctional folds and insertion of AChR into the folds even in the absence of the nerve terminal (Sanes et al., 1978; Burden et al., 1979; Glicksman and Sanes, 1983; McMahan and Slater, 1984; Hall and Sanes, 1993; Sanes, 2003).

The inductive and regulatory properties of the synaptic basal lamina depend on its molecular components. The synapse-specific components of the basal lamina include laminins, asymmetric AChE collagen, heparan sulfate proteoglycan, β-N-acetylgalactosamine (βGalNAc)-terminated glycoconjugates, and nerve-derived agrin and neuregulin (Sanes, 1995; Patton et al., 1997; Meier et al., 1998). Agrin and neuregulin will be discussed further in Section 3.7.5.

3.5.1. Asymmetric AChE

The synaptic basal lamina harbors the EP-specific asymmetric species of AChE at a density of ~2000 to $3000/\mu m^2$ (Salpeter, 1987). Asymmetric AChE consists of 1, 2, or 3 homotetrameric catalytic subunits ($AChE_T$) attached to a collagenic tail subunit formed by the triple helical association of three collagen-like strands, ColQ (Massoulié et al., 1993). ColQ has two major functions: it binds tetramers of $AChE_T$, and it anchors the enzyme to the synaptic basal lamina. An N-terminal proline-rich attachment domain of ColQ binds $AChE_T$ (Bon et al., 1997). Anchorage of the asymmetric enzyme in the synaptic space is assured by two cationic heparan sulfate proteoglycan binding domains within the collagen domain (Deprez and Inestrosa, 1995) together with essential residues in the C-terminal domain of ColQ (Ohno et al., 2000; Kimbell et al., 2004). The tail subunit is anchored to the synaptic basal lamina by two binding partners: the heparan sulfate proteoglycan perlecan (Arikawa-Hirasawa

et al., 2002), which, in turn, binds to α-dystroglycan, and by the extracellular domain of the muscle-specific kinase MuSK (Cartaud et al., 2004). Association with these binding partners predicts close proximity of the extracellular asymmetric enzyme to the postsynaptic membrane. The turnover rate of synaptic AChE is similar to that of AChR. Synaptic AChEs and AChRs removed from synapses colocalize in the same intracellular pool after being internalized (Krejci et al., 2006). Recessive mutations in ColQ cause disabling congenital myasthenic syndromes (see Chapter 10).

3.5.2. Synaptic laminins

Laminins are cruciform, heterotrimeric, ~1000 kDa glycoproteins composed of a central α and flanking β and γ subunits. The three identified NMJ-specific laminins, laminin-4 (α2β2γ1), laminin-9 (α4β2γ1), and laminin-11 (α5β2γ1), contain β2 subunits associated with different α and γ subunits. Laminin-9 is restricted to the primary synaptic cleft, whereas laminin-11 lines both the primary and secondary clefts. Laminins play multiple roles in the development and maintenance of the NMJ:

1. Extrajunctional laminins, and probably tenascin and fibronectin, together with junctional laminin-4, guide growing axons to the NMJ where junctional laminin-11 stops axon growth (Patton et al., 1997).
2. Laminin-11 actively prevents Schwann cells from entering the synaptic cleft (Patton et al., 1998).
3. Both synaptic and extrasynaptic laminins bind to α-dystroglycan (α-DG), the extracellular component of the dystrophin/utrophin-associated transmembrane glycoprotein complex that links the extracellular matrix to the intracellular cytoskeleton. The attachment of synaptic laminins to the postsynaptic cytoskeleton may contribute to the immobilization of AChR at the NMJ (Jacobson et al., 1998).
4. Junctional laminin-4 and extrajunctional laminin-2 (α2β1γ1) bind to the N-terminal domain of agrin and anchor it to the basal lamina (Denzer et al., 1997).
5. Laminin-1, present in very early muscle development, induces clustering of both α-DG (Cohen et al., 1997) and AChR (Sugiyama et al., 1997) independently of agrin. This could be a supplemental pathway for AChR clustering during myogenesis but it does not occur at the mature NMJ (Sugiyama et al., 1997).
6. Mice with targeted deletion of the β2-laminin gene fail to express the β2 and α5 subunits of

laminin, show simplified terminal branching of presynaptic motor axons, paucity of presynaptic active zones, no clustering of the synaptic vesicles at the active zones, decreased spontaneous and evoked quantal release, and increased intrusion of Schwann cell processes into the primary synaptic cleft (Noakes et al., 1995; Patton et al., 1997; Knight et al., 2003). Homozygous mutants are weak, suffer from severe proteinuria, and die 15–25 days after birth.

7. In detergent-solubilized synaptosomes of the fish electric organ, laminin-9 co-immunoprecipitates with the voltage-gated calcium channel and cytoskeletal spectrin. This suggests that laminin-9 links the synaptic basal lamina to the calcium channel, which in turn is attached by its α subunit to cytosolic spectrin in the nerve terminal. Spectrin then could play a role organizing synaptic vesicle clusters by binding to vesicle associated proteins (Sunderland et al., 2000).

3.6. The postsynaptic region

3.6.1. The junctional folds

The postsynaptic region consists of junctional folds and junctional sarcoplasm (Figs. 3.1 and 3.10). Junctional folds are found at no other synapse except the NMJ. At synapses that lack junctional folds the surface areas of the pre- and postsynaptic membranes are essentially identical. The junctional folds produce a severalfold amplification of the postsynaptic surface. For example, morphometric studies of human external intercostal (Engel and Santa, 1971) and rat limb muscles (Santa and Engel, 1973; Engel et al., 1976) show that the mean ratio of postsynaptic to presynaptic membrane areas ranges from 8:1 to 10:1, and the mean postsynaptic membrane profile density ranges from 5.8 $\mu m/m^2$ to 6.4 $\mu m/m^2$. Because the junctional folds are separated by secondary synaptic clefts, they also increase the volume of the synaptic space.

The degree of development, complexity and dimensions of the junctional folds varies according to species, stage of development, type of innervation, type of nerve ending, and muscle fiber type. For example, junctional folds are absent at newly formed NMJs and are relatively shallow or absent on multiply innervated muscle fibers (e.g., some extrafusal fibers in extraocular, facial, lingual, and laryngeal muscles, and some intrafusal fibers) (Bennett, 1983; Pachter, 1983). In mammals, fast twitch (type 2B) muscle fibers have better developed junctional folds than slow twitch (type 1) muscle fibers, but in humans these differences are difficult to discern (Engel, 1994).

The three-dimensional disposition of the junctional folds can be determined from serial sections (Anderson-Cedergren, 1959) or by scanning electron microscopy (Shotton et al., 1979; Desaki and Uehara, 1981; Fahim et al., 1983, 1984; Ogata and Yamasaki, 1985). At the linear frog NMJ the folds appear as a series of parallel ridges perpendicular to the long axis of the synaptic gutter. The folds become narrow and shallow at the end of the synaptic gutter, and are irregular near the entry of the axon into the synaptic groove (Shotton et al., 1979). At the mammalian NMJ the junctional folds lack regular orientation with respect to the long axis of the muscle fiber (Anderson-Cedergren, 1959; Desaki and Uehara, 1981), but the crests of the folds still tend to be oriented more or less perpendicularly to the long axis of the irregularly curving synaptic gutter (Fahim et al., 1983, 1984) (Fig. 3.11).

The junctional folds contain a varying complement of pinocytotic and other vesicles, small tubules and cisternae, microtubules, finer filaments, scattered ribosomes, and infrequent glycogen granules (Figs. 3.1 and 3.10). Some of the tubulovesicular structures in the folds are secondary lysosomes (Fumagalli et al., 1982). Coated vesicles appear in the junctional sarcoplasm during synaptogenesis, but are absent from the mature junctional folds.

The sarcolemma lining the terminal expansions of the junctional folds is packed with AChRs (10 000 receptors/μm^2) (Matthews-Bellinger and Salpeter, 1978) and also contains rapsyn, integrins, MuSK, ErbB receptors, and N-acetylgalactosaminyl transferase (Fischbach and Rosen, 1997). The troughs of the junctional folds are enriched in neural cell adhesion molecule (NCAM), and in voltage-sensitive Na^+ channels. The Na^+ channels are tethered to the membrane by ankyrin G and β-spectrin (Flucher and Daniels, 1989; Wood and Slater, 1998), and are linked to the cytoskeleton by syntrophins (Gee et al., 1998). The cytoskeletal components of the folds include utrophin as well as dystrophin, both linked to isoforms of dystrobrevin and syntrophin, and via β- and α-dystroglycans to the extracellular matrix (Flucher and Daniels, 1989; Hall and Sanes, 1993; Fischbach and Rosen, 1997; Sanes et al., 1998a) (see Fig. 3.12).

3.6.1.1. Functional significance of the junctional folds

The junctional folds enhance the safety margin of neuromuscular transmission by three mechanisms: 1. The terminal expansions and upper part of the stalks of the folds are "parking lots" for AChRs, increasing the surface harboring AChR ~3-fold over that available at synapses without junctional folds (Engel, 1994). 2. The folds increase the series resistance of the postsynaptic membrane, and thus enhance the

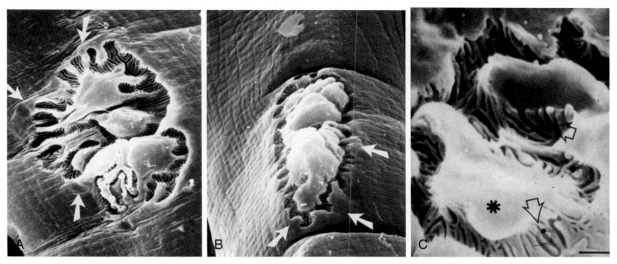

Fig. 3.11. Scanning electron micrograph of a NMJ of the mouse extensor digitorum muscle. (A and B). The elliptically shaped NMJ is surrounded by a raised area that corresponds to the underlying junctional sarcoplasm (arrows). The nerve terminal capped by Schwann cells hides most underlying junctional folds. (C). The junctional folds in the synaptic gutter become visible after the nerve terminal has been stripped from the junction. The folds are oriented perpendicularly to the long axis of the irregularly curving synaptic gutter. ×10 000. These micrographs were prepared by Dr. M.A. Fahim. (A and B are from Fahim et al., 1983; C is from Fahim et al., 1984, with permission.)

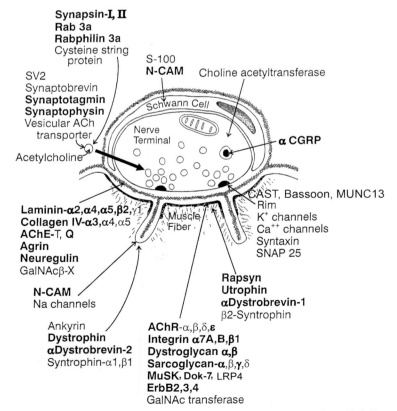

Fig. 3.12. Key molecular components of the neuromuscular junction. Most components for which "knock-out" mice have been generated are indicated in bold face. Additional components are described in the text. (Adapted from Sanes et al., 1998a, with permission.)

depolarization produced by the EPP (Martin, 1994). 3. A high concentration of AChRs on crests of the folds (Matthews-Bellinger and Salpeter, 1978) and of sodium channels in the depth of the folds (Flucher and Daniels, 1989; Ruff, 1996) ensures that the depolarizing effect of the EPP is greatest where the sodium channels are concentrated at high density (Martin, 1994; Wood and Slater, 2001). The combined effects of these mechanisms increase the safety factor of neuromuscular transmission at least 2- to 4-fold.

3.6.2. The acetylcholine receptor

The postsynaptic membrane on the terminal expansions of the junctional folds is thicker and denser than elsewhere, and its cytoplasmic surface is lined by a 20–40 nm layer of fuzzy material (Figs. 3.1 and 3.9). This subsynaptic density corresponds to the location of AChR and its cytoskeletal supporting elements.

AChR, localized with ^{125}I-αBGT (Matthews-Bellinger and Salpeter, 1983) or peroxidase-labeled αBGT (Engel et al., 1977), is concentrated on the terminal expansions of the folds where the electron dense thickened portions of the folds are located. At the mouse NMJ, the maximal concentration of αBGT binding sites is close to 20 000/μm^2, indicating the presence

of half as many AChR molecules per unit membrane area (Matthews-Bellinger and Salpeter, 1978). The binding site density on the junctional folds decreases to 3% of the peak value halfway down the folds, and is only 4% of the peak value on the extrajunctional muscle fiber surface at a distance of 1 μm from the edge of the nerve terminal (Fertuck and Salpeter, 1976). Although the autoradiographic method cannot exclude the presence of a small amount of presynaptic AChR, at least 95% of NMJ AChR is postsynaptic (Matthews-Bellinger and Salpeter, 1978). Further, no BGT binding is found on the nerve terminal when it is dissociated from the postsynaptic region (Jones and Salpeter, 1983).

Peroxidase labeled αBGT gives more precise light microscopic (Fig. 3.13) and ultrastructural (Fig. 3.14) localization of AChR than autoradiography with ^{125}I-αBGT. The peroxidase method reveals AChR on the terminal expansions of the junctional folds and for a variable distance along the stalks of the folds (Daniels and Vogel, 1975) (Fig. 3.14). Fainter reaction product also appears on the presynaptic membrane and Schwann cell processes facing reactive segments of the junctional folds. The staining of Schwann cell processes strongly suggests that any presynaptic localization is a diffusion artifact. That localization

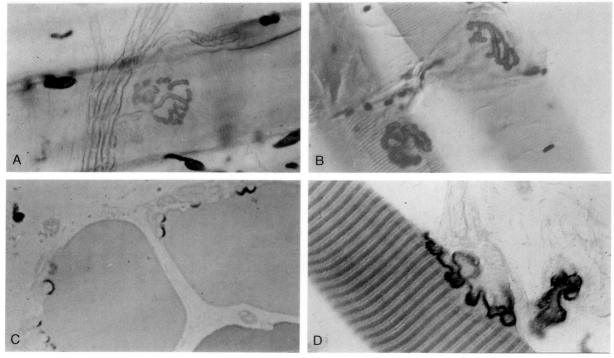

Fig. 3.13. Light microscopy visualization of AChR on dissected muscle fibers (A, B) and in transverse (C) and longitudinal (D) sections. Nerve fibers near the NMJ are seen in A, B, and D. A, B ×400; C, D ×1000. (From Engel, 2004, with permission.)

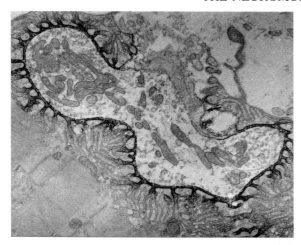

Fig. 3.14. Ultrastructural localization of AChR with peroxidase labeled αBGT. The electron dense reaction product is localized on terminal expansions of the junctional folds and extends onto the stalks of the folds. Original magnification ×18 400. (From Engel, 2004, with permission.)

of extracellular antigens by the immunoperoxidase procedure is associated with diffusion artifact is now well established (Courtoy et al., 1983).

At the human external intercostal NMJ approximately 30% of the postsynaptic membrane reacts for AChR (Engel et al., 1977). The length of the postsynaptic membrane reacting for AChR, normalized by the length of the primary synaptic cleft, gives a measure, or index, of the relative abundance of AChR at a NMJ. At the normal human NMJ the average AChR index is close to 3 (Engel et al., 1977). This means that the junctional folds increase the ACh-receptive membrane surface for each nerve terminal and each active zone. If the junctional folds are absent, as is the case at some NMJs, the AChR index must be <1 and the ACh receptive surface per nerve terminal, and per active zone, is only one-third or less of that found at NMJs with well-developed junctional folds.

Freeze-fracture studies of the NMJ demonstrate large (10- to 12-nm) intramembrane particles packed in double parallel rows on the P-face of the junctional folds (Dreyer et al., 1973; Heuser et al., 1974; Rash and Ellisman, 1974; Ellisman et al., 1976; Rash, 1983) (Figs. 3.15 and 3.16). This arrangement is probably secondary to dimerization of AChRs through their δ-subunit (Brisson and Unwin, 1984). The distribution of the particles is like that of αBGT binding sites, but the maximal particle density is one-half of that expected from ^{125}I-αBGT binding studies. However, the superior quick-freeze, deep-etch, rotary replication method reveals the expected maximal concentration of

10 000 particles/μm^2 on the outside surface of the postsynaptic membrane at the *Torpedo* electroplaque synapse (Heuser and Salpeter, 1979) and at the rat (Grohovaz et al., 1982; Hirokawa and Heuser, 1982), snake, and frog (Hirokawa and Heuser, 1982) NMJ. This value corresponds to the best autoradiographic and electrophysiologic estimates of the peak AChR packing density (Matthews-Bellinger and Salpeter, 1978; Heuser and Salpeter, 1979).

3.6.2.1. Structure–function correlations

The positioning of the presynaptic active zones in relation to the junctional folds (Figs. 3.8, 3.9 and 3.15), the density (10 000/μm^2) and distribution of AChRs on the terminal expansions of the junctional folds, and the lower density (2000–3000/μm^2) but uniform distribution of AChE in the synaptic basal lamina provide for effective interaction between the ACh quantum and a disk-like region of the postsynaptic membrane. These features form the basis of the "saturating disk model" of neuromuscular transmission (Matthews-Bellinger and Salpeter, 1978; Salpeter, 1987). ACh concentration is highest at the exocytotic site and gradually decreases as ACh spreads in the synaptic space. By the time ACh reaches the junctional folds its average concentration (about 3 mM) is still sufficiently high to swamp AChE and also hinder the action of AChE by substrate inhibition. ACh only needs to spread over a distance of 0.3 μm along the top and the same distance down the side of the folds before it encounters the number of AChRs it can saturate. These factors favor the occurrence of most collisions between ACh and AChR within a few microseconds after quantal release and account for the short rise time of the quantal conductance change. After ACh dissociates from AChR it diffuses laterally into the primary and radially into the secondary clefts and its concentration decreases. The depths of the secondary clefts, with sparse AChR (Figs. 3.14–3.16) and abundant AChE, serve as cul de sacs for trapping and hydrolyzing ACh, and for trapping choline so that most of it can be taken up by the nerve terminal. Further, as mentioned above in Section 3.6.1.1, the alternating arrangement of voltage-sensitive sodium channels in the troughs and of AChR on the crests of the junctional folds facilitates the initiation of the action potential (Flucher and Daniels, 1989).

The small size of the saturating disks of AChR assures that they do not overlap, and that only a small proportion of all available disks is saturated with ACh when up to several hundred quanta are released by a nerve impulse. Since the active zone sites that release ACh are discrete and vary from impulse to impulse (Heuser et al., 1974, 1979; Heuser and Reese, 1977,

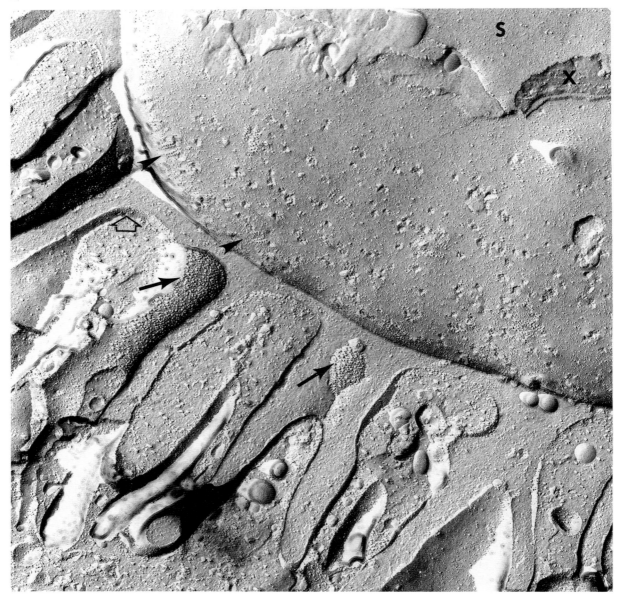

Fig. 3.15. Freeze-fractured human NMJ. The fracture plane traverses Schwann cell P face (S) and interior (X), the P face of the presynaptic membrane, the synaptic clef, and P faces (arrows), E faces (open arrow), and the interior of the junctional folds. The presynaptic membrane displays numerous active zones and exocytotic or endocytotic dimples. A number of active zones are in register with the secondary clefts (arrowheads). AChRs are represented by densely packed large particles on P faces of the junctional folds (arrows). The AChR particles extend more than halfway down the stalks of a junctional fold. Original magnification ×50 000. With permission from Engel, 2004.

1981), different sets of disks become saturated on repetitive stimulation. This prevents desensitization of AChR from continued exposure to ACh.

3.6.3. Postsynaptic cytoskeletal components

The junctional folds contain numerous cytoskeletal elements (Froehner, 1991; Hall and Sanes, 1993). Some of

these are topographically related to the AChR macromolecules, whereas others may confer rigidity on the folds. Numerous cytoskeletal proteins have been localized to the postsynaptic region (see Fig. 3.12): rapsyn (Sealock et al., 1984; LaRochelle et al., 1990; Krikorian and Bloch, 1992; Antolik et al., 2006), α1-, β1-, and β2-syntrophins (Ahn et al., 1996; Froehner et al., 1997; Peters et al., 1997), α-dystrobrevins-1 and -2 (Enigk

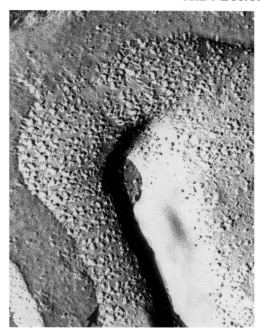

Fig. 3.16. AChR particles on a junctional fold revealed by freeze-fracture and imaged at high resolution. Original magnification ×103 000. With permission from Engel, 2004.

and Maimone, 2001; Newey et al., 2001), tropomyosin 2 (Marazzi et al., 1989), actin (Hall et al., 1981), talin (Sealock et al., 1986), vinculin (Bloch and Hall, 1983; Yorifuji and Hirokawa, 1989), an isoform of β-spectrin (Bloch and Morrow, 1989), paxilin (Turner et al., 1991), filamin (Bloch and Hall, 1983), α-actinin (Bloch and Hall, 1983), ankyrin G (Flucher and Daniels, 1989; Wood and Slater, 1998), desmin (Sealock et al., 1989; Askanas et al., 1990), α-tubulin (Jasmin and Cartaud, 1990), dystrophin (Sealock et al., 1991; Bewick et al., 1992), utrophin (Khurana et al., 1990; Bewick et al., 1992), plectin (Banwell et al., 1999) as well as NCAM, which associates with the postsynaptic spectrin scaffold (Sytnyk et al., 2006). β-amyloid precursor protein and amyloid-β protein are also present in the postsynaptic region, but their relation to the cytoskeleton and their functional significance is unclear (Askanas et al., 1992, 1998).

Although the above components are concentrated at the NMJ, all except rapsyn, utrophin and NCAM are also present extrajunctionally. Clustering of AChRs in the postsynaptic region is initiated by Dok-7, and by MuSK under the influence of neural agrin (discussed in Section 3.7.5).

Rapsyn, present in a 1:1 stoichiometry with AChR, appears early in synaptogenesis and crosslinks AChR at NMJ (Mitra et al., 1989). The molecule has distinct domains for membrane targeting, self-association, and

AChR clustering (Ramarao and Cohen, 1998). Rapsyn is attached to the sarcolemma as well as to the subsynaptic cytoskeleton by binding to the cytoplasmic tail of β-dystroglycan (Cartaud et al., 1998). Seven tetratricopeptide repeats of rapsyn subserve rapsyn self-association (Ramarao and Cohen, 1998) and bind directly to MuSK (Antolik et al., 2006). The coiled-coil domain near the C-terminus of rapsyn binds to AChR, effecting its clustering (Bartoli et al., 2001). Mutations in rapsyn cause endplate AChR deficiency and result in a congenital myasthenic syndrome (Ohno et al., 2002) (see Chapter 10).

Utrophin, an autosomal dystrophin homolog, is closely associated with AChR on the crests of the junctional folds, while dystrophin and Na$^+$ channels, together with β-spectrin and G-ankyrin, are concentrated in the depth of the folds (Bewick et al., 1996; Wood and Slater, 1998). Dystrophin is linked to the actin cytoskeleton, and also to the extracellular matrix via the cytoplasmic tail of β-dystroglycan; it also associates with α1- and β1-syntrophins and with α-dystrobrevin-2 (Peters et al., 1997; Enigk and Maimone, 2001). Syntrophins bind the neuronal form of nitric oxide synthase (nNOS) as well as Na$^+$ channels, and therefore act as modular adaptor proteins (Froehner et al., 1997). Since the density of AChR is not affected in patients with Duchenne dystrophy (Sakakibara et al., 1977), dystrophin does not participate in AChR clustering. Dystrophin, however, may regulate turnover of AChR, for in the dystrophin deficient *mdx* mouse the turnover of AChR is accelerated ($t_{1/2}$ ∼3–5 days instead of ∼10 days) (Xu and Salpeter, 1997). Utrophin, like dystrophin, is linked to the actin cytoskeleton and to the extracellular matrix via β-dystroglycan (Matsumura et al., 1992; Ervasti and Campbell, 1993), and also associates with β1- and β2-syntrophins (Ahn et al., 1996) and α-dystrobrevin-1. The associations of utrophin with cytoskeletal proteins suggest that it plays an important role in the organization of the postsynaptic region and in clustering AChRs on the junctional folds. Utrophin expression at the NMJ is reduced when the density of AChRs at the NMJ is reduced, as in autoimmune myasthenia gravis and in congenital myasthenic syndromes in which AChR expression is reduced (Slater et al., 1997). Utrophin null mice, however, only show mild AChR deficiency and somewhat simplified junctional folds, but no decrease in the packing density of AChR (Deconinck et al., 1997; Grady et al., 1997).

At the mammalian NMJ, high-voltage electron microscopy demonstrates 10-nm filaments that run parallel and at a distance of 50 nm from the AChR-rich portion of the postsynaptic membrane. A network of "connecting" filaments extends from the "parallel" filaments to the dense postsynaptic membrane (Ellisman et al., 1976). The quick-freeze, deep-etch, rotary replication procedure has been applied to the study of the subsynaptic cytoskeleton of the *Torpedo* electroplaque (Heuser and Salpeter, 1979), and to frog, snake and rat NMJs (Heuser and Salpeter, 1979; Hirokawa and Heuser, 1982; Yorifuji and Hirokawa, 1989). This approach reveals a sub-membranous meshwork of short, thin strands, which connects with more deeply positioned intermediate filaments that course parallel to the postsynaptic folds (Hirokawa and Heuser, 1982; Yorifuji and Hirokawa, 1989). If taxol is also used during the preparatory procedure, microtubules are often observed among the intermediate filaments (Hirokawa and Heuser, 1982). The thin strands and intermediate filaments in these preparations correspond to the "connecting" and "parallel" filaments, respectively, observed by high-voltage electron microscopy.

Although the biochemical identity and precise connections of the subsynaptic cytoskeleton are still not fully understood, the following scheme appears probable at the present time:

1. The AChRs are kept in compact arrays by a cross-linking network. This includes rapsyn that links AChRs via β-dystroglycan to utrophin, which is linked to actin, α2-syntrophin, and dystrobrevin.
2. The cross-linking network is in contact with, and is probably stabilized by, a network of spectrin tetramers which, in turn, are linked to actin oligomers (Bloch and Morrow, 1989). These components may be part of the 20–40 nm thick layer of fuzzy material that lines the AChR-rich portions of the postsynaptic membrane in routine preparations.
3. The meshwork of fine filaments is supported by a network of intermediate filaments and microtubules located in the deeper regions of the junctional folds.

3.6.4. The junctional sarcoplasm

In a longitudinally oriented fiber and with the NMJ on the upper surface of the fiber, the junctional sarcoplasm is limited inferiorly by the myofibrils; superiorly it extends to, and is continuous with, the base of the junctional folds and/or is limited by sarcolemma between adjacent junctional regions. In the scanning electron microscope, the presence of junctional sarcoplasm is indicated by a mound-like elevation beneath and/or around the synaptic gutter (Fahim et al., 1984) (Fig. 3.11). The amount of junctional sarcoplasm differs between different NMJs, and even between different regions at a given NMJ.

The junctional sarcoplasm contains a varying complement of mitochondria, smooth and rough endoplasmic reticulum, Golgi cisternae, lysosomal structures, small clear vesicles, microtubules, intermediate filaments, and scattered glycogen granules (Fig. 3.10). The region is traversed by transverse tubules that open into the secondary synaptic clefts. The known metabolic functions of the junctional sarcoplasm include the synthesis and degradation of AChR, synthesis of the end-plate specific species of AChE, and regulation of the subsynaptic ionic milieu. Multiple nuclei are adjacent to, or intermingle with, the junctional sarcoplasm at each NMJ (Fig. 3.1). At the mature NMJ, subsynaptic nuclei are specialized to selectively transcribe mRNA for AChR subunits and for other NMJ-specific proteins (Klarsfeld et al., 1991; Sanes et al., 1991; Simon et al., 1992). In mature muscle fibers, AChR gene expression is spatially restricted to the subsynaptic nuclei (Simon et al., 1992). The junctional sarcoplasm is also immunoreactive for cellular prion protein, ApoE, ubiquitin, superoxide dismutase, transforming growth factor -β1, and interleukins 1α, 1β and 6 (Askanas et al., 1998). The biological significance of these proteins at the NMJ is not known.

3.6.4.1. AChR synthesis and degradation

AChR synthesis has not been studied in detail at the mature NMJ; however, it probably resembles that described in model cell systems (Green, 1999; Keller and Taylor, 1999). AChR subunit messenger RNAs are inserted into endoplasmic reticulum (ER) membrane; the nascent peptides within the ER are cotranslationally glycosylated and undergo initial rapid folding. The nascent peptides are protected against degradation by chaperones, such as calnexin. Next, slower folding reactions and other types of processing, such as disulfide bond formation and proline isomerization, take place to allow oligomerization with other subunits. Amino acids positioned at homologous sites at subunit interfaces direct partnering during assembly of the pentameric receptor. The assembly process is not very efficient; it extends over 2–3 hours and only 20–30% of the synthesized subunits are assembled. The assembled receptor exits the ER to pass through Golgi cisternae and reaches the surface membrane along the secretory pathway on lipid rafts (Marchand et al., 2002). Unassembled subunits and intermediates dissociate from calnexin, become polyubiquinated at exposed lysines, enter the cytoplasm, and are degraded in proteasomes.

Observation of NMJs of living mice by reflected-light confocal microscopy over several days combined with periodic laser-flash induced unbinding of fluorescent BGTs from AChRs reveals that 1. extrajunctional receptors migrate into the postsynaptic membrane; 2. receptors within the postsynaptic membrane migrate from one spot to another, both directly and by moving in and out of the membrane; 3. AChRs are maintained for only ~8 h in any one spot. Thus during their 8–14 day half-life at the mature NMJ, AChRs display a remarkable wanderlust. In mice lacking α-dystrobrevin, the rates of AChR turnover and intermingling are increased ~4- to 5-fold. Thus, α-dystrobrevin emerges as a critical regulator of AChR mobility and turnover (Akaaboune et al., 2002).

The macroscopic half-life of AChR at the mature NMJ is approximately 8–14 days (Salpeter and Harris, 1983; Shyng and Salpeter, 1990). The loss of labeled AChR is monoexponential, indicating that the probability of degradation is the same for all NMJ AChRs. If any receptors turn over more rapidly than others, then their number must be less than 50 sites/μm^2 (Salpeter and Harris, 1983). AChR removal occurs randomly at a given NMJ (Weinberg et al., 1981) and on a given junctional fold (Fumagalli et al., 1982).

When rat forelimb NMJ AChR is labeled in vivo with peroxidase-labeled BGT, the degradative pathway of AChR can be monitored by electron microscopy (Fumagalli et al., 1982). Membrane segments containing AChR are internalized by endocytotic invagination (Fig. 3.17A–C). The labeled vesicles merge with other membrane-bound vesicles, tubules, saccules, or cisternae within the junctional folds and in the junctional sarcoplasm (Fig. 3.17C and D). Most of the membrane-bound structures containing the internalized label are lysosomes that react for both acid phosphatase and internalized AChR (Fig. 3.17E), and a lysosomal network of tubules and vesicles is present throughout the junctional folds and junctional sarcoplasm. These morphologic findings indicate that NMJ AChR is internalized by endocytosis and is then rapidly transferred to the lysosomal system where it can be degraded (Fumagalli et al., 1982).

3.7. Synaptogenesis

The developing NMJ provides an unusually favorable system for correlating morphologic and physiologic parameters of development, for investigating trophic interactions between nerve and muscle, and for exploring the developmental regulation and the regulatory effects of the basal lamina, AChR and AChE. Since 1966, the development of chick (Hirano, 1967; Atsumi, 1971; Bennett and Pettigrew, 1974a), frog (Letinsky and Morrison-Graham, 1980), *Xenopus* (Kullberg et al., 1977), rat (Terävainen, 1968; Kelly and Zacks, 1969; Bennett and Pettigrew, 1974a; Dennis et al.,

1981), mouse (Matthews-Bellinger and Salpeter, 1983), and human (Blechschmidt and Daikoku, 1966; Juntunen and Terävainen, 1972) NMJ has been studied in vivo. NMJ formation has also been investigated in organ cultures of fetal rat intercostal muscle (Ziskind-Conhaim and Dennis, 1981) and in cocultures of fetal spinal cord and skeletal muscle obtained from the chick (Frank and Fischbach, 1979), *Xenopus* (Anderson et al., 1977) and mouse (Crain and Peterson, 1974). Recent reviews summarize current understanding of the development of NMJ (Sanes and Lichtman, 1999, 2001; Marques et al., 2000).

3.7.1. General principles

Shortly before myoblasts fuse to form myotubes, developing muscle is penetrated by unmyelinated nerve fibers (Terävainen, 1968). The earliest nerve–muscle contacts occur soon after the appearance of myotubes. The pre- and postnatal developmental steps are similar in different species, but their onset and the intervals between them vary. For example, in human muscle, primitive NMJs appear between the 6th and 10th week (Juntunen and Terävainen, 1972), but in the mouse (Matthews-Bellinger and Salpeter, 1983) and rat (Dennis et al., 1981) they appear between the 14th and 16th day of embryonic life.

In focally innervated muscles (e.g., the rat diaphragm), the initial synaptic contact occurs at random along the length of the short myotube. As a result of subsequent bidirectional longitudinal growth of the myotube, the initial synaptic site eventually falls close to the center of the mature muscle fiber. As development proceeds, each synapse receives polyaxonal innervation that is lost during the latter part of embryonic life and in the early postnatal period (Bennett and Pettigrew, 1974c). In muscles that receive a distributed innervation (e.g., the chick anterior latissimus dorsi), a series of synaptic contacts are established along the length of the early myotube, but the distance between individual synaptic contacts is always greater than 170 μm; each junctional site subsequently receives polyaxonal innervation and then loses it, so that eventually all synaptic contacts on the mature muscle fiber are supplied by a single motor neuron. As the fiber becomes elongated, the spacing between the NMJs increases (Bennett and Pettigrew, 1974a).

3.7.2. The structural development of the NMJ

Kelly and Zacks (1969) described NMJ formation in rat intercostal muscle from day 16 in utero to day 10 postpartum. On day 16, groups of primitive myotubes are in close apposition to clusters of axons. Early

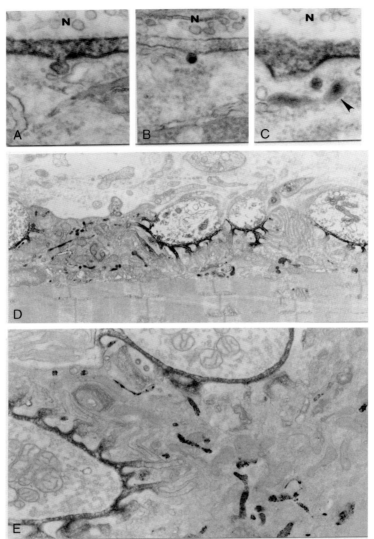

Fig. 3.17. Internalization and lysosomal uptake of AChR at the rat NMJ. The NMJ was labeled in vivo 24 h before biopsy by an intramuscular injection of peroxidase labeled αBGT. The label for AChR is present in panels A to E. Panel C also shows localization of acid phosphatase in the form of punctate highly electron dense granules. In A, B, and C, the nerve terminal (N) is on the top of the panel. Within a few hours after in vivo labeling with αBGT, AChR is present on the junctional folds, in endocytotic invaginations of the postsynaptic membrane (A, B, C) and in a few tubulovesicular structures (arrowhead in C). After 24 h, AChR appears in numerous tubulovesicular structures and larger cisternae in the junctional sarcoplasm (D). The tubulovesicular structures also react for acid phosphatase, indicating that they are lysosomes (E). Original magnification ×25 100. (From Fumagalli et al., 1982, with permission.)

axon–myotube contacts are marked by a shallow depression and a local thickening of the myotube membrane, and traces of basal lamina appear in the rudimentary synaptic space. The axon terminals contain a few clear and some dense-core synaptic vesicles.

On day 18 larger myotubes surrounded by and fusing with smaller myotubes and myoblasts are mutually innervated by clusters of axons. The axon terminals contain an increased number of synaptic vesicles. The synaptic gaps are 50–90 nm wide and are partially filled with basal lamina. AChE activity becomes detectable at the primitive NMJ.

On day 22, when birth occurs, adjacent small and large muscle fibers are mutually innervated by terminal axon networks covered by Schwann cells. The synaptic vesicles are relatively abundant but dense core vesicles are sparse. The primary synaptic clefts are short and the secondary clefts are rudimentary or absent. Incipient junctional sarcoplasm appears beneath or to one side of the postsynaptic membrane.

Ten days postpartum some NMJs begin to look mature. Axon terminals covered by Schwann cells lie in individual synaptic gutters. The junctional sarcoplasm is more abundant and contains nuclei that are distributed between neighboring synaptic clefts.

With continued maturation the synaptic site becomes larger, the ramifications of individual nerve terminals increase, the synaptic gutters become deeper, and the junctional folds become more elaborate (Juntunen, 1979).

3.7.3. Structure–function correlations

The morphologic development of the NMJ has been correlated with changes in the packing density, metabolic stability and gating properties of AChR, alterations in AChE, differentiation of the basal lamina, and changes in neuromuscular transmission (Dennis et al., 1981; Ziskind-Conhaim and Dennis, 1981; Matthews-Bellinger and Salpeter, 1983; Sanes and Chiu, 1983). The description below summarizes the findings at the developing rat and mouse NMJ.

Neuromuscular transmission begins on day 14 or 15 in utero. AChR accumulates at the NMJ one or two days later, and patches of thickened basal lamina are associated with the accumulating AChR. The initial packing density of AChR is about one-third of that found at the adult NMJ. AChR turnover rate is as fast as at extrajunctional sites. Synaptic AChE appears one or two days after AChR begins to accumulate.

Between day 16 in utero and birth, AChR half-life increases from about 1 day to 8–14 days, the half-life of AChR found at the mature NMJ. Junctional AChR increases and extrajunctional AChR gradually disappears (Bevan and Steinbach, 1977; Steinbach, 1981). Basal lamina covers the entire synaptic space; synapse specific basal lamina antigens appear, and some extrasynaptic basal lamina antigens are cleared from the synaptic space (Sanes and Chiu, 1983).

Polyaxonal innervation of the junctions peaks about day 17 and then begins to decline (Dennis et al., 1981). The quantum content (m) of the end-plate potential (EPP) and the MEPP frequency are low and remain low until birth. This can be attributed to the relative smallness of the nerve terminal and lack of available quanta for release (Bennett and Florin, 1974). The duration of the MEPP and EPP is prolonged because the open time of the AChR ion channel is also prolonged (Michler and Sakmann, 1980). This is due to the presence of γ-AChR, which has a lower conductance but longer open time than the mature ε-AChR (Gu and Hall, 1988; Sakmann et al., 1992). The polyaxonal innervation and the prolonged EPP facilitate synaptic transmission and compensate for the low m (Lomo, 1980).

During the first postnatal week, the junctions are still multiply innervated and show relatively little change. The MEPP frequency and m remain low (Matthews-Bellinger and Salpeter, 1983). During the second postnatal week the postsynaptic surface increases rapidly. Junctional folds develop and the fraction of the postsynaptic membrane occupied by AChR decreases. Polyaxonal innervation is now rapidly eliminated so that the number of nerve terminals per NMJ decreases. The MEPP frequency and m increase, due to an increase in nerve terminal size. The EPP and MEPP duration decrease, due to replacement of a γ-AChR by ε-AChR with a concomitant decrease in the open time and increase in the conductance of the AChR channel (Matthews-Bellinger and Salpeter, 1983; Gu and Hall, 1988; Sakmann et al., 1992).

Between the second postnatal week and adult life, the nerve terminals enlarge, the postsynaptic membrane surface increases 2-fold, and the AChR-enriched membrane area increases 1.6-fold. The continuing enlargement of the junction is proportional to the increase in muscle fiber diameter and is associated with an increase in m (Steinbach, 1981; Matthews-Bellinger and Salpeter, 1983). The enlargement of the nerve terminal is proportionate to the enlargement of the synaptic gutter. Repeated visualization of AChR at the same NMJ shows that previously labeled AChR spread apart in the membrane and new AChR are intercalated throughout the enlarging postsynaptic area (Balice-Gordon and Lichtman, 1990). Growth of the NMJ is not monotonic, however, for some nerve terminals retract and synaptic branches shorten as net lengthening proceeds (Hill and Robbins, 1991).

3.7.4. Trophic interactions

A detailed account of the trophic interactions at the NMJ is beyond the scope of this chapter. Excellent reviews of this subject were written by others (Sanes and Lichtman, 1999, 2001; Davis et al., 2001; Burden, 2002; Willman and Fuhrer, 2002; Fox and Umemori, 2006; Kummer et al., 2006). Only a brief summary of selected topics is presented here.

3.7.5. Agrin, MuSK, Rapsyn, and Dok-7

Agrin, a multidomain proteoglycan, named for its ability to aggregate AChR, is critically important in the organization and maintenance of the synapse (McMahan, 1990). Agrin occurs in different N- and C-terminal isoforms. Long and short N-terminal isoforms (LN and SN agrin) arise from different transcriptional start sites followed by a common sequence (Fig. 3.18). The amino terminus of LN agrin is essential

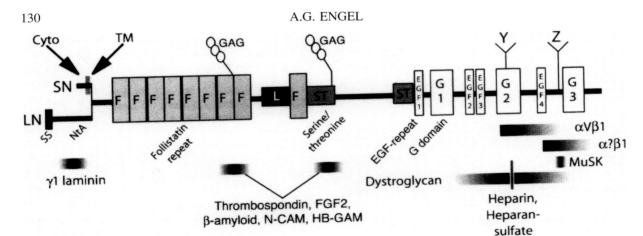

Fig. 3.18. The agrin protein and its interactions. The domain structure of agrin is shown at the top. SN and LN are distinct N-termini encoded by unique exons. The SN isoform has a cytoplasmic N-terminus and transmembrane domain for insertion into neuronal membranes. The LN isoform has a signal peptide and a laminin binding domain (NtA) and is secreted into the basal lamina of the NMJ. A and B are sites of alternative splicing. An 8 amino acid insert at B is essential for agrin to exert its effects at the NMJ. F, follistatin repeats; GAG, sites of glycosaminoglycan addition; L, laminin III domain; ST, serine/threonine rich regions; EGFs, EGF-like repeats; G, laminin-type G domain. Proteins that interact with agrin are shown at the bottom. Shaded boxes indicate their region of interaction with the agrin protein. (Based on Burgess et al., 2002, and reproduced with permission.)

for the secretion of agrin into the extracellular matrix of the NMJ. SN agrin is expressed only in the central nervous system where it is anchored to neuronal membranes through mediation of its unique amino terminus (Burgess et al., 2002).

Other agrin isoforms arise from alternative splicing at the second and third C-terminal laminin G domains, previously named as Y- and Z-sites in rodents but more recently designated as A- and B-sites (see Fig. 3.19). A conserved Asn-Glu-Ile tripeptide motif in the 8 amino acid insert at the B-site of LN agrin is necessary and sufficient for MuSK phosphorylation (Scotton et al., 2006), with consequent accumulation of AChR, neuregulin receptors, rapsyn, and utrophin in the postsynaptic region, and of neuregulin and AChE in the synaptic basal lamina (Glass and Yancopoulos, 1997; Meier et al., 1997; Burden, 1998; Sanes et al., 1998b). Binding of agrin to α-dystroglycan requires the presence of both LG domains but is negatively affected by inserts at the A- and B-sites (Scotton et al., 2006). Agrin null mice have severely disorganized NMJs with sparse, scattered AChR clusters, motor nerve branches forming no terminals, and undifferentiated presynaptic regions (Gautam et al., 1996). Fig. 3.18 shows a scheme of the agrin molecule, its binding domains, and molecules known to associate with it (Reist et al., 1987; Glass and Yancopoulos, 1997; Sanes and Lichtman, 2001; Burden, 2002; Burgess et al., 2002; Willman and Fuhrer, 2002). Muscle also expresses an agrin isoform but this isoform lacks the insert at the B-site (Ferns and Hall, 1992) and is 1000- to 10 000-fold less effective than neural LN agrin secreted into the synaptic space (Gesemann et al., 1995).

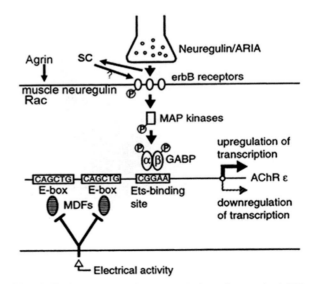

Fig. 3.19. Scheme showing upregulation of synaptic AChR transcription by the neuregulin signaling pathway, and its down-regulation at extrasynaptic nuclei by electrical activity. Although it was initially suggested that neuregulin released from the nerve terminal activates the muscle erbB family receptors directly, the activation may occur via a trophic influence on Schwann cells (SC), or through direct activation of muscle neuregulin by agrin. Once activated, erbB receptors initiate a mitogen-activated protein (MAP) kinase signaling cascade. MAP kinases phosphorylate the GA binding protein (GABPα/β) which activates transcription of the AChR-ε subunit gene via the Ets-binding site in the promoter of the AChR-ε subunit gene. Electrical activity of the innervated muscle causes phosphorylation of myogenin, a myogenic differentiation factor (MDF), by protein kinase C, which prevents stimulation of extrasynaptic AChR gene transcription by myogenin.

NCAM, HBGAM, βGalNAc, integrins, and laminins all potentiate the agrin-induced aggregation of AChR (Martin and Sanes, 1997; Burkin et al., 1998; Ruegg and Bixby, 1998; Sanes et al., 1998b) but are not the principal agrin receptor. Because agrin binds to α-DG (Campanelli et al., 1994; Sugiyama et al., 1994), initially α-DG was thought to be the principal agrin receptor. However, some agrin mutants can cluster AChR without binding to α-DG, or bind to α-DG but without clustering AChR (Glass and Yancopoulos, 1997). Subsequent studies implicated MuSK, a muscle-specific transmembrane protein with intrinsic tyrosine kinase activity, as the main agrin receptor. MuSK is expressed in close association with AChR in developing muscle, and agrin induces aggregation, phosphorylation, and dimerization of MuSK (Valenzuela et al., 1995). MuSK aggregation, in turn, is accompanied by the accumulation of β2-laminins and of AChE in the synaptic space. MuSK knock-out mice closely resemble agrin knock-out mice in that they lack differentiated NMJs, but myotubes cultured from the MuSK deficient mice do not respond to agrin (Glass et al., 1996, 1997). Agrin, however, does not bind to MuSK directly, but via a receptor complex that includes MuSK and a hypothetical muscle-associated specificity component, MASC (Glass et al., 1996; Meier and Wallace, 1998). The cytoplasmic domain of MuSK associates with the tetratricopeptide repeat domain of rapsyn which, in turn, enables an otherwise inactive tyrosine kinase (TrkA) to associate with rapsyn (Antolik et al., 2006).

Rapsyn clusters AChR by binding it to a postsynaptic scaffold (Froehner et al., 1990). Rapsyn knock-out mice cluster AChR poorly, and fail to accumulate dystroglycan, utrophin, and ErbB receptors at the NMJ. Thus, rapsyn is an effector of agrin-induced clustering. The absence of rapsyn, however, does not prevent accumulation of MuSK, β2-laminins, and AChE at the NMJs, nor does it abolish synapse-specific transcription by the junctional nuclei (Gautam et al., 1995; Apel et al., 1997; Sanes et al., 1998b). Thus, agrin acts indirectly on MuSK causing it to cluster postsynaptically, and a MuSK-rapsyn scaffold induces clustering of AChR, ErbB receptors, dystroglycan, and utrophin (Glass and Yancopoulos, 1997; Sanes et al., 1998b).

The MuSK ectodomain mediates the rapsyn-dependent aggregation of AChR via an unidentified rapsyn associated transmembrane linker (RATL) and the MuSK endodomain phosphorylates β- and δ-subunits of AChR via src-like kinases (Apel et al., 1997; Glass et al., 1997; Meier and Wallace, 1998) in a rapsyn-dependent manner (Lee et al., 2002). Phosphorylation of AChR increases its stability and promotes the cyto-

skeletal linkage of the AChR aggregates (Willman and Fuhrer, 2002).

AChR clusters first appear in central regions of developing noninnervated myotubes in a MuSK- and rapsyn-dependent, but agrin-independent, manner (pre-patterning). After arrival of the nerve terminal, agrin together with its postsynaptic effectors causes further clustering and stabilization of AChRs in the synaptic region (Lin et al., 2001; Yang et al., 2001). Moreover AChRs themselves are required for agrin-induced clustering of rapsyn and of some other postsynaptic proteins (Marangi et al., 2001; Ono et al., 2001). Interestingly, ACh tends to destabilize AChR clusters and agrin offsets this effect by stabilizing the clustered receptors (Misgeld et al., 2005).

It is now recognized that Dok-7, a NMJ protein in vertebrate skeletal muscle, is an essential aneural as well as agrin-dependent activator of MuSK, and a factor required for the growth and maturation of the NMJ. MuSK is activated by Dok-7 through interaction of the N-terminal phosphotyrosine-binding domain of Dok-7 with an Asn-Pro-X-Tyr motif in the juxtamembrane region of MuSK. Concomitantly there is intense autophosphorylation of MuSK (Okada et al., 2006).

Forced expression of Dok-7 in aneural myotubes induces the formation of elaborately branched pretzel-shaped clusters of AChR associated with Dok-7 (Okada et al., 2006). A recessive Val790Met mutation in MuSK impairs its interaction with Dok-7 (Okada et al., 2006) and causes a congenital myasthenic syndrome (Chevessier et al., 2004). Dok-7 is also essential for proper growth and differentiation of the NMJ: recessive missense mutations in Dok-7 result in a congenital myasthenic syndrome associated with small and often immature or unstable neuromuscular junctions (Beeson et al., 2006) (also see Chapter 10).

3.7.6. LDL-receptor-related protein 4 (LRP4)

LRP4 is expressed in multiple tissues and is important for the development and morphogenesis limbs, viscera and ectodermal organs. It is also expressed in the postsynaptic region of the NMJ and is required for the earliest events in formation of this region. LRP4 null mice die at birth with defects in pre- and postsynaptic protein clustering (Weatherbee et al., 2006).

3.7.7. Regulation of synapse specific transcription

Two candidates for regulation of synapse specific transcription have previously emerged. The first was the α-calcitonin gene related peptide (αCGRP) stored and released from dense-core vesicles in the nerve terminal (Matteoli et al., 1988). CGRP increases the synthesis and membrane insertion of AChR in cultured myotubes in a cAMP-dependent manner (New and Mudge, 1986; Fontaine et al., 1987). However, αCGRP null mice have normal NMJs and show no phenotypic abnormality (Lu et al., 1999).

The second candidate to regulate synapse specific transcription was neuregulin (previously called ARIA for AChR inducing activity), an isoform produced by the *NR-1* gene. Neuregulin, like agrin, is a motor nerve derived trophic factor, and member of a family of growth factors that are differentially distributed among functionally distinct classes of neurons (Falls et al., 1993; Sandrock et al., 1995). Mice homozygous for deletion of neuregulin die before birth; heterozygous animals survive, but with NMJs deficient in AChR and with a reduced safety margin of neuromuscular transmission (Sandrock et al., 1997). The postsynaptic receptor for neuregulin is formed by ErbB2, ErbB3, and ErbB4, members of the 185 kDa epidermal growth factor-related transmembrane receptor tyrosine kinases (Jo et al., 1995; Lemke, 1996; Meier and Wallace, 1998). In cultured muscle cells, liganded ErbB receptors activate mitogen activated protein (MAP) kinases (Si et al., 1996; Altiok et al., 1997). These, in turn, phosphorylate a heterodimeric GA binding protein (GABPα/β), a member of the Ets-binding family, which serves as a transcription activating factor (Schaffer et al., 1998). Phosphorylated GABPα/β binds to a specific neuregulin response element designated as the Ets binding site, or N-box, in the promoter regions of genes coding for utrophin and AChE, and for the AChR δ- and ε-, and possibly α-, subunits (Koike et al., 1995; Duclert et al., 1996; Fromm and Burden, 1998; Schaffer et al., 1998; Lu et al., 1999). Fig. 3.19 shows proposed pathways of neuregulin signaling at the NMJ.

A direct or exclusive role of *nerve derived* neuregulin on synapse-specific transcription has recently been questioned: 1. Neuregulin exerts a strong mitogenic effect on Schwann cells, which are required for differentiation of the nerve terminal. According to this scenario, neuregulin is primarily a trophic factor for Schwann cells. 2. Muscle, under the influence of agrin, also synthesizes neuregulin, which then can act downstream of agrin. Consistent with this, agrin in itself can augment AChR gene transcription in cultured myotubes via ErbB receptors (Sanes and Lichtman, 1999) and in mice after conditional inactivation of *NRG-1* (Jaworski and Burden, 2006). It is now believed that agrin has a dual effect: it induces assembly of the muscle derived neuregulin-1/ErbB pathway indirectly via

MuSK and directly by a shunt involving activation of Rac (Lacazette et al., 2003).

Regardless of how the ErbB path is activated, there is good evidence that the resultant binding of Ets factors GABPα/β to the N-box of selected postsynaptic genes enhances their transcription: 1. missense mutations in the N-box of the AChR ε-subunit reduce AChR transcription at the NMJ and result in a congenital myasthenic syndrome (Nichols et al., 1999; Ohno et al., 1999) (also see Chapter 10); 2. transgenic mice harboring a dominant-negative Ets mutation, which blocks binding of GABPα/β to the N-box, show a ~50% decrease in expression of genes for the AChR ε-subunit, AChE, β2-laminin, and utrophin A, and a ~30% decrease in expression of the gene for the AChR α-subunit. However, utrophin B, MuSK, and rapsyn gene expressions are unaffected (de Kerchove d'Exaerde et al., 2002). Neuregulin also has other inductive functions at the NMJ. One of these is to promote the accumulation of voltage-gated Na^+ channels in the depths of synaptic clefts (Fischbach and Rosen, 1997).

Shortly after neuregulin appears at the developing NMJ, fetal AChRs containing the γ-subunit (γ-AChRs) are replaced by adult AChRs harboring the ε-subunit (ε-AChRs). Continued expression of the ε-subunit at the NMJ depends on the presence of neuregulin in the synaptic basal lamina (Fischbach and Rosen, 1997; Sapru et al., 1998) or activation of muscle neuregulin by agrin.

3.7.8. The metabolic stability of NMJ AChR

The metabolic stability of NMJ AChR (i.e., its half-life) depends on innervation. At the mature innervated NMJ the AChR half-life is about 8–14 days while extrajunctional AChR on myotubes or in denervated muscle is only about 1 day (Shyng and Salpeter, 1990; Salpeter et al., 1992). At the denervated NMJ the degradation of the pre-existing AChR accelerates to a half-life of 3 days but returns to normal with reinnervation. Newly synthesized AChRs incorporated into the denervated NMJ have a half-life of about 1 day and their degradation rate is not slowed down by reinnervation (Shyng and Salpeter, 1990).

The stabilizing effect of innervation on AChR turnover is mediated by activity-dependent calcium influx into the muscle fiber. Stabilization of the turnover of junctional but not of extrajunctional AChR can be induced in the absence of activity if muscles are treated with the calcium ionophore A23187. Conversely, the activity-dependent stabilization of AChR is prevented if the muscle is stimulated in the presence of calcium channel blockers (Rotzler et al., 1991).

3.7.9. Regulation of the distribution and kinetic properties of AChR

Two hetero-oligomeric forms of muscle AChR exist: an immature extrajunctional form made up of $\alpha_2\beta\delta\gamma$-subunits ($\gamma$-AChR) and a mature junctional form consisting of $\alpha_2\beta\delta\epsilon$-subunits ($\epsilon$-AChR). AChR has a lower conductance and longer mean open time than AChR. Before innervation, γ-AChR is diffusely distributed over the entire fiber surface; during early synapse formation γ-AChR is concentrated at the NMJ and disappears from the extrajunctional sites. Subsequently (during the first 14 postnatal days in the rat), γ-AChR is replaced by ϵ-AChR at the NMJ (Sakmann and Brenner, 1978; Mishina et al., 1986; Schuetze and Role, 1987). Experimental studies have defined several regulatory influences underlying the appearance of ϵ-AChR at the NMJ, and the disappearance of γ-AChR from the rest of the muscle fiber (Sakmann et al., 1992). These influences act transiently as neural imprinting signals or continuously as inhibitory signals, and affect the different AChR subunit genes differently. The following interactions have been identified (Sakmann et al., 1992):

1. Neural agrin causes aggregation of AChR at the NMJ during early synapse formation and maintains this influence after it becomes imprinted on the basal lamina (Wallace et al., 1985).
2. A neural imprinting influence activates transcription by α-, β-, δ-, and ϵ-subunit genes at NMJ nuclei and also renders these nuclei independent of myogenic control signals. The γ-subunit gene expression at NMJ nuclei remains susceptible to myogenic and neural control signals.
3. Neural inhibiting factor acting on extrajunctional nuclei and electrical activity of the muscle fiber repress extrajunctional α-, β-, γ-, and δ-subunit gene transcription.
4. A neural imprinting signal activates transcription of the ϵ-subunit gene at NMJ nuclei and the ϵ-subunit gene and then becomes independent from other control mechanisms.
5. The γ-subunit gene is regulated by a myogenic influence, a neural inhibitory factor, and electrical activity. A neural influence inhibits γ-subunit gene transcription at NMJ nuclei. The neural inhibitory factor requires the presence of the nerve terminal, appears to be released by the clear synaptic vesicles, and could be ACh, ATP, a proteoglycan, or some other factor.

The net result is that the α-, β-, and δ-subunit genes are permanently activated at NMJ nuclei by a neural imprinting influence but remain subject to regulation by electrical activity and a neural inhibitory factor at extrajunctional nuclei.

The differential regulation of AChR subunit genes by a variety of signals is likely to be mediated by transcriptional factors acting on regulatory elements in the AChR subunit genes. MyoD1 sequence motifs, present in α-, δ- and γ-subunit genes, may serve as cis-acting regulatory elements. Myogenin and MyoD bind directly to α- and γ-subunit enhancers and the regulatory sequences of both genes contain two MyoD binding sites (Buonanno and Lautens, 1991; Salpeter et al., 1992). Myogenin, MyoD and Myf-5 transcript levels decrease during innervation and this precedes decreases in the corresponding AChR mRNAs (Salpeter et al., 1992) while increases in MRF4 transcript levels during development precede the expression of ϵ mRNA (Martinou and Merlie, 1991). However, in the rat the levels of α-, δ-, and γ-subunit transcripts correlate only weakly with changes in the level of myogenin mRNA and do not correlate with levels of MyoD1 mRNA (Sakmann et al., 1992).

3.7.10. AChE expression at the NMJ

Prior to innervation the asymmetric collagen-tailed form of AChE is formed along the entire muscle fiber. Within a few days after innervation there is increased synthesis and accumulation of this AChE at the NMJ and a decreased synthesis of extrajunctional AChE. AChE transcripts diffuse for only a short distance from their nuclei of origin (Salpeter et al., 1992). This suggests preferential transcription of AChE by subsynaptic nuclei and repression of AChE transcription by extrajunctional nuclei. The principal neural factor that augments AChE synthesis at the synapse is probably agrin (Hall and Sanes, 1993). If an ectopic synapse is denervated just at it is beginning to form and the muscle is stimulated, AChE still appears at the synaptic site. This indicates transfer of the neural signal to the basal lamina early during synaptogenesis and that muscle activity is also required for the appearance of AChE at the synaptic site (Lomo, 1980).

The above findings imply that activity and neural trophic factors work in concert during different stages of synaptogenesis (Lomo, 1983; Sanes and Chiu, 1983). Activity itself renders the denervated fiber refractory to innervation, but once innervation has taken place, activity is required for the appearance of AChE, metabolic stabilization of AChR, decrease of the AChR ion channel open time, and growth of junctional folds. Neural trophic factors are responsible for the early clustering of AChR at the synaptic site and induce synaptic differentiation of the basal lamina. These neural factors leave an "imprint," or "imprints," on the basal lamina and possibly the muscle fiber, which allow subsequent activity to exert its effect on AChE, AChR and synaptic architecture, and enable the basal lamina to bind AChE and to play a key role in synaptic regeneration (Lomo, 1983; Sanes and Chiu, 1983; Hall and Sanes, 1993).

3.8. Synaptic plasticity

Synaptic plasticity is evidenced by 1. the appearance and disappearance of polyaxonal inputs at the developing NMJ; 2. the sequential changes that occur in the fine structure and molecular architecture of nerve terminal, basal lamina and postsynaptic region at the developing and regenerating NMJ; 3. the appearance of collateral, ultraterminal, and intraterminal nerve sprouts in response to a variety of stimuli; and 4. remodeling of the NMJ during life and with aging. The sequential changes during synaptogenesis were discussed in the previous section. This section considers some aspects of the removal of polyaxonal innervation, nerve sprouting, and NMJ remodeling.

3.8.1. The withdrawal of polyaxonal innervation

The exact sequence of events associated with the withdrawal of some axon terminals from NMJs that receive multiple axons is still not fully understood. It has been generally accepted that axons from inappropriate segments of the spinal cord are withdrawn, that motor neuron death accompanies withdrawal of incorrect projections from motor neuron pools, and that loss of polyaxonal innervation of synaptic sites accompanies motor neuron death (Bennett and Raftos, 1977; Miyata and Yoshioka, 1980; Bennett, 1983). However, morphometric study of the mouse spinal cord cannot account for the prenatal loss of polyaxonal innervation by anterior horn cell death (Banker, 1982). Further, in mammals and birds, postnatal loss of polyaxonal innervation occurs even after correct spatial relationship between motor neuron pools and muscles has been established. At this time there is a decrease in the number of muscle fibers per motor unit, but not in the number of motor units per muscle (Korneliussen and Jansen, 1976; McGrath and Bennett, 1979; Mark, 1980). Therefore, the late loss of polyaxonal innervation results from the elimination of collateral sprouts rather than motor neuron cell death (McGrath and Bennett, 1979).

The factors that control withdrawal of the polyneuronal innervation are still not fully understood.

Activity or electric stimulation hastens and inactivity retards the elimination of polyaxonal innervation (O'Brien et al., 1978; Lomo, 1980; O'Brien, 1981). This suggests that inactive muscle releases a trophic "nerve growth factor" that maintains innervation and/or promotes nerve sprouting (Lomo, 1980; Bennett, 1983). O'Brien et al. suggest that activity hastens the elimination of multiple innervation through the release of proteolytic enzymes from muscle that attack susceptible nerve terminals (O'Brien et al., 1984). Oppenheim suggests that axonal branches compete for a soluble trophic factor released from muscle (Oppenheim, 1991). Sequential in vivo observation of BGT-labeled NMJ during the elimination of polyaxonal innervation reveals that AChR depletion of postsynaptic regions precedes the withdrawal of axon terminals from these regions. This might indicate that alterations in the postsynaptic region predetermine synaptic reorganization (Balice-Gordon and Lichtman, 1993). Alternatively, a given postsynaptic region fails to support an overlying nerve terminal because more dominant nerve terminals have enticed trophic factors away from that postsynaptic region (Rich and Lichtman, 1989).

3.8.2. Nerve sprouting

Excellent morphologic studies of nerve sprouting in denervated muscles were published more than three decades ago (Edds, 1950; Hoffman, 1950, 1951a, b). Hoffman distinguished between two types of sprouting: 1. ultraterminal, arising from nerve terminals at one NMJ and extending to a nearby denervated NMJ, or to a downstream newly formed junction on the same fiber; 2. collateral, arising from a preterminal nerve fiber at a node of Ranvier and reaching its target through the empty endoneurial sheath of the degenerated axon (Hoffman, 1951b). Reinnervation begins from ultraterminal branches because collateral sprouts can enter empty endoneurial sheaths only after Wallerian degeneration has taken place. Hoffman noted that growth of a foreign nerve implanted into a muscle was increased by denervating the muscle, and that growth of a foreign nerve into an innervated muscle was enhanced by denervation of a nearby muscle, suggesting a humoral mechanism for nerve growth (Hoffman, 1951a). Hoffman also found that an ether-soluble factor extracted from myelin stimulated collateral sprouting and postulated that such a factor is released from degenerating nerves (Hoffman, 1950).

A third type of sprouting, referred to as intraterminal sprouting, occurs within the confines of a single NMJ (Wernig et al., 1981). It may be a feature of local synaptic regeneration with aging, or may occur in pathologic states. However, the term "intraterminal sprouting" is misleading because an ultraterminal nerve sprout from a NMJ on a given muscle fiber can also establish a new synaptic contact on the same muscle fiber, but outside the confines of the original NMJ. This is the case in myasthenia gravis (Engel and Santa, 1971; Engel and Santa, 1973; Bowden and Duchen, 1976), some congenital myasthenic syndromes, and in botulinum intoxication (Duchen, 1971).

3.8.3. Candidates for muscle derived factors for nerve sprouting

Partial denervation of a corresponding contralateral muscle can induce intranodal and preterminal sprouting and increase in end-plate size (Pachter and Eberstein, 1991). Ultraterminal sprouting can occur with inactivity without any loss of innervation. It has been observed in hereditary motor end-plate disease of the mouse (Duchen, 1970), where the inactivity is attributed to a failure of the nerve action potential to invade the nerve terminal (Duchen and Stefani, 1971); after local injection of botulinum (Duchen, 1971) or tetanus (Duchen and Tonge, 1973) toxin into muscle; in human botulism; after prolonged tetrodotoxin blockade of nerve conduction (Brown and Ironton, 1977) or curarization of AChR (Wernig et al., 1980); and in inactive winter frogs (Wernig et al., 1980). Direct electric stimulation prevents motor nerve sprouting in botulinum poisoned mouse soleus muscle (Brown et al., 1977). All these observations support the notion that a humoral factor released by inactive muscle stimulates ultraterminal nerve sprouting.

The local administration of ciliary neurotrophic factor induces intranodal and terminal sprouting; this effect is potentiated by basic fibroblast growth factor, but treatment with the latter alone does not induce sprouting (Gurney et al., 1992). The subcutaneous injection of minute amounts of insulin-like growth factors induces nerve sprouting in innervated adult muscle. These growth factors are excellent candidates for muscle-derived sprouting activity because their mRNA levels in adult muscle increase severalfold after denervation or paralysis (Caroni and Grandes, 1990).

3.8.4. Remodeling of the NMJ

Remodeling of the NMJ during life is also a sign of plasticity in the nervous system (Young, 1952). A small proportion of the NMJs in normal human muscle have abnormal conformations. These include postsynaptic regions without nerve terminals, nerve terminals engorged by neurofilaments, abnormally small nerve terminals that fail to occupy the entire synaptic gutter, focal degeneration of the junctional folds, and abnormally simple postsynaptic regions that have no or only sparse and shallow synaptic clefts (Engel et al., 1975). These alterations probably reflect on the wear and tear of the NMJ in the normal state.

Conformational changes similar to those noted in normal human muscle and a decrease in synaptic vesicle density have been observed in aging mice (Banker et al., 1983). Scanning electron microscopy shows an increase in the total length and number of side branches of the synaptic gutter in the old mice (Fahim et al., 1983). These morphologic changes are associated with a decrease in NMJ AChR in some but not other muscles, with a decrease in the MEPP frequency, and an increase in m (Banker et al., 1983).

In the rat, the complexity of the NMJ increases with age and is associated by adaptation of terminal axons (Tweedle and Stephens, 1981). In diaphragm NMJs of aged rats m (Kelly, 1978), ACh released per nerve impulse (Smith, 1984), NMJ AChR (Courtney and Steinbach, 1981) and the safety margin of neuromuscular transmission all decrease (Smith, 1984).

Repeated in vivo visualization of NMJs in adult mice reveal that about 15% of the NMJ in gastrocnemius and 44% of the NMJ in soleus alter their configuration over 3–6 months. This suggests that remodeling of the NMJ increases with impulse activity (Wigston, 1990). Similar types of observations on the slow-twitch pectineus muscle of the mouse show that the nerve terminal is the dynamic entity, continually changing shape on a scale of micrometers, with nerve terminal outgrowths preceding the appearance of new AChR-positive postsynaptic regions. These alterations involve about 1–2% of the junctional area per month, but with relatively small permanent changes (Hill et al., 1991).

Acknowledgment

I thank Drs. John Heuser, M.A. Fahim, Josh Sanes, and Uel J. McMahan for permission to reproduce figures in this chapter.

References

Ahn AH, Freener CA, Gussoni E, et al. (1996). The three human syntrophin genes are expressed in diverse tissues, have distinct chromosomal localizations, and each bind to dystrophin and its relatives. J Biol Chem 271: 2724–2730.

Akaaboune M, Grady RM, Turney S, et al. (2002). Neurotransmitter receptor dynamics studied in vivo by reversible photo-unbinding of fluorescent ligands. Neuron 34: 865–876.

Alder J, Kanki H, Valtorta F, et al. (1995). Overexpression of synaptophysin enhances neurotransmitter release at *Xenopus* neuromuscular junctions. J Neurosci 15: 511–519.

Altiok N, Altiok K, Changeux J-P (1997). Heregulin-stimulated acetylcholine receptor gene expression in muscle—requirement for MAP kinase and evidence for parallel inhibitory pathway independent electrical activity. EMBO J 16: 717–725.

Anderson DC, King SC, Parsons SM (1982). Proton gradient linkage to active uptake of [³H]acetylcholine by *Torpedo* electric organ synaptic vesicles. Biochemistry 21: 3037–3043.

Anderson MJ, Cohen MW, Zorychta E (1977). Effects of innervation on the distribution of acetylcholine receptors on cultured muscle cells. J Physiol 268: 731–756.

Anderson-Cedergren E (1959). Ultrastructure of the motor endplate and sarcoplasmic components of mouse skeletal muscle fiber as revealed by three-dimensional reconstructions from serial sections. J Ultrastruct Res 1(Suppl.): 1–191.

Antolik C, Catino DH, Resnick WG, et al. (2006). The tetra-tricopeptide repeat domains of rapsyn bind directly to cytoplasmic sequences of the muscle-specific kinase. Neuroscience 141: 87–100.

Apel ED, Glass DJ, Moscosco LM, et al. (1997). Rapsyn is required for MuSK signaling and recruits synaptic components to a MuSK-containing scaffold. Neuron 18: 623–625.

Arikawa-Hirasawa E, Rossi SG, Rotundo RL, et al. (2002). Absence of acetylcholinesterase at the neuromuscular junction of perlecan-null mice. Nat Neurosci 5: 119–123.

Askanas V, Bornemann A, Engel WK (1990). Immunocytochemical localization of desmin at human neuromuscular junctions. Neurology 40: 949–953.

Askanas V, Engel WK, Alvarez RB (1992). Strong immunoreactivity of β-amyloid precursor protein, including the β-amyloid protein sequence, at human neuromuscular junctions. Neurosci Lett 143: 96–100.

Askanas V, Engel WK, Alvarez RB (1998). Fourteen newly recognized proteins at the human neuromuscular junctions—and their nonjunctional accumulation in inclusion—body myositis. Ann NY Acad Sci 841: 28–56.

Atsumi S (1971). The histogenesis of motor neurons with special reference to the correlation of their endplate formation. I. The development of endplates in the intercostal muscle in the chick embryo. Acta Anat 80: 161–182.

Balice-Gordon RJ, Lichtman JW (1990). In vivo visualization of the growth of pre- and post-synaptic elements of neuromuscular junctions in the mouse. J Neurosci 10: 894–908.

Balice-Gordon RJ, Lichtman JW (1993). In vivo observations of pre- and postsynaptic changes during transition from multiple to single innervation at developing neuromuscular junctions. J Neurosci 13: 834–855.

Banker BQ (1982). Physiologic death of neurons in the developing anterior horn of the mouse. Adv Neurol 473–485.

Banker BQ, Kelly SS, Robbins N (1983). Neuromuscular transmission and correlative morphology in young and old mice. J Physiol 339: 355–375.

Banwell BL, Russel J, Fukudome T, et al. (1999). Myopathy, myasthenic syndrome, and epidermolysis bullosa simplex due to plectin deficiency. J Neuropathol Exp Neurol 58: 832–846.

Bartoli M, Ramarao MK, Cohen JB (2001). Interactions of the rapsyn RING-H2 domain with dystroglycan. J Biol Chem 276: 24911–24917.

Bean AJ, Scheller RH (1997). Better late than never: a role for Rabs late in exocytosis. Neuron 19: 751–754.

Becherer U, Rettig J (2006). Vesicle pools, docking, priming, and release. Cell Tissue Res 326: 393–407.

Becherer U, Guatimosism C, Betz WJ (2001). Effects of staurosporine on exocytosis and endocytosis at frog motor nerve terminals. J Neurosci 217: 782–787.

Beeson D, Higuchi O, Palace J, et al. (2006). Dok-7 mutations underlie a neuromuscular junction synaptopathy. Science 313: 1975–1978.

Benfenati F, Valtorta F, Rubenstein JL, et al. (1992). Synaptic vesicle associated Ca^{2+}/calmodulin-dependent kinase II is a binding protein for synapsin I. NAT 359: 417–420.

Bennett MR (1983). Development of neuromuscular synapses. Physiol Rev 63: 915–1048.

Bennett MR, Florin T (1974). A statistical analysis of the release of acetylcholine at newly formed synapses in striated muscle. J Physiol 238: 93–107.

Bennett MR, Pettigrew A (1974a). The formation of synapses in striated muscle during development. J Physiol 241: 515–545.

Bennett MR, Pettigrew AG (1974b). The formation of synapses in reinnervated and cross-reinnervated striated muscle during development. J Physiol 241: 547–573.

Bennett MR, Pettigrew AG (1974c). The formation of synapses in striated muscle during development. J Physiol 241: 515–545.

Bennett MR, Raftos J (1977). The formation and regression of synapses during the reinnervation of axolotl striated muscles. J Physiol 265: 261–295.

Betz WJ, Bewick GS (1992). Optical analysis of synaptic vesicle recycling at the frog neuromuscular junction. Science 255: 200–203.

Betz WJ, Bewick GS (1993). Optical monitoring of transmitter release and synaptic vesicle recycling at the frog neuromuscular junction. J Physiol 460: 287–309.

Betz WJ, Mao F, Bewick GS (1992). Activity-dependent fluorescent staining and destaining of living vertebrate motor nerve terminals. J Neurosci 12: 363–375.

Bevan S, Steinbach JH (1977). The distribution of alpha-bungarotoxin binding sites on mammalian skeletal muscle developing "in vivo." J Physiol 267: 195–213.

Bewick GS, Nicholson LVB, Young C, et al. (1992). Different distributions of dystrophin and related proteins at nerve–muscle junctions. Neuroreport 3: 857–860.

Bewick GS, Young C, Slater CR (1996). Spatial relationships of utrophin, dystrophin, β-dystroglycan and β-spectrin to acetylcholine receptor clusters during postnatal maturation of the rat neuromuscular junction. J Neurocytol 25: 367–379.

Bi G-Q, Morris RL, Liao G, et al. (1997). Kinesin- and myosin-driven steps of vesicle recruitment for Ca^{2+}-regulated exocytosis. J Cell Biol 138: 999–1008.

Birks R, Huxley HE, Katz B (1960). The fine structure of the neuromuscular junction in the frog. J Physiol 150: 134–144.

Birnbaumer L, Campbell KP, Catterall WA, et al. (1994). The naming of voltage-gated calcium channels. Neuron 13: 505–506.

Blechschmidt E, Daikoku SH (1966). Die Entstehung der motorischen Innervation in der menschlichen Zungenmuskulatur. Elektronenmikroskopie der embryonalen Endplatte. Acta Anat 63: 179–198.

Bloch RJ, Hall ZW (1983). Cytoskeletal components of the vertebrate neuromuscular junction: vinculin, α-actinin, and filamin. J Cell Biol 97: 217–223.

Bloch RJ, Morrow JS (1989). An unusual β-spectrin associated with clustered acetylcholine receptors. J Cell Biol 108: 481–493.

Bon S, Coussen F, Massoulié J (1997). Quaternary associations of acetylcholinesterase. II. The polyproline attachment domain of the collagen tail. J Biol Chem 272: 3016–3021.

Bööj S, Larsson P-A, Dahllöf A-G, et al. (1986). Axonal transport of synapsin I and cholinergic synaptic vesicle-like material. Further immunohistochemical evidence for transport of axonal cholinergic transmitter vesicles in motor neurons. Acta Physiol Scand 128: 155–165.

Borst JGG, Sakmann B (1996). Calcium influx and transmitter release in a fast CNS synapse. NAT 383: 431–434.

Boudier JL, Jover E, Cau P (1988). Autoradiographic localization of voltage-dependent sodium channels on the mouse neuromuscular junction using ^{125}I-α scorpion toxin. I. Preferential labeling of glial cells on the presynaptic side. J Neurosci 8: 1469–1478.

Bowden REM, Duchen LW (1976). The anatomy and pathology of the neuromuscular junction. In: E Zaimis (Ed.), Neuromuscular Junction, Springer, N.Y. pp. 23–29.

Braun JEA, Wilbanks SM, Scheller RH (1996). The cysteine string secretory vesicle protein activates Hsc70 ATPase. J Biol Chem 271: 25989–25993.

Brigant JL, Mallart A (1982). Presynaptic currents in mouse motor endings. J Physiol 333: 619–636.

Brisson A, Unwin PNT (1984). Tubular crystals of acetylcholine receptor. J Cell Biol 99: 1202–1211.

Brodin L, Löw P, Gad H, et al. (1997). Sustained neurotransmitter release: new molecular clues. Eur J Neurosci 9: 2503–2511.

Brown MC, Ironton R (1977). Motor neuron sprouting induced by prolonged tetrodotoxin block of nerve action potentials. NAT 265: 459–461.

Brown MC, Goodwin GM, Ironton R (1977). Prevention of motor nerve sprouting in botulinum toxin poisoned mouse soleus muscles by direct stimulation of the mouse. J Physiol 267: 42P–43P.

Buchner E, Gundersen CB (1997). The DnaJ-like cysteine ring protein and exocytotic neurotransmitter release. Trends Neurosci 20: 223–227.

Buonanno A, Lautens L (1991). Regulation of nicotinic acetylcholine receptor gene transcription by myogenin and MyoD. J Cell Biochem 15C: 22–22.

Burden SJ (1998). The formation of neuromuscular synapses. Genes Dev 12: 133–148.

Burden SJ (2002). Building the vertebrate neuromuscular junction. J Neurobiol 53: 501–511.

Burden SJ, Sargent PB, McMahan UJ (1979). Acetylcholine receptors accumulate at original synaptic sites in the absence of the nerve. J Cell Biol 82: 412–425.

Burgess RW, Dickman DK, Nunez L, et al. (2002). Mapping sites responsible for agrin interactions with neurons. J Neurochem 83: 271–284.

Burkin DJ, Gu M, Hodges BL, et al. (1998). A functional role for specific spliced variants of the α7β1 integrin in acetylcholine receptor clustering. J Cell Biol 143: 1067–1075.

Burns ME, Sasaki T, Augustine GJ (1998). Rabphilin-3A: a multifunctional regulator of synaptic vesicle traffic. J Gen Physiol 111: 243–255.

Calakos N, Scheller RH (1996). Synaptic vesicle biogenesis, docking, and fusion: a molecular description. Physiol Rev 76: 1–29.

Campanelli JT, Roberds SL, Campbell KP, et al. (1994). A role for dystrophin-associated glycoproteins and utrophin in agrin-induced AChR clustering. Cell 77: 663–674.

Caroni P, Grandes P (1990). Nerve sprouting in innervated adult skeletal muscle induced by exposure to elevated levels of insulin-like growth factors. J Cell Biol 110: 1307–1317.

Cartaud A, Coutant S, Petrucci TC, et al. (1998). Evidence for in situ and in vitro association between β-dystroglycan and the subsynaptic 43K rapsyn protein. Consequence for acetylcholine receptor clustering at the synapse. J Biol Chem 273: 11321–11326.

Cartaud A, Strochlic L, Guerra M, et al. (2004). MuSK is required for anchoring acetylcholinesterase at the neuromuscular junction. J Cell Biol 165: 505–515.

Ceccarelli B, Hurlbut WP (1980). Vesicle hypothesis of the release of quanta of acetylcholine. Physiol Rev 60: 396–441.

Ceccarelli B, Hurlbut WP, Mauro A (1973). Turnover of transmitter and synaptic vesicles at the frog neuromuscular junction. J Cell Biol 57: 499–524.

Chamberlain LH, Burgoyne RD (1997). The molecular chaperone function of cysteine string proteins. J Biol Chem 272: 31420–31426.

Charvin N, Leveque C, Walker D, et al. (1997). Direct interaction of the calcium sensor protein synaptotagmin I with a cytoplasmic domain of the α_{1A} subunit of the P/Q-type calcium channel. EMBO J 16: 4591–4596.

Chen S, Zheng X, Schulze KL, et al. (2002a). Enhancement of presynaptic current by cysteine string protein. J Physiol 538: 383–389.

Chen X, Tomchick DR, Kovrigin E, et al. (2002b). Three-dimensional structure of the complexin/SNARE complex. Neuron 33: 397–409.

Chen YA, Scales SJ, Scheller RH (2001). Sequential SNARE assembly underlies priming and triggering of exocytosis. Neuron 30: 161–170.

Cheng TPO, Wood JG (1982). Compartmentalization of clathrin in synaptic terminals. Brain Res 239: 210–212.

Cheng TPO, Byrd FI, Whitaker JN, et al. (1980). Immunocytochemical localization of coated vesicles protein in rodent nervous system. J Cell Biol 86: 624–633.

Chevessier F, Faraut B, Ravel-Chapuis A, et al. (2004). MUSK, a new target for mutations causing congenital myasthenic syndrome. Hum Mol Genet 13: 3229–3240.

Clark AW, Hurlbut WP, Mauro A (1972). Changes in the fine structure of the neuromuscular junction of the frog caused by black widow spider venom. J Cell Biol 52: 1–14.

Cöers C (1967). Structure and organization of the myoneural junction. Int Rev Cytol 22: 239–267.

Cohen MW, Jacobson C, Yurchenko PD, et al. (1997). Laminin-induced clustering of dystroglycan on embryonic muscle cells: comparison with agrin induced clustering. J Cell Biol 136: 1047–1058.

Courtney S, Steinbach JH (1981). Age changes in neuromuscular junction morphology and acetylcholine receptor distribution on rat skeletal muscle fibers. J Physiol 320: 435–447.

Courtoy PJ, Picton DH, Farquhar MG (1983). Resolution and limitations of the immunoperoxidase procedure in localization of extracellular matrix antigens. J Histochem Cytochem 31: 945–951.

Couteaux R, Pécot-Dechavassine M (1970). Vésicules synaptiques et poches au niveau des zones actives de la jonction neuromusculaire. C R Seances Acad Sci D 271: 2346–2349.

Couteaux R, Pécot-Dechavassine M (1974). Les zones spécalisées des membranes présynaptiques. C R Seances Acad Sci D 278: 291–293.

Crain SM, Peterson ER (1974). Development of neural connections in culture. Ann N Y Acad Sci 228: 6–34.

Daniels MP, Vogel Z (1975). Immunoperoxidase staining of α-bungarotoxin binding sites in muscle end-plates shows distribution of acetylcholine receptors. NAT 254: 339–341.

David C, McPherson PS, Mundigl O, et al. (1996). A role of amphiphysin in synaptic vesicle endocytosis suggested by its binding to dynamin in nerve terminals. Proc Natl Acad Sci U S A 93: 331–335.

Davis GW, Eaton B, Paradis S (2001). Synapse formation revisited. Nat Neurosci 4: 558–560.

Deák F, Shin O-H, Tang J, et al. (2006). Rabphilin regulates SNARE-dependent re-priming of synaptic vesicle fusion. EMBO J 25: 2856–2866.

De Camilli P, Jahn R (1990). Pathways to regulated exocytosis of neurons. Annu Rev Physiol 52: 625–645.

De Camilli P, Takei K (1996). Molecular mechanisms in synaptic vesicle endocytosis and recycling. Neuron 16: 481–486.

Deconinck AE, Potter AC, Tinsley JM, et al. (1997). Postsynaptic abnormalities at the neuromuscular junction of utrophin-deficient mice. J Cell Biol 136: 883–894.

De Iraldi AP, De Robertis E (1968). The neurotubular system of the axon and the origin of granulated and nongranulated vesicles in regenerating nerves. Z Zellforsch Mikroskop Anat 87: 330–344.

de Kerchove d'Exaerde A, Cartaud J, Ravel-Chapuis A, et al. (2002). Expression of mutant Ets proteins at the neuromuscular synapse causes alterations in morphology and gene expression. EMBO Rep 3: 1075–1081.

Dennis MJ, Ziskind-Conhaim L, Harris AJ (1981). Development of neuromuscular junctions in rat embryos. Dev Biol 81: 266–279.

Denzer AJ, Brandenberger R, Gesemann M, et al. (1997). Agrin binds to the nerve-muscle basal lamina via laminin. J Cell Biol 137: 671–683.

Deprez PN, Inestrosa NC (1995). Two heparin-binding domains are present on the collagenic tail of asymmetric acetylcholinesterase. J Biol Chem 270: 11043–11046.

De Robertis EDP, Bennett HS (1955). Some features of the submicroscopic morphology of synapses in frog and earthworm. J Biophys Biochem Cytol 1: 47–58.

Desai RC, Vyas B, Earles CA, et al. (2000). The C2B domain of synaptotagmin is a Ca^{2+}-sensing module essential for exocytosis. J Cell Biol 150: 1125–1135.

Desaki J, Uehara Y (1981). The overall morphology of neuromuscular junctions as revealed by scanning electron microscopy. J Neurocytol 10: 101–110.

Dreyer F, Peper K, Akert K, et al. (1973). Ultrastructure of the "active zone" on the frog neuromuscular junction. Brain Res 62: 373–380.

Duchen LW (1970). Hereditary motor end-plate disease in the mouse: light and electron microscopic studies. J Neurol Neurosurg Psychiatry 33: 238–250.

Duchen LW (1971). An electron microscopic study of the changes induced by botulinum toxin in the motor end-plates of slow and fast skeletal muscle fibres of the mouse. J Neurol Sci 14: 47–60.

Duchen LW, Stefani E (1971). Electrophysiologic studies of neuromuscular transmission in hereditary "motor end-plate" disease in the mouse. J Physiol 212: 535–548.

Duchen LW, Tonge DA (1973). The effects of tetanus toxin on neuromuscular transmission and on the morphology of motor end-plates in slow and fast skeletal muscle of the mouse. J Physiol 228: 157–172.

Duclert A, Savatier N, Schaeffer L, et al. (1996). Identification of an element crucial for the sub-synaptic expression of the acetylcholine receptor epsilon-subunit gene. J Biol Chem 271: 17433–17438.

Dunaevsky A, Connor EA (2006). F-Actin is concentrated in nonrelease domains at frog neuromuscular junctions. J Neurosci 20: 6007–6012.

Düring M (1967). Über die Feinstruktur der motorischen Endplatte von höheren Wirbeltieren. Z Zellforsch Mikroskop Anat 81: 74–90.

Edds MV (1950). Collateral regeneration of residual motor axons in partially denervated muscles. J Exp Zool 113: 517–552.

Eiden LE (1998). The cholinergic gene locus. J Neurochem 70: 2227–2240.

Ellisman MH, Rash JE, Staehlin LA, et al. (1976). Studies of excitable membranes. II. A comparison of specializations at neuromuscular junctions and nonjunctional sarcolemmas of mammalian fast and slow twitch muscle fibers. J Cell Biol 68: 752–774.

Engel AG (1994). Quantitative morphological studies of muscle. In: AG Engel, C Franzini-Armstrong (Eds.), Myology. 2nd ed. McGraw-Hill, New York, pp. 1018–1045.

Engel AG (2004). The neuromuscular junction. In: AG Engel, C Franzini-Armstrong (Eds.), Myology. 3rd ed. McGraw-Hill, New York, pp. 325–372.

Engel AG, Santa T (1971). Histometric analysis of the ultrastructure of the neuromuscular junction in myasthenia gravis and in the myasthenic syndrome. Ann N Y Acad Sci 183: 46–63.

Engel AG, Santa T (1973). Motor end-plate fine structure Quantitative analysis in disorders of neuromuscular transmission. In: JE Desmedt, (Eds.), New Developments in Electromyography and Clinical Neurophysiology. Karger, Basel, pp. 196–228.

Engel AG, Tsujihata M, Jerusalem F (1975). Quantitative assessment of motor end-plate ultrastructure in normal and diseased muscle. In: PJ Dyck, PK Thomas, EH Lambert (Eds.), Peripheral Neuropathy. Saunders, Philadelphia, pp. 1404–1415.

Engel AG, Tsujihata M, Lindstrom JM, et al. (1976). The motor endplate in myasthenia gravis and in experimental autoimmune myasthenia gravis: a quantitative ultrastructural study. Ann N Y Acad Sci 274: 60–79.

Engel AG, Lindstrom JM, Lambert EH, et al. (1977). Ultrastructural localization of the acetylcholine receptor in myasthenia gravis and in its experimental autoimmune model. Neurology 27: 307–315.

Engel AG, Fukunaga H, Osame M (1982). Stereometric estimation of the area of the freeze-fractured membrane. Muscle Nerve 5: 682–685.

Enigk RE, Maimone MM (2001). Cellular and molecular properties of α-dystrobrevin in skeletal muscle. Front Biosci 6: d53–64.

Ervasti JM, Campbell KP (1993). A role for the dystrophin-glycoprotein complex as a transmembrane linker between laminin and actin. J Cell Biol 122: 809–823.

Eshkind LG, Leube RE (1995). Mice lacking synaptophysin reproduce and form typical synaptic vesicles. Cell Tissue Res 282: 423–433.

Evans GJ, Morgan A (2002). Phosphorylation-dependent interaction of the synaptic vesicle proteins cysteine string protein and synaptotagmin I. Biochem J 364: 343–347.

Fahim MA, Holley JA, Robbins N (1983). Scanning and light microscopic study of age changes at a neuromuscular junction in the mouse. J Neurocytol 12: 13–25.

Fahim MA, Holley JA, Robbins N (1984). Scanning electron microscopic comparison of neuromuscular junctions of slow and fast twitch mouse muscles. Neuroscience 13: 227–235.

Falls DL, Rosen KM, Corfas G, et al. (1993). ARIA, a protein that stimulates acetylcholine receptor synthesis, is a member of the Neu ligand family. Cell 72: 801–815.

Fasshauer D, Bruns D, Shen B, et al. (1997a). A structural change occurs upon binding of syntaxin to SNAP-25. J Biol Chem 272: 4582–4590.

Fasshauer D, Eliason WK, Brunger AT, et al. (1997b). Identification of the minimal core of the synaptic SNARE complex sufficient for reversible assembly and disassembly. Biochemistry 37: 10354–10362.

Fasshauer D, Otto H, Eliason WK, et al. (1997c). Structural changes are associated with soluble N-ethylmaleimide-sensitive fusion protein attachment protein receptor complex formation. J Biol Chem 272: 28036–28041.

Fernandez-Chacon R, Wölfel M, Nishimune H, et al. (2004). The synaptic vesicle protein CSPα prevents synaptic degeneration. Neuron 42: 237–251.

Ferns MJ, Hall ZW (1992). How many agrins does it take to make a synapse? Cell 70: 1–3.

Fertuck HC, Salpeter MM (1976). Quantitation of junctional and extrajunctional acetylcholine receptors by electron microscope autoradiography after ^{125}I-α-bungarotoxin binding at mouse neuromuscular junctions. J Cell Biol 69: 144–158.

Fischbach GD, Rosen KM (1997). ARIA: a neuromuscular junction neuregulin. Annu Rev Neurosci 20: 429–458.

Flucher BE, Daniels MP (1989). Distribution of Na$^+$ channels and ankyrin in neuromuscular junctions is complementary to that of acetylcholine receptors and the 43 kd protein. Neuron 3: 163–175.

Fontaine B, Klarsfeld A, Changeux J-P (1987). Calcitonin-gene-related peptide and muscle activity regulate acetylcholine receptor α-subunit mRNA levels by distinct intracellular pathways. J Cell Biol 105: 1337–1342.

Fox MA, Umemori H (2006). Seeking long-term relationship: axon and target communicate to organize synaptic differentiation. J Neurochem 97: 1215–1231.

Frank E, Fischbach GD (1979). Early events in neuromuscular junction formation in vitro. J Cell Biol 83: 143–158.

Fraterman S, Khurana TS, Rubinstein NA (2006). Identification of acetylcholine receptor subunits differentially expressed in singly and multiply innervated fibers of extraocular muscles. Invest Ophthalmol Vis Sci 47: 3828–3834.

Froehner SC (1991). The submembrane machinery for nicotinic acetylcholine receptor clustering. J Cell Biol 114: 1–7.

Froehner SC, Luetje CW, Scotland PB, et al. (1990). The postsynaptic 43K protein clusters muscle nicotinic acetylcholine receptors in Xenopus oocytes. Neuron 5: 403–410.

Froehner SC, Adams ME, Peters MF, et al. (1997). Syntrophins: modular adapter proteins at the neuromuscular junction and the sarcolemma. In: SC Froehner, V Bennett (Eds.), Cytoskeletal Regulation and Membrane Function. Rockefeller University Press, New York, pp. 197–207.

Fromm L, Burden SJ (1998). Synapse-specific and neuregulin-induced transcription require an Ets site that binds GABPα/GAPBβ. Genes Dev 12: 3074–3083.

Fukunaga H, Engel AG, Osame M, et al. (1982). Paucity and disorganization of presynaptic membrane active zones in the Lambert–Eaton myasthenic syndrome. Muscle Nerve 5: 686–697.

Fukunaga H, Engel AG, Lang B, et al. (1983). Passive transfer of Lambert–Eaton myasthenic syndrome with IgG from man to mouse depletes the presynaptic membrane active zones. Proc Natl Acad Sci U S A 80: 7636–7640.

Fumagalli G, Engel AG, Lindstrom J (1982). Ultrastructural aspects of acetylcholine receptor turnover at the normal end-plate and in autoimmune myasthenia gravis. J Neuropathol Exp Neurol 41: 567–579.

Gaffield MA, Rizzoli SO, Betz WJ (2006). Mobility of synaptic vesicles in different pools in resting and stimulated frog motor nerve terminals. Neuron 51: 317–325.

Gautam M, Noakes PG, Mudd J, et al. (1995). Failure of postsynaptic specialization to develop at neuromuscular junctions of rapsyn-deficient mice. NAT 377: 232–236.

Gautam M, Noakes PG, Moscoso L, et al. (1996). Defective neuromuscular synaptogenesis in agrin-deficient mutant mice. Cell 85: 525–535.

Gee SH, Madhavan R, Levinson SR, et al. (1998). Interaction of muscle and brain sodium channels with multiple members of the syntrophin family of dystrophin-associated proteins. J Neurosci 18: 128–137.

Geppert M, Goda Y, Hammer RE, et al. (1994). Synaptotagmin I: a major Ca^{2+} sensor for transmitter release at a central synapse. Cell 79: 717–727.

Geppert M, Goda Y, Stevens CF, et al. (1997). The small GTP-binding protein Rab3A regulates a late step in synaptic vesicle fusion. NAT 387: 810–814.

Gesemann M, Denzer AJ, Ruegg MA (1995). Acetylcholine receptor aggregating activity of agrin isoforms and mapping of the active site. J Cell Biol 128: 625–636.

Ginzel D, Shoshan-Barmatz V (2002). The synaptic vesicle protein synaptophysin: purification and characterization of its channel activity. Biophys J 83: 3223–3229.

Giraudo CG, Eng WS, Melia TJ, et al. (2006). A clamping mechanism involved in SNARE-dependent exocytosis. Science 313: 676–680.

Glass DJ, Yancopoulos GD (1997). Sequential roles of agrin, Musk and rapsyn during neuromuscular junction formation. Curr Opin Neurobiol 7: 379–384.

Glass DJ, Bowen DC, Stitt TN, et al. (1996). Agrin acts via MuSK receptor complex. Cell 85: 513–523.

Glass DJ, Apel ED, Shah H, et al. (1997). Kinase domain of the muscle-specific receptor tyrosine kinase (MuSK) is sufficient for phosphorylation but not clustering of acetylcholine receptors. Required role for the MuSK ectodomain? Proc Natl Acad Sci U S A 94: 8848–8853.

Glicksman MA, Sanes JR (1983). Differentiation of motor nerve terminals in the absence of muscle fibers. J Neurocytol 12: 661–671.

Gorio A, Hurlbut WP, Ceccarelli B (1978). Acetylcholine compartments in mouse diaphragm: a comparison of the effects of black widow spider venom, electrical stimulation, and high concentration of potassium. J Cell Biol 78: 716–733.

Götte M, von Mollard FG (1998). A new beat for the SNARE drum. Trends Cell Biol 8: 215–218.

Grady RM, Merlie JP, Sanes JR (1997). Subtle neuromuscular defects in utrophin-deficient mice. J Cell Biol 136: 871–882.

Granseth B, Odermatt B, Royle SJ, et al. (2006). Clathrin-mediated endocytosis is the dominant mechanism of vesicle retrieval at hippocampal synapses 1. Neuron 51: 773–786.

Green WN (1999). Ion channel assembly: creating structures that function. J Gen Physiol 113: 163–169.

Greengard P, Valtorta F, Czernik AJ, et al. (1993). Synaptic vesicle phosphoproteins and regulation of synaptic vesicle function. Science 259: 780–785.

Grohovaz F, Limbrick AR, Miledi R (1982). Acetylcholine receptors at the rat neuromuscular junction as revealed by deep etching. Proc R Soc Lond B Biol Sci 215: 147–154.

Gu Y, Hall ZW (1988). Immunological evidence for a change in subunits of the acetylcholine receptor in developing and denervated rat muscle. Neuron 1: 117–125.

Gurney ME, Yamamoto H, Kwon Y (1992). Induction of motor neuron sprouting in vivo by ciliary neurotrophic factor and basic fibroblast growth factor. J Neurosci 12: 3241–3247.

Hall ZW, Sanes JR (1993). Synaptic structure and development: the neuromuscular junction. Cell 72(Suppl.): 99–121.

Hall ZW, Lubit BW, Schwartz JH (1981). Cytoplasmic actin in postsynaptic structures at the neuromuscular junction. J Cell Biol 90: 789–792.

Hanson PI, Roth R, Morisaki H, et al. (1997). Structure and conformational changes in NSF and its membrane receptor complexes visualized by quick-freeze/deep-etch electron microscopy. Cell 90: 523–525.

Harlow ML, Ress D, Stoschek A, et al. (2001). The architecture of active zone material at the frog's neuromuscular junction. NAT 409: 479–484.

Hess A (1970). Vertebrate slow muscle fibers. Physiol Rev 50: 40–62.

Heuser JE (1974). A possible origin of the "giant" spontaneous potentials that occur after prolonged transmitter release at frog neuromuscular junctions. J Physiol 239: 106–108.

Heuser JE (1977). Synaptic vesicle exocytosis revealed in quick-frozen frog neuromuscular junctions treated with 4-aminopyridine and given a single electrical shock. In: M Cowan, JA Ferendelli (Eds.), Neuroscience Symposia. Society for Neuroscience, Bethesda, Md., pp. 215–239.

Heuser JE (1978). Synaptic vesicle exocytosis and recycling during transmitter discharge from the neuromuscular junction. In: SC Silverstein (Eds.), Transport of Macromolecules in Cellular Systems. Dahlem Coferenze, Berlin, pp. 445–464.

Heuser JE (1980a). 3-D visualization of membrane and cytoplasmic specializations at the frog neuromuscular junction. In: J Taxi (Eds.), Ontogenesis and Functional Mechanisms of Peripheral Synapses. Elsevier, North Holland, pp. 139–155.

Heuser JE (1980b). Three-dimensional visualization of coated vesicle formation in fibroblasts. J Cell Biol 84: 560–583.

Heuser JE, Miledi R (1971). Effect of lanthanum ions on function and structure of frog neuromuscular junctions. Proc R Soc Lond [Biol] 179: 247–260.

Heuser JE, Reese TS (1973). Evidence for recycling of synaptic vesicle membrane during transmitter release at the frog neuromuscular junction. J Cell Biol 57: 315–344.

Heuser JE, Reese TS (1977). Structure of the synapse. In: JR Pappenheimer (Ed.), Handbook of Physiology - The Nervous System. American Physiological Society, Bethesda, Md., pp. 261–294.

Heuser JE, Reese TS (1981). Structural changes after transmitter release at the frog neuromuscular junction. J Cell Biol 88: 564–580.

Heuser JE, Salpeter SR (1979). Organization of acetylcholine receptors in quick-frozen, deep-etched, and rotary-replicated *Torpedo* postsynaptic membrane. J Cell Biol 82: 150–173.

Heuser JE, Reese TS, Landis DMD (1974). Functional changes in frog neuromuscular junctions studied with freeze-fracture. J Neurocytol 3: 109–131.

Heuser JE, Reese TS, Dennis MJ, et al. (1979). Synaptic vesicle exocytosis captured by quick freezing and correlated with quantal transmitter release. J Cell Biol 81: 275–300.

Hilfiker S, Pieribone VA, Czernik AJ, et al. (1999). Synapsins as regulators of neurotransmitter release. Phil Trans R Soc Lond B 354: 269–279.

Hill RR, Robbins N (1991). Mode of enlargement of young mouse neuromuscular junctions observed repeatedly in vivo with visualization of pre- and postsynaptic borders. J Neurocytol 20: 183–194.

Hill RR, Robbins N, Fang ZP (1991). Plasticity of presynaptic and postsynaptic elements of neuromuscular junctions repeatedly observed in living adult mice. J Neurocytol 20: 165–182.

Hines M (1932). Studies in the innervation of skeletal muscle. IV. Of certain muscles of the boa constrictor. J Comp Neurol 56: 105–133.

Hirano H (1967). Ultrastructural study of the morphogenesis of the neuromuscular junction in the skeletal muscle of the chick. Z Zellforsch Mikroskop Anat 79: 198–208.

Hirokawa N, Heuser JE (1982). Internal and external differentiations of the postsynaptic membrane at the neuromuscular junction. J Neurocytol 11: 487–510.

Hirokawa N, Sobue K, Kanda K, et al. (1989). The cytoskeletal architecture of the presynaptic terminal and molecular structure of synapsin. J Cell Biol 108: 111–126.

Hoffman H (1950). Local re-innervation in partially denervated muscle: a histophysiological study. Aust J Exp Biol Med Sci 28: 383–397.

Hoffman H (1951a). A study of the factors influencing innervation of muscles by implanted nerves. Aust J Exp Biol Med Sci 29: 289–308.

Hoffman H (1951b). Fate of interrupted nerve-fibers regenerating into partially denervated muscles. Aust J Exp Biol Med Sci 29: 211–219.

Hosaka M, Südhof TC (1998). Synapsin III, a novel synapsin with an unusual regulation by Ca^{2+}. J Biol Chem 273: 13371–13374.

Hu K, Carroll J, Fedorovich S, et al. (2000). Vesicular restriction suggests a role for calcium in membrane fusion. NAT 415: 646–650.

Jacobson C, Montanaro F, Lindenbaum MH, et al. (1998). α-Dystroglycan functions in acetylcholine receptor aggregation but is not a coreceptor for agrin—Musk signaling. J Neurosci 18: 6340–6348.

Jahn R, Hanson PI (1998). SNAREs line up in new environment. NAT 393: 14–15.

Jahn R, Scheller RH (2006). SNAREs—engines for membrane fusion. Nature Rev Mol Cell Biol 7: 631–643.

Jahn R, Hanson PI, Otto H, et al. (1995). Botulinum and tetanus neurotoxins: emerging tools for the study of membrane fusion. Cold Spring Harb Symp Quant Biol 40: 329–335.

Janz R, Goda Y, Geppert M, et al. (1999). SV2A and SV2B function as redundant Ca^{2+} regulators in neurotransmitter release. Neuron 24: 1003–1016.

Jasmin BJ, Cartaud J (1990). Compartmentalization of cold-stable and acetylated microtubules in the subsynaptic domain of chick skeletal muscle fiber. NAT 344: 673–675.

Jaworski A, Burden SJ (2006). Neuromuscular synapse formation in mice lacking motor neuron- and skeletal muscle-derived neuregulin—1. J Neurosci 26: 655–661.

Jena BP, Webster P, Geibel JP, et al. (1997). Localization of SH-PTP1 to synaptic vesicles: a possible role in neurotransmission. Cell Biol Int 21: 469–475.

Jessell TM, Kandel ER (1993). Synaptic transmission: a bidirectional and self-modifiable form of cell–cell communication. Cell 72(Suppl.): 1–30.

Jo SA, Zhu X, Marchionni MA, et al. (1995). Neuregulins are concentrated at nerve–muscle synapses and activate Ach-receptor gene expression. NAT 373: 158–161.

Jones SW, Salpeter MM (1983). Absence of [^{125}I]α-bungarotoxin binding to motor nerve terminals of frog, lizard and mouse muscle. J Neurosci 3: 326–331.

Juntunen J (1979). Morphogenesis of the cholinergic synapse in striated muscle. Prog Brain Res 49: 351–358.

Juntunen J, Teräväinen H (1972). Structural development of myoneural junctions in the human embryo. Histochemie 32: 107–112.

Kao H-T, Song H-J, Porton B, et al. (2002). A protein kinase A-dependent molecular switch in synapsins regulates neurite outgrowth. Nat Neurosci 5: 431–437.

Katz B, Kuffler SW (1941). Multiple motor innervation of the frog's sartorius muscle. J Neurophysiol 4: 209–223.

Keller SH, Taylor P (1999). Determinants responsible for assembly of the nicotinic acetylcholine receptor. J Gen Physiol 113: 171–176.

Kelly AM, Zacks SI (1969). The fine structure of motor end-plate myogenesis. J Cell Biol 42: 154–169.

Kelly RB (1993). Storage and release of neurotransmitters. Cell 72(Suppl.): 43–53.

Kelly SS (1978). The effect of age on neuromuscular transmission. J Physiol 274: 51–62.

Khurana TS, Hoffman EP, Kunkel LM (1990). Identification of a chromosome 6-encoded dystrophin-related protein. J Biol Chem 256: 16717–16720.

Kiene L-M, Stadler H (1987). Synaptic vesicles in electromotoneurones. I. Axonal transport, site of transmitter uptake and processing of a core proteoglycan during maturation. EMBO J 6: 2209–2215.

Kimbell LM, Ohno K, Rotundo RL, et al. (2004). C-terminal and heparin-binding domains of collagenic tail subunit are both essential for anchoring acetylcholinesterase at the synapse. J Biol Chem 279: 10997–11005.

Klarsfeld A, Bessereau J-L, Salmon A-M, et al. (1991). An acetylcholine receptor α-subunit promoter conferring preferential synaptic expression in muscle of transgenic mice. EMBO J 10: 625–632.

Knight D, Tolley LK, Kim DK, et al. (2003). Functional analysis of neurotransmission at β2-laminin deficient terminals. J Physiol 546: 789–800.

Koike S, Schaeffer L, Changeux J-P (1995). Identification of a DNA element determining synaptic expression of the mouse acetylcholine receptor delta-subunit gene. Proc Natl Acad Sci USA 92: 10624–10628.

Korneliussen H, Jansen JKS (1976). Morphological aspects of the elimination of polyneuronal innervation of skeletal muscle fibres in new-born rats. J Neurocytol 5: 591–604.

Korneliussen H, Waerhaug O (1973). Three morphological types of motor nerve terminals in the rat diaphragm, and their possible innervation of different muscle fiber types. Z Anat Entwickl Gesch 140: 73–84.

Krejci E, Valenzuela IM-P, Ameziane R, et al. (2006). Acetylcholinesterase dynamics at the neuromuscular junction of live animals. J Biol Chem 281: 10347–10354.

Krikorian JG, Bloch RJ (1992). Treatments that extract the 43K protein from acetylcholine receptor clusters modify the conformation of cytoplasmic domains of all subunits of the receptor. J Biol Chem 267: 9118–9128.

Kühne W (1887). Neue Untersuchunge über die motorische Nervenendigungen. Z Biol 23: 1–148.

Kullberg RW, Lentz TL, Cohen MW (1977). Development of the myotomal neuromuscular junction in Xenopus laevis: an electrophysiological and fine-structural study. Dev Biol 60: 101–129.

Kummer TT, Misgeld T, Sanes JR (2006). Assembly of the postsynaptic membrane at the neuromuscular junction: a paradigm lost. Curr Opin Neurobiol 16: 74–82.

Kuromi H, Kidokoro Y (2000). Tetanic stimulation recruits vesicles from reserve pool via a Camp-mediated process in Drosophila synapses. Neuron 27: 133–143.

Lacazette E, Le Calvez S, Gajendran N, et al. (2003). A novel pathway for MuSK to induce key genes in neuromuscular synapse formation. J Cell Biol 161: 727–736.

Landis DMD, Reese TS (1983). Cytoplasmic organization in cerebellar dendritic spines. J Cell Biol 97: 1169–1178.

LaRochelle WJ, Witzeman V, Fiedler W, et al. (1990). Developmental expression of the 43K and 58K postsynaptic membrane proteins and nicotinic acetylcholine receptors in Torpedo electrocytes. J Neurosci 10: 3460–3467.

Laskowski MB, Sanes JR (1987). Topographic mapping of motor pools onto skeletal muscles. J Neurosci 7: 252–260.

Lee YI, Swope SL, Ferns MJ (2002). Rapsyn's C-terminal domain mediates MuSK-induced phosphorylation of the AChR. Mol Biol Cell 13: 395a.

Lemke G (1996). Neuregulins in development. Mol Cell Neurosci 7: 247–262.

Letinsky MS, Morrison-Graham K (1980). Structure of developing frog neuromuscular junctions. J Neurocytol 9: 321–342.

Leveque C, Pupier S, Marqueze B, et al. (1998). Interaction of cysteine string proteins with the $\alpha_1 A$ subunit of the P/Q type calcium channel. Proc Natl Acad Sci U S A 273: 13488–13492.

Lin RC, Scheller RH (1997). Structural organization of the synaptic exocytosis core complex. Neuron 19: 1087–1094.

Lin W, Burgess RW, Dominguez B, et al. (2001). Distinct roles of nerve and muscle in postsynaptic differentiation of the neuromuscular synapse. NAT 410: 1057–1064.

Llinás R, Sugimori M, Lin J-W, et al. (1989). ATP-dependent directional movement of rat synaptic vesicles injected into the presynaptic terminal of squid giant synapse. Proc Natl Acad Sci USA 86: 5656–5660.

Llinas RR, Sugimori M, Silver RB (1995). The concept of calcium concentration microdomains in synaptic transmission. Neuropharmacology 34: 1443–1451.

Lomo T (1980). What controls the development of neuromuscular junctions? Trends Neurosci 3: 126–129

Lomo T (1983). Trophic factors and postsynaptic activity in synapse formation. NAT 305: 576.

Lu JT, Son Y-J, Lee J, et al. (1999). Mice lacking α-calcitonin gene-related peptide exhibit normal cardiovascular regulation and neuromuscular development. Mol Cell Neurosci 14: 99–120.

Marangi PA, Forsayeth JR, Mittaud P, et al. (2001). Acetylcholine receptors are required for agrin-induced clustering of postsynaptic proteins. EMBO J 20: 7060–7073.

Marazzi G, Bard F, Klymkowsky MW, et al. (1989). Microinjection of a monoclonal antibody against a 37-kD protein (tropomyosin 2) prevents the formation of new acetylcholine receptor clusters. J Cell Biol 1097: 2337–2344.

Marchand S, Devillers-Thiéry A, Pons S, et al. (2002). Rapsyn escorts the nicotinic acetylcholine receptor along the exocytic pathway via association with lipid rafts. J Neurosci 22: 8891–8901.

Mark RF (1980). Synaptic repression at neuromuscular junctions. Physiol Rev 60: 355–395.

Marques MJ, Conchello JA, Lichtman JW (2000). From plaque to pretzel: fold formation and acetylcholine receptor loss at the developing neuromuscular junction. J Neurosci 20: 3663–3675.

Martin AR (1994). Amplification of neuromuscular transmission by postjunctional folds. Proc R Soc Lond B Biol Sci 258: 321–326.

Martin PT, Sanes JR (1997). Integrins mediate adhesion to agrin and modulate agrin signaling. Development 124: 3909–3917.

Martin TFJ (2003). Prime movers of synaptic vesicle exocytosis. Neuron 34: 9–12.

Martinou JC, Merlie JP (1991). Nerve-dependent modulation of acetylcholine receptor ε-subunit gene expression. J Neurosci 11: 1291–1299.

Massoulié J, Pezzementi L, Bon S, et al. (1993). Molecular and cellular biology of cholinesterases. Prog Neurobiol 41: 31–91.

Matsumura K, Ervasti JM, Ohlendieck K, et al. (1992). Association of dystrophin-related protein with dystrophin-associated proteins in mdx mouse muscle. NAT 360: 588–591.

Matteoli M, Haimann C, Torri-Tarrelli F, et al. (1988). Differential effect of alpha-latrotoxin on exocytosis of acetylcholine-containing small synaptic vesicles and CGRP-containing large dense-core vesicles at the frog neuromuscular junction. Proc Natl Acad Sci U S A 85: 7366–7370.

Matthews G (1996). Neurotransmitter release. Annu Rev Neurosci 19: 219–233.

Matthews-Bellinger J, Salpeter MM (1978). Distribution of acetylcholine receptors at frog neuromuscular junctions with a discussion of some physiological implications. J Physiol 279: 197–213.

Matthews-Bellinger JA, Salpeter MM (1983). Fine structural distribution of acetylcholine receptors at developing mouse neuromuscular junctions. J Neurosci 3: 644–657.

McEwen JM, Madison JN, Dybbs M, et al. (2006). Antagonistic regulation of synaptic vesicle priming by tomosyn and UNC-13. Neuron 51: 303–315.

McGrath PA, Bennett MR (1979). Development of the synaptic connections between different segmental motoneurons and striated muscles in an axolotl limb. Dev Biol 69: 133–145.

McMahan UJ (1990). The agrin hypothesis. Cold Spring Harb Symp Quant Biol 55: 407–418.

McMahan UJ, Slater CR (1984). The influence of basal lamina on the accumulation of acetylcholine receptors at synaptic sites in regenerating muscle. J Cell Biol 98: 1453–1473.

McMahan UJ, Spitzer JJ, Peper K (1972). Visual identification of nerve terminals in living isolated skeletal muscle. Proc R Soc Lond B Biol Sci 181: 421–430.

McMahon HT, Nicholls DG (1991). The bioenergetics of neurotransmitter release. Biochim Biophys Acta 1059: 243–264.

Meier T, Wallace BG (1998). Formation of the neuromuscular junction. BioEssays 20: 819–829.

Meier T, Hauser DM, Chiquet M, et al. (1997). Neural agrin induces ectopic postsynaptic specializations in innervated muscle fibers. J Neurosci 17: 6534–6544.

Meier T, Masciulli F, Moore C, et al. (1998). Agrin can mediate acetylcholine receptor gene expression in muscle by aggregation of muscle-derived neuregulins. J Cell Biol 141: 715–726.

Michler A, Sakmann B (1980). Receptor stability and channel conversion in the subsynaptic membrane of the developing mammalian neuromuscular junction. Dev Biol 80: 1–17.

Misgeld T, Kummer TT, Lichtman JW, et al. (2005). Agrin promotes synaptic differentiation by counteracting an inhibitory effect of neurotransmitter. Proc Natl Acad Sci U S A 102: 11088–11093.

Mishina M, Takai T, Imoto K, et al. (1986). Molecular distinction between fetal and adult forms of muscle acetylcholine receptor. NAT 321: 406–411.

Mitra K, McCarthy MP, Stroud RM (1989). Three-dimensional structure of the nicotinic acetylcholine receptor and location of the major associated 43-kD cytoskeletal protein, determined at 22 Å by low dose electron microscopy and x-ray diffraction to 12.5 Å. J Cell Biol 109: 755–774.

Miyata Y, Yoshioka K (1980). Selective elimination of motor nerve terminals in the rat soleus muscle during development. J Physiol 309: 631–646.

Monck JR, Fernandez J (1992). The exocytotic fusion pore. J Cell Biol 119: 1395–1404.

Murthy VN, De Camilli P (2003). Cell biology of the presynaptic nerve terminal. Annu Rev Neurosci 26: 701–728.

Nakata T, Terada S, Hirokawa N (1998). Visualization of the dynamics of synaptic vesicle and plasma membrane proteins in living axons. J Cell Biol 140: 659–674.

New HV, Mudge AW (1986). Calcitonin gene-related peptide regulates muscle acetylcholine receptor synthesis. NAT 323: 809–811.

Newey SA, Gramolini AO, Wu J, et al. (2001). A novel mechanism for modulating synaptic gene expression: differential localization of α-dystrobrevin transcripts in skeletal muscle. Mol Cell Neurosci 17: 127–140.

Nichols PR, Croxen R, Vincent A, et al. (1999). Mutation of the acetylcholine receptor ε-subunit promoter in congenital myasthenic syndrome. Ann Neurol 45: 439–443.

Nickel E, Vogel A, Waser PG (1967). Coated Vesicles in der Umgebung der neuromuskularen Synapsen. Z Zellforsch Mikroskop Anat 78: 261–266.

Noakes PG, Gautam M, Mudd J, et al. (1995). Aberrant differentiation of neuromuscular junctions in mice lacking s-laminin β2. NAT 374: 258–262.

Nunes P, Haines N, Kuppuswamy V, et al. (2006). Synaptic vesicle mobility and presynaptic F-actin are disrupted in an NSF allele of Drosophila. Mol Biol Cell 17: 4709–4719.

Nystrom RR, Ko C-P (1988). Disruption of active zones in frog neuromuscular junctions following treatment with proteolytic enzymes. J Neurocytol 17: 63–71.

O'Brien RAD (1981). A difference in transmitter release between surviving and non-surviving nerve terminals in developing rat skeletal muscles. J Physiol 371: 89P–90P.

O'Brien RAD, Östberg AJC, Vrbova G (1978). Observations on the elimination of polyneuronal innervation in developing mammalian skeletal muscle. J Physiol 282: 571–582.

O'Brien RAD, Östberg AJC, Vrbova G (1984). Protease inhibitors reduce the loss of nerve terminals induced by activity and calcium on developing rat soleus muscles in vitro. Neuroscience 12: 637–646.

Ogata T, Yamasaki Y (1985). The three-dimensional structure of motor end-plates in different fiber types of rat intercostal muscle. A scanning electron-microscopic study. Cell Tissue Res 241: 465–472.

Ohno K, Anlar B, Engel AG (1999). Congenital myasthenic syndrome caused by a mutation in the Ets-binding site of the promoter region of the acetylcholine receptor ε subunit gene. Neuromuscul Disord 9: 131–135.

Ohno K, Engel AG, Brengman JM, et al. (2000). The spectrum of mutations causing endplate acetylcholinesterase deficiency. Ann Neurol 47: 162–170.

Ohno K, Tsujino A, Brengman JM, et al. (2001). Choline acetyltransferase mutations cause myasthenic syndrome associated with episodic apnea in humans. Proc Natl Acad Sci U S A 98: 2017–2022.

Ohno K, Engel AG, Shen X-M, et al. (2002). Rapsyn mutations in humans cause endplate acetylcholine receptor deficiency and myasthenic syndrome. Am J Hum Genet 70: 875–885.

Ohtsuka T, Takao-Rikitsu E, Inoue E, et al. (2002). CAST: a novel protein of the cytomatrix at the active zone of synapses that forms a ternary complex with RIM12 and Munc13-1. J Cell Biol 158: 577–590.

Okada K, Inoue A, Okada M, et al. (2006). The muscle protein Dok-7 is essential for neuromuscular synaptogenesis. Science 312: 1802–1805.

Okada Y, Yamazaki H, Sekine-Aizawa Y, et al. (1995). The neuron-specific kinesin superfamily protein KIF1A is a unique monomeric motor for anterograde axonal transport of synaptic vesicle precursors. Cell 81: 769–780.

Ono F, Higashijima S, Shcherbatko A, et al. (2001). Paralytic zebrafish lacking acetylcholine receptors fail to localize rapsyn clusters to the synapse. J Neurosci 21: 5439–5448.

Oppenheim RW (1991). Cell death during development of the nervous system. Annu Rev Neurosci 14: 453–501.

Pachter BR (1983). Rat extraocular muscle. I. Three dimensional cytoarchitecture, component fibre populations and innervation. J Anat 137: 143–159.

Pachter BR, Eberstein A (1991). Nerve sprouting and endplate growth induced in normal muscle by contralateral partial denervation of rat plantaris. Brain Res 560: 311–314.

Palay SL (1958). The morphology of synapses in the central nervous system. Exp Cell Res 5(Suppl.): 275–293.

Pang ZP, Shin OH, Meyer AC, et al. (2006). A gain-of-function mutation in synaptotagmin-1 reveals a critical role of Ca2+-dependent soluble N-ethylmaleimide-sensitive factor attachment protein receptor complex binding in synaptic exocytosis. J Neurosci 26: 12556–12565.

Parsons SM, Carter RS, Koenigsberger R, et al. (1982). Transport in the cholinergic synaptic vesicle. Fed Proc 41: 2765–2768.

Patton BL, Miner JL, Chiu AY, et al. (1997). Distribution and function of laminins in the neuromuscular system of developing, adult, and mutant mice. J Cell Biol 139: 1507–1521.

Patton BL, Chiu AY, Sanes JR (1998). Synaptic laminin prevents glial entry into the synaptic cleft. NAT 393: 698–701.

Peachey LD, Takeichi M, Nag AC (1974). Muscle fiber types and innervation in adult cat extraocular muscles. In: AT Milhorat (Eds.), Exploratory Concepts in Muscular Dystrophy. II. Control Mechanisms. Excerpta Medica, Amsterdam, pp. 246–254.

Pécot-Dechavassine M (1982). Synaptic vesicle openings captured by cooling and related to transmitter release at the frog neuromuscular junction. Biol Cell 46: 43–50.

Pécot-Dechavassine M, Couteaux R (1975). Modifications structurales des terminaisons motrices des muscles de grenouille soumis à l'action de la vinblastine. C R Seances Acad Sci D 280: 1099–1101.

Peters MF, Adams ME, Froehner SC (1997). Differential association of syntrophin pairs with the dystrophin complex. J Cell Biol 138: 81–93.

Phillips GR, Huang JK, Wang Y, et al. (2001). The presynaptic particle web: ultrastructure, composition, dissolution, and reconstitution. Neuron 32: 63–77.

Pobbati AV, Stein A, Fasshauer D (2006). N- to C-terminal SNARE complex assembly promotes rapid membrane fusion. Science 313: 673–676.

Polo-Parada L, Bose CM, Landmesser LT (2001). Alterations in transmission, vesicle dynamics, and transmitter release machinery at NCAM-deficient neuromuscular junctions. Neuron 32: 815–828.

Polo-Parada L, Bose CM, Plattner F, et al. (2004). Distinct roles of different neural cell adhesion molecule (NCAM) isoforms in synaptic maturation revealed by analysis of NCAM 180 kDa isoform-deficient mice. J Neurosci 24: 1852–1864.

Polo-Parada L, Plattner F, Bose C, et al. (2005). NCAM 180 acting via a conserved C-terminal domain and MLCK is essential for effective transmission with repetitive stimulation. Neuron 46: 917–931.

Poskanzer KE, Fetter RD, Davis GW (2006). Discrete residues in the C2B domain of Synaptotagmin I independently specify endocytic rate and synaptic vesicle size. Neuron 50: 49–62.

Pow DV, Morris XY (1989). Dendrites and hypothalamic magnocellular neurons release neurohypophyseal peptides. Neuroscience 32: 435–439.

Propst JW, Ko C-P (1987). Correlation between active zone ultrastructure and synaptic function studied by freeze-fracture of physiologically identified neuromuscular junctions. J Neurosci 7: 3654–3664.

Pyle R, Schivell AE, Hikada H, et al. (2000). Phosphorylation of synaptic vesicle protein 2 modulates binding to synaptotagmin. J Biol Chem 275: 17195–17200.

Ramarao MK, Cohen JB (1998). Mechanism of nicotinic acetylcholine receptor cluster formation by rapsyn. Proc Natl Acad Sci USA 95: 4007–4012.

Ranjan R, Bronk P, Zinsmaier KE (1998). Cysteine string protein is required for calcium secretion coupling of evoked neurotransmission in Drosophila but not for vesicle recycling. J Neurosci 18: 956–964.

Rash JE (1983). Ultrastructure of normal and myasthenic endplates. In: EX Albuquerque, AT Eldefrawi (Eds.), Myasthenia Gravis. Chapman and Hall, London, pp. 395–421.

Rash JE, Ellisman MH (1974). Studies of excitable membranes. I. Macromolecular specializations of the neuromuscular junction and the non-junctional sarcolemma. J Cell Biol 63: 567–586.

Reist NE, Magill C, McMahan UJ, et al. (1987). Agrin-like molecules at synaptic sites in normal, denervated, and damaged skeletal muscles. J Cell Biol 105: 2457–2469.

Renden R, Berwin B, Davis W, et al. (2001). Drosophila CAPS is an essential gene that regulates dense-core vesicle release and synaptic vesicle fusion. Neuron 31: 421–437.

Rettig J, Neher E (2002). Emerging roles of presynaptic proteins in Ca++-triggered exocytosis. Science 298: 781–785.

Rettig J, Sheng Z-H, Kim DK, et al. (1996). Isoform-specific interaction of the α_{1A} subunits of brain Ca2+ channels with the presynaptic proteins syntaxin and SNAP-25. Proc Natl Acad Sci USA 93: 7363–7368.

Rettig J, Heinemann C, Ashery U, et al. (1997). Alteration of Ca2+ dependence of neurotransmitter release by disruption of Ca2+ channel/syntaxin interaction. J Neurosci 17: 6647–6656.

Retzius G (1892). Zur Kenntnis der motorischen Nervenen-digungen. Biol Untersuch (NS) 3: 41–52.

Rich MM, Lichtman JW (1989). In vivo visualization of pre- and postsynaptic changes during synapse elimination in reinnervated mouse muscle. J Neurosci 9: 1781–1805.

Richards DA, Guatimosim C, Betz WJ (2002). Two endocytotic recycling routes selectively fill two vesicle pools in frog motor nerve terminals. Neuron 27: 551–559.

Richards DA, Guatimosim C, Rizzoli SO, et al. (2003). Synaptic vesicle pools at the frog neuromuscular junction. Neuron 39: 529–541.

Rizzoli SO, Betz WJ (2004). The structural organization of the readily releasable pool of synaptic vesicles. Science 303: 2037–2039.

Rizzoli S, Betz WJ (2005). Synaptic vesicle pools. Nat Rev Neurosci 6: 57–69.

Robinson L, Martin TFJ (1998). Docking and fusion in cell biology. Curr Opin Cell Biol 10: 483–492.

Robitaille R, Adler EM, Charlton MP (1990). Strategic location of calcium channels at transmitter release sites of frog neuromuscular synapses. Neuron 5: 773–779.

Rotzler S, Schramek H, Brenner HR (1991). Metabolic stabilization of end-plate acetylcholine receptors regulated by Ca^{2+} influx associated with muscle activity. NAT 349: 337–339.

Ruegg MA, Bixby JL (1998). Agrin orchestrates synaptic differentiation at the vertebrate neuromuscular junction. Trends Neurosci 21: 22–27.

Ruff RL (1996). Sodium channel slow inactivation and the distribution of sodium channels on skeletal muscle fibres enable the performance properties of different skeletal muscle fibre types. Acta Physiol Scand 156: 159–168.

Ryan TA (2001). Inhibitors of myosin light-chain kinase block synaptic vesicle pool mobilization during action potential firing. J Neurosci 19: 1317–1323.

Saito A, Zacks SI (1969). Ultrastructure of Schwann and perineural sheaths at the mouse neuromuscular junction. Anat Rec 164: 379–390.

Sakakibara H, Engel AG, Lambert EH (1977). Duchenne dystrophy: ultrastructural localization of the acetylcholine receptor and intracellular microelectrode studies of neuromuscular transmission. Neurology 27: 741–745.

Sakmann B, Brenner HR (1978). Change in synaptic channel gating during neuromuscular development. NAT 276: 401–402.

Sakmann B, Witzemann V, Brenner H (1992). Developmental changes in acetylcholine receptor channel structure and function as a model for synaptic plasticity. Fidia Foundation Neuroscience Award Lectures 6: 51–103.

Salpeter MM (1987). Vertebrate neuromuscular junctions: general morphology, molecular organization, and functional consequences. In: MM Salpeter (Ed.), The Verebrate Neuromuscular Junction. Alan Liss, New York, pp. 1–54.

Salpeter MM, Harris R (1983). Distribution and turnover rate of acetylcholine receptors throughout the junction function folds at a vertebrate neuromuscular junction. J Cell Biol 96: 1781–1785.

Salpeter MM, Buonanno A, Eftimie R, et al. (1992). Regulation of molecules at the neuromuscular junction. In: AM Kelly, HM Blau (Eds.), Neuromuscular Development and Disease. Raven, New York, pp. 251–283.

Sandrock AW, Goodearl ADJ, Yin Q-W, et al. (1995). ARIA is concentrated in nerve terminals at neuromuscular junctions and at other synapses. J Neurosci 15: 6124–6136.

Sandrock AW, Dryer SE, Rosen KM, et al. (1997). Maintenance of acetylcholine receptor number by neuregulins at the neuromuscular junction in vivo. Science 276: 599–603.

Sanes JR (1995). The synaptic cleft of the neuromuscular junction. Semin Dev Biol 6: 163–173.

Sanes JR (2003). The basement membrane/basal lamina of skeletal muscle. J Biochem 278: 12601–12604.

Sanes JR, Chiu AY (1983). The basal lamina of the neuromuscular junction. Cold Spring Harbor Symp Quant Biol 48: 667–678.

Sanes JR, Lichtman JW (1999). Development of the vertebrate neuromuscular junction. Annu Rev Neurosci 22: 389–442.

Sanes JR, Lichtman JW (2001). Induction, assembly, maturation and maintenance of a postsynaptic apparatus. Nat Rev Neurosci 2: 791–805.

Sanes JR, Marshall LM, McMahan UJ (1978). Reinnervation of muscle fiber basal lamina after removal of myofibers. Differentiation of axons at original synaptic sites. J Cell Biol 78: 176–198.

Sanes JR, Johnson YR, Kotzbauer PT, et al. (1991). Selective expression of an acetylcholine receptor-lacZ transgene in synaptic nuclei of adult muscle fibers. Development 113: 1181–1191.

Sanes JR, Apel ED, Burgess RW, et al. (1998a). Development of the neuromuscular junction: genetic analysis in mice. J Physiol (Paris) 92: 167–172.

Sanes JR, Apel ED, Gautam M, et al. (1998b). Agrin receptors at the skeletal neuromuscular junction. Ann N Y Acad Sci 841: 1–13.

Santa T, Engel AG (1973). Histometric analysis of neuromuscular junction ultrastructure in rat red, white and intermediate muscle fibers. In: JE Desmedt (Ed.), New Developments in Electromyography and Clinical Neurophysiology. Karger, Basel, pp. 41–54.

Sapru MK, Florance SK, Kirk C, et al. (1998). Identification of a protein-tyrosine kinase phosphatase response element in the nicotinic acetylcholine receptor ε subunit gene: regulatory role of an Ets transcription factor. Proc Natl Acad Sci U S A 95: 1289–1294.

Schaffer L, Duckert N, Huchet-Dymanus M, et al. (1998). Ets related transcription factor in synaptic expression of the nicotinic acetylcholine receptor. EMBO J 17: 3078–3090.

Schivell AE, Batchelor RH, Bajjalieh SM (1996). Isoform-specific, calcium-regulated interaction of the synaptic vesicle proteins SV2 and synaptotagmin. J Biol Chem 271: 27770–27775.

Schmidt SL, Braell WA, Schlossman DM, et al. (1984). A role for clathrin light chains in the recognition of clathrin cages by "uncoating ATPase." NAT 311: 228–231.

Schoch S, Gundelfinger ED (2006). Molecular organization of the presynaptic active zone. Cell Tissue Res 326: 379–391.

Schuetze SM, Role LW (1987). Developmental regulation of nicotinic acetylcholine receptors. Annu Rev Neurosci 10: 403–457.

Scotton P, Bleckmann D, Stebler M, et al. (2006). Activation of muscle-specific receptor tyrosine kinase and binding to dystroglycan are regulated by alternative mRNA splicing of agrin. J Biol Chem 281: 36835–36845.

Sealock R, Wray BE, Froehner SC (1984). Ultrastructural localization of the M_r 43,000 protein and the acetylcholine receptor in *Torpedo* postsynaptic membranes using monoclonal antibodies. J Cell Biol 98: 2239–2244.

Sealock R, Paschal B, Beckerle M, et al. (1986). Talin is a postsynaptic component of the rat neuromuscular junction. Exp Cell Res 163: 143–150.

Sealock R, Murnane AA, Pauline D, et al. (1989). Immunochemical identification of desmin in the *Torpedo* postsynaptic membranes and at the rat neuromuscular junction. Synapse 3: 315–324.

Sealock R, Butler MH, Kramarcy NR, et al. (1991). Localization of dystrophin relative to acetylcholine receptor domains in electric tissue and adult and cultured skeletal muscle. J Cell Biol 113: 1133–1144.

Shao X, Davletov BA, Sutton RB, et al. (1996). Bipartite C^{2+}-binding motif in C_2 domains of synaptotagmin and protein kinase C. Science 273: 248–251.

Shao X, Li C, Fernandez I, et al. (1997). Synaptotagmin–syntaxin interaction: the C_2 domain as a Ca^{2+} dependent electrostatic switch. Neuron 18: 133–142.

Sheng Z-H, Westenbroek RE, Catterall WA (1998). Physical link and functional coupling of presynaptic calcium channels and the synaptic docking/fusion machinery. J Bioenerg Biomembr 30: 335–345.

Shotton DM, Heuser JE, Reese BS, et al. (1979). Postsynaptic membrane folds at the frog neuromuscular junction visualized by scanning electron microscopy. Neuroscience 4: 427–435.

Shyng S-L, Salpeter MM (1990). Effect of reinnervation on the degradation rate of junctional acetylcholine receptors synthesized in denervated skeletal muscles. J Neurosci 10: 3905–3915.

Si J, Luo Z, Mei L (1996). Induction of acetylcholine receptor gene expression by ARIA requires activation of mitogen-activated protein kinase. J Biol Chem 271: 19752–19759.

Siebert A, Lottspeich F, Nelson N, et al. (1994). Purification of the synaptic vesicle binding protein physophilin. Identification as 39-kDa subunit of the vacuolar H(+)-ATPase. J Biol Chem 269: 28329–28334.

Simon AM, Hoppe P, Burden SJ (1992). Spatial restriction of AChR gene expression to subsynaptic nuclei. Development 114: 545–553.

Siri MDR, Uchitel OD (1999). Calcium channels coupled to neurotransmitter release at neonatal rat neuromuscular junctions. J Physiol 514: 533–540.

Slater CR, Young C, Wood SJ, et al. (1997). Utrophin abundance is reduced at neuromuscular junctions of patients with both inherited and acquired acetylcholine receptor deficiencies. Brain 120: 1513–1531.

Smith DO (1984). Acetylcholine storage, release and leakage at the neuromuscular junction of mature adults and aged rats. J Physiol 347: 161–176.

Smith S, Augustine GJ (1988). Calcium ions, active zones and synaptic transmitter release. Trends Neurosci 11: 458–465.

Söllner T, Whitehart S, Brunner M, et al. (1993). SNAP receptors implicated in vesicle targeting and fusion. NAT 362: 318–324.

Stadler H, Kiene ML (1987). Synaptic vesicles in electromotoneurones. II. Heterogeneity of populations is expressed in uptake properties; exocytosis and insertion of a core proteoglycan into the extracellular matrix. EMBO J 6: 2217–2221.

Steinbach JH (1981). Developmental changes on acetylcholine receptor aggregates in rat skeletal neuromuscular junctions. Dev Biol 84: 267–276.

Südhof TC (1995). The synaptic vesicle cycle: a cascade of protein–protein interactions. NAT 375: 645–653.

Südhof TC (2006). Synaptic vesicles: an organelle comes of age. Cell 127: 671–673.

Südhof TC, Jahn R (1991). Proteins of synaptic vesicles involved in exocytosis and membrane recycling. Neuron 6: 665–677.

Südhof TC, Rizo J (1996). Synaptotagmins: C_2-domain proteins that regulate membrane traffic. Neuron 17: 379–388.

Sugiyama JE, Bowen DC, Hall ZW (1994). Dystroglycan binds nerve and muscle agrin. Neuron 13: 103–115.

Sugiyama JE, Glass DJ, Yancopoulos GD, et al. (1997). Laminin-induced acetylcholine receptor clustering: an alternative pathway. J Cell Biol 139: 181–191.

Sunderland WJ, Son YJ, Miner JH, et al. (2000). The presynaptic calcium channel is part of a transmembrane complex linking a synaptic laminin ($\alpha4\beta2\gamma1$) with nonerythroid spectrin. J Neurosci 20: 1009–1019.

Sutton RB, Fasshauer D, Jahn R, et al. (1998). Crystal structure of a SNARE complex involved in synaptic exocytosis at 2.4 Å resolution. NAT 395: 347–353.

Sytnyk V, Leshchyns'ka I, Nikonenko AG, et al. (2006). NCAM promotes assembly and activity-dependent remodeling of the postsynaptic signaling complex. J Cell Biol 174: 1071–1085.

Takamori S, Holt M, Stenius K, et al. (2006). Molecular anatomy of a trafficking organelle. Cell 127: 831–846.

Takao-Rikitsu E, Mochida S, Inoue E, et al. (2004). Physical and functional interaction of the active zone proteins, CAST, RIM1, and Bassoon, in neurotransmitter release. J Cell Biol 164: 301–311.

Tarelli FT, Passafaro M, Clementi F, et al. (1991). Presynaptic localization of omega-conotoxin-sensitive calcium channels at the frog neuromuscular junction. Brain Res 547: 331–334.

Tarelli FT, Bossi M, Fesce R, et al. (1992). Synapsin I partially dissociates from synaptic vesicles during exocytosis induced by electrical stimulation. Neuron 9: 1143–1153.

Teräväinen H (1968). Development of the myoneural junction in the rat. Z Zellforsch Mikroskop Anat 87: 249–265.

Tobaben S, Thakur P, Fernàdez-Chacón R, et al. (2001). A trimeric protein complex functions as a synaptic chaperone machine. Neuron 31: 987–999.

Torri-Tarrelli F, Grohovaz F, Fesce R, et al. (1985). Temporal coincidence between synaptic vesicle fusion and quantal secretion of acetylcholine. J Cell Biol 101: 1386–1399.

Tschiriew MS (1879). Sur les terminaisons nerveuses dans les muscle striés. Arch Physiol Norm Pathol 6: 89–116.

Turner C, Kramarcy N, Sealock R, et al. (1991). Localization of paxilin, a focal adhesion protein, to smooth muscle dense plaques and the myotendinous and neuromuscular junction of skeletal muscle. Exp Cell Res 192: 651–655.

Tweedle CD, Stephens KE (1981). Development of complexity in motor nerve endings at the rat neuromuscular junction. Neuroscience 6: 1657–1662.

Ungewickell E (1984). First clue to biological role of clathrin light chains. NAT 311: 213.

Urbano FJ, Uchitel OD (1999). L-type calcium channels unmasked by cell-permeant Ca^{2+} buffer at mouse motor nerve terminals. Pflügers Archiv—Eur J Physiol 437: 523–528.

Valenzuela DM, Stitt TN, Distefano PS, et al. (1995). Receptor tyrosine kinase specific for the skeletal muscle lineage: expression in embryonic muscle, at the neuromuscular junction, and after injury. Neuron 15: 573–584.

Valtorta F, Jahn R, Fesce R, et al. (1988a). Synaptophysin (p38) at the frog neuromuscular junction: its incorporation into the axolemma and recycling after intense quantal secretion. J Cell Biol 107: 2719–2730.

Valtorta F, Villa A, Jahn R, et al. (1988b). Localization of synapsin I at the frog neuromuscular junction. Neuroscience 24: 593–603.

Valtorta F, Benfenati F, Greengard P (1992). Structure and function of the synapsins. J Biol Chem 267: 7195–7198.

Varochi H, Eriksson A (1998). The cytoplasmic tail of the vesicular acetylcholine transporter contains a synaptic vesicle targeting signal. J Biol Chem 273: 9094–9098.

Verma V, Reese TS (1984). Structure and distribution of neuromuscular junctions on slow muscle fibers in the frog. Neuroscience 12: 647–662.

Voets T, Toonen RF, Brian EC, et al. (2001). Munc18-1 promotes large dense-core vesicle docking. Neuron 31: 581–591.

Voglmaier SM, Kam K, Yang H, et al. (2006). Distinct endocytic pathways control the rate and extent of synaptic vesicle protein recycling. Neuron 51: 71–84.

Volnandt W, Zimmermann H (1986). Acetylcholine, ATP, and proteoglycan are common to synaptic vesicles isolated from the electric organ of eel and electric catfish as well as from rat diaphragm. J Neurochem 47: 1449–1462.

von Mollard FG, Südhof TC, Jahn R (1991). A small GTP-binding protein dissociates from synaptic vesicles during exocytosis. NAT 349: 79–81.

von Wedel RJ, Carlson SS, Kelly RB (1981). Transfer of synaptic vesicle antigens to the presynaptic plasma membrane during exocytosis. Proc Natl Acad Sci U S A 78: 1014–1018.

Wagner JA, Carlson SC, Kelly RB (1978). Chemical and physical characterization of cholinergic synaptic vesicles. Biochemistry 17: 1199–1206.

Wallace BG, Nitkin RM, Reist NE, et al. (1985). Aggregates of acetylcholinesterase induced by acetylcholine receptor-aggregating factor. NAT 315: 574–577.

Wang C-T, Grishanin R, Earles CA, et al. (2001). Synaptotagmin modulation of fusion pore kinetics in regulated exocytosis of dense-core vesicles. Science 294: 1111–1115.

Wang Y, Okamoto M, Schmitz F, et al. (1997). RIM is a putative Rab3 effector in regulating synaptic vesicle fusion. NAT 388: 593–598.

Washbourne P, Schiavo G, Montecucco C (1995). Vesicle-associated membrane protein-2 (synaptobrevin-2) forms a complex with synaptophysin. Biochem J 305: 721–724.

Weatherbee SD, Anderson KV, Niswander LA (2006). LDL-receptor-related protein 4 is crucial for formation of the neuromuscular junction. Development 133: 4993–5000.

Weber T, Zemelman BV, McNew JA, et al. (1998). SNAREpins: minimal machinery for membrane fusion. Cell 92: 759–772.

Weinberg CB, Reiness CG, Hall EW (1981). Topographical segregation of old and new acetylcholine receptors at developing ectopic endplates in adult rat muscle. J Cell Biol 88: 215–218.

Weis WI, Scheller RH (1998). SNARE the rod, coil the complex. NAT 395: 328–329.

Wernig A, Pécot-Dechavassine M, Stover H (1980). Sprouting and regression of nerve at the frog neuromuscular junction in normal conditions and after prolonged paralysis with curare. J Neurocytol 9: 277–303.

Wernig A, Anzil AP, Bieser A (1981). Formation and regression of synaptic contacts in the adult muscle. In: H Flohr, and W Precht (Eds.), Lesion Induced Plasticity in Sensorimotor Systems. Springer, Berlin, pp. 38–50.

Whittaker VP (1984). The structure and function of cholinergic synaptic vesicles. Biochem Soc Trans 12: 561–576.

Wiedenmann B, Franke WW (1985). Identification and localization of synaptophysin, an integral membrane glycoprotein of M_r38,000 characteristic of presynaptic vesicles. Cell 41: 1017–1028.

Wigge P, McMahon HT, Vallis Y, et al. (1997). Amphiphysin heterodimers: potential role in clathrin-mediated endocytosis. Mol Biol Cell 8: 2003–2015.

Wigston DJ (1990). Repeated in vivo visualization of neuromuscular junctions in adult mouse lateral gastrocnemius. J Neurosci 10: 1753–1761.

Wilkinson RS, Cole JC (2001). Resolving the Heuser–Ceccarelli debate. Trends Neurosci 24: 195–197.

Willman R, Fuhrer C (2002). Neuromuscular synaptogenesis. Cell Mol Life Sci 59: 1296–1316.

Wood SJ, Slater CR (2001). Safety factor at the neuromuscular junction. Prog Neurobiol 64: 393–429.

Wood SJ, Slater CR (1998). β-Spectrin is colocalized with both voltage-gated sodium channels and ankyrin G at the adult rat neuromuscular junction. J Cell Biol 140: 675–684.

Wucherpfennig KW, Wilsch-Brauninger M, Gonzalez-Gaitan M (2003). Role of *Drosophila* Rab 5 during endosomal trafficking at the synapse and evoked neurotransmitter release. J Cell Biol 161: 609–624.

Xu R, Salpeter MM (1997). Acetylcholine receptor in innervated muscles of dystrophic mdx mice degrade as after denervation. J Neurosci 17: 8194–8200.

Xu T, Bajjalieh SM (2001). SV2 modulates the size of the readily releasable pool of secretory vesicles. Nature Cell Biol 3: 691–698.

Yang X, Arber S, William C, et al. (2001). Patterning of muscle acetylcholine receptor gene expression in the absence of motor innervation. Neuron 30: 399–410.

Yorifuji H, Hirokawa N (1989). Cytoskeletal architecture of neuromuscular junction. I. Localization of vinculin. J Electron Microsc Tech 12: 160–171.

Yoshihara M, Littleton JT (2002). Synaptotagmin functions as a calcium sensor to synchronize neurotransmitter release. Neuron 36: 897–908.

Young JZ (1952). Growth and plasticity in the nervous system. Proc R Soc Lond B Biol Sci 139: 18–37.

Zacks SI, Saito A (1969). Uptake of exogenous horseradish peroxidase by coated vesicles in mouse neuromuscular junctions. J Histochem Cytochem 17: 161–170.

Zacks SI, Saito A (1970). Direct connections between the T-system and the subneural apparatus in mouse neuromuscular junctions demonstrated by lanthanum. J Histochem Cytochem 18: 302–304.

Zhang B, Koh YH, Beckstead RB, et al. (1998). Synaptic vesicle size and number are regulated by a clathrin adaptor protein required for endocytosis. Neuron 21: 1465–1475.

Zhang X, Kim-Miller MJ, Fukuda M, et al. (2002). Ca^{2+}-dependent synaptotagmin binding to SNAP-25 is essential for Ca^{2+}-triggered exocytosis. Neuron 34: 599–611.

Ziskind-Conhaim L, Dennis MJ (1981). Development of rat neuromuscular junctions in organ culture. Dev Biol 85: 243–251.

Handbook of Clinical Neurology, Vol. 91 (3rd series)
Neuromuscular junction disorders
A.G. Engel, Editor

Chapter 4

Electromyographic aspects of neuromuscular junction disorders

C. MICHEL HARPER *

Mayo Clinic College of Medicine, Department of Neurology, Mayo Clinic, Rochester, MN, USA

4.1. Introduction

The motor unit is the basic anatomical and physiological unit of the peripheral nervous system. Clinical electrodiagnosis utilizes electrophysiologic techniques to localize and understand the pathophysiology of diseases affecting the peripheral nervous system. Standardized techniques with well established normal values are available for sensory and motor nerve conduction studies (NCS), standard concentric needle electromyography (EMG), single fiber EMG, and autonomic studies (Daube, 1996). Electrodiagnostic localization is based on defining the spinal segments, systems and individual components of the functional unit involved in the disease process. Neuromuscular junction (NMJ) diseases are diffuse disorders of the motor unit associated with impaired neuromuscular transmission (NMT). Motor NCS, in particular repetitive stimulation studies, and needle EMG are useful in the evaluation of NMJ disorders. They help detect the presence of a NMT disorder and provide additional information related to the mechanism and severity of the disorder. The clinical history and examination, serological tests, and electrodiagnostic studies provide complementary diagnostic information in patients with NMJ disorders. In selected cases specialized morphological and microelectrode studies performed on intercostal muscle biopsy specimens or genetic studies are required to determine the molecular basis for NMJ diseases (Engel, 2004; Engel and Sine, 2005).

4.2. Molecular anatomy and physiology of the NMJ

The NMJ is an integral part of the motor unit and is composed of the nerve terminal (presynaptic component), synaptic cleft, and a specialized section of the muscle fiber membrane (postsynaptic component) (Fig. 4.1). The nerve terminal is responsible for synthesis, storage, and release of acetylcholine (ACh) (Engel, 1999; Ruff, 2003; Hughes et al., 2006). Choline acetyltransferase is the rate limiting enzyme in the synthesis of ACh from acetyl-CoA and choline. ACh is packaged at a concentration of 8000–10 000 per vesicle by an energy dependent proton pump that exchanges hydrogen ions for ACh. ACh vesicles are functionally compartmentalized within the nerve terminal. Vesicles that are immediately available for release are clustered in active zones closely associated with P/Q-type and N-type voltage-gated calcium channels (VGCC) embedded in the terminal membrane. Vesicles are transported into the active zones by an energy dependent process involving vesicle associated proteins (e.g., synapsin) and elements of the cytoskeleton (e.g., actin).

The terminal motor axon becomes devoid of myelin just proximal to the neuromuscular junction, but retains a rich concentration of membrane associated voltage-gated ion channels (Ruff, 2003). Chloride and "leak" potassium channels help maintain the resting membrane potential. Sodium channel activation initiates the action potential, while inactivation of the sodium channel and voltage-activated delayed rectifier

---

*Correspondence to: C. Michel Harper, MD, Department of Neurology, Mayo Clinic, 200 First Street S.W., Rochester, MN 55905, USA. E-mail: mharper@mayo.edu, Tel: 1-507-284-4409, Fax: 1-507-266-4419.

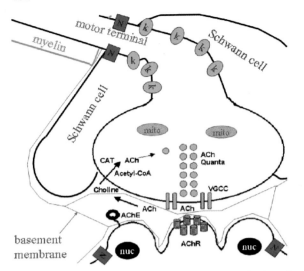

Fig. 4.1. Graphic representation of neuromuscular junction. ACh, acetylcholine; AChE, acetylcholine esterase; AChR, acetylcholine receptor; CAT, choline acetyltransferase; CoA, co-enzyme A; k, potassium channel; mito, mitochondria; N, sodium channel; nuc, nucleus; VGCC, voltage-gated calcium channel.

potassium channels limit action potential duration. When an action potential invades the nerve terminal, P/Q-type and N-type VGCC facilitate the release of ACh. The VGCC are strategically distributed in the active zones where they are arranged in double parallel rows separated by 20 nm and located immediately opposite the crests of the postsynaptic folds (Engel, 2004).

Neuronal VGCC channels consist of five subunits (Jones, 1998; Black and Lennon, 1999). The $\alpha 1$ subunit is largest and contains the voltage-sensor and cation pore. It has four domains, each with six transmembrane segments. The M4 segment contains the voltage sensor, and loops between M5 and M6 segments in each domain form the ion channel and determine calcium selective permeability. The $\alpha 1$ subunit contains high affinity binding sites for channel antagonists and for regulatory G-proteins and SNARE proteins and determines the family of the VGCC (L, N, P/Q, R, T). The auxiliary subunits, β, $\alpha 2-\delta$ and γ, influence the insertion and stability of $\alpha 1$ in the plasma membrane, and modify the conductance and kinetics of the channel.

The process of synaptic vesicle docking, membrane fusion, release of contents, and vesicle reformation involves a complex interaction between multiple cytoplasmic, vesicular and nerve terminal membrane associated glycoproteins and enzymes as well as cytoplasmic co-factors (Hughes et al., 2006). Influx calcium through the VGCC channel is triggered by nerve terminal depolarization. The local rise in calcium concentration in

the nerve terminal is sensed by synaptotagmin, a vesicular membrane soluble N-ethylmaleimide-sensitive factor (NSF) attachment receptor (v-SNARE) protein. The binding of synaptotagmin to the synaptic core complex formed by the association of vesicular synaptobrevin (v-SNARE) and nerve terminal proteins syntaxin-1 and SNAP-25 (t-SNAREs) destabilizes the vesicular and nerve terminal membranes creating a fusion pore leading to exocytosis of ACh. The VGCC channel interacts in a calcium-dependent manner with t-SNAREs and synaptotagmin. The t-SNARE proteins interact noncovalently with the synaptic core complex and with soluble cytoplasmic factors, including NSF and α–SNAP, to facilitate formation of the fusion pore. Following exocytosis, vesicle membranes are recycled from the plasma membrane by clathrin-dependent and independent processes. Synaptotagmin plays a role in the former, which involves sequential interaction of dynamin and amphiphysin with other highly conserved cytoplasmic proteins (Boonyapisit et al., 1999; Hughes et al., 2006).

Once released, the entire quantum (8000–10 000 molecules) of ACh diffuses into the synapse. The synaptic cleft is a 70–100 nm space located between the nerve terminal and the muscle fiber filled with an electron-dense ground substance (Engel, 1999). Acetylcholine esterase (AChE), the enzyme responsible for the degradation of ACh, is found in high concentrations in this region. The catalytic subunits of AChE are anchored into the basal lamina of the postsynaptic membrane by a collagen-like tail (Ohno et al., 2000). AChE activity is inhibited by high concentrations of its substrate, ACh. Thus, only a small amount of ACh is metabolized before it reaches the postsynaptic receptors.

The 3-dimensional configuration of the endplate is uniquely designed to maximize the safety margin of neuromuscular transmission. The postsynaptic membrane is highly convoluted, which increases the surface area of the endplate region and brings the acetylcholine receptors (AChRs) into close proximity to the active zones on the nerve terminal membrane. AChRs are concentrated on the crests of the post-junctional folds at a density of approximately $10\,000/\mu m^2$ with a total number approximated at 1.5×10^7 per endplate (Ruff, 2003).

The AChR is a 250 kilodalton pentameric glycoprotein ligand-gated receptor embedded into the postsynaptic membrane (Karlin and Akabas, 1994). The immature fetal receptor is composed of two α-subunits along with one β, δ, and γ-subunit. The mature adult AChR contains an ϵ-subunit in place of the γ-subunit. The fetal receptor is normally replaced by the adult receptor just before birth but may also be expressed in normal premature infants, certain congenital myasthenic syndromes associated with ϵ-subunit mutations, and in muscle that is denervated or in the early stages of reinnervation (Sine et al., 2004). All of the AChR sub-units share the same basic structure. The N-terminus forms the large extracellular domain where, in the α-sub-unit, the ACh binding site is located (amino acids 192 and 193). There are four transmembrane domains (M1–M4), with the M2 domain forming the major channel-lining segment. The large cytoplasmic loop between M3 and M4 contains phosphorylation sites that affect channel conductance and bind AChR to rapsyn. Rapsyn is a membrane associated muscle protein that is necessary for AChR clustering and anchors AChR to dystroglycan forming structural and functional linkage between AChRs and the muscle cytoskeleton (Ohno et al., 2002). AChR clustering on the crests of the postsynaptic folds is induced by the interaction of agrin, released from the nerve terminal, with muscle specific kinase (MuSK) and myotube associated specific component (MASC), which are associated with the muscle membrane in the endplate region (Hughes et al., 2006).

4.3. Physiology of neuromuscular transmission

The neuromuscular junction is uniquely designed to produce tight coupling of nerve and muscle action potentials at discharge frequencies ranging from 1–50 Hz for extended periods of activity (Harper, 1999; Ruff, 2003). Under physiological conditions, central nervous system and muscle fatigue lead to loss of contractile force long before NMT fails. Even under experimental conditions, the safety margin of NMT allows for tight coupling of nerve and muscle action potentials at rates of electrical stimulation up to 100 Hz. Repetitive discharge of the muscle fiber in response to a single nerve action potential is prevented at the normal NMJ by the rapid decay constant of the endplate potential and the catalytic activity of AChE. Neuromuscular transmission failure or endplate "blocking" occurs when the amplitude of the endplate potential (EPP) falls below the threshold for muscle action potential generation.

4.3.1. Single channel events

The basic physiological event that underpins NMT is the interaction of ACh with the AChR. ACh binding to the α-subunit changes the configuration of the extra-cellular AChR vestibule allowing cations (primarily sodium but also calcium) to flow through the channel (Zhang et al., 1995). Different agonists or alterations of the receptor (genetic or pharmacological) change the total amount of current conducted by an individual channel by alteration of the single channel open time or the total burst duration (Zhang et al., 1995). Mutations that cause the slow channel congenital myasthenic syndrome (SCCMS) produce prolonged individual

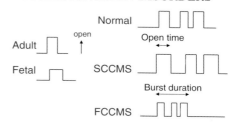

Fig. 4.2. Acetylcholine receptor (AChR) channel currents in normal and pathological states. Adult and fetal AChR are compared on the left. Height of each bar is related to rate of current flow. Length of each bar is related to open time of the AChR. FCCMS, fast channel congenital myasthenic syndrome; SCCMS, slow channel congenital myasthenic syndrome.

open times or prolong the burst durations (Fig. 4.2) (Engel et al., 1996). The "mirror image" of SCCMS is the fast channel congenital myasthenic syndrome (FCCMS), which is produced by mutations that shorten channel openings or burst duration (Sine et al., 2002). Congenital or acquired endplate acetylcholinesterase deficiency prolongs the endplate current without having any effect on the burst duration (Hutchinson et al., 1993). Prolonged synaptic currents produce muscle weakness by three mechanisms (Sine et al., 2002). First, prolonged currents bring excess calcium into the muscle, which activates proteases and other enzymes, and produces degeneration of the endplate region (i.e., 'endplate' myopathy) (Engel et al., 1982). Second, the prolonged endplate potentials arising in each other's wake at physio-logic rates of stimulation can produce a depolarization block. Third, prolonged channel openings may desensitize AChR and make it refractory to further stimulation, particularly at high rates of activation as occurs during exertion or repetitive electrical stimulation.

4.3.2. Endplate potentials and the safety margin of NMT

The temporal and spatial summation of a single quanta of ACh on postsynaptic AChRs produces a small depolarization of the muscle membrane, the miniature endplate potential (MEPP), which is best measured with an intracellular microelectrode (Ruff, 2003; Engel, 2004). The MEPP arises from the spontaneous and random release of ACh quanta in the absence of a nerve action potential. The MEPP is of insufficient size to trigger a muscle fiber action potential. The amplitude and duration of the MEPP are determined by the miniature endplate current (MEPC) and the cable properties of the muscle membrane. The MEPC is determined by the number of ACh per quanta, the 3-dimensional configuration of the synaptic cleft, density and channel kinetics of the AChR, and the concentration and catalytic activity of the AChE (Engel, 2004). Abnormalities of MEPP amplitude and duration usually reflect "postsynaptic" disturbances of NMT.

When a nerve action potential invades the nerve terminal, 60–300 quanta are released. The resulting depolarization of the normal postsynaptic membrane is approximately 40 mV and is called the endplate potential (EPP) (Ruff, 2003; Engel, 2004). The amplitude and duration of the EPP are determined by the same postsynaptic factors that determine the MEPP, and in addition, by the quantal release of ACh from the presynaptic terminal. The quantal release is in turn determined by two important presynaptic factors. The first is the concentration and kinetics of the P/Q-type and N-type voltage-gated calcium channel. This factor is also referred to as the "probability" of ACh release. The second is the size of the immediately available store of ACh vesicles. The immediately available store represents those in or near the active zones of the nerve terminal membrane.

Presynaptic factors that influence the amplitude of the EPP are manipulated by altering the discharge frequency of the nerve terminal (Harper, 1999; Engel, 2004). At firing rates less than 2 Hz, the amplitude of the EPP remains constant but at rates of 2–5 Hz, the amplitude of the EPP falls for the first 3–5 impulses and then gradually returns to normal. The decrement of the EPP is caused by depletion of the immediate stores of ACh. The repair of the EPP after the first 3–5 impulses is caused by mobilization of additional ACh stores and accumulation of calcium in the nerve terminal. At rates of 10–50 Hz the EPP is initially unchanged, but will eventually fall if stimulation persists for several minutes. This is especially true in disorders that impair reuptake, synthesis, packaging and mobilization of ACh (e.g., hemicholinium administration or congenital choline acetyltransferase deficiency) (Schmidt et al., 2003). If the EPP is reduced in size by disease, then high frequency stimulation will increase the EPP amplitude (facilitation) for several seconds. Post-activation facilitation of the EPP results from an influx and accumulation of calcium within the nerve terminal. Facilitation lasts less than 1 min and is followed by a 2–10 min depressed EPP called post-activation exhaustion. During the exhaustion phase VGCCs are desensitized and ACh stores are depleted (Jones, 1998; Ruff, 2003). The EPP gradually returns to baseline with resynthesis and mobilization of additional ACh.

4.3.3. Endplate potentials and the safety margin of NMT in NMJ disorders

Abnormalities of the EPP amplitude and duration translate directly into the clinical manifestations and electrodiagnostic abnormalities observed in NMJ disorders.

The safety margin of NMT is defined as the difference between the EPP and the amount of depolarization required to bring the muscle membrane to action potential threshold (Harper, 1999; Ruff, 2003; Engel, 2004; Hughes et al., 2006). When the EPP amplitude drops below threshold, the muscle fiber action potential is blocked. The safety margin of neuromuscular transmission is large enough to prevent blocking at normal endplates. The characteristic abnormality observed in NMJ disease of either presynaptic or postsynaptic origin is blocking of NMT at multiple endplates. This produces fatigable weakness and correlates with increased jitter and blocking on single fiber EMG studies, motor unit potential (MUP) amplitude variation on standard concentric needle EMG, and a decrement of the compound muscle action potential (CMAP) observed at slow rates of repetitive stimulation (Harper, 1999).

Conditions that abnormally prolong the duration of the EPP are associated with repetitive compound muscle action potentials (R-CMAP) following single stimuli on standard NCS, a rate-dependent CMAP decrement on repetitive stimulation studies, and small MUPs on standard concentric needle EMG (Harper, 2004). The R-CMAP occurs because the EPP remains above threshold beyond the muscle fiber action potential refractory period in selected fibers. This triggers a second muscle fiber action potential 3–6 ms after the main component of the CMAP. Prolonged EPPs are produced by inhibition of AChE, congenital deficiency of endplate AChE or altered AChR channel kinetics (e.g., SCCMS). An increase in the CMAP decrement with increasing rates of repetitive stimulation (rate-dependent decrement) is observed in conditions with prolonged EPPs because the muscle fiber membrane remains depolarized and refractory to further stimuli (Harper, 1999). Small MUPs on concentric needle EMG are observed when there is an endplate myopathy produced by excessive calcium influx due to prolonged EPP duration or when severe blocking occurs from any disorder of NMT (Harper, 1999). Fibrillation potentials occur in severe NMJ diseases when there is blocking of all impulses at the endplate (i.e., "functional denervation") or when there is structural damage to the motor nerve terminal or physical disruption of the synaptic cleft.

4.4. Electrodiagnostic techniques used to evaluate NMJ disease

4.4.1. Standard motor NCS

The amplitude and negative area of the CMAP recorded with surface electrodes is directly related to the number of muscle fibers electrically activated by the stimulus (Daube, 1996). Disorders that reduce the number of functioning axons, nerve terminals or muscle fibers will reduce the amplitude and area of the CMAP proportionally. In mild disorders of NMT the size of the CMAP on standard motor NCS is normal. In severe disorders the CMAP is reduced as EPP falls below threshold in the majority of muscle fibers in the resting baseline state.

R-CMAPs are typically observed in patients exposed to exogenous AChE inhibitors, in congenital AChE deficiency and in SCCMS (Harper, 1999; Engel, 2004). In each of these disorders the decay constant of the EPP is significantly prolonged. R-CMAPs follow the main CMAP by 3–6 ms and may recur several times at similar intervals, particularly in AChE inhibitor intoxication or severe SCCMS. They are more easily detected in small hand and foot muscles that have relatively short duration CMAPs (Harper, 1999, 2004). In muscles with longer duration CMAPs (e.g., biceps, tibialis anterior) the repetitive discharge is typically buried in the negative tail of the main potential. R-CMAPs are sometimes mistaken for artifacts caused by limb movement or activity picked up by the reference electrode in normal motor NCS recordings. These normal variations of CMAP configuration are unchanged in size or appearance by brief isometric exercise or repetitive stimulation. In contrast R-CMAPs are abolished by a few seconds of exercise or by 2–3 stimuli of low frequency repetitive stimulation (i.e., 0.5–2.0 Hz) (Fig. 4.3). If a decrement is present in the main CMAP with repetitive stimulation at 2–3 Hz, the R-CMAP decrement is invariably greater. Administration of a short acting AChE inhibitor like edrophonium can be used to distinguish congenital AChE deficiency from other causes of R-CMAP. When AChE is congenitally deficient, administration of a cholinesterase inhibitor has no effect on the R-CMAP (Harper, 2004). In contrast, when a cholinesterase inhibitor is administered to subjects already exposed to an exogenous AChE inhibitor or in SCCMS patients, the number and size of R-CMAPs is increased (Harper, 2004).

4.4.2. Repetitive stimulation

Repetitive stimulation is a reliable technique that accurately reflects the severity of NMT defect in moderate to severe disease of the NMJ (Daube, 1996; Harper, 1999). Its sensitivity is limited in mild disorders but is increased by performing repetitive stimulation after exercise. In normal subjects of any age (newborns to adults), repetitive stimulation at 2–5 Hz fails to produce a decrement in the amplitude or area of the CMAP. No change in the area of the CMAP is observed with rapid repetitive stimulation (>5 Hz) or

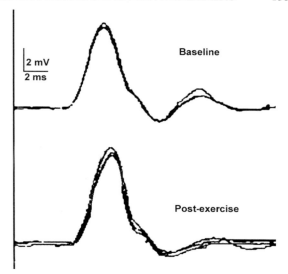

Fig. 4.3. Repetitive stimulation of the median nerve at 2 Hz recording over the abductor pollicis brevis muscle in a patient with slow channel congenital myasthenic syndrome (SCCMS). The top group of traces demonstrates a well defined repetitive compound muscle action potential (R-CMAP) following the main CMAP by approximately 6 ms. The bottom group of traces demonstrates disappearance of the R-CMAP immediately following 10 s of exercise.

brief exercise in normal adults but a decrement can occur in newborns or premature infants. Mild "pseudo-facilitation" is frequently observed in normal subjects. Pseudofacilitation is identified as an increased CMAP amplitude but not area (due to shortened CMAP duration) and is caused by increased synchronization of motor unit firing at higher firing frequencies.

The sensitivity and specificity of repetitive stimulation is affected by technical factors and the distribution of clinical weakness. Maintaining supramaximal stimulation, and minimizing discomfort and voluntary patient movement, are technical variables that impact the reliability of repetitive stimulation. These technical factors are best controlled when repetitive stimulation is performed on nerves and muscles in distal regions of the extremities. If repetitive stimulation is normal in distal regions then repetitive stimulation should be done on nerves and muscles in regions that are affected most by symptoms and signs of weakness. Table 4.1 lists the advantages and disadvantages of commonly tested nerve and muscle combinations. A reproducible abnormality should be seen in at least two muscles before a definite NMT defect is diagnosed.

4.4.2.1. Repetitive stimulation technique

Surface electrodes are attached to the skin with the active electrode over the motor endplate zone and the

Table 4.1

Common muscles used for repetitive stimulation

Nerve	Muscle	Stimulation site	Advantages	Disadvantages
Ulnar	Abuctor digiti minimi	Wrist	Readily immobilized	May be uninvolved
Median	Abductor pollicis brevis	Wrist	Well tolerated	Difficult to immobilize
				May be uninvolved
Radial	Extensor indicis proprius or Anconeus	Radial groove	Relatively sensitive for distal muscle	Volume conduction from other forearm muscles
Musculo-cutaneous	Biceps	Axilla	Proximal muscle	Difficult to immobilize
				Painful
Axillary	Deltoid	Supraclavicular	Proximal muscle	Unstable stimulus
Accessory	Trapezius	Posterior neck triangle	Proximal muscle; Well tolerated	Same as musculo-cutaneous
Facial	Nasalis	Angle of jaw	Proximal muscle	Difficult to immobilize
Trigeminal	Masseter	Pterygoid fossa*	Proximal muscle	Poor relaxation
Peroneal	Anterior tibial	Knee	Leg	Unable to immobilize; Masseter contraction
Femoral	Rectus femoris	Inguinal ligament*	Proximal leg muscle	Unstable stimulus
				Painful
				May be uninvolved
				Unable to immobilize
				Painful

*Needle stimulation routinely used.

reference electrode over the distal tendon. Routine nerve conduction studies are done to ensure that the nerve and muscle are normal and that there are no artifacts that could alter the test results. Stimulation rates of 2–3 Hz with supramaximal stimulation (about 25% above maximal stimulation) should be used because these rates will produce maximal depression of the EPP and thus be most likely to show a decrement. Between three and seven stimuli are given. If a decrement is present, the greatest relative change occurs between the first and second CMAPs and the greatest maximal change occurs between the first and fourth response. Slow repair of the CMAP is observed by the 5th–10th potential. Thus, the typical decrement observed in disorders of NMT follows a smooth tapering course that peaks by the 3rd–5th response and is repaired with continued repetitive stimulation or exercise (Fig. 4.4).

Technical problems are identified by instability of the baseline or by an atypical pattern of decrement. Muscle channelopathies associated with clinical myotonia produce atypical patterns of decrement as well. Normal muscle shows no decrement so the presence of any reliable, reproducible decrement without technical difficulties is indicative of a NMT defect. In order to enhance specificity of the repetitive stimulation, typically a minimum decrement of 10% is required to establish a definite abnormality (Daube, 1996; Harper, 1999).

After 2–3 trials of repetitive stimulation are completed at rest, 2 Hz stimulation is repeated at regular intervals following exercise of the target muscle. Exercise enhances the EPP (post-activation facilitation) for 10–60 s, but by 2–4 min post-exercise, depression of the EPP (post-activation exhaustion) causes the decrement to be greater than that observed at rest. Therefore, repetitive stimulation after exercise reveals abnormalities that are not obvious at rest. Stimulation at high rates (20–50 Hz) produces the same effect as exercise but because high frequency stimulation is

painful, it is used only when the target muscle can not be exercised adequately.

Repetitive stimulation of resting muscles, and at intervals after muscle exercise, is performed in several muscles until a well-defined abnormality is seen in at least two muscles (Daube, 1996; Harper, 1999). Although many abnormalities of NMT can be elucidated by repetitive stimulation studies, the absence of a defect does not preclude a mild NMJ disease.

4.4.2.2. Technical factors relevant to repetitive stimulation

Technical factors play a major role in the reliability of repetitive stimulation studies (Daube, 1996; Harper, 1999). The two major factors that can produce false-negative results (absence of a decrement despite the presence of NMT defect) are temperature and anticholinesterase medications. As the temperature is lowered, the amplitude and duration of the MEPP and EPP increase, the duration of the nerve action potential is prolonged releasing more ACh, and the metabolism of ACh by AChE is slowed. All of these consequences improve the safety margin and can lessen or eliminate an otherwise obvious decrement. Anticholinesterase medications may partially or completely obscure the underlying defect of NMT. Medications of this nature should be discontinued at least 4–6 h before electrophysiological testing is done.

Factors that produce a false impression of a defect of NMT include recording electrode movement, inadequate immobilization of the muscle, and submaximal nerve stimulation due to inadequate stimulus intensity or movement of the stimulating electrodes. Changes in the area under the negative phase of the compound muscle action potential or changes in the configuration, with or without changes in the amplitude, should alert one to the possibility of a technical problem.

4.4.2.3. Repetitive stimulation studies in nerve and muscle disorders

Although repetitive stimulation is typically used to study NMJ diseases, primary disorders of nerve and muscle can occasionally produce abnormalities on repetitive stimulation studies (Daube, 1996). Failure to recognize these disorders can lead to the incorrect diagnosis. A decrement on repetitive stimulation is often observed in neurogenic disorders that produce severe denervation and active reinnervation of muscle. The most common disease of this type is amyotrophic lateral sclerosis, but a mild decrement on repetitive stimulation studies can also be seen in acute demyelinating neuropathies and poliomyelitis (Daube, 1996). Myotonic disorders are frequently associated with a

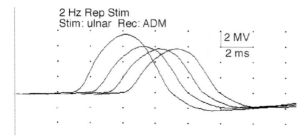

Fig. 4.4. Typical smooth tapering decrement in myasthenia gravis. ADM, abductor digiti minimi; Rec, record; Rep Stim, repetitive stimulation; Stim, stimulate.

variable decrement on repetitive stimulation because of altered muscle membrane excitability induced by electrical stimulation or exercise.

4.4.3. Concentric and single fiber EMG

Concentric needle EMG is used to record activity inducted by needle movement, spontaneous muscle action potentials, and motor unit potentials generated by voluntary muscle contraction (Daube, 1996). In normal muscle, needle movement elicits very brief self limited depolarization by mechanical irritation of the muscle membrane. Denervated muscle fibers spontaneously discharge at a regular firing rate. This activity is recorded as fibrillation potentials with a concentric needle electrode. Fibrillation potentials are observed most commonly in primary nerve and muscle disease but can be seen in NMJ disorders that are associated with complete block of NMT at the motor endplate or when there is physical disruption of either the motor nerve terminal or synaptic cleft. Fibrillation potentials are observed in some severe cases of auto-immune myasthenia gravis and are common in botulism (Cornblath, 1986). They are very rarely found in Lambert–Eaton myasthenic syndrome or in congenital myasthenic syndromes (Harper, 2004).

The motor unit is the basic physiological unit of the peripheral nervous system, consisting of all muscle fibers innervated by a single lower motor neuron. The MUP recorded with a concentric needle EMG electrode represents the extracellular summation of muscle action potentials produced by fibers belonging to an individual motor unit (Daube, 1996). Force is produced during voluntary activation by increasing the firing rate of individual MUPs and recruitment of additional higher threshold MUPs. Disorders of NMT that result in inter-mittent blocking at the endplate are associated with "instability" or variation in size of individual MUPs on concentric needle EMG due to intermittent loss of individual muscle fiber action potentials. Small MUPs are observed in NMJ disease when there is severe blocking of multiple endplates or when there is an associated endplate myopathy. Small varying MUPs are common in botulism (Cornblath, 1986), moderately severe autoimmune myasthenia gravis (Benatar, 2006), Lambert–Eaton syndrome and most congenital myasthe-nic syndromes (Harper, 2004). MUP variation can only be detected reliably at minimal levels of activation and when there is no movement of the recording elec-trode within the muscle. MUP variation is nonspecific and gives no information about the site or underlying mechanism of the NMT defect.

Single fiber EMG (SFEMG) is the most sensitive clin-ical neurophysiological test available for the detection of mild disorders of NMT (Sanders, 1979; Oh, 1992). Sin-gle fiber EMG utilizes restricted filter settings and a small recording surface to selectively and simulta-neously record 2–4 muscle fiber action potentials from a single MUP. Jitter is measured as variability in the latency of time-locked firing of individual muscle action potentials. Increased jitter results from a delay in the rise time of the EPP, which occurs even in very mild disor-ders of NMT making single fiber very sensitive in the diagnosis of NMJ disease. Blocking is recorded on SFEMG when time-locked muscle fiber action poten-tials fail to appear intermittently. Blocking occurs when the EPP falls below the safety margin of NMT for one of the muscle fibers being recorded. Blocking is the SFEMG equivalent of MUP variation recorded with concentric needle EMG. In voluntary SFEMG, record-ings are made with voluntary activation, while stimu-lated SFEMG utilizes electrical stimulation to produce individual muscle fiber action potentials. SFEMG requires specialized equipment, a skilled examiner and a cooperative patient. It is sensitive enough to detect a mild defect in NMT in muscles that are not clinically weak. Abnormalities in SFEMG are commonly detected in myopathies, motor neuron disease and peripheral neuropathies because of impaired NMT in immature reinnervated endplates. Because of this, SFEMG is very sensitive but not specific for the diagnosis of primary dis-eases of the NMJ. The specificity of SFEMG is greatly enhanced if the study is restricted to those patients with normal nerve conduction studies and concentric needle EMG. Single fiber EMG is abnormal in all disorders of NMT. In autoimmune myasthenia gravis, sensitivity has been reported to be has high as 98% (Sanders, 1979; Oh, 1992; Sanders and Stalberg, 1996). Although techni-cally challenging, changes in jitter and blocking with increasing discharge frequencies can be used to distin-guish presynaptic and postsynaptic disorders of NMT (Sanders and Stalberg, 1996). In presynaptic disorders, jitter and blocking temporarily improve with increasing discharge frequencies whereas the opposite is observed in postsynaptic disorders.

Table 4.2 summarizes the general findings and interpretation of nerve conduction studies, repetitive stimulation at various rates, concentric needle EMG, and SFEMG in primary disorders of NMT. These tech-niques are better at quantifying the severity of the disorder than accurately predicting the site or type of NMT defect. Nonetheless, when used in conjunction with findings on clinical examination and serological studies, accurate diagnosis of a specific NMJ disease is possible. Rarely, additional specialized microelec-trode, morphological and genetic studies are required to make a specific diagnosis, especially in cases of congenital myasthenia.

Table 4.2

Summary of electrodiagnostic findings in disorders of neuromuscular transmission

Electrodiagnostic parameter	Severity of neuromuscular transmission disorder		
	Mild	Moderate	Severe
Baseline CMAP size	Normal	Normal	Reduced
2–5 Hz repetitive stimulation	Decrement only after exercise	Decrement, repairs with exercise; mild facilitation	Decrement, prominent facilitation
20–50 Hz repetitive stimulation	Normal	Mild facilitation	Prominent facilitation
Concentric needle EMG	Normal	MUP amplitude variation	Fibrillation potentials, small MUP, MUP amplitude variation
Single fiber EMG	Mild increased jitter with minimal blocking	Increased jitter and blocking	Severe increased jitter and blocking

CMAP, compound muscle action potential; EMG, electromyography; MUP, motor unit potential.

4.5. Electrodiagnostic evaluation of specific neuromuscular junction disorders

4.5.1. Autoimmune myasthenia gravis

Autoimmune myasthenia gravis (MG) is caused by an antibody mediated reduction in the number of functioning postsynaptic AChRs at the neuromuscular junction (Engel and Hohlfeld, 2004). Antibodies directed against the AChR have been shown to act by three separate mechanisms: 1. Complement mediated destruction of the receptor following binding of antibodies to extracellular receptor epitopes. 2. Cross-linking of adjacent AChRs by the Fab fragments of AChR antibodies with enhanced turnover (modulation) of the receptors. 3. Allosteric interference (blocking) of the ACh–AChR interaction by antibodies binding to the alpha chain of the AChR.

Clinically, autoimmune MG is characterized by fluctuating fatigable weakness of skeletal muscles (Romi, 2005). Early in the course of the disease, the weakness can be mild or confined to ocular muscles. In moderate disease, extraocular, bulbar and proximal muscles are typically involved. Although 50% of patients with MG present with ocular involvement, 85% eventually developed generalized disease within 2 years of symptom onset. In severe cases, any skeletal muscle including those controlling respiration can be affected. In addition to clinical manifestations, the diagnosis of autoimmune MG depends on demonstrating autoimmunity against the nicotinic AChR and physiological evidence for a disorder of NMT. The diagnostic sensitivity of a combination of clinical manifestations, serological tests and electrodiagnostic testing is nearly 100%. AChR antibodies are detected in the sera of 70% of patients with mild early generalized or ocular disease and in 90% of those with generalized MG of at least 6 months' duration (Lindstrom et al., 1975).

Repetitive stimulation is the most widely used electrodiagnostic test to diagnose MG. It is less sensitive than serologic testing, but gives an accurate measure of the severity and distribution of the neuromuscular transmission defect, and often helps establish a diagnosis early in the course of MG when serological studies are negative (Oh et al., 1992; Zivkovic and Shipe, 2005). In mild MG, the baseline CMAP is normal and there is no decrement at rest with slow rates of stimulation. Under these circumstances isometric exercise of 1 min duration frequently elicits a decrement through post-activation exhaustion (Fig. 4.5). The decrement may take 1–5 min to reach maximal levels in this setting. Within a train of responses, the decrement reaches its maximum 2–5 min after exercise and returns to normal within 15 min. In moderately severe MG, the baseline CMAP is normal and there is a decrement with repetitive stimulation from 2–5 Hz in weakest muscles, even at rest. Brief exercise elicits repair, followed by an increased decrement even over baseline levels due to post-activation exhaustion. In severe MG, the endplate potential falls below the safety margin of NMT in some muscle fibers, reducing the amplitude CMAP at rest and resulting in facilitation of 110–300% following brief exercise or 50 Hz stimulation. In this setting MG is difficult to differentiate from moderately severe Lambert–Eaton myasthenic syndrome (Fig. 4.6). Clinical and serological studies can usually clarify the diagnosis in these cases.

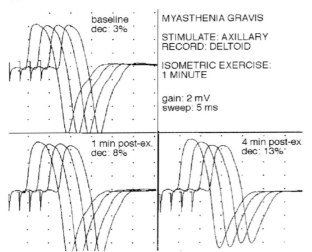

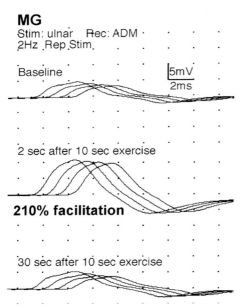

Fig. 4.5. Increased decrement after exercise in patient with myasthenia gravis (post-exercise exhaustion). Dec, decrement; ex, exercise; min, minute.

Fig. 4.6. Repetitive stimulation of the ulnar nerve at 2 Hz recording over the abductor digiti minimi muscle in a patient with severe myasthenia gravis. The amplitude of the compound muscle action potential is reduced at rest (top group of traces) and demonstrates 210% facilitation with exercise (bottom group of traces). ADM, abductor digiti minimi; MG, myasthenia gravis; Rec, record; Rep Stim, repetitive stimulation; sec, seconds; Stim, stimulate.

The sensitivity of repetitive stimulation depends on the severity of myasthenia, the distribution of weakness, the number of nerves tested, and the use of exercise (Oh et al., 1992; Costa et al., 2004; Benatar, 2006). In moderate to severe disease about 65% of patients show a decrement in hand muscles and 85% show a decrement in proximal muscles. The yield is much lower in mild myasthenia where the absence of a decrement at rest or after exercise does not exclude the diagnosis. In this situation, other physiological tests can enhance diagnostic sensitivity. The edrophonium test is frequently positive in ocular myasthenia; however, false positives are not uncommon. Single fiber EMG is universally abnormal in autoimmune MG when a clinically involved region of the body is examined (Sanders and Stalberg, 1996; Farrugia et al., 2006). In patients with ocular or bulbar symptoms a cranial muscle (e.g., frontalis) is examined, while a limb muscle is tested (e.g., extensor digitorum communis) when limb weakness predominates. Since single fiber EMG is frequently abnormal in myopathies and neurogenic diseases, it is typically done only in patients suspected of myasthenia gravis with documented normal findings on standard nerve conduction studies (including repetitive stimulation) and concentric needle EMG. It is most useful in making the diagnosis of MG in very mild cases or excluding it in patients with atypical features or nonspecific chronic fatigue (Sanders and Stalberg, 1996).

Cholinesterase inhibitors repair abnormalities on repetitive stimulation and lessen the severity of findings on concentric SFEMG in patients with myasthenia gravis. Regular acting pyridostigmine (Mestinon®) should be discontinued 6 h and time-release pyridostigmine (Mestinon Timespan®) 12 h prior to electrodiagnostic testing. Immunosuppressive therapy may also render a patient seronegative and improve abnormalities in electrodiagnostic testing, although mild changes in SFEMG usually persist.

4.5.2. Seronegative autoimmune myasthenia gravis

Approximately 10–15% of patients with the diagnosis of autoimmune myasthenia gravis based on clinical and electrodiagnostic criteria do not have detectable serum levels of AChR antibodies, even when serological tests are repeated 6–12 months after the diagnosis (Vincent et al., 2004). These patients typically respond to one or more types of immunotherapy. Approximately 40% of "seronegative" myasthenia gravis patients have serological evidence of antibodies to MuSK (Vincent and Leite, 2005). Another small subset of seronegative cases is associated with an unidentified factor that phosphorylates the AChR through a secondary messenger (Plested et al., 2002). MuSK interacts with agrin and rapsyn to induce AChR clustering on the postsynaptic folds of the neuromuscular junction (Hughes et al., 2006). The mechanism of weakness in anti-MuSK antibody positive patients has not been completely elucidated. One study failed to demonstrate a reduction in AChR density in a patient with anti-MuSK MG (Selcen et al., 2004).

Anti-MuSK antibody associated MG may manifest as several different phenotypes (Stickler et al., 2005; Vincent and Leite, 2005; Padua et al., 2006). One sub-type is indistinguishable clinically and electrophysiologically from classical AChR antibody MG. A more distinctive subtype has preferential and severe involvement of ocular, facial, bulbar and respiratory muscles. Patients with this form experience a mixture of exertional weakness as well as "myopathic" features with static muscle weakness and atrophy. Younger females are over-represented in this phenotype. Patients with anti-MuSK antibody MG typically have normal thymic histology and do not benefit from thymectomy. Intolerance to or at least minimal benefit from treatment with cholinesterase inhibitors is also typical. Plasmapheresis is beneficial, but responsiveness to prednisone, azathioprine and mycophenolate is less predictable and dramatic than classical autoimmune MG. The findings on electrodiagnostic studies in the "myopathic" phenotype of anti-MuSK antibody associated myasthenia are relatively characteristic and support the diagnosis based on clinical and serological grounds. On routine motor NCS, the CMAP is usually reduced in amplitude when recorded over weak and atrophic muscles. In addition, like other myopathies, repetitive stimulation typically produces minimal if any decrement. Likewise, concentric needle EMG typically reveals fibrillation potentials and small polyphasic MUP in the "myopathic" form of anti-MuSK MG. Single fiber EMG is abnormal in all patients even when performed on muscles that are unaffected by atrophy or severe clinical weakness (Stickler et al., 2005; Farrugia et al., 2006; Padua et al., 2006). The "myopathic" form of anti-MuSK antibody associated MG may be mistaken for a congenital myopathy or congenital myasthenia. Serological testing for anti-MuSK antibodies should be performed in any patient fitting the "myopathic" phenotype described above and in patients with the more typical phenotype of autoimmune MG who have repeatedly negative serologic tests for AChR antibodies.

4.5.3. Lambert–Eaton myasthenic syndrome

Lambert–Eaton myasthenic syndrome is associated with impaired release of ACh from the nerve terminal. It occurs as a paraneoplastic syndrome secondary to small cell lung carcinoma (SCLC) in 60% of patients and rarely with other carcinomas (O'Neill et al., 1988). The neuromuscular syndrome may precede the discovery of SCLC by up to 8 years. Lambert–Eaton myasthenic syndrome also occurs as an idiopathic chronic autoimmune disease with a similar natural history to autoimmune myasthenia gravis. Serum antibodies directed against P/Q-type VGCC that impair ACh release are present in up to 90% of cases (Lennon et al., 1995). In the setting of SCLC, it is likely that Lambert–Eaton myasthenic syndrome results from a cross-reaction with antigenically similar VGCC expressed on the surface of SCLC cells. In the mildest form of the disorder weakness and fatigue are confined to the proximal muscles of the lower extremities. When fully developed, the manifestations are generalized weakness and fatigue, mainly of proximal muscles, reduced or absent tendon reflexes, dryness of mouth, and male impotence. Ptosis, diplopia, dysarthria, dysphagia, and decreased sweating are relatively common but not prominent symptoms. Other paraneoplastic syndromes (e.g., limbic encephalitis, subacute cerebellar degeneration, sensory neuronopathy and gut or generalized dysautonomia) may occur concomitantly making the diagnosis of Lambert–Eaton syndrome more difficult. The idiopathic form of the syndrome can occur at any age, with the paraneoplastic form being more frequent beyond the 5th decade (O'Neill, 1988).

Serologic and electrophysiological tests confirm the diagnosis of Lambert–Eaton syndrome. Anti-P/Q VGCC antibodies are detected in the serum of 90% of patients at the time of presentation. Initial seronegativity has been observed when the syndrome occurs in the setting of non-small cell cancers or when testing is done in the setting of immunosuppressive therapy (Oh et al., 2007). Anti-VGCC antibodies can also be seen in SCLC in the absence of Lambert–Eaton syndrome, in other paraneoplastic disorders, and rarely in patients with autoimmune myasthenia gravis or amyotrophic lateral sclerosis. Electrodiagnostic studies are needed to make the diagnosis in these cases and complement serologic studies in antibody positive patients. They can also be used to judge the severity of the disorder and monitor the effects of treatment. In classic cases, the baseline CMAP is reduced in amplitude in clinically involved muscles. Repetitive stimulation shows a decrement of the CMAP at rates of 2–5 Hz with facilitation of 200% (doubling the size of the CMAP) or greater induced by brief (e.g., 10 s) exercise or a brief train of 30–50 Hz repetitive stimulation (Fig. 4.7). In mild cases the baseline CMAP may be normal in size, the decrement greater than in severe cases and the degree of facilitation in the range of 120–190%. These cases can be mistaken for myasthenia gravis if clinical features and serological studies are not considered (Fig. 4.8).

In patients presenting with subacute exertional weakness CMAP facilitation greater than 200%

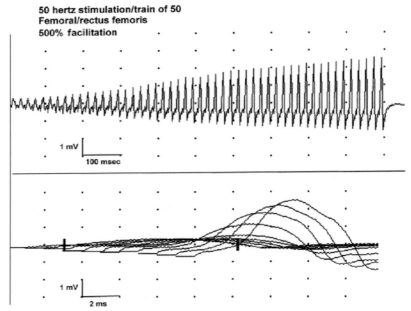

Fig. 4.7. Stimulation of the femoral nerve at 50 Hz recording over the rectus femoris muscle in a patient with Lambert–Eaton syndrome. The femoral compound muscle action potential facilitates by 500% with 1 s of high frequency stimulation.

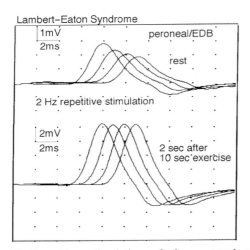

Fig. 4.8. Repetitive stimulation of the peroneal nerve recording over the extensor digitorum brevis muscle in a patient with mild Lambert–Eaton syndrome. The amplitude of the compound muscle action potential is within normal limits at rest and exercise produces less than 200% facilitation. This pattern can be mistaken for myasthenia gravis. EDB, extensor digitorum brevis; sec, seconds.

suggests the diagnosis of Lambert–Eaton myasthenic syndrome rather than MG. However, because repetitive stimulation is a better measure of the severity than the mechanism of neuromuscular transmission defect, there is considerable overlap between mild Lambert–Eaton myasthenic syndrome and severe MG (Harper and Lennon, 2003). A normal baseline CMAP ampli-

tude and facilitation of <200% can be observed in either mild early Lambert–Eaton myasthenic syndrome or severe MG. The distribution of weakness, facilitation of reflexes and presence of autonomic dysfunction in Lambert–Eaton syndrome as well as serologic tests help differentiate these disorders when physiological abnormalities overlap (Harper and Lennon, 2003). Like MG, the findings of motor nerve conduction studies, including repetitive stimulation, in Lambert–Eaton myasthenic syndrome vary with the distribution and severity of clinical involvement. The ulnar CMAP, recorded over the hypothenar region, is used most frequently, and is both reliable and sensitive, particularly in disease of moderate or greater severity. In mild early cases, examination of weaker muscles in the lower extremities (e.g., peroneal CMAP recorded from the tibialis anterior or femoral CMAP recorded from the rectus femoris muscle) is more likely to demonstrate abnormalities (Harper and Lennon, 2003).

4.5.4. Congenital myasthenic syndromes

The congenital myasthenic syndromes are a group of neuromuscular junction diseases caused by genetic defects of endplate molecules involved in neuromuscular transmission (Engel and Sine, 2005). The genetic defect is present at birth but may not manifest until later in life because of compensatory mechanisms in recessive disorders and variable expression in autosomal dominant forms. Some patients do not present until adulthood because they have never recognized their life-long symptoms as "abnormal." The congenital myasthenic syndromes are not autoimmune diseases. Thus serologic tests for AChR and MuSK antibodies are negative. The pathogenesis of congenital myasthenic syndromes has been elucidated utilizing a combination of clinical studies, standard electrodiagnostic examination, microelectrode and morphological studies on intercostal or anconeus muscle biopsy specimens, and molecular genetic studies (Engel, 2004). Definition of pathogenesis at the molecular level has been correlated with clinical manifestations and findings from clinical neurophysiological testing. As a result, many patients with congenital myasthenic syndromes can be accurately diagnosed without sophisticated microelectrode, morphological or molecular genetic analysis. Following is a popular classification for congenital myasthenic syndromes based on the site and mechanism of the neuromuscular transmission abnormality:

Presynaptic defects
   Choline acetyltransferase deficiency
   Paucity of synaptic vesicles
   Congenital Lambert–Eaton-like syndrome
Synaptic defect (basal lamina)
   Congenital endplate acetylcholine esterase
Postsynaptic defects
   Reduced AChR expression without significant kinetic
       abnormality
   AChR mutations
   • Rapsyn mutations
   • MuSK mutations
   AChR kinetic abnormality
   • Slow channel syndrome
   • Fast channel syndrome
   Sodium channel mutations

4.5.4.1. Congenital choline acetyltransferase deficiency

This is an autosomal recessive disorder caused by mutations in choline acetyltransferase (ChAT), the rate-limiting cytoplasmic neuronal enzyme for ACh synthesis at the neuromuscular junction (Ohno et al., 2001). The syndrome presents in infancy or early childhood with intermittent hypotonia and fatigable generalized weakness, ptosis, dysphagia, weak suck and cry, and respiratory insufficiency. Episodic severe crises associated with severe weakness and respiratory failure, and precipitated by infection or excitement, typifies ChAT deficiency. The crises lessen in frequency and severity in early to mid-childhood and give way to a clinical syndrome that is very similar to autoimmune myasthenia gravis. The symptoms respond to cholinesterase inhibitors.

NCS in ChAT deficiency demonstrate normal amplitude of the baseline CMAP and no R-CMAPs. The results of repetitive stimulation are variable. In clinically weak muscles, there is a decrement of the CMAP at rest that repairs with brief exercise or high frequency stimulation, shows post-activation exhaustion for 2–5 min, and then gradually recovers over 5–10 min (Harper, 1999; Schmidt et al., 2003; Engel et al., 2004). In infants that are between crises or in older patients that are mildly affected, exercise or repetitive stimulation at 10 Hz may have to be continued for 5–10 min before a decrement of the CMAP is observed (Fig. 4.9). The decrement induced by prolonged stimulation recovers very slowly over 15–30 min and also improves following administration of cholinesterase inhibitors.

Microelectrode studies in ChAT deficiency demonstrate a normal miniature endplate current and quantal content at rest but a gradual fall in both with 10 Hz stimulation for 5–10 min (Engel and Sine, 2005). A similar pattern of decrement is seen when hemicholinium, an inhibitor of choline uptake, is added to normal muscle. Ultrastructural and histochemical studies have shown normal morphology of the synapse and normal concentration of both AChE and AChR. Impaired function of the ChAT molecule leads to impaired resynthesis of ACh within the nerve terminal.

4.5.5. CMS with paucity of synaptic vesicles

This is a rare autosomal recessive disorder characterized by a reduced density of nerve terminal synaptic vesicles on ultrastructural studies of the endplate (Walls et al., 2003). The onset of symptoms is in the infantile period with generalized hypotonia and feeding difficulties. Ptosis, bulbar and limb weakness develops by early childhood with an overall clinical picture similar to seronegative autoimmune myasthenia gravis. The symptoms are moderately responsive to cholinesterase inhibitors.

The findings on NCS and needle EMG in CMS associated with paucity of synaptic vesicles are indistinguishable from moderately severe seronegative autoimmune myasthenia gravis with a normal baseline CMAP, a decrement at slow rates of repetitive stimulation and partial repair of the decrement with exercise or high frequency stimulation (Walls et al., 2003). Edrophonium produces partial repair of the decrement as well. Needle examination reveals small, rapidly recruited motor unit potentials that are simple in configuration and display prominent amplitude variation on consecutive discharges. Single fiber EMG findings have not been reported. Ultrastructural studies are normal except for an 80% reduction in the density of

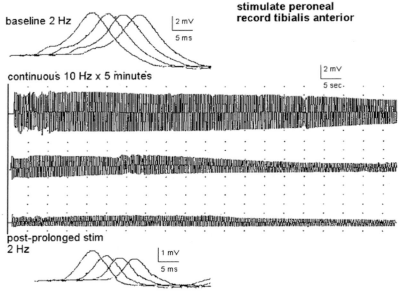

Fig. 4.9. Repetitive stimulation of peroneal nerve recording over the tibialis anterior muscle in a patient with choline acetyltransferase deficiency. Top insert shows no decrement with 2 Hz stimulation on baseline recordings. Middle traces show gradual steady decline of compound muscle action potential amplitude with prolonged continuous stimulation at 10 Hz for 5 min. Immediately after prolonged stimulation, brief 2 Hz stimulation produces a decrement (bottom insert).

synaptic vesicles in the motor nerve terminal. Micro-electrode studies show a commensurate 80% decrease in the quantal content of the EPP and the number of readily releasable quanta, with normal probability of release. The presumed pathogenesis of this disorder lies in impaired synthesis or recycling of synaptic vesicles.

4.5.6. Congenital "Lambert–Eaton-like" myasthenic syndrome

This is an ill-defined group of rare autosomal recessive or sporadic disorders that share a common pattern on electrophysiologic studies with autoimmune Lambert–Eaton syndrome (Albers et al., 1984; Bady et al., 1987; Harper, 2004). All cases reported to date have presented in the infantile period. Manifestations include hypotonia and severe generalized weakness with poor motor development. Respiratory muscle weakness can be severe enough to require mechanical ventilation. Patients usually do not survive the infantile period.

In congenital Lambert–Eaton-like syndrome, the amplitude of baseline CMAP is reduced, a decrement of the CMAP occurs with low rates of repetitive stimulation and facilitation of 200% or more is observed with high frequency stimulation (Harper, 2004). Needle examination shows small varying motor unit potentials with increased jitter and blocking that may improve at higher rates on stimulated single fiber EMG. When studied, intercostal muscle biopsies have demonstrated normal morphology of the endplate. Microelectrode

studies demonstrate abnormalities similar to those observed in autoimmune Lambert–Eaton syndrome with reduced release of ACh quanta per nerve action potential. Attempts to identify a mutation in the P/Q VGCC have been unsuccessful. Defects in other components of the synaptic vesicle release complex could produce the same type of defect as a calcium channel mutation. Cholinesterase inhibitors, guanidine and 3, 4-diaminopyridine have been used for treatment without consistent improvement.

4.5.7. Endplate acetylcholine esterase deficiency

This disorder is an autosomal recessive disease characterized by a deficiency of AChE in the basement membrane of muscle in the endplate region. Congenital AChE deficiency is caused by mutations of the *COLQ* gene that codes for ColQ, the collagen-like tail of AChE, which anchors the catalytic subunits of the enzyme to the basal lamina (Hutchinson et al., 1993; Ohno et al., 2000; Engel and Sine, 2005). Clinical manifestations are usually present in the neonatal period but may be delayed into later infancy or childhood in mild cases. Infants with severe congenital AChE deficiency present with severe generalized weakness and hypotonia, poor feeding, weak cry and respiratory insufficiency requiring mechanical ventilation. Developmental delay of motor milestones is common. In older children and adults manifestations include fatigable asymmetric ptosis, ophthalmoparesis, dysarthria, dysphagia and weakness of both axial and limb musculature. The extraocular muscles can be spared and distal upper extremity muscles (wrist and finger extensors) can be involved. There is often a diffuse reduction in muscle bulk with either normal or hypoactive reflexes. Scoliosis and lumbar lordosis, which worsen after standing for 30–60 s, unresponsiveness to AChE inhibitors, and a delay in the pupillary response to light are characteristic findings in congenital AChE deficiency.

Standard motor NCS reveal the presence of a R-CMAP in the majority of cases of congenital endplate AChE deficiency (Fig. 4.10). This phenomenon occurs in congenital AChE deficiency, drugs that inhibit AChE, and in the congenital myasthenic syndrome associated with a prolonged open-time of the AChR (slow channel syndrome) (Hutchinson et al., 1993). All of these conditions are associated with prolonged duration of the endplate potential which, in a subset of muscle fibers, remains above threshold beyond the refractory period and produces one or more additional action potentials.

The R-CMAPs in congenital or acquired AChE deficiency, or in SCCMS, are lower in amplitude than the main M-wave and follow it by 3–6 ms intervals. With repetitive stimulation at rates of 0.2–2 Hz, the second CMAP decrements more rapidly than the main M-wave, falling to zero by the second to sixth stimulus (Fig. 4.11). The second CMAP is easily missed when stimuli are delivered every 1–2 s in the routine process of obtaining a supramaximal response. This is avoided by delivering a single supramaximal stimulus 5–10 s after the initial supramaximal stimulus intensity is

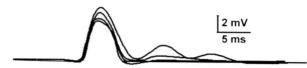

Fig. 4.11. Repetitive stimulation of the median nerve recording over abductor pollicis brevis muscle in slow channel congenital myasthenic syndrome. Train of four stimuli at 2 Hz with four consecutive traces superimposed. Initial trace demonstrates two well defined repetitive compound muscle action potentials that disappear on all subsequent traces.

determined. Administration of cholinesterase inhibitors produce no change in the R-CMAP in congenital AChE deficiency, but increase the number and amplitude of R-CMAPs in SCCMS (Fig. 4.12) (Harper, 2004). The R-CMAP is absent in some young, severely affected infants with congenital AChE deficiency, possibly secondary to a severe compensatory reduction in ACh release overshadowing the effect of the prolonged EPP duration. Repetitive stimulation at 2 Hz congenital AChE deficiency produces a 10–50% decrement of the main CMAP, which shows minimal repair with exercise and no repair following the administration of AChE inhibitors. Stimulation at rates >20 Hz for more than 10–15 s typically produces a decrement that worsens with increasing rates (i.e., "rate-dependent decrement") caused by progressive depolarization block caused by a "stair-step" depolarization of the muscle membrane caused by prolonged endplate currents as

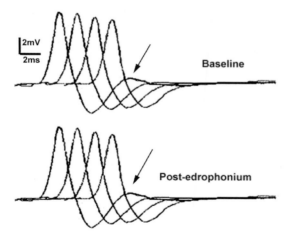

Fig. 4.10. Repetitive stimulation at 2 Hz of the ulnar nerve recording over the adductor digiti minimi muscle in a patient with congenital acetylcholine esterase deficiency. No change in size or number of repetitive compound muscle action potentials (arrows) after administration of edrophonium.

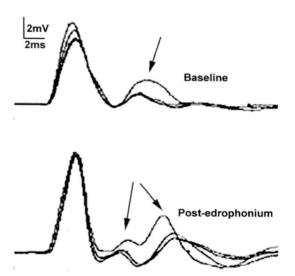

Fig. 4.12. Repetitive stimulation at 2 Hz of the median nerve recording over the abductor pollicis brevis muscle in a patient with slow channel congenital myasthenic syndrome. There is an increase in the size or number of repetitive compound muscle action potentials (arrows) after administration of edrophonium.

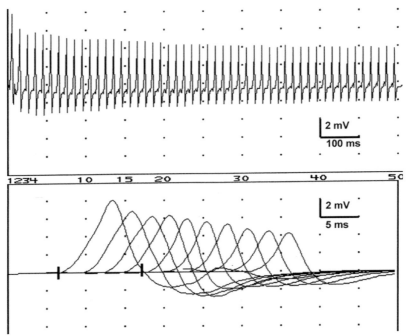

Fig. 4.13. Repetitive stimulation of the peroneal nerve at 20 Hz recording over the tibialis anterior muscle in congenital acetylcholine esterase deficiency. The decrement at 20 Hz was greater in magnitude than with 2 Hz stimulation.

well as desensitization of the AChR (Fig. 4.13) (Harper, 2004; Engel and Sine, 2005).

As with many of the congenital myasthenic syndromes, the findings on needle EMG in AChE deficiency are nonspecific (Harper, 2004). Standard concentric needle examination reveals normal insertional activity with no fibrillation potentials or other abnormal spontaneous discharges. With voluntary muscle activation, low amplitude short duration polyphasic motor unit potentials that vary in amplitude and morphology are recorded diffusely. Small motor unit potentials result from a combination of blocking of neuromuscular transmission and an endplate myopathy. The latter is caused by excess calcium influx into the muscle resulting from prolonged endplate currents. Single fiber EMG shows increased jitter and blocking. An abnormal delay in contraction of the iris using quantitative pupillography is present in some patients with AChE deficiency (Hutchinson et al., 1993). Other tests of autonomic function including QSART and cardiovascular reflexes have been performed in a small number of patients and have been normal (Hutchinson et al., 1993).

4.5.8. Slow channel congenital myasthenic syndrome

SCCMS is an autosomal dominant disorder with variable expression caused by AChR mutations that increase the rate of channel opening, slow the rate of

channel closure, or increase the affinity of acetylcholine for the receptor (Engel et al., 1996). The net effect is a gain of function that prolongs channel opening events, slows the decay of endplate currents, and permits cationic overload of the synaptic region of the muscle fiber. The age of presentation varies from childhood to the third decade. Some patients are asymptomatic but manifest R-CMAP on standard nerve conduction studies due to mild prolongation of endplate potentials. Fluctuating and fatigable ptosis, ophthalmoparesis, and trunk and extremity weakness are common. Prominent weakness and atrophy of neck muscles, wrist and finger extensor muscles, and intrinsic hand muscles is characteristic of SCCMS. The muscle weakness may be asymmetric and does not respond to AChE inhibitors.

Like AChE deficiency, one or more R-CMAPs are typically observed in SCCMS (Harper and Engel, 1998; Engel et al., 2004; Harper, 2004). Stimulation at 2 Hz produces a decrement of 5–50% of the main CMAP with little or no repair or post-activation exhaustion following exercise or high frequency stimulation. AChE inhibitors produce an increased size and number of repetitive CMAPs (Fig. 4.12). As with congenital AChE deficiency, repetitive stimulation at higher frequencies in SCCMS elicits a rate dependent decrement due to progressive depolarization block and AChR desensitization triggered by prolonged endplate currents.

Needle EMG in SCCMS reveals normal spontaneous activity with short duration low amplitude varying MUPs. Although the electrodiagnostic findings are similar, the slow channel syndrome and congenital AChE deficiency can usually be distinguished by the pattern of inheritance, age of onset and clinical distribution of weakness, and by the effect of cholinesterase inhibitors on the size and number of repetitive CMAPs.

Microelectrode studies in SCCMS show prolonged duration of endplate potentials due to prolonged open-time of the AChR (Engel and Sine, 2005). The single channel conductance is altered by one or more structural mutations of the AChR that delay closure of the channel once activation has occurred. In addition to sodium, excess calcium influx through the AChR leads to activation of catabolic enzymes and degeneration of the junctional folds and junctional sarcoplasm, leading to an endplate myopathy (Engel, 2004). The endplate myopathy is responsible for the static weakness and atrophy noted in patients with SCCMS. SCCMS responds favorably to quinidine or fluoxetine, which act as long lived dose-dependent blockers of AChR opening. Therapy with either of these drugs reduces the severity of electrophysiologic abnormalities and leads to improved strength and functional activities in SCCMS patients (Harper and Engel, 1998; Harper et al., 2003).

4.5.9. Fast channel congenital myasthenic syndrome

The FCCMS is the mirror image of SCCMS. FCCMS is an autosomal recessive disorder caused by mutations in the AChR that shorten the opening episodes of the receptor by decreasing its affinity for ACh, destabilizing the open state, or stabilizing the closed state of the receptor (Sine et al., 2003; Engel and Sine, 2005). Patients with the FCCMS typically present in infancy or early childhood with generalized weakness, fatigue, dysphagia, dysarthria, ptosis and ophthalmoparesis. The picture is indistinguishable from autoimmune myasthenia gravis or many other subtypes of AChR deficiency syndromes. The symptoms respond to cholinesterase inhibitors and 3,4-diaminopyridine (Engel and Sine, 2005).

Electrodiagnostic abnormalities in FCCMS are indistinguishable from mild to moderately severe autoimmune myasthenia gravis (Harper, 2004). There are no R-CMAPs and with repetitive stimulation there is a decrement of the main CMAP at low rates that shows post-activation repair and exhaustion following exercise or higher rates of repetitive stimulation. No rate-dependent decrement has been reported in FCCMS. The needle examination is non-specific with small varying motor unit potentials on standard EMG and increased jitter and blocking on single fiber EMG.

4.5.10. Congenital AChR deficiency

This is a heterogeneous group of autosomal recessive disorders that have in common a congenital deficiency in the number of AChRs at the endplate. Mutations of genes coding for one or more AChR subunits are the most common cause of AChR deficiency (Engel et al., 2003). These mutations typically affect AChR expression with little or no effect on receptor kinetics. Mutations in genes coding for ε-subunit AChR mutations are most common (Engel and Sine, 2005). These mutations are typically non-lethal because the γ-subunit can substitute for the ε-subunit leading to expression of fetal AChR. Mutations of rapsyn, a muscle protein that is needed for AChR clustering and linkage to the muscle cytoskeleton, also cause AChR deficiency with little or no kinetic abnormality (Ohno et al., 2002). The age of onset ranges from infancy to adulthood. Clinical manifestations include hypotonia, respiratory insufficiency, weakness of ocular and bulbar muscles, and skeletal deformities. The majority of patients with congenital AChR deficiency respond to AChE inhibitors.

The findings of electrodiagnostic studies on congenital AChR deficiency are indistinguishable from autoimmune myasthenia gravis (Harper, 2004). The amplitude of the CMAP at rest is normal. There are no R-CMAPs observed with single stimuli. With repetitive stimulation at low rates there is typically a decrement of the CMAP at rest in weak muscles. The decrement is partially repaired with exercise, tetanic stimulation or AChE inhibitors. Mild cases, particularly certain kindreds with rapsyn deficiency, may have normal repetitive stimulation studies (Ohno et al., 2002). Needle examination shows normal spontaneous activity with rapidly recruited short, low amplitude varying motor unit potentials. In mild cases single fiber EMG is required to establish the diagnosis of a NMT disorder.

4.5.11. Congenital MuSK deficiency

A single patient has been described with a congenital myasthenic syndrome caused by mutations in the gene encoding the muscle-specific receptor tyrosine kinase (Chevessier et al., 2004). MuSK interacts with agrin and rapsyn to promote AChR aggregation during synaptic development (Hughes et al., 2006). The patient with congenital MuSK deficiency was symptomatic from birth with ptosis, generalized weakness and respiratory difficulties requiring tracheostomy. When she was definitively studied in her 20s, the clinical manifestations were similar to generalized autoimmune myasthenia gravis. Partial clinical improvement was noted following treatment with cholinesterase inhibitors and 3,4-diaminopyridine. The only electrodiagnostic study reported was repetitive stimulation, which was performed at a frequency of 3 Hz on facial and spinal accessory nerves, revealing a CMAP decrement of 17% and 56%, respectively. Results of standard NCS, concentric needle or single EMG were reported. Morphological studies showed reduced expression of MuSK and AChR at the NMJ. Mutational analysis identified two heteroallelic mutations, a frameshift mutation (c.220insC) and a missense mutation (V790M) in the *MuSK* gene. Expression studies confirmed reduced expression of MuSK and agrin-induced AChR aggregation.

4.5.12. Congenital sodium channel myasthenia

One patient has been reported with a congenital myasthenic syndrome caused by mutations of the perijunctional muscle voltage-gated sodium channel ($Na_v1.4$) (Tsujino et al., 2003). Acute episodes of bulbar and respiratory weakness started shortly after birth and persisted, requiring apnea monitoring and intermittent ventilatory support. Other manifestations included ptosis, ophthalmoparesis and weakness of facial, axial and appendicular muscles that worsened with exertion. High arched palate and lumbar lordosis were also noted.

Standard motor NCS including repetitive stimulation at 2 Hz were normal (Tsujino et al., 2003). However, prolonged stimulation of 1 min duration at 10 Hz or brief high frequency stimulation at 50 Hz elicited severe CMAP decrements of 50% and 85%, respectively. Morphological studies of the endplate were essentially normal but microelectrode studies showed significant elevation of the threshold for muscle fiber action potential generation, despite normal endplate currents. Molecular genetic analysis revealed two heteroallelic missense mutations in *SCN4A*, the gene that codes for perijunctional $Na_v1.4$ (Tsujino et al., 2003). Expression studies later confirmed that mutant sodium channels produced a hyperpolarizing shift in the voltage dependence of fast inactivation, leading to reduced excitability at baseline with further reduction induced by brief trains of 50 Hz stimulation of the muscle membrane (Tsujino et al., 2003).

4.5.13. Botulism

Botulinum intoxication is associated with impaired release of acetylcholine from the nerve terminal with a low quantal content and very small postsynaptic endplate potentials (Maselli, 1998). The toxin interferes with the vesicle docking and fusion by irreversibly binding to, and inactivating, several vesicular and neuronal membrane proteins (Cherington, 1998). Electrodiagnostic studies are characterized by low amplitude CMAPs with a small decrement at slow rates of stimulation (Vali, 1983; Cornblath, 1986; Maselli, 1998; Bolton et al., 2000; Maselli and Bakshi, 2000). Unlike the myasthenic syndrome, exercise and rapid repetitive stimulation produce only mild facilitation (typically 110–150%). The needle EMG features of botulism are short duration motor unit potentials and widespread fibrillation potentials, the density of which correlates closely with the severity of weakness (Cronblath, 1986; Maselli and Bakshi, 2000). Single fiber EMG shows increased jitter, blocking and, when severe, reduction in fiber density (Chaudhry, 1999; Padua et al., 1999). The electrodiagnostic findings in botulism mimic acute motor axonal neuropathy or an acute severe myopathy (Bolton et al., 2000). A high index of clinical suspicion should prompt one to perform repetitive stimulation at 40–50 Hz in these patients. Repetitive stimulation may have to be continued for a longer interval (30 s or more) than is typically used in Lambert–Eaton myasthenic syndrome.

References

Albers JW, Faulkner JA, Dorovini-Zis K, et al. (1984). Abnormal neuromuscular transmission in an infantile myasthenic syndrome. Ann Neurol 16: 28–34.

Bady B, Chauplannaz G, Carrier H (1987). Congenital Lambert–Eaton myasthenic syndrome. J Neurol Neurosurg Psychiatry 50: 476–478.

Benatar M (2006). A systematic review of diagnostic studies in myasthenia gravis. Neuromuscul Disord 16: 459–467.

Black JL, Lennon VA (1999). Identification and cloning of human neuronal high voltage-gated calcium channel γ-2 and γ-3 subunits: neurological implications. Mayo Clin Proc 74: 357–361.

Bolton CF, Zifko U, Bird SJ (2000). Clinical neurophysiology in the intensive care unit. Suppl Clin Neurophysiol 53: 29–37.

Boonyapisit K, Kaminski HJ, Ruff RL (1999). The molecular basis of neuromuscular transmission disorders. Am J Med 106: 97–113.

Chaudhry V, Crawford TO (1999). Stimulation single-fiber EMG in infant botulism. Muscle Nerve 22: 1698–1703.

Cherington M (1998). Clinical spectrum of botulism. Muscle Nerve 21: 701–710.

Chevessier F, Faraut B, Ravel-Chapuis A, et al. (2004). MUSK, a new target for mutations causing congenital myasthenic syndrome. Hum Mol Genet 13: 3229–3240.

Cornblath DR (1986). Disorders of neuromuscular transmission in infants and children. Muscle Nerve 9: 606–611.

Costa J, Evangelista T, Conceicao I, et al. (2004). Repetitive nerve stimulation in myasthenia gravis—relative sensitivity of different muscles. Clin Neurophysiol 115: 2776–2782.

Daube JR (1996). Clinical Neurophysiology. FA Davis, Philadelphia.

Engel AG (1999). Anatomy and molecular architecture of the neuromuscular junction. In: AG Engel (Ed.), Myasthenia Gravis and Myasthenic Disorders (Contemporary Neurology Series). Oxford University Press, Oxford, pp. 3–39.

Engel AG (2004). The neuromuscular junction. In: AG Engel, C Franzini-Armstrong (Eds.), Myology. 3rd ed. McGraw-Hill, New York, pp. 325–372.

Engel AG, Hohlfeld R (2004). Acquired autoimmune myasthenia gravis. In: AG Engel, C Franzini-Armstrong (Eds.), Myology. 3rd ed. McGraw-Hill, New York, pp. 1755–1790.

Engel AG, Sine SM (2005). Current understanding of congenital myasthenic syndromes. Curr Opin Pharmacol 5: 306–321.

Engel AG, Lambert EH, Mulder DM, et al. (1982). A newly recognized congenital myasthenic syndrome attributed to a prolonged open time of the acetylcholine-induced ion channel. Ann Neurol 11: 553–569.

Engel AG, Ohno K, Milone M, et al. (1996). New mutations in acetylcholine receptor subunit genes reveal heterogeneity in the slow-channel congenital myasthenic syndrome. Hum Mol Genet 5: 1217–1227.

Engel AG, Ohno K, Shen XM, et al. (2003). Congenital myasthenic syndromes: multiple molecular targets at the neuromuscular junction. Ann N Y Acad Sci 998: 138–160.

Engel AG, Ohno K, Sine SM (2004). Congenital myasthenic syndromes. In: AG Engel, C Franzini-Armstrong (Eds.), Myology. 3rd ed. McGraw-Hill, New York, pp. 1755–1790.

Farrugia ME, Kennett RP, Newsom-Davis J, et al. (2006). Single-fiber electromyography in limb and facial muscles in muscle-specific kinase antibody and acetylcholine receptor antibody myasthenia gravis. Muscle Nerve 33: 568–570.

Harper CM (1999). Electrodiagnosis of endplate disease. In: AG Engel (Ed.), Myasthenia Gravis and Myasthenic Disorders (Contemporary Neurology Series). Oxford University Press, Oxford, pp. 65–86.

Harper CM (2004). Congenital myasthenic syndromes. Semin Neurol 24: 111–124.

Harper CM, Engel AG (1998). Quinidine sulfate therapy for the slow-channel congenital myasthenic syndrome. Ann Neurol 43: 480–484.

Harper CM, Lennon VA (2003). Lambert–Eaton syndrome. In: HJ Kaminski (Ed.), Myasthenia Gravis and Related Disorders. Humana Press, Totowa, pp. 269–292.

Harper CM, Fukodome T, Engel AG (2003). Treatment of slow-channel congenital myasthenic syndrome with fluoxetine. Neurology 60: 1710–1713.

Hughes BW, Kusner LL, Kaminski HJ (2006). Molecular architecture of the neuromuscular junction. Muscle Nerve 33: 445–461.

Hutchinson DO, Walls TJ, Nakano S, et al. (1993). Congenital endplate acetylcholinesterase deficiency. Brain 116: 633–653.

Jones SW (1998). Overview of voltage-dependent calcium channels. J Bioenerg Biomembr 30: 299–312.

Karlin A, Akabas MH (1994). Toward a structural basis for the function of nicotinic acetylcholine receptors and their cousins. Neuron 15: 1231–1244.

Lennon VA, Kryzer TJ, Griesmann GE, et al. (1995). Calcium-channel antibodies in the Lambert–Eaton syndrome and other paraneoplastic syndromes. N Engl J Med 332: 1467–1471.

Lindstrom JM, Seybold ME, Lennon VA, et al. (1975). Antibody to acetylcholine receptor in myasthenia gravis: prevalence, clinical correlates, and diagnostic value. Neurology 51: 933–939.

Maselli RA (1998). Pathogenesis of human botulism. Ann N Y Acad Sci 841: 1221–1239.

Maselli RA, Bakshi N (2000). AAEM case report 16. Botulism. American Association of Electrodiagnostic Medicine. Muscle Nerve 23: 1137–1144.

Oh SJ, Kim DE, Kuruoglu R, et al. (1992). Diagnostic sensitivity of the laboratory tests in myasthenia gravis. Muscle Nerve 15: 720–724.

Oh SJ, Hatanaka Y, Claussen GC, et al. (2006). Electrophysiological differences in seropositive and seronegative Lambert–Eaton myasthenic syndrome. Muscle Nerve 35: 178–183.

Ohno K, Engel AG, Brengman JM, et al. (2000). The spectrum of mutations causing end-plate acetylcholinesterase deficiency. Ann Neurol 47: 162–170.

Ohno K, Tsujino A, Brengman JM, et al. (2001). Choline acetyltransferase mutations cause myasthenic syndrome associated with episodic apnea in humans. Proc Natl Acad Sci U S A 98: 2017–2022.

Ohno K, Engel AG, Shen XM, et al. (2002). Rapsyn mutations in humans cause endplate acetylcholine-receptor deficiency and myasthenic syndrome. Am J Hum Genet 70: 825–835.

O'Neill JH, Murray NM, Newsom-Davis J (1988). The Lambert–Eaton myasthenic syndrome. A review of 50 cases. Brain 111: 577–596.

Padua L, Aprile I, Monaco ML, et al. (1999). Neurophysiological assessment in the diagnosis of botulism: usefulness of single-fiber EMG. Muscle Nerve 22: 1388–1392.

Padua L, Tonali P, Aprile I, et al. (2006). Seronegative myasthenia gravis: comparison of neurophysiological picture in musk+ and musk− patients. Eur J Neurol 13: 273–276.

Plested CP, Tang T, Spreadbury I, et al. (2002). AChR phosphorylation and indirect inhibition of AChR function in seronegative MG. Neurology 59: 1682–1688.

Romi F, Gilhus NE, Aarli JA (2005). Myasthenia gravis: clinical, immunological, and therapeutic advances. Acta Neurol Scand 111: 134–141.

Ruff RL (2003). Neuromuscular junction physiology and pathophysiology. In: HJ Kaminski (Ed.), Myasthenia Gravis and Related Disorders. Humana Press, Totowa, pp. 1–14.

Sanders DB, Stalberg E (1996). AAEM minimonograph #25: single fiber electromyography. Muscle Nerve 19: 1069–1083.

Sanders DB, Howard JF, Johns TR (1979). Single-fiber electromyography in myasthenia gravis. Neurology 29: 68–76.

Schmidt C, Abicht A, Krampfl K, et al. (2003). Congenital myasthenic syndrome due to a novel missense mutation in the gene encoding choline acetyltransferase. Neuromuscul Disord 13: 245–251.

Selcen D, Fukuda T, Shen XM, et al. (2004). Are musk antibodies the primary cause of myasthenic symptoms? Neurology 62: 1945–1950.

Sine SM, Shen XM, Wang HL, et al. (2002). Naturally occurring mutations at the acetylcholine receptor binding site independently alter ACh binding and channel gating. J Gen Physiol 120: 483–496.

Sine SM, Wang HL, Ohno K, et al. (2003). Mechanistic diversity underlying fast channel congenital myasthenic syndromes. Ann N Y Acad Sci 998: 1128–1237.

Sine SM, Engel AG, Wang HL, et al. (2004). Molecular insights into acetylcholine receptor structure and function revealed by mutations causing congenital myasthenic syndromes. In: RA Maue (Ed.), Molecular and Cellular Insights to Ion Channel Biology. Elsevier, New York, pp. 95–119.

Stickler DE, Massey JM, Sanders DB (2005). Musk-antibody positive myasthenia gravis: clinical and electrodiagnostic patterns. Clin Neurophysiol 116: 2065–2068.

Tsujino A, Maertens C, Ohno K, et al. (2003). Myasthenic syndrome caused by mutation of the SCN4A sodium channel. Proc Natl Acad Sci U S A 100: 7377–7382.

Valli G, Barbieri S, Scarlato G (1983). Neurophysiological tests in human botulism. Electromyogr Clin Neurophysiol 23: 3–11.

Vincent A, Leite MI (2005). Neuromuscular junction autoimmune disease: muscle specific kinase antibodies and treatments for myasthenia gravis. Curr Opin Neurol 18: 519–525.

Vincent A, McConville J, Farrugia ME, et al. (2004). Seronegative myasthenia gravis. Semin Neurol 24: 125–133.

Walls TJ, Engel AG, Nagel AS, et al. (1993). Congenital myasthenic syndrome associated with paucity of synaptic vesicles and reduced quantal release. Ann N Y Acad Sci 681: 461–468.

Zhang Y, Cheng J, Auerbach A (1995). Activation of recombinant mouse acetylcholine receptor by acetylcholine, carbamylcholine, and tetraethylamonium. J Physiol 486: 189–206.

Zivkovic SA, Shipe C (2005). Use of repetitive nerve stimulation in the evaluation of neuromuscular junction disorders. Am J Electroneurodiagnostic Technol 45: 248–261.

Handbook of Clinical Neurology, Vol. 91 (3rd series)
Neuromuscular junction disorders
A.G. Engel, Editor

Chapter 5

The immunopathogenesis of myasthenia gravis

NORBERT SOMMER [1,2][†], BJÖRN TACKENBERG [1][†] AND REINHARD HOHLFELD [3]*

[1]*Clinical Neuroimmunology Group, Philipps-University, Marburg, Germany*

[2]*Department of Neurology, Christophsbad, Göppingen, Germany*

[3]*Institute for Clinical Neuroimmunology, Ludwig-Maximilians University,
Munich and Department of Neuroimmunology, Max-Planck-Institute of Neurobiology, Martinsried, Germany*

5.1. Introduction

Myasthenia gravis (MG) is one of the best studied human autoimmune diseases. The history of seminal discoveries has been reviewed recently (Vincent, 2002), providing an outstanding example of translational research. Autoantibodies against neuromuscular antigens play a key role in the pathogenesis of MG, and the detection and monitoring of these antibodies is essential for the clinical management of myasthenic patients. The role of anti-acetylcholine receptor (AChR) antibodies was elucidated in the 1970s (Patrick and Lindstrom, 1973; Engel et al., 1977a,b; Pinching et al., 1977; Toyka et al., 1977), whereas research on the role of other, less frequent autoantibodies, including those against muscle specific kinase (MuSK), is ongoing.

Thymic abnormalities in MG patients have long been reported, and thymectomy for MG has been performed since the first half of the 20th century (Schumacher and Roth, 1912; Blalock, 1944). Thymectomy was in fact introduced long before the central immunological role of the thymus was recognized (Miller, 1961, 2001). An enormous amount of data has since been generated on the role of the thymus and T cells in the pathogenesis of MG. Although a straightforward unifying pathogenetic concept is still lacking, MG has served as an extremely useful model for the study of human autoimmune mechanisms (Hohlfeld et al., 1984; Brocke et al., 1988; Sommer et al., 1990; Spuler et al., 1994; Wang et al., 1997; Hoffacker et al., 2000; Buckley et al., 2001; Balandina et al., 2005; Tackenberg et al., 2007).

Closely related to cellular immune responses is the function of the major histocompatibility gene complex (MHC), which is called the human leukocyte antigen (HLA) region in humans. Similar to other autoimmune diseases, MG is associated with certain HLA-haplotypes, depending on the patient population and clinical subtype. Moreover, in MG the HLA type—in combination with immunogical features—is considered relevant for treatment decisions (Compston et al., 1980; Matsuki et al., 1990; Zisman et al., 1995; Hill et al., 1999b; Niks et al., 2006).

In this chapter, we review the immunopathogenesis of MG. We begin with a short overview of some fundamental principles of immunology, and then systematically address the role of antibodies, T cells, immunogenetic aspects, and thymus. In the final sections of the chapter, we discuss the relevant animal models of MG, and finally, the risk factors of MG and associations with other immunological diseases.

5.2. Immunological principles

The immune system consists of many different types of cells and molecules with specialized roles in defending infections. It can be divided into an innate (antigen-nonspecific, natural or native) and adaptive (antigen-specific) arm. The innate immune response is the forefront of defense against infection. It includes mechanisms that exist before infection occurs, such as epithelial barriers, blood proteins and phagocytic cells.

[†]Equal contribution to this work.

*Correspondence to: Reinhard Hohlfeld, MD, Institute for Clinical Neuroimmunology, Ludwig-Maximilians University, Marchioninistr. 15, D-81366 Munich, Germany. E-mail: Reinhard.Hohlfeld@med.uni-muenchen.de, Tel: 49-89-7095-4780, Fax: 49-89-7095-4782.

It reacts in the same way to repeated infections, i.e., it has no memory. The effector mechanisms of innate immunity are often used as a primary line of defense to eliminate microbes before the adaptive, usually secondary, immune response has fully developed.

5.2.1. The complement system

One of many components of the innate immune system is the complement system. It is relevant for MG because it mediates destruction of the postsynaptic membrane of the neuromuscular junction. The complement system includes approximately 25 different plasma glycoproteins (Medzhitov and Janeway, 2000; Parkin and Cohen, 2001). The complement components are named by a capital C and a number, the most abundant protein being C3 with a plasma concentration of 1 g/L. Most complement proteins are zymogens (i.e., proenzymes), which become active only after their cleavage. Their cleavage products are named by adding a lower case letter (e.g., C3b). They can be triggered by one of three pathways and are activated in a cascade sequence. The classical pathway is triggered directly by pathogen or indirectly by antibody binding to the pathogen surface. The alternative pathway is stimulated by polysaccharides from yeasts and gram-negative bacteria. The more recently identified mannan binding lectin pathway feeds into the classical sequence by activating it independently of the C1rs complex and is stimulated by mannose containing proteins and carbohydrates on microbes, including viruses and yeasts. Irrespective of the source of activation, the outcome is the generation of a number of immunologically active substances. For example, the proteolytic-cleavage fragment C3b becomes deposited on the surface of microorganisms, which in turn enhances (opsonizes) phagocytosis of the microbe. The complement components C3a, C4a, and C5a cause release of inflammatory mediators from mast cells, and C5a also acts as a strong neutrophil chemoattractant. The complement components C5b, C6, C7, C8, and C9 form the membrane-attack complex, which perforates cell surface membranes leading to subsequent cell death by osmotic lysis.

5.2.2. Cellular components of the innate immune system

The main cellular components of the innate immune system are the natural killer cells (NKCs). Owing to their capability to present antigens via their MHC/HLA and their concomitant functions in unspecific immunity, dendritic cells (DCs) and monocytes are one of the most important connecting elements of the innate and adaptive immune system (Janeway et al., 2005).

NKCs are large granular lymphoid-like cells, but they do not express somatically rearranged antigen-specific receptors. However, NKCs are able to (co-) regulate immune responses and seem to be involved in autoimmunity (Zhang et al., 2006). In the context of autoimmunity they may show a "Janus-like" character, because on the one hand, they may increase vulnerability, and on the other hand, they may act in concert with regulatory T cells (see below) to dampen immune reactions (Zhang et al., 2006). Common precursors of NKCs and T-cells can be found in the fetal thymus and spleen. Mature NKCs are characterized by CD161 (NKR-P1A)/CD56 (NCAM)/CD16 (IgG-Fc receptor IIIa). NKCs recognize abnormal cells in two ways. First, they bind to antibody-coated targets via Fc receptors, leading to antibody-dependent cellular cytotoxity. Second, they have various surface receptors that recognize molecular flags on target cells, indicating that the target cell is potentially dangerous and needs to be eliminated. NKC activity is stimulated by cytokines, such as interferons and IL-12.

NKCs are functionally identified by their ability to kill certain lymphoid tumor cell lines in vitro without prior immunization or activation. Their mechanism of killing is thought to be identical to that used by cytotoxic T cells (CTLs) in the adaptive immune response. However, in contrast to CTLs, NKC killing is triggered not by variable, antigen-specific receptors, but by invariant receptors. The NKC receptors may be stimulatory or inhibitory (Lodoen and Lanier, 2006). Two families of NKC receptors have been characterized: 1. The immunoglobulin-like receptors [NCR and killer inhibitory receptors (KIR)], which need adapter proteins like immunoreceptor tyrosine-based activation motifs (ITAMs) or immunoreceptor tyrosine-based inhibitory motifs (ITIMs) for signaling. KIRs are able to recognize HLA molecules. However, their ligands are not well characterized. 2. The NKC lectin-like receptors (CD94/NKG2) are involved in probing the presence and integrity of HLA class I molecules on the target cell (Janeway et al., 2005).

5.2.3. Pattern recognition receptors of the innate immune system

In contrast to the antigen-specific receptors of B- and T-lymphocytes (see below), which are somatically rearranged, the receptors of the innate immune system are encoded in the germ line. They are expressed on many cells of the innate immune system, especially macrophages, dendritic cells, and the "innate subdivision" of B cells. These receptors recognize a few, highly conserved structures present in large groups of microorganisms, and are therefore called "pattern-recognition receptors." Among them, toll-like receptors (TLRs) are an immunologically highly relevant receptor family, which are involved especially in Th1 specific immunity (Ehlers and Ravetch, 2007). TLRs can be viewed as eyes of the innate immune cells turned outward to identify conserved molecular patterns of pathogens and danger signals originating from stressed or injured cells (Wagner, 2001). Therefore, they usually have protecting functions. However, data from animal models suggest that TLR signaling might be involved in autoimmunity induced by or associated with the presence of microbial antigens, like cytomegalovirus or *B. burgdorferi* (Ehlers and Ravetch, 2007). In addition, a reduced expression of, e.g., TLR5 was demonstrated to be associated with resistance to systemic lupus erythemtosus (Hawn et al., 2005).

5.2.4. The adaptive immune system: B cells and their receptors

The adaptive immune system is characterized by the antigen specificity of its responses. An antigen is recognized by antigen-specific receptors, which initiate a chain of signals, leading to cell priming, activation and differentiation. In most immune reactions B and T cells cooperate closely. The antigen receptor of a B cell is a surface-associated immunoglobulin (Ig). Immunoglobulins consist of two identical heavy chains and two identical light chains that are held together by disulfide bonds and form the typical Y-shape of the protein. The N-terminals of the chains possess variable domains that bind antigens through three hypervariable complementarity-determining regions (CDRs). The C-terminal domain of the chains forms the constant region, which defines the type (kappa or lambda), the class (IgG, IgA, IgM, IgD or IgE), and subclass (IgG1–4, IgA1–2) of the antibody. The basic antibody "monomer" (which is biochemically in fact a tetramer) is bivalent. The secretory IgA at mucosal surfaces is a tetravalent "dimer"; the circulating IgM is a decavalent "pentamer." IgG is the most abundant immunoglobulin in human serum comprising 75% of all Ig. The normal serum IgG concentration is 8–16 g/L of which IgG1 is 66%, IgG2 23%, IgG3 7% and IgG4 4%. IgG1 and IgG3 are the most effective complement activators. IgG1, IgG3 and IgG4 cross the placenta easily. Maintenance of a specific serum antibody level requires continuous secretion of antibodies, because the half-life of an antibody molecule in serum is approximately 3 weeks. On the other hand, plasma cells, the terminal differentiation stage of B cells, can synthesize and secrete several thousand antibody molecules per second (Manz et al., 2005).

In relation to autoimmunity it is especially noteworthy that more than half of the nascent B cells in humans initially express autoreactive antibodies. However, most of these autoantibodies are removed from the repertoire before maturation into naive B cells. Nevertheless, low-affinity self-reactive antibodies are frequently found in the serum of normal humans. Self-reactive antibodies, including anti-nuclear antibodies, are frequently expressed by IgG+ memory B cells in healthy donors (Tiller et al., 2007). Most of these antibodies are created de novo by somatic hypermutation during the transition between mature naive and IgG+ memory B cells. It is therefore likely that deregulation of self-reactive IgG+ memory B cells contributes to the pathogenesis of autoimmune dieases. The presence of autoreactive lymphocytes in the healthy immune system has been firmly established not only for B cells but also for T cells.

5.2.5. The adaptive immune system: T-cell receptor and antigen presentation

The antigen receptor of a T cell is a heterodimer, usually consisting of an alpha and beta chain (alpha/beta T-cell receptor, TCR), or rarely (<5% of all T cells in blood), of a gamma and delta chain (the gamma/delta TCR). B- and T-cell receptors recognize antigens in fundamentally different ways. B cells and immunoglobulins recognize soluble antigens, whereas T cells recognize antigen fragments only if they are presented, in a processed form, on the surface of antigen presenting cells in the context of an HLA class I or II molecule (Fig. 5.1). Though virtually every cell in the body can present an antigen in the context of HLA class I molecules, the spectrum of cells that also express HLA class II and therefore may act as "professional antigen-presenting cells" (APCs) is much more restricted. The professional APCs are very efficient at internalizing and processing antigens, the prototypes being B cells, dendritic cells and macrophages. The two principal pathways of antigen processing are referred to as the MHC class I ("endogenous") and MHC class II ("endocytic") pathway. The former leads to presentation of endogenously synthesized antigens in the context of HLA class I molecules, which in a complex with self or foreign (e.g., viral) antigens are recognized by CD8 T cells. The endocytic pathway leads to presentation of HLA-class II associated-antigens to CD4 T cells. For the activation of T cells two signals are necessary, one of which is provided by the trimolecular complex, i.e., T-cell receptor, antigen fragment peptide and HLA molecule. The "second signal" is antigen-independent, and mediated through co-stimulatory molecules such as CD28 on T cells, which interacts with CD80 and CD86 on the APC. Two major subsets of T cells are defined by expression of the CD4 and CD8 differentiation antigens (Fig. 5.2).

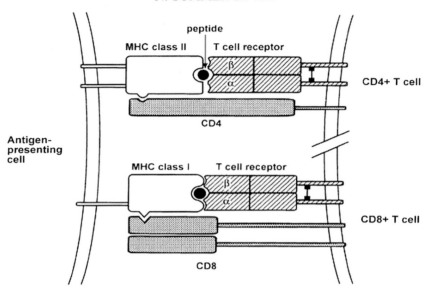

Fig. 5.1. Antigen recognition by CD4+ T cells (top) and CD8+ T cells (bottom). The T-cell receptor of CD4+ T cells recognizes an antigen peptide (indicated by black dot) bound to an MHC class II molecule on the surface of an antigen-presenting cell. The T-cell receptor of CD8+ T cells recognizes an antigen peptide bound to an MHC class I molecule. CD4 and CD8 act as co-receptors. (After Hohlfeld, 1997.)

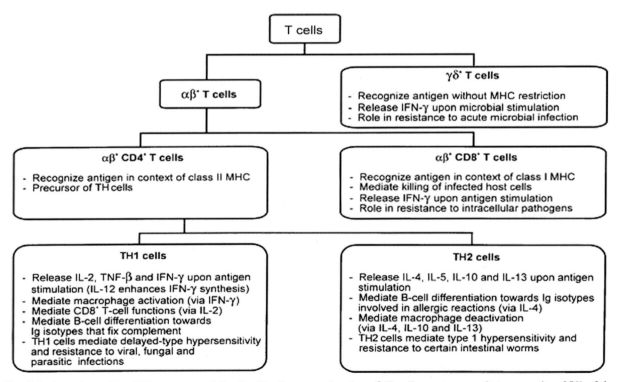

Fig. 5.2. Overview of the different types of T cells. T cells expressing the α/β T-cell receptor constitute more than 95% of the T cells in blood. They can be divided into CD4+ and CD8+ cells, and the CD4+ T cells can be divided into TH1 and TH2 cells. (After Hohlfeld, 1997.)

The majority of CD4+ T cells act as antigen-specific helper (TH2) or pro-inflammatory (TH1) cells. The two cell types can be distinguished by their pattern of cytokine secretion: TH1 cells produce interleukin-2 and interferon-γ, whereas TH2 cells produce interleukins 4, 5, 10 and related "TH2-type" cytokines (Mosmann and Coffman, 1989). Although the concept of a functional dichotomy of TH1 and TH2 cells has served well for over 35 years, it is becoming more and more obvious that this idea is an oversimplification. For example, TH1 cells—long thought to mediate tissue damage—might be involved in the initiation of damage, but they do not sustain or play a decisive role in many commonly studied models of autoimmunity, allergy and microbial immunity. A major role for the cytokine interleukin-17 (IL-17) has emerged in various models of immune-mediated tissue injury. A pathway named TH17 is now credited for causing and sustaining tissue damage in many diverse situations. The TH1 pathway antagonizes the TH17 pathway in an intricate fashion. The evolution of our understanding of the TH17 pathway reflects an important shift in immunologists' perspectives regarding the basis of tissue damage, where for over 20 years the role of TH1 cells was considered paramount (Steinman, 2007).

CD8+ T cells act as antigen-specific killer cells. A small minority of T cells, the gamma-delta T cells, are predominantly CD3+CD4−CD8−. Most gamma-delta T cells have cytotoxic potential in vitro, but their in vivo functions are largely unknown.

5.2.6. Generation of antigen receptor diversity

An extraordinary property of the antigen receptors, immunoglobulins and T-cell receptors is their amazingly large diversity. There are probably 10^8–10^{10} (some estimates say 10^{15}) different specificities. One T cell and one B cell and their progeny (one clone) normally, with few exceptions, carry one single type of antigen-specific receptors. Their diversity originates from fewer than 400 genes and is generated by a unique recombination process of cutting, splicing, and modifying variable-region genes (Tonegawa, 1983). Each B- or T-cell clone selects one gene segment from each of several pools of germ-line segments (Rowen et al., 1996), and combines these segments into the functional genes coding for the protein chains of B-cell receptors (immunoglobulin light and heavy chains) or T-cell receptors (α and β, or γ and δ chains) (Fig. 5.3). Part of the diversity of the rearranged immunoglobulin and T-cell receptor genes results from random combinatorial joining of the different gene segments. Additional diversity results from the deletion or insertion of nucleotides at the junctional borders between the different rearranged gene segments.

5.2.7. T-cell–B-cell cooperation

Four types of signaling contribute to B-cell activation or differentiation: 1. direct activation of the B-cell receptor by a microbial antigen, 2. activation via TLR7 and TLR9 on the plasma membrane or in the endosomal compartment of the B cell, 3. cytokines (e.g., IFN, IL6, IL12) or membrane receptors (e.g., via the B-cell activation factor from the TNF superfamily (BAFF)), which are induced or produced by T cells, DC or epithelial cells, and finally 4. T-cell help for B cells via the CD40–CD40L system (Lanzavecchia and Sallusto, 2007). In the context of T-cell dependent antibody-mediated autoimmune diseases, like MG, the latter mechanism is of fundamental importance.

Perhaps the most important example of the reciprocal interaction between B and T cells is the immunoglobulin class (isotype) switching that occurs in B cells when they are "helped" by antigen-specific T cells. In this collaboration, the B cell uses IgM molecules on its surface to capture the antigen and presents the processed antigen to the T cell. Contact between the collaborating lymphocytes is enhanced by complementary pairs of adhesion molecules.

T-cell help for B cells occurs in secondary lymphoid tissue in the presence of dendritic and follicular dendritic cells. The main structure for T-/B-cell contact are the germinal centers, which usually arise after antigen contact. They provide a milieu for B-cell proliferation, somatic hypermutation of immunoglobulins, and class-switch recombination. A sophisticated system of interactions finally leads to an efficient B-cell response. B-helper T cells are characterized by the expression of CD4, the CXC-chemokine receptor 5 on their surface (CXCR5), CD57 and ICOS (Vinuesa et al., 2005; Rasheed et al., 2006; Tackenberg et al., 2007). CXCR5 and its ligand CXCL13 is critically involved in stabilizing lymphoid follicles. Expression of CD40L on the surface of follicular/germinal center B-helper T cells increases dramatically after antigen stimulation, facilitating close contact with B cells (Vinuesa et al., 2005). The B cell itself upregulates B7, the natural ligand for CD28 or CTLA4, which either provides the second proliferation signal, or a suppressive signal back to the T cell. These cooperative interactions between the T cell and B cell induce the secretion of cytokines, such as interleukin-2 and interleukin-4. Isotype switching requires two signals. The first is delivered by an interleukin and the second by the binding of CD40 to its ligand on the T cell.

After receptor-mediated endocytosis of the antigen, the immunoglobulin may sterically influence the rate

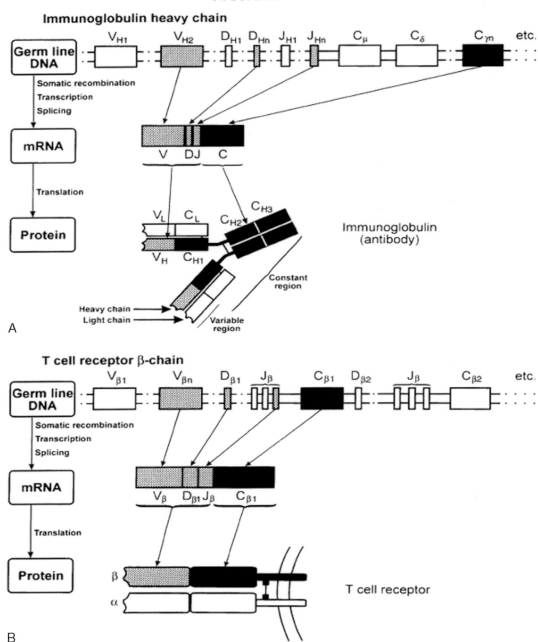

Fig. 5.3. Genetic organization and expression of Ig and T-cell receptor genes. (A) The germ line DNA encoding the variable region of the Ig heavy chain contains 51 variable (V_H), 27 diversity (D_H) and six joining (J_H) functional gene segments. The constant-region genes code for the different Ig isotypes (e.g., C_μ for IgM, C_δ for IgD etc.). A complete heavy-chain variable-region gene is assembled by somatic recombination events that first join the D and J segments, and then join the V gene segment to the combined DJ sequence. The heavy-chain constant-region sequences are spliced to the variable domain sequences during processing of the heavy-chain gene RNA transcript. The mRNA coding for the two types of Ig light chain (κ and λ) is constructed by similar mechanisms (not shown). (B) The germ line DNA encoding the T-cell receptor β chain genes contains 65 (64 functional) V_β, 13 J_β (not all here shown), two D_β, and two C_β segments. Like the Ig heavy chain, the variable domain of the T-cell receptor β-chain is encoded by three gene segments, V_β, D_β, and J_β. Rearrangement of these gene segments generates a functional exon that is transcribed, spliced to join VDJ to C, and the resulting mRNA translated to yield the T-cell receptor β-chain protein. The mRNA coding for the T-cell receptor α-chain is constructed by similar mechanisms (not shown). (After Hohlfeld, 1997.)

at which different parts of the antigen are processed in the B cell (Lanzavecchia, 1990). Thus, different B cells bearing different surface immunoglobulin would process the antigen differently, in contrast to antigen-nonspecific antigen presenting cells, which process antigens in a uniform manner. By these mechanisms, B-cell specificity could lead to selective antigen presentation to helper T cells, and therefore to selective T-cell help for certain specific epitopes. Thus, helper T cells and B cells can reciprocally influence each other's specificity.

5.2.8. Thymus function

The thymus plays a special role in myasthenia gravis pathogenesis and therefore structure and function of the normal thymus deserves particular mention. The thymus is a central (primary) immune organ, and is the key site of T-cell maturation. The thymic cortex is populated by blood-borne precursor cells that originate from bone-marrow stem cells. These immature T-cell progenitors proliferate rapidly, interact sequentially with various components of the thymic stroma reaching the medulla, and eventually leave the organ as immunocompetent T cells. The fact that the "thymus at birth may be essential for life" was first realized in the early 1960s. Neonatally thymectomized mice were severely depleted of lymphocytes, were highly susceptible to infection and failed to reject allogeneic skin, a prototypical function of cellular immunity (Miller, 1961, 2001). An impressive example of human thymic function is the restoration of T-cell function with thymic transplantation, as exemplified in DiGeorge syndrome. This is a rare congenital disorder caused by developmental defects in the third pharyngeal pouch and fourth pharyngeal arch. It results in defects of the thymus, heart, and parathyroid glands and is often associated with chromosomal changes at 22q11. Newborns with complete DiGeorge syndrome have no detectable thymus function and basically no measurable T-cell count (fewer than 50/mm^3). Recent trials show that transplantation with allogeneic cultured thymus can restore thymus function in these children and dramatically improve survival of patients with this otherwise fatal disorder (Markert et al., 2004).

5.2.9. Changes of thymus function in life

In a newborn child the thymus consists of two lobes located in the upper anterior mediastinum. Aging is associated with anatomical and functional involution of the thymus, leading to a reduction of its contribution to the naive T-cell pool (Aspinall and Andrew, 2000). Macroscopically the thymus decreases in size with increasing age. It can usually be recognized by computed tomography in individuals below age 30, but cannot be identified in 27% between 30 and 49 years, and in as many as 83% of those over 49 years old (Baron et al., 1982). Also, there is a marked sensitivity of (normal and myasthenic) thymic tissue to corticosteroids and stress in humans, though there seems to be an individual, perhaps genetically determined heterogeneity (Dourov, 1986; Willcox et al., 1989). On the other hand, in severe immune deficiency situations (e.g., HIV infection, or chemotherapy for malignant tumors), there is an astonishing potential for immune recovery in parallel with an increase in thymic size in adults (Smith et al., 2000; Kolte et al., 2002).

5.2.10. Thymus microenvironments

The thymus is composed of cells of diverse origin (Fig. 5.4). The thymic microenvironments are determined by the nature of the local stromal cells, and, vice versa, the composition and the character of the stromal cells is controlled by the local T cells. The factors that characterize each thymic microenvironment have not been fully identified. Clearly, epithelial cells must act in concert with bone marrow-derived stroma cells, such as thymic interdigitating cells and macrophages. Consistent with diverse microenvironments, monoclonal antibody studies indicate regional diversity among thymic epithelial cells (van Ewijk et al., 1994). Phenotypic analysis of lymphocyte development in the thymus is usually performed by multicolor flow cytometry. This work has led to a large amount of data concerning T-cell developmental stages (Fig. 5.5). The vast majority of thymocytes (>95%) undergo apoptotic, programmed cell death, indicated by fragmentation of their nuclei, and never reach the periphery. Productive rearrangement of the TCR genes is an initial key event in T-cell differentiation, and the progressive changes in TCR expression are closely linked to the induction and surface expression of the CD4 and CD8 markers on the differentiating T cells. Progenitor T cells arriving from the bone marrow lack rearranged TCRs and express neither the CD4 nor the CD8 marker. At this stage, the structural genes of the TCR are still located in germline formations at separate chromosomal loci. Components of the TCR β-chain gene rearrange first. The TCR β-chain proteins appear on the cell membrane together with a primitive surrogate α-chain. This is the signal for several differentiation steps. The first of these steps is the induction of CD4 and CD8 expression, which is followed by rearrangement of the TCR α-genes and the appearance of CD4/CD8 double-positive thymocytes expressing the TCR. These cells are now ready to

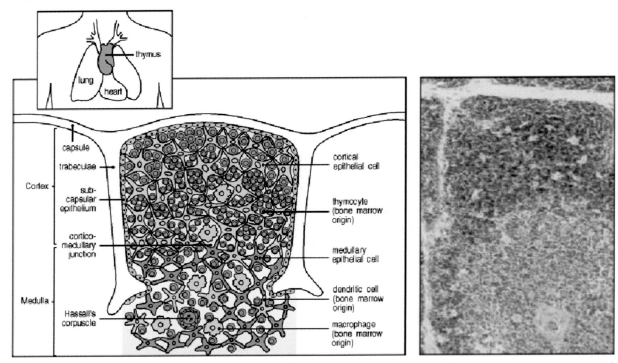

Fig. 5.4. The cellular organization of the human thymus. The thymus, which lies in the midline of the body, above the heart, is made up of several lobules, each of which contains discrete cortical (outer) and medullary (central) regions. As shown in the diagram on the left, the cortex consists of immature thymocytes (dark blue), branched cortical epithelial cells (pale blue), with which the immature cortical thymocytes are closely associated, and scattered macrophages (yellow), which are involved in clearing apoptotic thymocytes. The medulla consists of mature thymocytes (dark blue), and medullary epithelial cells (orange), along with macrophages (yellow) and dendritic cells (yellow) of bone marrow origin. Hassall's corpuscles are probably also sites of cell destruction. The thymocytes in the outer cortical cell layer are proliferation immature cells, whereas the deeper cortical thymocytes are mainly immature T cells undergoing thymic selection. The photograph shows the equivalent section of a human thymus, stained with hematoxylin and eosin. The cortex is darkly stained; the medulla is lightly stained. The large body in the medulla is a Hassall's corpuscle. (From Janeway et al., 2001).

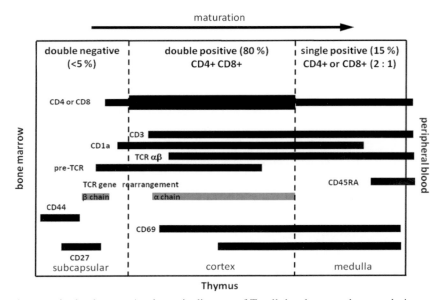

Fig. 5.5. T-cell development in the thymus. A schematic diagram of T-cell developmental stages during maturation in the thymus. Double positive cells make up approximately 80% of all thymocytes. The thymic maturation status of T cells depends on differential expression of surface markers. Their detailed function is not yet clear. (After Vanhecke et al., 1995.)

undergo further maturational steps that eventually produce an intact, functional T-cell repertoire composed of CD4 or CD8 single-positive lymphocytes (Robey and Fowlkes, 1994; Spits, 2002).

5.2.11. Positive and negative selection of thymocytes

Generation of the mature T-cell repertoire involves intensive interactions between the TCR of the developing T cells and the self-peptides expressed in the context of MHC molecules on the surface of thymic stroma cells. Two separate global rounds of T-cell selection take place. First, there is positive selection: all thymocytes are pushed into proliferation and express TCRs that bind to self-peptide/MHC complexes available within the thymus gland. During this phase of the self-recognition process, thymocytes that bind with low affinity to a readily available self-peptide/MHC complex, or with higher affinity to a rare self-peptide/MHC complex, are positively selected; high-avidity binding to a self-peptide is not a selective advantage (von Boehmer, 1993; Spits, 2002). This is followed by negative selection: now all T-cell clones that bind with high affinity to highly concentrated self-antigen/MHC complexes are eliminated. Obviously, this is to prevent the generation of autoreactive T cells that would attack the body's own tissues upon activation in the peripheral immune system (Allen, 1994). Both positive and negative selections constitute the core of "central tolerance" (see below). Thus, T-cell maturation and differentiation in the thymus is an extremely complex process. It ultimately results in a T-cell population that efficiently reacts against foreign antigens but tolerates self-antigens. Any defect in the structure of any thymic compartment could cause, or be a consequence of, an immunological aberration.

5.2.12. Peripheral tolerance, immunoregulatory mechanisms and autoimmunity

One of the main tasks of the thymus is to enable T cells to discriminate intrinsic (self) from extrinsic (foreign) antigens (see above; "central tolerance"). The mechanisms of how the immune system develops and controls self-tolerance are still not completely understood, though this is one of the fundamental questions of immunology. It is clear, however, that a detailed understanding of the principles of self-tolerance is essential for the development of specific immunotherapies for autoimmune disorders. A number of recent discoveries have offered promising new opportunities for therapy, as briefly summarized below.

The cells mainly responsible for immunoregulation and maintenance of immune tolerance are the T-lymphocytes. T cells become activated in a two-step scenario. The first is the TCR specific signal after recognition of a certain peptide and MHC on an antigen presenting cell. This usually leads to an upregulation of CD25 and production of IL-2, followed by T-cell proliferation. The latter step is critically controlled by a co-stimulatory signal via CD28–CD80/86, which leads to a stabilization of IL-2 mRNA with a 20–30 fold increase of IL-2 synthesis (Janeway et al., 2005). Absence of CD80/86 co-stimulation renders T cells anergic. Therefore, lack of CD80/86 expression on a self-tissue allows self-antigens to induce peripheral tolerance. Other mechanisms are clonal ignorance, which means that a T cell never "sees" its antigen, or conal deletion by Fas-mediated apoptosis (Abbas et al., 2004; Gonzalez-Rey et al., 2007). The degree of "degeneracy" or polyspecificity of the TCR is still a matter of discussion (Hemmer et al., 1998; Mason, 1998; Felix et al., 2007). It seems that the TCR is characterized by a high level of cross-reactivity against antigens (Mason, 1998), as well as "polyspecific" antigen activation (Felix et al., 2007). Different subpopulations of T cells may differ in their cross-reactive potential. Therefore, the stringency of tolerance and the need for active immune regulation may critically depend on the antigenic epitope.

An emerging field of great interest for research into autoimmunity is the role of "regulatory" cells (previously called "suppressor" cells), and the contribution of "neuropeptidergic modulation" (Lohr et al., 2006; Romagnani, 2006; Afzali et al., 2007; Gonzalez-Rey et al., 2007). Figure 5.6 summarizes some mechanisms of T-helper cell-dependent immune regulation. At least four CD4+ T-helper cell subtypes seem to be of particular relevance. Regulatory T cells (T_{reg}) have a CD4+CD25^{high} phenotype and comprise different subpopulations (Romagnani, 2006; Gonzalez-Rey et al., 2007). They represent a kind of immunological meta-level, primarily controlling excessive immune responses against non-self-antigens (Romagnani, 2006). T_{reg} cells that express the transcription factor FoxP3 are directly involved in CTLA-4 dependent downregulation of T-cell proliferation. A minor group of T_{reg}, lacking FoxP3, evolve their immunosuppressive activity via the synthesis of IL-10 or TGF-β (Gonzalez-Rey et al., 2007). As mentioned above, the paradigm of CD4+ TH1 and TH2 cells, which are proinflammatory (TH1) via their index cytokines IFN-γ and IL-2 or anti-inflammatory (TH2) via IL-4 and IL-13, has been amended by the discovery of IL-17 producing TH17 cells (Afzali et al., 2007). TH17 cells seem to represent a link between proinflammatory TH1 and immunosuppressive T_{reg} cells (Romagnani, 2006; Afzali et al., 2007).

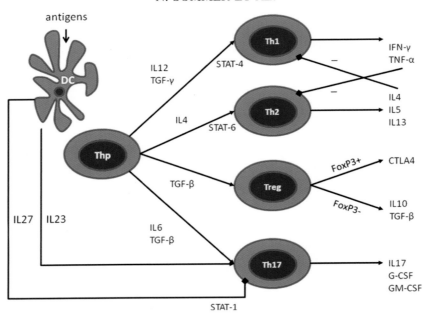

Fig. 5.6. T-helper cell dependent immune regulatory network. T-helper precursors (Thp) can expand into Th1, Th2, Th17 or regulatory T-cell (Treg) phenotypes dependent on the cytokine milieu around. Th1 and Th2 cells balance each other via IL4 or TNF-α. Signal transducer and activators of transcription (STAT) proteins are known for Th1 (STAT-4) and Th2 (STAT-6), and IL27 controls Th17 cells via STAT-1. Note that TGF-β is required for both Th17 and Treg expansion, but Th17 needs IL6 additionally. Neuropeptides, like VIP or PACAP, interfere at different stages with this system and lead in summary to an anti-inflammatory response. (For further details, see text; after Afzali et al., 2007; Gonzalez-Rey et al., 2007; Neufert et al., 2007.)

Besides regulation via cytokine networks, neuro-peptidergic regulation gradually comes into the focus of immunologists. One promising concept includes the effect of neuropeptides of the vasointestinal polypeptide (VIP) family. Amongst others this peptide family comprises VIP, pituitary adenylate cyclase activating polypeptide (PACAP), secretin, and glucagon. VIP showed anti-inflammatory effects in innate and adaptive immunity (Gonzalez-Rey et al., 2007), and VIP inhibits the production of the TH1-associated cytokine IL-12 by activated macrophages (Delgado et al., 1999). Furthermore, VIP induces CD86 upregulation in dendritic cells and macrophages with a consecutive TH1→TH2 shift (Gonzalez-Rey et al., 2007).

Among other effects, homing of TH2 cells, and therefore their recruitment for inflammatory action, is mediated by decreased CXC-chemokine ligand 10 (CXCL10) expression, which is downregulated on dendritic cells by VIP/PACAP (Delgado et al., 2004). The survival of TH2 but not TH1 cells can be supported by VIP/PACAP (Delgado et al., 2002). VIP/PACAP significantly induces FoxP3+ or FoxP3− T_{reg} cells and transfer of these VIP expanded T_{reg} cells into naive hosts inhibits antibody production (Gonzalez-Rey et al., 2007).

5.3. Autoantibodies and their target antigens in MG

5.3.1. Clinical relevance of AChR antibodies

The detection of autoantibodies against AChR is a key element for making the diagnosis of autoimmune MG. Approximately 85–90% of patients with generalized disease and 65% (45–71%) with purely ocular MG have an increased serum antibody titer (Lindstrom et al., 1976a; Lefvert et al., 1978; Oda et al., 1980; Tindall, 1981; Limburg et al., 1983; Vincent and Newsom-Davis, 1985; Sommer et al., 1993). There is no clear-cut correlation between disease severity and antibody titer in general. However, in an individual patient, the relative, longitudinally measured titers usually correlate with the clinical course. Accordingly, there is a relative decrease of the antibody titer in patients with a good clinical response to thymectomy and during effective immunosuppressive therapy, and a rise in titer may precede a clinical relapse (Tindall, 1980; Vincent et al., 1983; Schumm et al., 1984; Hohlfeld et al., 1985; Tindall et al., 1987). AChR antibodies are highly specific for MG. They may be rarely observed in patients with thymoma without muscle weakness, and essentially never in healthy subjects

(Cuénoud et al., 1980). For clinical purposes, AChR antibodies are usually measured by immunoprecipitation of iodine-125 α-bungarotoxin-labeled AChR extracted from human amputated leg muscle or from human muscle-like cell lines (Beeson et al., 1996).

The discovery of autoantibodies against AChR was one of the milestones in myasthenia research. This was made possible by two previous, unrelated discoveries which turned out to be extremely relevant to neurobiology in general. The myogenic electric organ of electrogenic fish provided a rich source of AChR, and the alpha-neurotoxins of venomous snakes (Elapidae) were found to bind to AChR with high affinity. Shortly after discovery of the technique for producing monoclonal antibodies (Köhler and Milstein, 1975), Patrick and Lindstrom immunized rabbits with AChR in order to produce antisera for further biochemical characterization of the protein (Patrick and Lindstrom, 1973). Vanda Lennon, who worked in their laboratory at the time, observed that the immunized rabbits had a kind of myasthenic weakness that could be reversed with anti-cholinesterase drugs. These seminal observations opened a whole new field of antibody studies.

5.3.2. AChR and the neuromuscular junction

The neuromuscular junction is a complex structure communicating the electrical impulse from the motor neuron to the skeletal muscle to induce contraction (Hughes et al., 2006). It consists of the nerve terminal, synaptic cleft and postsynaptic surface (Slater et al., 1992). The presynaptic region is capped by a terminal Schwann cell. The nerve terminal contains synaptic vesicles that are located precisely opposite the AChR-rich synaptic folds and are aligned near release sites (called active zones), where voltage-gated calcium channels (the target antigens of autoantibodies in the Lambert–Eaton myasthenic syndrome) are arranged in parallel double rows. When an action potential arrives, calcium enters, fusion of the synaptic vesicle membrane with the plasma membrane is triggered, and ACh is released into the synaptic cleft. The cleft is approximately 50 nm wide, and is filled with a basal lamina, which among other proteins (e.g., collagen IV, laminin, and fibronectin) contains acetylcholine esterase, the enzyme that breaks down ACh immediately after release. The postsynaptic membrane has deep infoldings, synaptic folds, at the crests of which the AChR, functionally the most important protein of the neuromuscular junction, is clustered (Engel et al., 1977a; Matthews-Bellinger and Salpeter, 1983).

The muscle nicotinic AChR is a ligand-gated ion channel that mediates synaptic transmission at the vertebrate neuromuscular junction. Channel opening results in an influx of cations, mainly sodium. The AChR is a pentamer consisting of five subunits in the stoichiometry $\alpha_2\beta\delta\gamma$ in the fetal striated muscle. In mature, adult muscle, the γ subunit is replaced by an ε subunit. The genes that code for AChR are well characterized and belong to a gene superfamily of ligand-gated ion channels, which also includes receptors for glycine, 5-hydroxy tryptamine, and γ-aminobutyric acid. There is extensive homology between the AChR subunits and across species (Noda et al., 1983). Prior to muscle development, the fetal AChR is expressed along the entire fiber surface. With innervation, fetal AChR is downregulated and the adult receptor is expressed at the synapse. Adult channels have shorter open times and a larger single channel conductance (Mishina et al., 1986). Extraocular muscles and other bulbar muscles of adults may express fetal AChR.

The high-resolution crystal structure of the extracellular domain of the mouse nicotinic AChR, bound to α-bungarotoxin, was recently solved at 1.94 Å resolution (Dellisanti et al., 2007). This structure, the first atomic-resolution view of an AChR subunit extracellular domain, revealed receptor-specific features such as the main immunogenic region (MIR), the signature Cys-loop and the N-linked carbohydrate chain. The toxin binds to the receptor through extensive protein–protein and protein–sugar interactions. Surprisingly, the structure showed a well-ordered water molecule and two hydrophilic residues deep in the core of the alpha subunit. The two hydrophilic core residues are highly conserved in nAChRs, but correspond to hydrophobic residues in the nonchannel homolog acetylcholine-binding proteins. Site-directed mutagenesis and electrophysiology analyses helped to assess the functional role of the glycosylation and the hydrophilic core residues, providing new insights into the gating mechanism (Dellisanti et al., 2007).

5.3.3. Functional effects of AChR antibodies

Several pieces of evidence showed that the AChR antibodies are responsible for the muscle weakness of MG. As mentioned, immunization of rabbits induced myasthenia-like muscle weakness that was reversible with anti-cholinesterase drugs (Patrick and Lindstrom, 1973). Furthermore, injection of patients' IgG into mice transferred myasthenic weakness (Toyka et al., 1977). Conversely, the removal of serum antibodies by plasmapheresis led to dramatic improvement of myasthenic symptoms of treated patients (Pinching et al., 1977). Immune complexes of IgG and C3 were demonstrated on the postsynaptic membrane of MG patients' muscle (Engel et al., 1977), and AChR isolated from myasthenic muscle was complexed with IgG (Lindstrom and Lambert, 1978).

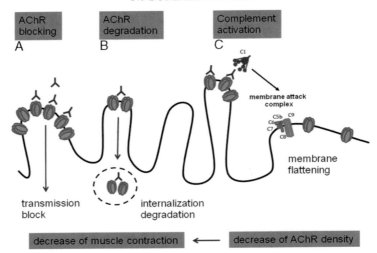

Fig. 5.7. Mechanisms of action of AChR autoantibodies. Neuromuscular synapse in myasthenia gravis. AChR antibodies interfere with signal transduction by direct blocking of AChR (A), by cross-linking and increased degradation (B), or by immune mediated destruction including complement activation (C).

There are three different mechanisms by which AChR antibodies impair neuromuscular transmission (Fig. 5.7):

1. Direct blocking of activation of the ion channel is one antibody-mediated effector mechanism in MG, but its overall contribution is minor. AChR antibodies that prevent α-bungarotoxin binding, and therefore presumably also ACh binding, were detected in 10–88% of patients' sera (Mittag et al., 1981; Drachman et al., 1982; Pachner, 1989). In most patients blocking antibodies account for only a minor fraction (Tzartos et al., 1982; Vincent et al., 1983), and fewer than 1% of patients have blocking antibodies only, which inconsistently correlate with the clinical status (Lennon, 1982; Besinger et al., 1983).

2. AChR antibodies may cross-link AChR, leading to their accelerated internalization and degradation. The normal receptor half-life at the neuromuscular junction has been estimated to be approximately 8 days (Fumagalli et al., 1982a; Stanley and Drachman, 1983). Compensatory mechanisms exist, but they are usually insufficient to prevent clinical symptoms from occurring. For example, when human rhabdomyoma cells or cultured myotubes are exposed to monoclonal anti-AChR antibodies, the cultured muscle cells upregulate transcription of AChR subunit mRNA (Guyon et al., 1998).

3. Complement-mediated effects seem to play a central role in endplate destruction. AChR antibodies readily fix complement and destroy myotubes in

the presence of complement (Ashizawa and Appel, 1985; Childs et al., 1987). At the myasthenic neuromuscular junction, complement fixation, activation of the lytic phase of the complement reaction sequence, and membrane-attack complex deposition are consistent findings (Engel et al., 1977; Sahashi et al., 1980; Fazekas et al., 1986; Engel and Arahata, 1987). Also, in experimental autoimmune MG (EAMG) complement fixation leads to opsonization of the junctional folds for destruction by macrophages. However, macrophage invasion at or near the neuromuscular junction was detected in only a minority of MG patients (Engel et al., 1981; Nakano and Engel, 1993).

5.3.4. Properties of AChR antibodies

AChR antibodies are polyclonal, and bind to a variety of sites on the AChR, but the majority recognize epitopes in a circumscribed extracellular portion of the α-subunit. This site, designated as the main immunogenic region (MIR), maps to residues 67–76 on the α-subunit and is distinct from the ACh/bungarotoxin binding site (Tzartos and Lindstrom, 1980; Tzartos et al., 1988a; Beroukhim and Unwin, 1995). Other antibodies are directed against other AChR subunits, but only a few bind to sites on the α-subunit outside the MIR. AChR antibodies are very variable in their light chains and IgG subclasses, but are highly specific and have a high affinity for the AChR. Therefore it was suggested that the antibodies are induced by a form of native AChR.

Most of the antibodies are of the IgG1 or IgG3 subclass, which activate complement (Vincent et al., 1998).

AChR antibodies from patients with ocular MG react better with ocular and normal muscle than with denervated muscle. How these characteristics contribute to the clinical state is unclear, especially in view of the observation that ocular MG sera do not react better with ocular than with normal limb muscle (Vincent and Newsom-Davis, 1982). Also, antibody reactivity with AChR can vary depending on whether AChR is extracted from myasthenic, denervated, or normal human muscle (Lefvert, 1982). Because some antibodies are directed primarily against epitopes present only on embryonic extrajunctional AChR (containing the γ rather than ε-subunit) or on myasthenic AChR, it was suggested that the fetal form of AChR is the primary autoantigen in MG (Vincent et al., 1998; Matthews et al., 2002). Also it has been proposed that antibodies to fetal AChR bind preferentially to extraocular muscle, which could explain why extraocular muscle weakness is often an initial and persisting symptom (Horton et al., 1993; Kaminski and Ruff, 1997). On the other hand, a subsequent study of AChR subunit expression in extraocular muscle showed that γ-subunit mRNA levels were comparable with those in other innervated muscle types and the ε-subunit was expressed at higher levels in extraocular muscle than in other muscles (MacLennan et al., 1997).

5.3.5. Placenta-crossing autoantibodies, neonatal MG and arthrogryposis multiplex congenita

Transient neonatal myasthenia is a well-known phenomenon. Because of trans-placenta antibody transfer from pregnant women to their fetuses, AChR antibodies are detected in nearly half of the newborn babies, and approximately 1 in 10 babies have signs of myasthenia that may be severe, but abate over the following weeks (Vernet-der Garabedian et al., 1994). There is no close association between neonatal MG and the severity of the maternal disease. Even if the mother is in remission, neonatal signs of MG may occur (Batocchi et al., 1999). It has been suggested that AChR antibodies against the fetal receptor might play a dominant role in this syndrome (Vernet-der Garabedian et al., 1994).

Arthrogryposis multiplex congenita (AMC) is characterized by multiple joint contractures developing in utero as a result of lack of fetal movement. Some cases are genetically determined, e.g., a mutation in the AChR genes (Brownlow et al., 2001), but in others the cause is unknown. AMC may also be associated with AChR-antibody positive MG and was found in 3 of 176 children born to MG mothers (Hoff et al.,

2006). Sera from five mothers of children with AMC from another series had high titer antibodies against fetal AChR, strongly suggesting that these are relevant for the development of the fetal deformities (Riemersma et al., 1996). Importantly, antibodies against fetal AChR were detected in a mother with repeated AMG pregnancies without clinical MG but with (retrospectively detected) antibodies against fetal AChR (Vincent et al., 1995). Also, in sera from anti-AChR negative AMC mothers fetal AChR function was inhibited (Riemersma et al., 1996). This suggests that placental transfer of antibodies against fetal antigens may be involved in fetal and perinatal disorders.

5.3.6. MuSK-antibodies and "seronegative" MG

When antibodies against AChR were detected in MG, it was soon clear that they were highly specific and sensitive for MG. In 10–15% of patients with generalized MG, however, anti-AChR antibodies are not detectable with standard assays (Lindstrom et al., 1976a). This was considered to be due to very low titers, possibly because most antibodies are not circulating but rather bound to endplates. Alternatively, endplate dysfunction in "AChR antibody-negative patients" might be caused by antibodies directed against other target molecules of the neuromuscular junction.

A number of interesting observations gradually led to a better understanding of "antibody-negative MG." Patients with so-called "seronegative" myasthenia responded to plasma exchange and to immunosuppressive therapy (Oosterhuis et al., 1983; Mossmann et al., 1986; Thorlacius et al., 1988; Kuks and Skallebaek, 1998). A mother transferred myasthenic symptoms to her newborn baby, while neither had AChR antibodies in their serum (Mier and Havard, 1985). After adoptive transfer into mice, antibodies from seronegative patients led to a reduction in miniature endplate potential amplitudes and also reduction of quantal content of the endplate potential (Mossmann et al., 1986). Furthermore, IgG from seronegative MG patients bound to a human muscle-like cell line (TE671), but not to human AChR (Blaes et al., 2000). Eventually, detection of antibodies against a muscle-specific receptor tyrosine kinase (termed MuSK) in 2001 was an important and far-reaching discovery (Hoch et al., 2001). MuSK mediates the agrin-induced clustering of AChRs during synapse formation, and is also expressed at the mature neuromuscular junction (Fig. 5.8). Subsequently, MuSK antibodies turned out to be present in approximately 40% of AChR antibody negative patients with generalized MG, though their prevalence may vary between populations (Evoli et al., 2003; McConville et al., 2004; Yeh et al.,

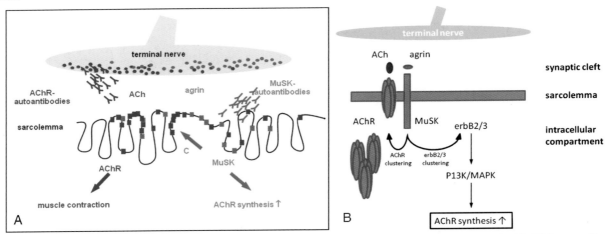

Fig. 5.8. (A) Role of anti-MuSK autoantibodies in neuromuscular transmission. The physiological task for MuSK is to mediate the agrin-induced postsynaptic clustering of AChR. Furthermore, MuSK increases the intracellular synthesis of AChR. Left (blue): acetylcholine receptor function; right (red): MuSK function. C: clustering; MuSK: muscle specific kinase; AChR: acetylcholine receptor; ACh: acetylcholine. (After Liyanage et al., 2002.) (B) Molecular function of MuSK. The nerve terminal secretes diffusable factors like acetylcholine or agrin into the synaptic cleft. Their postsynaptical targets are MuSK or the AChR, respectively. Activation of MuSK leads to a rapsyn-dependent increase in both AChR and erbB2/3 clustering, the latter activating the P13 kinase/MAP kinase pathway, leading to AChR transcription by the nucleus.

2004; Zhou et al., 2004; Niks et al., 2007; Zhang et al., 2007) (Table 5.1). MuSK antibodies are IgG (basically IgG4 isotype), bind to extracellular domains of MuSK and inhibit agrin-induced clustering of extrajunctional AChR in myotubes. This suggests that they could also decrease the density of AChR at the NMJ (Hoch et al., 2001).

Patients with anti-MuSK MG are usually anti-AChR negative, though two exceptions have been reported, one in a Japanese population using a different assay method (Ohta et al., 2004), the second in a female patient with anti-VGKC abs positive Morvan's syndrome (Diaz-Manera et al., 2007). The clinical manifestation of MG in patients with anti-MuSK antibodies is different from that in anti-AChR-positive patients, or patients who neither have anti-MuSK nor anti-AChR antibodies. Patients with anti-MuSK MG have prominent facial, bulbar, neck, and respiratory muscle involvement. They are younger and more frequently female compared to the anti-AChR patients (Zhou et al., 2004; Stickler et al., 2005).

MRI investigation showed that bulbar and facial muscle weakness was associated with significant muscle atrophy and fatty replacement in anti-MuSK MG, but not anti-AChR MG (Farrugia et al., 2006a). Electrodiagnostic patterns are also different to anti-AChR MG. Repetitive nerve stimulation is less often abnormal in anti-MuSK MG patients (Padua et al., 2006). Anti-MuSK patients are less likely to have abnormal jitter in single-fiber EMG (Stickler et al., 2005; Farrugia et al., 2006b), and may have electromyographic signs of myopathy (Rostedt Punga et al., 2006a). Anti-MuSK

Table 5.1

Prevalence of MuSK antibodies in generalized MG in different populations published between 2001 and 2006

Authors	Country	% AChR-antibody negative of all generalized MG		% MuSK-positive of generalized AChR-antibody negative	
Hoch et al., 2001	(European)			71%	(17/24)
Niks et al., 2007	Netherlands, regional	15%	(26/179)	22%	(5/23; F:M = 1:5)
	Netherlands, nationwide			36%	(35/97; F:M = 3:4)
Zhang et al., 2007	China	25%	(41/161)	2%	(1/43)
Yeh et al., 2004	China	10%	(38/385)	4%	(1/26)
Evoli et al., 2003				47%	(37/78; F:M = 3:6)
McConville et al., 2004	UK			41%	(27/66; F:M = 5:8)
Zhou et al., 2004	US			40%	(10/25; F:M = 2:3)

MG patients respond to immunosuppression (Zhou et al., 2004), but their response to cholinesterase drugs is unreliable, often with an abnormal sensitivity to cholinesterase inhibitors (Rostedt Punga et al., 2006b). In patients with purely ocular MG, MuSK antibodies are rarely found (Hanisch et al., 2006).

It has been a matter of discussion whether or not antibodies against MuSK are the primary cause of myasthenic symptoms (Lindstrom, 2004; Vincent et al., 2005). At present this issue cannot be settled conclusively. Anti-MuSK antibodies correlate, in individual cases as well as in the population, with clinical severity (Bartoccioni et al., 2006). Anti-MuSK positive sera can inhibit the proliferation of TE671 muscle cells (Boneva et al., 2006). Immunization of various mouse strains with recombinant rat-MuSK extracellular domain led to exercise-induced fatigue, decrement after repetitive nerve stimulation and a decrease in miniature endplate potentials (Jha et al., 2006). In a patient with anti-MuSK antibodies and also a family history of facial weakness, an intercostal muscle biopsy specimen was examined. His endplates showed no AChR or MuSK deficiency, but the amplitudes of the miniature endplate potentials and currents were reduced. Endplate structure was preserved, but the junctional folds stained faintly for IgG. The authors concluded that the circulating anti-muscle-specific tyrosine kinase antibodies caused neither muscle-specific tyrosine kinase nor acetylcholine receptor deficiency at the endplates; the reduced intercostal miniature endplate potential and current amplitudes were not accounted for by acetylcholine receptor deficiency; the faint immunoglobulin G deposits at the endplates may or may not represent anti-muscle-specific tyrosine kinase antibodies; and the anti-muscle-specific tyrosine kinase antibodies may not be the primary cause of myasthenic symptoms in this patient (Selcen et al., 2004).

C3 was visualized in muscle biopsies from anti-MuSK MG patients. AChR density was not significantly decreased, as compared with anti-AChR endplates, and C3 was detected in only two of eight patients (Shiraishi et al., 2005). Thus, MuSK antibodies do not appear to cause substantial AChR loss, complement deposition, or morphological damage.

The pathogenesis of MG in patients who have neither anti-AChR nor anti-MuSK antibodies remains unclear. The antibodies may be sub-threshold, as in patients with ocular MG who often have no detectable AChR antibodies but test positively for AChR antibodies when their disease becomes generalized (Seybold, 1999). Some seronegative patients may have a genetically determined congenital myasthenic syndrome. Further, it has been suggested that plasma factors, distinct from anti-MuSK IgG antibodies, bind to a muscle membrane receptor and activate a second messenger pathway leading to AChR phosphorylation and reduced AChR function (Plested et al., 2002).

5.3.7. Antibodies to other neuromuscular antigens

A number of AChR-positive patients harbor additional autoantibodies directed against neuromuscular antigens. They belong to a group of striational antibodies, which were first described by Strauss and colleagues in the 1960s using fluorescent antibody staining of striated muscle structures with MG patients' sera (Strauss et al., 1960; Strauss and Kemp, 1967). In 1981 Aarli and colleagues demonstrated that antibodies binding to a citric acid extractable striated muscle antigen correspond in part to the known striational immunofluorescence-defined antibodies and are closely associated with thymoma (Aarli et al., 1981). However, evidence for a pathogenetic role of the striational antibodies in MG is sparse.

The most relevant striational antibody is anti-titin IgG, because it is tightly associated with thymoma in patients under age 60 (Yamamoto et al., 2001). This antibody can be clinically used as a negative predictor for thymoma in young patients (negative predictive value 99%; Romi et al., 2005). However, it is not predictive for a specific thymoma histology (Voltz et al., 2003). Titin is the third most abundant filamentous muscle protein and, despite its huge size of about 3000 kD, most antibodies recognize a restricted main immunogenic region (Gautel et al., 1993), called MGT30 (i.e., MG thymoma 30 kD). This might be due to the redundancy of its molecular structure; 90% of titin is composed of 244 to 297 copies of two different 100-residue repeats: 112–165 immunoglobulin superfamily domains, and 132 fibronectin-like domains (Romi et al., 2005).

The ryanodine receptor (RyR) is another muscle antigen against which autoantibodies of MG patients are directed. This is a calcium release channel protein located in the sarcoplasmatic reticulum that exists in two isoforms (RyR1, skeletal muscle; RyR2, heart muscle). RyR-antibodies of MG patients react with both isoforms (Romi et al., 2005). The receptor consists of four homologous subunits building a central channel, which is expressed mainly in striated muscle tissue, but also rarely in neurons and epithelium. The receptor is critically involved in the cytoplasmatic calcium influx during muscle contraction (Coronado et al., 1994).

Rapsyn is another muscle protein targeted by autoantibodies. It is an intracellular 43 kDa scaffold protein, which precisely colocalizes, and is therefore equimolar with AChRs at the neuromuscular synapse.

Rapsyn is essentially involved in anchoring and clustering the AChR and other NMJ proteins (Liyanage et al., 2002). Anti-rapsyn antibodies were detected in MG patients. The antibodies colocalize with the β-subunit of the AChR (Agius et al., 1998). They are not specific for MG, but also found in lupus and toxic myopathies (Agius et al., 1998). Antibodies against skeletal muscle myosin, α-actinin, actin, or connectin were also described in MG patients (Yamamoto et al., 2001), but their pathogenic relevance remains obscure.

5.3.8. Anti-cytokine and anti-TCR antibodies

Antibodies against cytokines or TCR have been described in human MG and experimental settings. These include autoantibodies directed against interferon-α, interferon-Ω, IL-12 (Meager et al., 2003), IFN-γ (Zhang et al., 2003), TNF-α (Duan et al., 2002), and TCR Vβ chains (Jambou et al., 2003). Some of these antibodies may have immunoregulatory effects, and therefore could be involved in the pathogenesis of MG (see below).

5.4. The cellular immune response in myasthenia gravis

5.4.1. General aspects of the T-cell response

It has long been established that CD4+ helper T cells are crucially involved in the immunopathogenesis of MG. In humans and animals the AChR is a CD4+ T-cell dependent antigen (Lennon et al., 1976; Hohlfeld et al., 1984; Sommer et al., 1990; Wang et al., 1999; Tackenberg et al., 2007) and the production of anti-AChR antibodies requires the cooperation of T and B cells (Hohlfeld et al., 1986). Data from animal studies suggest that the interaction of AChR-specific T cells with B cells first leads to low-affinity anti-AChR antibodies, and in a second step, to high-affinity anti-AChR antibodies (Vincent, 2002; Conti-Fine et al., 2007). The mechanism of this affinity maturation might be related to somatic hypermutation of Ig genes in germinal centers (Conti-Fine et al., 2007), or to molecular mimicry, or epitope spreading (Vincent et al., 1998; Vincent, 2002). During the 1970s and 1980s, it was thought that a "perturbation of regulation of (anti-)idiotypic networks of immunoglobulins" was involved in the pathogenesis of autoimmune diseases in general, and MG in particular, but this area of research has been largely abandoned (Dwyer et al., 1983; Jerne, 1985).

MG patients harbor AChR-specific TH cells in their blood and thymus (Melms et al., 1988; Sommer et al., 1990). Circumstantial evidence for their pathogenic importance includes the beneficial effects of thymectomy (Morgutti et al., 1979), improvement after treatment with anti-CD4 (Ahlberg et al., 1994), and transient improvement in MG patients who have AIDS with reduced numbers of CD4+ TH cells (Nath et al., 1990). Mice deficient in CD4+ T cells, and immunodeficient severe combined immunodeficiency (SCID) mice engrafted with CD4-depleted lymphocytes from MG patients, do not develop anti-AChR antibodies (Kaul et al., 1994; Wang et al., 1999). Furthermore, HLA class II alleles, which are critically needed for antigen presentation to CD4+ T cells, are associated with MG susceptibility in human subjects and animals (see Section 5.5).

5.4.2. AChR-specific T-cell lines

AChR-specific human T cells were first demonstrated in 1984, using AChR isolated from electric ray (Torpedo californica) as the stimulating antigen (Hohlfeld et al., 1984). Subsequently, a huge amount of data was collected from T-cell stimulation experiments with synthetic peptides or recombinant polypeptides of human or rodent AChR. This work revealed a remarkable extent of intra- and interindividual heterogeneity of the anti-AChR T-cell response. T-cell epitopes were identified on all (α, β, δ, or ε(γ)) AChR chains (Brocke et al., 1988; Harcourt et al., 1988; Hohlfeld et al., 1988; Oshima et al., 1990; Zhang et al., 1990; Berrih-Aknin et al., 1991; Sommer et al., 1991; Milani et al., 2003; Oshima et al., 2005b; Ragheb et al., 2005).

The majority of stimulatory epitopes were found in the α-subunit of the AChR (Hohlfeld et al., 1987). Although several dominant epitopes could be defined, there were significant interindividual differences (reviewed by Hawke et al., 1996). Furthermore, there was some cross-reactivity between different subunits (Krolick and Urso, 1987; Tami et al., 1987). Overall, it has not been possible to identify a T-cell equivalent of the "main immunogenic region" recognized by antibodies. This is not surprising in view of the distinct nature of antigen recognition by T cells, and especially the genetic heterogeneity of the HLA molecules, which need to bind the AChR peptides before they can be recognized by T cells. The presence of AChR-specific T cells is by no means unique to MG patients. In fact, T cells from healthy subjects may recognize very similar α-subunit epitopes as T cells from MG patients (Salvetti et al., 1991; Sommer et al., 1991).

Several AChR-specific T-cell lines responded preferentially to embryonic γ-subunit epitopes, which are expressed in the thymus (Protti et al., 1991).

The δ-subunit seems to be less immunogenic than the other subunits (Wang et al., 1998), which may or may not be related to reduced or absent expression of this subunit in the thymus (Navaneetham et al., 2001). There is evidence that during the course of disease AChR-specific T cells undergo an intraindividual evolution of their spectrum of recognized AChR epitopes (Milani et al., 2003). Longitudinal follow-up studies using overlapping 20-mer synthetic AChR peptides indicated that the AChR-specific T-cell response, which was initially restricted to a few epitopes, spread to all subunits with increasing disease duration. This is consistent with the general concept of epitope spreading (Vincent et al., 1998). It appears likely, although not certain, that the human AChR itself is the ultimate autoantigenic target of both the B- and T-cell response (Vincent, 2002). Alternatively, some cross-reacting self or foreign antigen could initiate the response.

5.4.3. CD8+ T cells in MG

For many years attention was focused on the role of CD4+ T-helper cells. There was little evidence that CD8+ cytolytic T cells played any role in the pathogenesis of MG. More recently, however, there has been renewed interest in the CD8+ subset of T cells. Data from EAMG cast another light on these cells. EAMG was found to be suppressed by CD8+ depletion (Zhang et al., 1995), and CD8$^{-/-}$ KO mice were resistant to EAMG (Zhang et al., 1996). On the other hand, after engrafting both human CD4+ and CD8+ cells into SCID mice (Wang et al., 1999), CD8+ cells were found not to be necessary to induce myasthenic weakness or AChR antibody production.

Regarding human anti-AChR T-cell responses, analyses of the T-cell repertoire by CDR3 spectratyping revealed that about half of the investigated MG patients showed evidence for clonal restriction and expansion in the CD8+ T-cell compartment (Tackenberg et al., 2007). Specifically, the T-cell receptor Vβ usage was investigated in blood from 118 MG patients. Major expansions (≥ 5 standard deviations above the mean of 118 healthy, individually age- and sex-matched controls) of diverse Vβ were found in 21 patients (17.6%, p<0.001) among CD4+ T cells, and in 45 patients (38.1%, p<0.001) among CD8+ T cells. In informative probands, the expanded CD4+ cells consistently showed a TH cell phenotype (CD57+CXCR5+) and expressed TH1 cytokines. Furthermore, their expression of markers for activation, lymphocyte trafficking and B-cell-activating ability persisted for ≥ 3 years. Although these data primarily support the evidence for persistent clonally expanded CD4+ B-helper T-cell populations in the blood of MG patients, they are consistent with an as yet undefined, perhaps regulatory, role of CD8+ T cells.

5.4.4. Regulation of the T-cell response

Tight regulation of the T-cell response is essential for maintenance of peripheral self-tolerance. Immune regulation involves an intricate network of cell interactions, most notably between TH1, TH2, T$_{reg}$ and TH17 cells. All these cells interact with each other, as well as with antigen-presenting cells and other cells. It appears that both TH1 and TH2 cells and their secreted cytokines contribute to regulation of the T-cell response in MG. IFN-γ, a classical TH1 cytokine, seems to be necessary for EAMG induction and also for development of the human disease. MG patients have abundant anti-AChR TH1 cells in their blood, which recognize many AChR epitopes (Moiola et al., 1994). AChR-specific T-cell clones from MG patients show either a TH1 or TH0 profile (Nagvekar et al., 1998a; Hill et al., 1999b). Clonally expanded TCR Vβ+ T cells show a TH1 cytokine pattern (Tackenberg et al., 2007). In IFN-γ$^{-/-}$ KO, STAT6$^{-/-}$ KO and STAT4$^{-/-}$ KO mice, EAMG cannot be induced (Moiola et al., 1998; Balasa and Sarvetnick, 2000; Wang et al., 2004). TH1 cells usually induce IgG subclasses that bind and activate complement efficiently. Moreover, IFN-γ can induce MHC class II expression in muscle cells, raising the possibility that muscle cells can directly present AChR epitopes to CD4+ T cells (Hohlfeld and Engel, 1990). In animals IFN-γ can increase the cytoplasmatic AChR concentration in thymic epithelial cells (Poea-Guyon et al., 2005), which could favor thymic presentation of AChR.

Apart from TH1 cells, AChR-specific TH2 and TGF-β-secreting TH3 cells can also be found in the blood of MG patients (Yi et al., 1994). Whereas TH1 cytokines seem to foster the autoimmune response, data from EAMG indicate that TH2 cells have complex tasks. On the one hand, they can be protective; on the other hand they can worsen EAMG if they produce IL5, IL6 or IL10 (Conti-Fine et al., 2007). Furthermore, TH2 cytokines reduce germinal center formation and anti-AChR IgG synthesis (Deng et al., 2002).

Recently a role for TH17 cells is beginning to emerge (see Section 5.2 for discussion of this "novel" subset of T cells). TH17 cells are stimulated by IL23, IL6, and TGF-β, and presumably by other cytokines. As far as it is known to date, TH17 cells produce IL17, G-CSF, and GM-CSF. IL27-producing dendritic cells inhibit their functions. Future experiments and data from human patients will clarify whether the preliminary but interesting results from EAMG (Wang et al., 2007), concerning a possible role of TH17 cells in MG, can be confirmed.

Apart from these cytokines, there is increasing evidence for the importance of chemokines in MG and EAMG (Feferman et al., 2005). The chemokine IFN-γ-inducible protein 10 (IP-10; CXCL10), a CXC chemokine, and its receptor, CXCR3, were found to be overexpressed in lymph node cells of EAMG rats. Quantitative real-time PCR confirmed these findings and revealed upregulated mRNA levels of another chemoattractant that activates CXCR3, a monokine induced by IFN-γ (Mig; CXCL9). TNF-α and IL-1β, which act synergistically with IFN-γ to induce IP-10, were also upregulated. These upregulations were observed in immune response effector cells, namely lymph node cells, and in the target organ of the autoimmune attack, the muscle of myasthenic rats, and were significantly reduced after suppression of EAMG by mucosal tolerance induction with an AChR fragment. The relevance of IP-10/CXCR3 signaling in myasthenia was validated by similar observations in MG patients. A significant increase in IP-10 and CXCR3 mRNA levels in both thymus and muscle was observed in myasthenic patients compared with age-matched controls. CXCR3 expression in peripheral blood mononuclear cells (PBMC) of MG patients was markedly increased in CD4(+), but not in CD8(+), T cells or in CD19(+) B cells. These results demonstrated a positive association of IP-10/CXCR3 signaling with the pathogenesis of EAMG in rats as well as in human MG patients.

Several studies have addressed the role of co-stimulatory molecules in the regulation of anti-AChR autoimmunity. For example, CTLA-4 plays a crucial role in controlling T-cell responses. The first evidence that the CTLA-4/CD28 system may be perturbed in MG came from the identification of a functionally relevant polymorphism in the CTLA-4 gene of thymoma patients (Huang et al., 1998a). This was associated with CD28 dysfunction, and a higher proliferation of CD4+ T cells in patients carrying the mutation (Huang et al., 2000). Subsequently, other functionally relevant polymorphisms were described in MG (Ligers et al., 2001; Wang et al., 2002a, b). At least indirect evidence from EAMG shows that CTLA-4 function is important to limit determinant spreading and clinical signs of weakness (Wang et al., 2001), and that the B7-ligand for CTLA-4 is critical in EAMG (Poussin et al., 2003). CD40L, which is necessary for T cells to provide B-cell help, seems to be linked to CTLA-4, because CTLA-1 is upregulated after CD40L blockade with monoclonal antibodies (Im et al., 2001a).

As mentioned above, potentially autoreactive T cells are a part of the physiological immune repertoire.

Thymus-derived CD4+CD25+ regulatory T (T$_{reg}$) cells are essential for the maintenance of immunologic self-tolerance. In thymocyte suspensions of hyperplastic thymuses the proportion of T$_{reg}$ seems to be similar to healthy newborn or adult controls, but there is evidence for a functional deficit of MG T$_{reg}$, which shows a decreased expression of the transcription factor FoxP3, and a decreased capacity to suppress cocultured CD25-negative T cells in vitro (Balandina et al., 2005). By contrast, in MG-associated thymomas both the number of T$_{reg}$ and the proportion of T$_{reg}$ emigrants, but not the export of other T-cell subsets, is reduced (Ströbel et al., 2004; Luther et al., 2005). In blood the number of circulating T$_{reg}$ cells is lower in MG patients than in controls. Directly after thymectomy, the number of T$_{reg}$ cells decreases, but tends to recover after 12–16 months (Fattorossi et al., 2005).

Data from animals with EAMG also suggest a protective role for T$_{reg}$ and provide evidence for their regulation via GM-CSF (Sheng et al., 2006) and NK T cells (Liu et al., 2005). Furthermore, subcutaneous application of myasthenogenic AChR epitopes as "altered peptide ligands" down-regulates the myasthenogenic T-cell response in EAMG, and is accompanied by an increase of T$_{reg}$ cells, which show upregulation of CTLA-4, intracellular and surface TGF-β, FoxP3 (Ben-David et al., 2005), and the Fas–FasL mediated apoptosis path (Aruna et al., 2006). Besides T$_{reg}$ cells, natural antibodies against individual TCR Vβ chains might act as immunomodulators in autoimmunity (Jambou et al., 2003). In HLA-DR3 positive MG patients, anti-TCR Vβ5.1 IgG antibodies were found at higher levels than in HLA-DR3 negative patients. These antibodies seemed to be related to the clinical course. They were directed against the TCR of Vβ5.1 expressing cells, and inhibited IFN-γ secretion and proliferation of the corresponding T cells (Jambou et al., 2003). Whether these antibodies are induced by T$_{reg}$ cells is unknown.

5.4.5. B- and T-cell cooperation in MG

There is ample direct and indirect evidence that the B-cell response in MG is T cell-dependent. Although it seems likely that a disturbance of T/B-cell cooperation is a key factor in the pathogenesis of MG, the precise mechanisms that lead to pathological B-cell activation remain unknown. The site of the initial "autosensitization" is also unknown. Possible sites of B-cell activation include the germinal centers in the thymus (lymphofollicular hyperplasia; see below), regional lymph nodes, and spleen (Vinuesa et al., 2005). So far, limited data about the initiation and regulation of the B-cell response in MG are available.

As discussed above, AChR antibodies recognize a main immunogenic region (MIR) of the AChR consisting of the α-subunit residues 67–76 (Tzartos and Lindstrom, 1980; Vincent et al., 1998). Interestingly, in a given patient AChR-specific T cells recognize epitopes that are different from the B-cell epitopes (Hohlfeld et al., 1987), especially with respect to the MIR (Hughes et al., 2004). Like the T-cell response to AChR antigens, the B-cell response is polyclonal (Engel, 1992). The T-helper cells that provide help to B cells in germinal centers usually express the chemokine receptor CXCR5 (together with CD57 and/or ICOS) and the chemokine CXCL13, the latter of which guides B cells into the follicle. CXCR5 is increased on T cells of treatment naive MG patients with thymic hyperplasia or thymoma (Saito et al., 2005).

B-cell help in general and in EAMG in particular seems to depend on the costimulatory molecule ICOS (Scott et al., 2004; Rasheed et al., 2006). The generation of high-affinity antibody-secreting plasma cells critically depends on the presence of CD4 T cells during the germinal center (GC) reaction. GC T cells are so far incompletely characterized in terms of phenotype and function. Human follicular B helper T (T(FH)) cells are characterized by high expression of the homeostatic chemokine receptor CXCR5 and the costimulatory molecule ICOS, but not CD57 expression (Rasheed et al., 2006). CXCR5(hi)ICOS(hi) CD4 T cells are the most potent inducers of IgG production that also secrete large amounts of the B cell-attracting chemokine CXCL13. CXCR5(hi)ICOS(hi) CD4 T cells differ from other tonsillar CD4 T-cell subsets in their stimulatory activity, proliferative capacity and susceptibility to apoptosis. T(FH) cells are only distantly related to CXCR5(−) and CXCR5(+) central memory T (T(CM)) as well as effector memory T (T(EM)) cells present in the periphery. CXCR5(hi)ICOS(hi) CD4 T cells appear to be terminally differentiated T-helper cells that express a unique set of transcription factors related to the Notch signaling pathway and thus differentiate independent of other T-helper cell populations (Rasheed et al., 2006).

It is interesting in this regard that in many MG patients, T-helper cells with a CXCR5+CD57+ B phenotype were found in a clonally expanded TCR Vβ+ population, pointing to their antigen-specific pathogenic relevance (Tackenberg et al., 2007). The phenotypical features of these T cells, including activation status, homing receptors, and CD40L surface expression, were stable over a 3-year period. A decrease of these expanded cells was followed by clinical improvement (Tackenberg et al., 2007). In a few MG patients CD4+CXCR5+ T-cell clones could be followed for up to 17 months using TCR Vβ CDR3

spectratyping (Matsumoto et al., 2006). Furthermore, CXCL13 was increased in thymic germinal centers and in sera of 24 MG patients, and decreased after initiation of immunosuppressive treatment (Meraouna et al., 2006). CXCL10, a chemokine regulating the growth of immature hematopoetic cells, is also increased in CD4+, but not CD8+ T cells or B cells, of MG patients (Feferman et al., 2005). The CXCL10 receptor, CXCR3, is decreased on CD4+ TH cells when disease severity is high, but increases during treatment (Suzuki et al., 2006), suggesting a possible protective effect.

Another interesting molecule relevant to T/B-cell cooperation is the B-cell activation factor of the tumor necrosis factor family (BAFF), a key factor for B-cell maturation. BAFF is expressed on classical APCs, like dendritic cells, monocytes and to a lesser extent on T cells. BAFF can be upregulated by IFN-γ, IL-10, GCSF and CD40L. Upregulation of BAFF is associated with an increased susceptibility for autoimmune diseases (Mackay et al., 2007). In human thymic hyperplasia germinal centers, BAFF and its receptor on B cells is upregulated (Thangarajh et al., 2006). IFN-γ treated (Adikari et al., 2004), or AChR-pulsed (Xiao et al., 2003) dendritic cells improve EAMG via downregulation of BAFF.

5.4.6. Cellular responses of the innate immune system in MG

The role of the innate immune system in MG pathogenesis is largely unexplored. However, a number of intriguing hints exist that the innate immune system might be involved. First, it was shown that in thymitis and in atrophic thymus, but not in thymoma, the toll-like receptor TLR4 was significantly upregulated (Bernasconi et al., 2005), raising the possibility that an endogenous or exogenous "danger signal" is involved. Second, NK T cells and NK cells of untreated MG patients with thymoma, but not thymic hyperplasia, were increased and returned to normal after therapy (Suzuki et al., 2005; Takahashi et al., 2007). Third, activation of NK T cells with a synthetic glycolipid improved EAMG in C57B/6 mice. This effect might be mediated by an increased T_{reg} population of a CD4+CD25+FoxP3+ phenotype in treated mice (Liu et al., 2005), suggesting that NK T cells participate in maintaining self-tolerance in EAMG. However, NK cells contribute to EAMG induction by their capability to secrete IFN-γ (Shi et al., 2000), perhaps in conjunction with the pro-inflammatory role of IL-18 in EAMG, increasing both NK cell and TH1 cell function (Im et al., 2001b). On the other hand, excessive NK cell function in EAMG seems to be inhibited by IL-21 and the IL21-R (Liu et al., 2006).

5.5. Immunogenetics of myasthenia gravis

Inheritance of human autoimmune MG is complex (Willcox, 1993; Garchon, 2003). Population-based data concerning the risk of relatives of MG patients are limited (Namba et al., 1971; Bundey, 1972; Pirskanen, 1977; Allen et al., 1984; Provenzano et al., 1988; Szobor, 1991). Recent data from a nationwide Swedish database estimated the sibling risk ratio for MG surprisingly high at about 22 when one sibling was diagnosed with any neuromuscular junction or muscle disorder (Hemminki et al., 2006), indicating that the genetic risk might be higher than previously assumed.

MG is associated with other autoimmune diseases (e.g., rheumatoid arthritis, thyroid disease) (Pirskanen, 1977; Kerzin-Storrar et al., 1988), pointing to a general "autoimmune predisposition" of MG patients conferred by unknown genes. Several surveys of twins (Allen et al., 1984; Murphy and Murphy, 1986; Agafonov et al., 1997) indicate that the concordance rate in monocygotic twins might be around or less than 50% and therefore similar to other autoimmune diseases (Olmos et al., 1988; Deapen et al., 1992; Silman et al., 1993; Hyttinen et al., 2003).

Though family studies suggest a complex mode of inheritance, several candidate genes have been identified, most importantly genes of the HLA region, which was recently sequenced (The MCH Sequencing Consortium, 1999). Genome sequencing and interspecies mapping revealed the highest density of genes in the entire human genome. HLA can be subdivided into class I, class II and class III regions, the latter encoding proteins with essential immune functions, e.g., complement factors, heat shock proteins, TNF, lymphotoxins, and NK cell receptors (Vandiedonck et al., 2005). The HLA class II region encodes the molecules most relevant for antigen presentation to CD4+ TH cells. These HLA class II molecules, expressed on the surface of antigen presenting cells, bind peptide fragments of antigens and present them to helper T cells. Recognition of a peptide fragment in the context of the HLA class II molecule by the T-cell antigen receptor results in T-cell activation, and activated antigen-specific T cells stimulate antibody production by B cells. From this, one can infer that disease-associated HLA class II molecules are particularly prone to bind and present pathogenic peptides, leading to activation of autoreactive T cells.

In MG, the association with HLA class I and II alleles was discovered first. In Caucasians the HLA class I alleles B8 and A1, and subsequently class II alleles DR3 and Dw3, were found to be associated with higher MG susceptibility (Feltkamp et al., 1974; Fritze et al., 1974; Pirskanen, 1976; Carlsson et al., 1990;

Dönmez et al., 2004). The 3 Mb 8.1 haplotype is stably inherited across Caucasian generations and comprises not only the HLA A1 and B8 DR3 alleles, but also many other HLA loci, like complement factor or TNF alleles (Vandiedonck et al., 2004). Besides MG, this locus is associated with numerous other autoimmune diseases, including rheumatoid arthritis, Graves disease, type I diabetes, celiac disease, and systemic lupus erythematosus (SLE) (Price et al., 1999). Thymic hyperplasia in early-onset MG is also associated with the 8.1 haplotype (Fritze et al., 1974; Compston et al., 1980), thus defining the so-called MYAS1 locus on chromosome 6 (Giraud et al., 2001). The 8.1 haplotype, HLA-DQ, and CHRNA1 (see below) are associated with increased AChR-autoantibody titers (Giraud et al., 2004a; Vandiedonck et al., 2004). Evidence for a functional relevance of HLA associations also comes from in vitro experiments with antibodies against HLA-DQ B1 peptides, which suppressed the proliferation of AChR-specific T cells from MG patients (Oshima et al., 2005b).

Some HLA haplotypes are partly associated with a specific type of thymic pathology and/or the presence of anti-titin antibodies in MG (Giraud et al., 2001; Garchon, 2003). HLA-DR16 and -DR9 are positively associated with thymic hyperplasia and early-onset MG. Patients with late-onset MG (i.e., onset >60 years) without evidence for a thymoma or a thymic hyperplasia showed an association with HLA-DR7 in the absence of anti-titin antibodies, and with HLA-DR3 in the presence of anti-titin antibodies (Giraud et al., 2001). Also thymoma-associated MG, which is usually accompanied by high titers of anti-titin antibodies (Yamamoto et al., 2001; Somnier and Engel, 2002; Voltz et al., 2003), seems to be associated with the HLA-DR7 haplotype (Giraud et al., 2001). About half of anti-MuSK positive Caucasian MG patients had an HLA-DR14 haplotype (in comparison to 5% of healthy controls), and the odds ratio of an association with DR14 DQ5 was 8.5 (Niks et al., 2006).

Because the antigenic target of the autoimmune reaction in MG is known, the influence of AChR polymorphisms can be investigated. The main immunogenic region for antibody binding is located on the AChR α-subunit (Tzartos et al., 1998). The AChR α-subunit encoding gene (CHRNA1), combined with the DQA1*0101 and DR3 haplotype, but not the AChR β-subunit encoding gene (CHRNB1), seems to contribute to MG susceptibility (Djabiri et al., 1997a, b). Polymorphisms in the AChR δ-subunit encoding gene (CHRND) seem to be interesting candidates for MG susceptibility (Giraud et al., 2004b).

Studies of HLA associations in ethnic groups other than Caucasians are sparse. They seem to be markedly different from the HLA associations noted in Caucasians. HLA-DR9 was associated with mild ocular forms of MG in Chinese or Japanese patients, whereas HLA-Bw46 was associated with generalized MG in China (Hawkins et al., 1986; Chiu et al., 1987; Hawkins et al., 1989; Matsuki et al., 1990). In 87 Japanese patients with childhood-onset, HLA genotypes DRB1*1302 (DRBI*1302/DQA1*0102/DQB1*0604 and DRB1*0901/DQA1*0301/DQB1*0303) were significantly more frequent than in healthy controls (Shinomiya et al., 2004). In middle and south Americans, HLA-DR11 was associated with thymoma (Garcia-Ramos et al., 2003), and HLA-A31, -B8, -B39, -B40, -C15, -C17, and -DRB1*09 (DR9) with MG in general (Fernandez-Mestre et al., 2004).

Apart from HLA I and II, numerous additional candidate loci were described to be associated with MG. Among them immunoglobulin polymorphisms (Nakao et al., 1980; Smith et al., 1983, 1984; Chiu et al., 1988; Gilhus et al., 1990; Demaine et al., 1992), notably the κ-chain Km allotype that correlates with autoantibody serum levels (Dondi et al., 1994) and the Fc gamma receptor IIA-R/R131 with MG in general (van der Pol et al., 2003). Others are T-cell receptor loci, cytokines, like IL1β, IL4, IL6, and IL10, or the β-adrenergic receptor (Huang et al., 1998b,c, 1999a,b; Xu et al., 2000). Mutations of the CD45 gene (exon 4; 77 C>G), which is a candidate gene in other autoimmune diseases like MS (Jacobsen et al., 2000), were not found to be associated with MG (Tackenberg et al., 2003). Three polymorphisms in the CTLA-4 gene, which is involved in downregulation of T-cell activation, were described and could have functional relevance in MG (Huang et al., 1998a, 2000; Wang et al., 2002a,b), especially in thymoma patients (Chuang et al., 2005). Furthermore, a polymorphism in the gene of the intracellular tyrosine phosphatase (PTPN22* R620W) confers an about twofold risk for "titin antibody-negative" MG (Vandiedonck et al., 2006).

5.6. The thymus in myasthenia gravis

The thymus is thought to play an important role in MG pathogenesis, but the precise mechanisms of the intriguing association between thymic pathology and MG have remained unsolved.

5.6.1. Early notions of the role of the thymus in MG

Thymic changes in patients with myasthenia gravis were observed in the early 20th century by Karl Weigert and Farquhar Buzzard (Weigert, 1901; Buzzard, 1906). At that time neither the immunological origin of MG nor the immune function of the thymus were

anticipated. A beneficial therapeutic effect of thymectomy was noticed by Alfred Blalock, first in patients with thymic tumors, and later also in MG without thymoma (Blalock, 1944). The autoimmune pathogenesis of MG was first proposed by Simpson, who argued that the association of MG with systemic lupus erythematosus, the transmission of symptoms from mother to the newborn baby, response to corticosteroids and pathological changes in muscle and thymus all pointed to an immunological mechanism (Simpson, 1960). Thymus abnormalities are present in 70–80% of MG patients (Castleman and Norris, 1949; Genkins et al., 1961; Castleman, 1966; Marx et al., 2003). The most frequent thymic abnormality is lympho-follicular hyperplasia, whereas about 10% of all MG patients have a thymic tumor, and the remaining patients have normal thymus involution.

Thymus pathology, clinical features and immunogenetic data were integrated into a scheme of pathogenetic heterogeneity, which has been useful for clinical and research purposes. Compared to earlier schemes (Compston et al., 1980), the current classification incorporates new findings regarding ocular MG, AChR-negative MG, and late onset MG. Late onset MG is now the most frequent subgroup (Phillips and Torner, 1996; Vincent et al., 2003; Somnier, 2005), whereas in the 1980s early onset MG was the most frequent type (Newsom-Davis et al., 1987).

5.6.2. Histology of thymic changes

Lymphofollicular hyperplasia (LFH), also called thymitis, was reported to occur in approximately two thirds of MG patients (Müller-Hermelink and Marx, 1999). It represents the most typical histological alteration in young onset patients with generalized, AChR-antibody positive MG (i.e., group A in Table 5.2). It is therefore likely that the relative frequency of LFH will change with the recently reported increase of incidence of old onset MG, which is usually associated with thymic atrophy. LFH has also been reported in patients with purely ocular MG (Schumm et al., 1985), but there is insufficient data on this subgroup, because usually these patients are not thymectomized. In LFH the thymus contains numerous lymphoid follicles with germinal centers, which are absent or at least very rare in normal thymus, but have occasionally been reported in other autoimmune diseases (Burnet and Holmes, 1962; Murakami et al., 1996; Nicolle, 1999; Budavari et al., 2002). Lymphoid follicles with germinal centers expand the perivascular spaces (PVSs) and disrupt the surrounding membrane. This results in fusion of the thymic medulla (i.e., a part of the thymus parenchyma) and the PVSs (thought to belong to the peripheral

Table 5.2

Pathogenetic heterogeneity of myasthenia gravis

Group	A Early onset MG	B Late onset MG	C Thymoma associated MG	D Ocular MG	E Seronegative MG	F MuSK-antibody associated MG
Approximate frequency	20%	45%	10%	15%	5%	5%
Course and manifestation	Generalized	Generalized	Generalized	Generalized	Generalized	Generalized, mainly facio-pharyngeal
Age at onset	≤45	>45	Any age, mostly 40–60	Any age	Any age	Any, often young adults
Male:female ratio	1:3	1.5:1	1	1	1	M<F
MHC-association	B8 A1 DR3 Strong	B7 DR2 Less strong Anti-titin abs with DR7	No association	?	?	Some reported
Associated autoantibodies	Anti-AChR, often other antibodies, such as anti-thyroid or anti-nuclear	Anti-AChR, often anti-titin or anti-ryanodine-receptor	Anti-AChR, often anti-titin, anti-ryanodine-receptor, or anti-cytokine antibodies	Anti-AChR in 50–70%	No	Anti-MuSK, no anti-AChR
Typical thymus pathology	Lympho-follicular hyperplasia	Involution	Thymoma Type A 5% Type AB, B1–3 95%	Usually not available, may be lympho-follicular hyperplasia	No typical LFH, but T-cell zones	No
Response of MG symptoms to thymectomy	Usually good	Few data	Often poor	Few data, may be good	May be good, but few data	Poor
Response to immunosuppressive drugs	Usually good	Good	Positive, but often not as good as in the other groups	Good	Usually good	Sometimes less

immune system) (Kirchner et al., 1986a; Flores et al., 1999). In the medulla there is an increase of dendritic cells (Kirchner et al., 1988). By contrast, the number of thymic myoid cells (TMCs) in the thymus of MG patients (both with hyperplasia and thymoma) is not significantly different from that of healthy controls (van de Velde and Friedman, 1970; Schluep et al., 1987; Kornstein et al., 1995; Wakkach et al., 1999). TMC usually do not express HLA II molecules, so that "AChR" would have to be presented by some other, presumably professional APC, provided this mechanism plays a part in MG pathogenesis (Schluep et al., 1987; Kirchner et al., 1988; Wakkach et al., 1999). In thymic hyperplasia TMCs are often seen in close relation to germinal centers, supporting the hypothesis that an early autoantibody attack on myoid cells provokes local GC formation (Roxanis et al., 2002). Further, myoid cells in thymitis are frequently located in intimate apposition to dendritic cells (Kirchner et al., 1986). Such contacts are rarely seen in normal thymus. The thymic cortex in thymitis shows the normal age-dependent morphology.

Thymitis in seronegative myasthenia gravis has been reported to be a separate entity (Williams et al., 1992), since germinal centers are rare and the number of B cells is almost normal (Schluep et al., 1987). By contrast, mature T cells extend the perivascular spaces, but whether the basal membrane between PVSs and medulla is disrupted as in seropositive MG-associated thymitis has not been reported.

Thymic atrophy is a typical finding in late onset MG (Table 5.2). The role of the thymus in these patients, if any, has not been clarified. Except for a slight increase in medullary B cells and dendritic cells (Kirchner et al., 1988), the thymuses of these patients are very similar to age-matched controls, and therefore probably do not represent an end stage of thymitis (Kirchner et al., 1988; Müller-Hermelink and Marx, 1999; Sempowski et al., 2000).

About 10% of MG patients with suspicious radiological findings (chest CT or MRI) have histologically confirmed thymoma, and 40% of all patients with thymoma have concomitant MG (Marx et al., 2003). There are rare reports of MG in single cases of epithelial or mesenchymal tumors, and hematopoietic neoplasms (Marx et al., 1996; Sciamanna et al., 1997; Gattenloehner et al., 1998; Burns et al., 1999; Müller-Hermelink and Marx, 2000). However, for MG-associated thymomas (Kirchner et al., 1992) it is undisputed that they play a role in the pathogenesis of MG (Willcox, 1993; Vincent, 1994; Marx et al., 1997, 1998; Nagvekar et al., 1998b; Vincent, 2002).

Criteria for the histological diagnosis of thymomas have been defined in the WHO thymoma classification (Marx and Müller-Hermelink, 1999; Rosai, 1999), distinguishing type A (medullary), AB (mixed), B1 (organoid), B2 (cortical) and B3 thymoma subtypes (the latter was also called "well differentiated thymic carcinoma" previously) (Kirchner et al., 1992). Interestingly, tumors of the thymus without "thymus-like features," i.e., type C thymomas (e.g., squamous cell or adenocarcinomas of the thymus) (Rosai, 1999) or thymic neuroendocrine or mesenchymal tumors, are virtually never associated with MG (Marx et al., 1997; Levy et al., 1998; Marx and Müller-Hermelink, 1999; Müller-Hermelink and Marx, 2000). Regarding the observation that only thymomas A–B3 are able to promote intratumorous T-cell development (Marx et al., 2003), their causal involvement in MG seems very likely. Nevertheless, type A thymomas are very rare in MG (<5%), and the majority of cases show a AB or B1–3 histology (Marx et al., 2003). In contrast to LFH-associated MG, neither AChR expressing myoid cells nor antibody production can be detected in thymomas (Newsom-Davis et al., 1987).

5.6.3. Severe combined immunodeficiency mice as a model of MG pathogenesis

Severe combined immunodeficiency (SCID) mice, which can tolerate xenografts, can be used as recipient organisms to study the immunopathogenetic role of human thymus or T cells (Schönbeck et al., 1992; Wang et al., 1999). After human thymic tissue fragments from MG patients with histological thymic hyperplasia had been grafted under kidney capsules of SCID mice, the animals developed high titers of human autoantibodies against the AChR and showed Ig deposits at the neuromuscular junction (Schönbeck et al., 1992). The number of thymic myoid cells, which are sparsely distributed in normal thymus, as well as their AChR surface expression, increased significantly and they differentiated into striated muscle fibers (Spuler et al., 1994). Interestingly, the same experiment did not work with fragments of human MG thymomas (Spuler et al., 1996), strongly suggesting that in contrast to lymphofollicular hyperplasia, the site of antibody production is extrathymic in thymoma-associated MG.

It has long been postulated that B cells in MG need help by CD4+ T cells. Experiments in SCID helped to support this concept. Autoantibody production occurred only if CD4+ T cell-containing peripheral blood lymphocytes from MG patients were engrafted into SCID mice, but not if CD4+ T cell-depleted samples were engrafted (Wang et al., 1999). Other investigators used anti-TCR Vβ specific antibodies, in the context of a specific HLA haplotype, as a tool to study the TH dependent regulation of the AChR antibody response after human thymocyte engraftment into SCID mice (Aissaoui et al., 1999; Jambou and Cohen-Kaminsky, 2003). The SCID mouse model should remain useful for future studies on the role of the myasthenic thymus, especially regarding T-cell dependent regulatory mechanisms, or regarding the possible role of "atrophic thymus."

5.6.4. Myogenesis in the thymus

One of the most important unsolved questions regarding the immunopathogenesis of MG is whether the site of autoimmunization is in the thymus or in the periphery, that is whether MG is caused by a breakdown of central or peripheral tolerance mechanisms. A huge body of evidence points to thymic alterations in MG, but to date a unifying concept is conjectural (see below). If the thymus is the primary site of autoimmunization, the antigenic target, the AChR must be presented there. In this regard, the AChR expressed by thymic myoid cells (TMCs) could be important. TMCs are a regular thymic stromal medullary compound in all vertebrates (van de Velde and Friedman, 1970). They derive either from pluripotent stem cells, from myoepithelial thymic cells, or from endodermal reticular cells (Wekerle et al., 1981; Dardenne et al., 1987). They are sparse, muscle-like cells expressing important muscle proteins like actin, myosin (Drenckhahn et al., 1979), creatine kinase, myogenin (Sato and Tamaoki, 1989), troponin T, desmin, and AChR (Kao and Drachman, 1977; Schluep et al., 1987). Results from SCID mice experiments (see above) demonstrated their potential for further differentiation into muscle cells (Spuler et al., 1994). They have therefore the antigenic characteristics of muscle tissue within the thymus (Seifert and Christ, 1990). TMCs in vitro and in situ express the full AChR (Schluep et al., 1987), especially the fetal isoform that is preferentially recognized by many autoantibodies in early onset MG patients (reviewed by Schluep et al., 1988; Vincent et al., 1998). Direct evidence for involvement of TMC in thymic AChR presentation is lacking for MG. In rat experiments, however, transfer of TMC into syngeneic rats seemed to induce anti-rat AChR antibody production (Matsumoto et al., 2004).

5.6.5. The role of the human thymus for the immunopathogenesis of MG

The majority of MG patients show thymic pathology, but the histological features vary remarkably. Evidence from SCID mice experiments also suggests that the immunopathogenesis of thymoma-associated MG is different from that of LFH-associated MG (Marx et al., 2003), although the pathogenic effector mechanisms are similar. The role of the thymus in late onset MG patients (with thymus atrophy) and in seronegative MG remains completely enigmatic (Andrews et al., 1993, 1994; Beeson et al., 1998; Christensen et al., 1998; Wilkins and Bulkley, 1999), despite the discovery of anti-MuSK antibodies (Hoch et al., 2001). The present knowledge on the thymus in anti-MuSK antibody-related MG is insufficient (Saka et al., 2005). Therefore, the following sections will focus on thymitis (thymic hyperplasia) and thymoma.

5.6.6. Pathogenesis of MG with thymic lymphofollicular hyperplasia

LFH occurs very frequently in MG (Vincent, 1994), not uncommonly in other autoimmune diseases (Müller-Hermelink et al., 1996), but rarely in healthy persons (Middleton and Schoch, 2000). Its etiology is not known, but a genetic contribution has been demonstrated for several polymorphic genes (see above). In particular it is unknown whether hyperexpressions of bcl-2 in thymic germinal centers (Onodera et al., 1996), of FAs in mature thymic T cells (Masunaga et al., 1994; Moulian et al., 1998, BAFF upregulation (Thangarajh et al., 2006), CXCR3 induction (Suzuki et al., 2006), or increased toll-like receptor 4 expression (Bernasconi et al., 2005) are involved in the etiology of thymitis.

Some authors consider thymitis a secondary phenomenon following the sensitization of T cells in the periphery, with recirculation to the thymus followed by local restimulation. However, the weight of evidence seems to favor a primary intrathymic pathogenesis of MG, as suggested by Wekerle many years ago (Wekerle and Ketelsen, 1977). According to this hypothesis AChRs on thymic myoid cells are primarily involved in the triggering of MG by thymitis as supported by a number of findings. 1. A substantial percentage of autoantibodies in thymitis-associated MG specifically recognize the fetal type of the AChR (Weinberg and Hall, 1979). 2. Fetal AChRs (i.e., AChRs with a γ-subunit instead of an ε-subunit) are expressed on thymic myoid cells but not on extrathymic muscle (Schluep et al., 1987; Geuder et al., 1992) except for a few extraocular muscle endplates (Kaminski et al., 1996). 3. TMCs were mainly seen close to Hassall's corpuscles in healthy subjects. In early onset MG with thymic hyperplasia they could be found frequently near to the laminin fenestrations, next to germinal center-like structures (Roxanis et al., 2002). It is tempting to speculate that AChR expressing TMCs come under attack by "early" autoantibodies, resulting in local injury and germinal center formation. 4. In germinal centers TH1 cytokines seem to play a dominant role in regulating the anti-AChR autoimmune response (see above), and those cytokines are indeed able to increase AChR expression on the TMC surface (Poea-Guyon et al., 2005). 5. The thymus with thymitis is the most important organ where anti-AChR autoantibodies are produced both in absolute terms and on a per plasma cell basis (Scadding et al., 1981). Upregulation of BAFF in the hyperplastic germinal centers (Thangarajh et al., 2006) suggests that this intrathymic environment might be favorable for B-cell survival. This may help to explain the clinical benefit of thymectomy (Nieto et al., 1999; Tsuchida et al., 1999). 6. Extrathymic immunization with AChR can induce experimental autoimmune MG (EAMG) in animals, but it does not elicit lymphofollicular thymitis (Meinl et al., 1991). 7. By contrast, the transplantation of thymitis-affected thymus fragments into SCID mice results in prolonged production of human anti-AChR autoantibodies, showing that thymitis tissue contains all the necessary constituents of a self-sustaining autoimmune reaction (Schönbeck et al., 1993; Spuler et al., 1994, 1996).

In support of the concept of intrathymic pathogenesis of MG, abnormally frequent clusters of myoid cells and antigen presenting dendritic cells were observed in thymitis (Kirchner et al., 1986). Because myoid cells remain negative for MHC class II in MG they are probably unable to present antigens to CD4+ T cells (Baggi et al., 1993). Therefore, it is thought that abnormal clustering enables dendritic cells to more efficiently take up AChR released from myoid cells. Processing of engulfed AChR in dendritic cells might result in a quantitatively improved presentation of AChR peptides to potentially AChR reactive T cells (Marx et al., 1997). Indeed, AChR reactive T cells are part of the normal T-cell repertoire (Melms et al., 1992a; Jermy et al., 1993; Salmon et al., 1998) and have been found in increased numbers in thymitis (Melms et al., 1988; Sommer et al., 1990). Such autoreactive T cells might provide help to B cells for autoantibody production (Hohlfeld and Wekerle, 1999b). Once produced, the autoantibodies may react with peripheral muscle AChR and with AChR on thymic myoid cells (see above). Whether the increased frequency of apoptotic thymic myoid cells observed in MG patients with thymitis (Bornemann and Kirchner, 1996) is caused by autoantibodies, cytotoxic attack or endogenous instability is not known. Therefore, it is unknown whether increased myoid cell apoptosis has any pathogenic significance or is just an epiphenomenon that occurs after initiation of MG.

There is some evidence that biochemical changes of thymic epithelial cells (TECs) might play a role in "remodeling" of the thymus in thymitis. Specifically, in TEC cultures derived in vitro from normal or hyperplastic age-matched MG thymuses, gene profiling analysis showed that MG-TECs basally overexpress genes coding for p38 and ERK1/2 MAPKs and for components of their signaling pathways (Colombara et al., 2005). Immunoblotting experiments confirmed that p38 and ERK1/2 proteins were overexpressed in MG-TEC and, in addition, constitutively activated. Pharmacological blockade with specific inhibitors confirmed their role in the control of IL-6 and RANTES gene expression. IL-6 and RANTES levels were abnormally augmented in MG-TEC, either basally or upon induction by adhesion-related stimuli. The finding that IL-6 and RANTES modulate, respectively, survival and migration of peripheral lymphocytes of myasthenic patients points to MAPK transcriptional and post-transcriptional abnormalities of MG-TEC as a key step in the pathological remodeling of myasthenic thymus (Colombara et al., 2005).

An interesting new twist in the concepts of thymic pathogenesis of MG relates to the role of the auto-immune regulator (AIRE), a nuclear protein loss-of-function mutation that causes the type 1 autoimmune polyendocrine syndrome (Giraud et al., 2007). Promiscuous expression of tissue-restricted auto-antigens in the thymus imposes T-cell tolerance and provides protection from autoimmune diseases. Promiscuous expression of a set of self-antigens occurs in medullary thymic epithelial cells and is partly controlled by AIRE. However, additional factors must be involved in the regulation of this promiscuous expression. One such mechanism relates to the control of thymic transcription of CHRNA1, which encodes the α-subunit of the muscle acetylcholine receptor. On re-sequencing the CHRNA1 gene, a functional bi-allelic variant in the promoter was identified that is associated with early onset of disease in two independent human populations (France and UK). This variant prevents binding of interferon regulatory factor 8 (IRF8) and abrogates CHRNA1 promoter activity in thymic epithelial cells in vitro. Notably, both the CHRNA1 promoter variant and AIRE modulate CHRNA1 messenger RNA levels in human medullary thymic epithelial cells ex vivo and also in a transactivation assay. These findings reveal a critical function of AIRE and the interferon signaling pathway in regulating quantitative expression of this auto-antigen in the thymus, suggesting that together they set the threshold for self-tolerance versus autoimmunity (Giraud et al., 2007).

5.6.7. Pathogenesis of thymoma-associated MG

There is evidence that the pathogenesis of thymoma-associated MG (TAMG) is different from LFH-associated MG (Marx et al., 1997; Vincent et al., 1998; Müller-Hermelink and Marx, 2000). About 60% of thymomas are not associated with MG (Marx et al., 2003). Some types of thymoma have multiple genetic alterations, especially on chromosome 2 or 6, but the functional role of these changes and their relation to the WHO classification subtypes are unknown (Zettl et al., 2000; Inoue et al., 2002, 2003; Chuang et al., 2005).

For several reasons, the pathogenesis of thymoma-associated MG is difficult to conceptualize. AChR expressing myoid cells, intrathymic antibody production (with some exceptions (Fujii et al., 1984)), and germinal centers are all absent from thymomas (Newsom-Davis et al., 1987; Marx et al., 2003). In contrast to patients with early onset MG, patients with TAMG typically do not benefit from thymectomy. For these and other reasons, it has been postulated that in TAMG there is a disturbance of both central and peripheral tolerance.

The majority of MG-associated thymomas show an AB or B1–3 histological pattern (Marx et al., 2003). In such cases, the following observations might relate to the pathogenesis. 1. Thymomas from TAMG patients contain *immature* T cells and promote their maturation. 2. In contrast to non-MG-associated thymomas, MG-related thymomas export mature CD4+ T cells (Ströbel et al., 2001; Marx et al., 2003). The hyothesis that these exported mature, but naive, T cells include potentially autoreactive TH was substantiated by Buckley and collegues by quantifying "T-cell receptor excision circles" (TRECs), which help in the detection of "recent thymic emigrants" in the blood (Buckley et al., 2001). 3. Thymomas express reduced levels of MHC class II molecules on epithelial cells (Ströbel et al., 2001). In addition, loss of one MHC locus on chromosome 6p21 in most TAMG cases may result in a qualitatively altered MHC/peptide repertoire on thymoma epithelial cells (Inoue et al., 2002). 4. Autoreactive T cells directed against the AChR α- or ε-subunits seem to be enriched in MG-associated thymomas (Sommer et al., 1991; Conti-Fine et al., 1998; Nagvekar et al., 1998a; Nenninger et al., 1998; Schultz et al., 1999). These T cells presumably escaped thymic negative selection (Nagvekar et al., 1998; Schultz et al., 1999) and are exported into the periphery. 5. Intratumor activation of mature T cells seems to occur only in rare type A thymomas (<5%), and 6. intratumor autoantibody production is exceptionally rare (Fujii et al., 1984; Newsom-Davis et al., 1987). 7. Several antigens seem to be relevant for the pathogenesis of TAMG. They include AChR, striational muscle antigens (e.g., titin; see above), neuronal antigens (e.g., neurofilaments; Marx et al., 1992), and cytokines, especially IL-12 and IFN-α (Meager et al., 1997, 2003). Though mRNA coding for a broad spectrum of possible antigens was observed in thymomas, few of the corresponding proteins could be detected (reviewed by Marx et al., 2003). 8. Lack of decline of antibody titers after

thymectomy of TAMG patients suggests that secondary lymphoid organs have a key role in perpetuating TAMG (Somnier, 1994). 9. Furthermore, it was shown in mice that the outcome of T-cell selection with respect to tolerance induction is influenced by the quantity and quality of MHC/peptide complexes presented by thymic epithelial cells (Ashton-Rickardt and Tonegawa, 1994; Hogquist et al., 1994; Barton and Rudensky, 1999), and the level of epithelial MHC expression (Fukui et al., 1997). The MHC level is particularly important when medullary structures (involved in negative selection under physiological conditions) are reduced (Laufer et al., 1999; van Meerwijk and MacDonald, 1999), which is the case in thymomas.

Putting the above mentioned findings together, one can envisage a two-step secenario of autoimmunization in TAMG with type AB or B histology. In the first step, non-tolerogenic thymopoiesis allows the export of naive but mature and potentially autoreactive T cells to the periphery. To become pathogenetically relevant, autoantigen-specific T cells must provide help to autoantibody-producing B cells outside the thymoma, after adequate activation (Marx et al., 2003). The mechanisms that activate and maintain the postulated peripheral autoimmunization process have yet to be defined, though unspecific infectious or traumatic stimuli have been favored (Müller-Hermelink and Marx, 2000). Loss of peripheral self-tolerance is probably amplified by reduced export of T_{reg} cells (Ströbel et al., 2004). Whether cytolytic CD8+ T cells (Vincent and Willcox, 1999; Palmieri et al., 2006; Tackenberg et al., 2007), perivascular memory T cells (Nagane et al., 2005), or genetic susceptibility (Machens et al., 1999) contribute to the pathogenesis is also not yet clear.

The molecular basis for the disturbance of intrathymic T-cell selection in thymoma has also remained enigmatic (Nagvekar et al., 1998b; Müller-Hermelink and Marx, 2000). Some interesting recent data concern the role of the autoimmune regulator, which regulates the presentation of self-antigens in the thymus (Mathis and Benoist, 2007). AIRE has a strong influence on the induction of T-cell tolerance in the thymus. It is mainly expressed by dendritic and thymic epithelial cells (Anderson et al., 2005). The latter presents peripheral tissue antigens to thymocytes during negative selection (Liston et al., 2003), leading to apoptotic clonal deletion. Animals lacking AIRE have a relatively normal immune response against foreign antigens, but they are highly susceptible to autoimmunity (Jiang et al., 2005). Furthermore, transplantation of thymus from AIRE$^{-/-}$ KO mice into athymic nude mice induced autoimmunity (Mathis and Benoist, 2007). In MG it has been shown that thymic epithelial cells express self-antigens, including insulin, AChR subunits, and thyroid antigens (reviewed by Shiono et al., 2003). Indeed, AIRE expression is nearly completely lost in thymomas of type A, AB, B2, or B3 (53.6% with TAMG), and only very few AIRE+ cells could be found in type B1 thymomas (Ströbel et al., 2007). Others found AIRE to be reduced in thymoma, compared to non-neoplastic thymi (Scarpino et al., 2007).

5.7. Relevant aspects of experimental autoimmunue myasthenia gravis

5.7.1. General considerations

The features of experimental autoimmune myasthenia gravis (EAMG) vary with the species and strain, source of AChR, use of adjuvants, and immunization schedules. EAMG was first induced in rabbits by direct immunization with AChR and Freund's adjuvant (Patrick and Lindström, 1973). Two years later the same group transferred EAMG into guinea pigs and rodents, the latter becoming the standard model, because rats developed both acute and chronic disease (Lennon et al., 1975). It is the chronic form of EAMG, not the acute form, that most closely resembles human MG, although some features of acute EAMG might apply at some endplates in some patients during the course of disease (Pascuzzi and Campa, 1988). Among rodents, Lewis rats are among the most susceptible to EAMG. In contrast, even the most susceptible mouse strain (C57Bl/6) develops myasthenic weakness only after repeated injections of AChR in Freund's adjuvant, and rarely in all injected animals (Milani et al., 2003).

Chronic EAMG adequately reflects many features of human MG. 1. Clinical weakness is most prominent in the upper proximal muscles. 2. Muscles show pathological decrement in repetitive electrical stimulation tests. 3. The edrophonium test is positive in EAMG-mice. 4. 90% of the animals develop autoantibodies against the AChR. 5. IgG and C3 deposits can be found at the NMJ. 6. Loss of endplate AChR occurs. 7. EAMG is MHC II (H-2) dependent. 8. Antigen presentation is also MHC II (H-2) dependent. 9. Antibody production is T-cell dependent as it is in human patients (for a detailed review see Christadoss et al., 2000). Because of these similarities, EAMG has been used to investigate new pathogenetic hypotheses not only in MG, but also in autoimmunity in general.

Experiments in transgenic and knock-out mice helped to postulate essential components of the autoimmune reaction against AChR in vivo, especially regarding the role of the MHC, antibodies, cytokine networks or receptors for cell–cell interaction. For example, mice deficient in IL-5 (Deng et al., 2002; Poussin et al., 2002) or TNF-receptor (Goluszko et al., 2002) are relatively resistant, whereas absence of IL-4 facilitates the induction of EAMG (Ostlie et al., 2003). Partially humanized mice have allowed in vivo studies of the role of human HLA molecules (Raju et al., 2001; Yang et al., 2002) and immunoglobulin loci (Stassen et al., 2003). An additional focus of interest are the mechanisms of T-cell–B-cell cooperation in EAMG and MG (Milani et al., 2006). This is of special interest, because the immunological dogma of TH2 dependence of T-cell help is challenged by (1) the observed IFN-gamma dependence of EAMG (Balasa and Sarvetnick, 2000), (2) the TH0 or TH1 cytokine profile of AChR-specific human CD4+ T-cell clones (Hill et al., 1999b; Nagvekar et al., 1998a), and (3) the clonal expansion of such CD4+ in MG patients (Tackenberg et al., 2007). Recent studies in EAMG focused on regulatory T cells (Liu et al., 2005; Sheng et al., 2006), NK cells (Liu et al., 2005), and the potential role of NMJ antigens, e.g., rapsyn (Losen et al., 2005).

Furthermore, EAMG has served as a useful tool for preclinical testing of new immunotherapies, including monoclonal antibodies against complement factors or T-cell surface molecules (Xu et al., 2005; Tuzun et al., 2007), cytokine-receptor antagonists (Yang et al., 2005), growth factors (Sheng et al., 2006), syngeneic AChR fragments (Maiti et al., 2004), altered peptide ligands (Ben-David et al., 2006), vaccination against immunologically relevant targets (Oshima et al., 2006), and new immunomodulators like fingolimod or phosphodiesterases (Kohno et al., 2005; Aricha et al., 2006).

5.7.2. Acute EAMG

In the rat, a single immunization with Torpedo electric organ AChR plus adjuvants induces acute EAMG accompanied by severe weakness after 7–11 days (Lennon et al., 1975; Lindstrom et al., 1976c). One of the first ultrastructural changes is the disintegration of the terminal expansions of the junctional folds. Shortly thereafter, degenerating postsynaptic regions split away from the underlying muscle fibers and are removed by macrophages (Engel et al., 1976a). This results in functional denervation of the affected muscle fibers; many NMJs become electrically silent and the apparent quantal content of the EPP is reduced owing to the inability of many released quanta to reach their postsynaptic target (Lambert et al., 1976). Some fibers undergo segmental necrosis, which is centered on the NMJ. After day 11, the macrophages leave the NMJ, the nerve terminals return to highly simplified postsynaptic regions, and the postsynaptic folds gradually regenerate (Engel et al., 1976a). Antibody against rat AChR is first detected in serum 3 days after immunization (Lindstrom et al., 1976a). The antibody titer is relatively low during the acute phase. It increases slowly until day 20 and then very rapidly until it exceeds the body content of AChR many times. The concentration of antibodies directed against electric organ AChR is always higher than antibodies directed against rat AChR.

5.7.3. Chronic EAMG

Following the acute phase animals regain their strength but again become weak with the onset of the chronic phase at about day 30 after immunization (Lennon et al., 1975). The junctional folds again degenerate and the postsynaptic regions become simplified (Engel et al., 1976a). The ultrastructural changes now resemble those observed in human MG (Engel et al., 1976b). During chronic EAMG the muscle AChR content declines and 70% or more of what remains is complexed with antibody (Lindstrom et al., 1976a). Ultrastructural studies also showed decreased AChR (Engel et al., 1977) and localized antibody and complement at the NMJ in chronic EAMG (Sahashi et al., 1980). AChR, IgG and C3 are found on the terminal expansions of the remaining junctional folds, over patches of the simplified postsynaptic membrane, and on fragments of the folds shed into the synaptic space (Engel et al., 1977; Sahashi et al., 1980). Therefore, shedding of AChR-rich fragments of the junctional folds into the synaptic space represents a mechanism of AChR loss in chronic EAMG. That lytic complement components are important in causing AChR deficiency in EAMG is indicated by the fact that C5 deficient mice immunized with AChR produce anti-AChR antibodies but show no clinical signs of EAMG (Christadoss, 1988). Accelerated internalization and destruction of AChR cross-linked with antibody (modulation) may also contribute to the AChR deficiency in chronic EAMG (Merlie et al., 1979; Fumagalli et al., 1982a,b).

5.7.4. Passive transfer of EAMG

IgG from rats with chronic EAMG induces acute passive-transfer EAMG in recipient rats (Lindstrom et al., 1976c). The weakness begins within 24 h after the transfer, peaks in 2–3 days, and improves in 5–10 days. As in acute EAMG, the NMJs are invaded by macrophages at the onset of weakness. Immunocytochemical studies reveal IgG, C3, C6, and C9 at the NMJ (Engel et al., 1979; Biesecker and Gomez, 1989). The macrophages do not contribute to the AChR loss but are attracted to the NMJ secondary to tissue damage (Hoedemaekers et al., 1997). Depletion

of C3 with cobra venom factor (Lennon et al., 1978) or of C6 by anti-C6 Fab antibody fragments (Biesecker and Gomez, 1989) prevents acute passive-transfer EAMG. Parenteral administration of a soluble recombinant form of human complement receptor 1 mitigates the effects of passive transfer and suppresses clinical disease (Piddlesden et al., 1996). Inhibition of EAMG by these agents indicates that the effects of the passive transfer model are closely linked to activation of the complement membrane attack complex (MAC), and on the MAC-mediated focal disruption of the postsynaptic membrane (Biesecker and Gomez, 1989).

A still unresolved question is why IgG from rats with chronic EAMG should induce acute passive-transfer EAMG. One possible explanation is that the extremely rapid destruction of the junctional folds in EAMG requires a high density of antigen (i.e., AChR) for fixing IgG and complement, and that this condition is met only at previously undamaged NMJs (Dupont and Richman, 1987).

5.8. Risk factors for myasthenia gravis and association with other immunological diseases

Patients with *thymic tumors* carry a markedly increased risk of developing myasthenia gravis. The role of thymoma was discussed in previous sections, but a few points deserve a special mention. Approximately one-third of patients with thymoma develop MG. The classical clinical context is detection of an asymptomatic mass lesion in the anterior mediastinum by chest CT or MRI. Remarkably, MG may appear after removal of the thymoma. Thymoma can occur up to 15 years after thymectomy for non-thymomatous MG (Hirabayashi et al., 2002). This implies that long-term follow up by imaging is required.

Regarding *association of thymoma-related MG* with other diseases, thymoma-associated MG occurred together with giant cell polymyositis and cardiomyopathy (Pascuzzi et al., 1986). In another series of 13 patients with giant cell polymyositis, all had thymoma and myocarditis and 6 had MG (Namba et al., 1974). Inflammatory changes in muscle and heart in fatal cases of MG were noted more than 100 years ago (Buzzard, 1906; Rowland et al., 1956; Mendelow, 1958). In autopsy studies Mendelow (1958) detected foci of inflammation and necrosis in the heart in 7 of 25 cases. Furthermore, thymomas with or without MG have been reported in association with such diverse conditions as red blood cell aplasia, hypogammaglobulinemia, aplastic, pernicious or hemolytic anemia, neutropenia or agranulocytosis, Addison's disease, Cushing syndrome, intestinal pseudo-obstruction, alopecia areata, encephalitis, neuromyotonia, stiff-person syndrome, and peripheral neuropathy (Vincent and Willcox, 1999; Marx et al., 2003).

Several conditions may be associated with non-thymoma-related MG, modifying its course or susceptibility. The occasional *association of MG with autoimmune disorders* was one of the tenets of Simpson's autoimmune hypothesis (Simpson, 1960). In 440 cases of MG Simpson observed 16 cases associated with rheumatoid arthritis, 4 with pernicious anemia, 1 with systemic lupus erythematosus and 1 with sarcoidosis. Subsequent studies added Sjögren syndrome (Ito et al., 1999), polymyositis (Gilhus et al., 1992), dermatomyositis (van de Warrenburg et al., 2002), systemic vasculitis (Cohle and Lie, 1996), inflammatory bowel disease (Lossos et al., 1995), primary biliary cirrhosis (Kiechl et al., 1996), hepatitis C virus infection (Eddy et al., 1999), pemphigus (Izumi et al., 2002), hyperthyroidism (Osserman et al., 1967), Hashimoto disease (Tsao et al., 2000), adrenocortical insufficiency (Dumas et al., 1985), allogeneic bone marrow transplantation (Grau et al., 1990), febrile neutrophilic dermatosis (Sweet syndrome) associated with myelofibrosis, thymoma, and immunodeficiency (Altomare et al., 1996), Castleman syndrome (Pasaoglu et al., 1994; Chorzelski et al., 1999), chronic inflammatory polyradiculopathy (Kimura et al., 1998), Lambert–Eaton myasthenic syndrome (Newsom-Davis et al., 1991), neuromyotonia (Heidenreich and Vincent, 1998; Newsom-Davis et al., 2003), red blood cell aplasia (Bailey et al., 1988), eosinophilia (Avni et al., 2006), rippling muscle disease (Ansevin and Agamanolis, 1996) or scleroderma (Zivkovic and Medsger, 2007). In a series of 220 Danish MG patients, the prevalence of associated autoimmune diseases was 14% (Christensen et al., 1995), but the percentage might be as high as 25 or 30%, as other studies suggest (Thorlacius et al., 1989; Tackenberg et al., 2001, 2007).

The *relationship between hyperthyroidism and MG* has been of interest to neurologists for many years (Engel, 1961). Careful case studies, together with experimental induction of hyperthyroidism in MG patients (Engel, 1961), showed that hyperthyroidism worsened myasthenia. Patients with *hematologic disorders* and especially those who had *bone marrow transplantation* have a relatively high incidence of anti-AChR antibodies without clinical MG (Lefvert and Björkholm, 1987). About one-third of bone marrow transplant recipients develop chronic graft versus host disease, but only 0.5% of the latter develop clinical MG (Bolger et al., 1986; Grau et al., 1990; Melms et al., 1992b).

Drug induced MG is an example of how an external risk factor can induce MG. For example, *penicillamine treatment* is known to induce MG in up to 30% of treated patients (Komal Kumar et al., 2004). Interestingly, the fine antigenic specificities of the anti-AChR antibodies are similar to those found in idiopathic MG (Tzartos et al., 1988b). This indicates that tolerance to self-AChR is broken in susceptible individuals (Masters et al., 1977). Penicillamine dependent MG, however, provides no clue as to what triggers the autoimmune response in idiopathic MG. D-penicillamine, which has a reactive sulfhydryl group, is capable of modifying self-antigens, including the AChR (Penn et al., 1998). It appears that the agent directly binds to antigenic peptides presented on macrophages or dendritic cells, especially in HLA-DR1-positive subjects (Hill et al., 1999a). Multiple sclerosis (MS) may be very rarely associated with MG (Somer et al., 1989), and glatiramer acetate, an immunomodulatory agent used for the treatment of MS, may enhance the risk of MG (Frese et al., 2000). Concerning the risk of MG in interferon-β treated MS patients, there are inconstistent data from case reports. Three MS patients developed clinical MG onset after initiation of interferon-β treatment, but it was not known whether these patients had AChR antibodies before treatment (Shimizu et al., 2007).

Epidemiological data indicate that the prevalence of late onset MG is increasing (Vincent et al., 2003; Somnier, 2005). The immunopathology of late onset MG is unknown (Tackenberg et al., 2007). Whether aging is an independent risk factor for the development of MG is yet to be determined.

References

Aarli JA, Lefvert AK, Tonder O (1981). Thymoma-specific antibodies in sera from patients with myasthenia gravis demonstrated by indirect haemagglutination. J Neuroimmunol 1: 421–427.

Abbas AK, Lohr J, Knoechel B, et al. (2004). T cell tolerance and autoimmunity. Autoimmun Rev 3: 471–475.

Adikari SB, Lian H, Link H, et al. (2004). Interferon-gamma-modified dendritic cells suppress B cell function and ameliorate the development of experimental autoimmune myasthenia gravis. Clin Exp Immunol 138: 230–236.

Afzali B, Lombardi G, Lechler RI, et al. (2007). The role of T helper 17 (Th17) and regulatory T cells (Treg) in human organ transplantation and autoimmune disease. Clin Exp Immunol 148: 32–46.

Agafonov BV, Tsuman VG, Shagal DI, et al. (1997). Twin studies of myasthenia. Zh Nevrol Psikhiatr Im S S Korsakova 97: 18–21 [article in Russian].

Agius MA, Zhu S, Kirvan CA, et al. (1998). Rapsyn antibodies in myasthenia gravis. Ann N Y Acad Sci 841: 516–521.

Ahlberg R, Yi Q, Pirskanen R, et al. (1994). Treatment of myasthenia gravis with anti-CD4 antibody: improvement correlates to decreased T-cell autoreactivity. Neurology 44: 1732–1737.

Aissaoui A, Klingel-Schmitt I, Couderc J, et al. (1999). Prevention of autoimmune attack by targeting specific T-cell receptors in a severe combined immunodeficiency mouse model of myasthenia gravis. Ann Neurol 46: 559–567.

Allen N, Kissel P, Pietrasiuk D, et al. (1984). Myasthenia gravis in monozygotic twins. Clinical follow-up nine years after thymectomy. Arch Neurol 41: 994–996.

Allen PM (1994). Peptides in positive and negative selection. Cell 76: 593–596.

Altomare G, Capella GL, Frigerio E (1996). Sweet syndrome in a patient with idiopathic myelofibrosis and thymoma-myasthenia gravis-immunodeficiency complex: efficacy of treatment with etretinate. Haematologica 81: 54–58.

Anderson MS, Venanzi ES, Chen Z, et al. (2005). The cellular mechanism of Aire control of T cell tolerance. Immunity 23: 227–239.

Andrews PI, Massey JM, Sanders DB (1993). Acetylcholine receptor antibodies in juvenile myasthenia gravis. Neurology 43: 977–982.

Andrews PI, Massey JM, Howard JF Jr, et al. (1994). Race, sex, and puberty influence onset, severity, and outcome in juvenile myasthenia gravis. Neurology 44: 1208–1214.

Ansevin CS, Agamanolis DP (1996). Rippling muscles and myasthenia gravis with rippling muscles. Arch Neurol 53: 197–199.

Aricha R, Feferman T, Souroujon MC, et al. (2006). Overexpression of phosphodiesterases in experimental autoimmune myasthenia gravis: suppression of disease by a phosphodiesterase inhibitor. FASEB J 20: 374–376.

Aruna BV, Ben-David H, Sela M, et al. (2006). A dual altered peptide ligand down-regulates myasthenogenic T cell responses and reverses experimental autoimmune myasthenia gravis via up-regulation of Fas-FasL-mediated apoptosis. Immunology 118: 413–424.

Ashizawa T, Appel SH (1985). Complement-dependent lysis of cultured rat myotubes by myasthenic immunoglobulins. Neurology 35: 1748–1753.

Ashton-Rickardt PG, Tonegawa S (1994). A differential-avidity model for T-cell selection. Immunol Today 15: 362–366.

Aspinall R, Andrew D (2000). Thymic involution in aging. J Clin Immunol 20: 250–256.

Avni I, Sharabi Y, Sadeh M, et al. (2006). Eosinophilia, myositis, and myasthenia gravis associated with a thymoma. Muscle Nerve 34: 242–245.

Baggi F, Nicolle M, Vincent A, et al. (1993). Presentation of endogenous acetylcholine receptor epitope by an MHC class II-transfected human muscle cell line to a specific CD4+ T cell clone from a myasthenia gravis patient. J Neuroimmunol 46: 57–65.

Bailey RO, Dunn HG, Rubin AM, et al. (1988). Myasthenia gravis with thymoma and pure red blood cell aplasia. Am J Clin Pathol 89: 687–693.

Balandina A, Lecart S, Dartevelle P, et al. (2005). Functional defect of regulatory CD4(+)CD25+ T cells in the thymus of patients with autoimmune myasthenia gravis. Blood 105: 735–741.

Balasa B, Sarvetnick N (2000). Is pathogenic humoral autoimmunity a Th1 response? Lessons from (for) myasthenia gravis. Immunol Today 21: 19–23.

Baron RL, Lee JKT, Sagel SS, et al. (1982). Computed tomography of the normal thymus. Radiology 142: 121–125.

Bartoccioni E, Scuderi F, Minicuci GM, et al. (2006). Anti-musk antibodies: correlation with myasthenia gravis severity. Neurology 67: 505–507.

Barton GM, Rudensky AY (1999). Evaluating peptide repertoires within the context of thymocyte development. Semin Immunol 11: 417–422.

Batocchi AP, Majolini L, Evoli A, et al. (1999). Course and treatment of myasthenia gravis during pregnancy. Neurology 52: 447–452.

Beeson D, Jacobson L, Newsom-Davis J, et al. (1996). A transfected human muscle cell line expressing the adult subtype of the human muscle acetylcholine receptor for diagnostic assays in myasthenia gravis. Neurology 47: 1552–1555.

Beeson D, Bond AP, Corlett L, et al. (1998). Thymus, thymoma, and specific T cells in myasthenia gravis. Ann N Y Acad Sci 841: 371–387.

Ben-David H, Sela M, Mozes E (2005). Down-regulation of myasthenogenic T cell responses by a dual altered peptide ligand via CD4+CD25+-regulated events leading to apoptosis. Proc Nat Acad Sci USA 102: 2028–2033.

Ben-David H, Aruna BV, Seger R, et al. (2006). A 50-kDa ERK-like protein is up-regulated by a dual altered peptide ligand that suppresses myasthenia gravis-associated responses. Proc Nat Acad Sci USA 103: 18232–18237.

Bernasconi P, Barberis M, Baggi F, et al. (2005). Increased toll-like receptor 4 expression in thymus of myasthenic patients with thymitis and thymic involution. Am J Pathol 167: 129–139.

Beroukhim R, Unwin N (1995). Three-dimensional location of the main immunogenic region of the acetylcholine receptor. Neuron 15: 323–331.

Berrih-Aknin S, Cohen-Kaminsky S, Lepage V, et al. (1991). T-cell antigenic sites involved in myasthenia gravis: correlations with antibody titre and disease severity. J Autoimmun 4: 137–153.

Besinger UA, Toyka KV, Homberg M, et al. (1983). Myasthenia gravis: long-term correlation of binding and bungarotoxin-blocking antibodies against acetylcholine receptors with changes in disease severity. Neurology 33: 1316–1321.

Biesecker G, Gomez CM (1989). Inhibition of acute passive transfer experimental autoimmune myasthenia gravis with Fab antibody to complement C6. J Immunol 142: 2654–2659.

Blaes F, Beeson D, Plested P, et al. (2000). Igg from "seronegative" myasthenia gravis patients binds to a muscle cell line, te671, but not to human acetylcholine receptor. Ann Neurol 47: 504–510.

Blalock A (1944). Thymectomy in the treatment of myasthenia gravis: report of twenty cases. J Thorac Surg 13: 316.

Bolger GB, Sullivan KM, Spence AM, et al. (1986). Myasthenia gravis after allogeneic bone marrow transplantation: relationship to chronic graft-versus-host disease. Neurology 36: 1087–1091.

Boneva N, Frenkian-Cuvelier M, Bidault J, et al. (2006). Major pathogenic effects of anti-musk antibodies in myasthenia gravis. J Neuroimmunol 177: 119–131.

Bornemann A, Kirchner T (1996). An immuno-electron-microscopic study of human thymic b cells. Cell Tissue Res 284: 481–487.

Brocke S, Brautbar C, Steinman L, et al. (1988). In vitro proliferative responses and antibody titers specific to human acetylcholine receptor synthetic peptides in patients with myasthenia gravis and relation to hla class ii genes. J Clin Invest 82: 1894–1900.

Brownlow S, Webster R, Croxen R, et al. (2001). Acetylcholine receptor delta subunit mutations underlie a fast-channel myasthenic syndrome and arthrogryposis multiplex congenita. J Clin Invest 108: 125–130.

Buckley C, Douek D, Newsom-Davis J, et al. (2001). Mature, long-lived CD4+ and CD8+ T cells are generated by the thymoma in myasthenia gravis. Ann Neurol 50: 64–72.

Budavari AI, Whitaker MD, Helmers RA (2002). Thymic hyperplasia presenting as anterior mediastinal mass in 2 patients with Graves disease. Mayo Clin Proc 77: 495–499.

Bundey S (1972). A genetic study of infantile and juvenile myasthenia gravis. J Neurol Neurosurg Psychiatry 35: 41–51.

Burnet FM, Holmes MC (1962). Thymus lesions in an autoimmune disease of mice. Nature 194: 146.

Burns TM, Juel VC, Sanders DB, et al. (1999). Neuroendocrine lung tumors and disorders of the neuromuscular junction. Neurology 52: 1490–1491.

Buzzard EF (1906). The clinical history and post-mortem examination of five cases of myasthenia gravis. Brain 28: 438–483.

Carlsson B, Wallin J, Pirskanen R, et al. (1990). Different HLA DR-DQ associations in subgroups of idiopathic myasthenia gravis. Immunogenetics 31: 285–290.

Castleman B (1966). The pathology of thymus gland in myasthenia gravis. Ann N Y Acad Sci 135: 496–503.

Castleman B, Norris EH (1949). The pathology of the thymus gland in myasthenia gravis. Medicine 28: 27–58.

Childs LA, Harrison R, Lunt GG (1987). Complement-mediated muscle damage produced by myasthenic sera. Ann N Y Acad Sci 505: 180–193.

Chiu HC, Hsieh RP, Hsieh KH, et al. (1987). Association of HLA-DRw9 with myasthenia gravis in Chinese. J Immunogenet 14: 203–207.

Chiu HC, de Lange GG, Willcox N, et al. (1988). Immunoglobulin allotypes in caucasian and Chinese myasthenia gravis: differences from Japanese patients. J Neurol Neurosurg Psychiatry 51: 214–217.

Chorzelski T, Hashimoto T, Maciejewska B, et al. (1999). Paraneoplastic pemphigus associated with Castleman tumor, myasthenia gravis and brochiolitis obliterans. J Am Acad Dermatol 41: 393–400.

Christadoss P (1988). C5 gene influences the development of murine myasthenia gravis. J Immunol 140: 2589–2592.

Christadoss P, Poussin M, Deng C (2000). Animal models of myasthenia gravis. Clin Immunol 94: 75–87.

Christensen PB, Jensen TS, Tsiropoulos I, et al. (1995). Associated autoimmune diseases in myasthenia gravis. Acta Neurol Scand 91: 192–195.

Christensen PB, Jensen TS, Tsiropoulos I, et al. (1998). Mortality and survival in myasthenia gravis: a Danish population based study. J Neurol Neurosurg Psychiatry 64: 78–83.

Chuang WY, Ströbel P, Gold R, et al. (2005). A CTLA4high genotype is associated with myasthenia gravis in thymoma patients. Ann Neurol 58: 644–648.

Cohle SD, Lie JT (1996). Myasthenia gravis-associated systemic vasculitis and myocarditis with involvement of the cardiac conducting tissue. Cardiovasc Pathol 5: 159–162.

Colombara M, Antonini V, Riviera AP, et al. (2005). Constitutive activation of p38 and ERK1/2 MAPKs in epithelial cells of myasthenic thymus leads to IL-6 and RANTES overexpression: effects on survival and migration of peripheral T and B cells. J Immunol 175: 7021–7028.

Compston DA, Vincent A, Newsom-Davis J, et al. (1980). HLA antigen and immunological evidence for disease heterogeneity in myasthenia gravis. Brain 103: 579–601.

Conti-Fine BM, Navaneetham D, Karachunski PI, et al. (1998). T cell recognition of the acetylcholine receptor in myasthenia gravis. Ann N Y Acad Sci 841: 283–308.

Conti-Fine BM, Milani M, Kaminski HJ (2007). Myasthenia gravis: past, present, and future. J Clin Invest 116: 2843–2854.

Coronado R, Morrissette J, Sukhareva M, et al. (1994). Structure and function of ryanodine receptors. Am J Physiol 266: C1485–1504.

Cuénoud S, Feltkamp TEW, Fulpius BE, et al. (1980). Antibodies to acetylcholine receptor in patients with thymoma but without myasthenia gravis. Neurology 30: 201–203.

Dardenne M, Savino W, Bach JF (1987). Thymomatous epithelial cells and skeletal muscle share a common epitope defined by a monoclonal antibody. Am J Pathol 126: 194–198.

Deapen D, Escalante A, Weinrib L, et al. (1992). A revised estimate of twin concordance in systemic lupus erythematosus. Arthritis Rheum 35: 311–318.

Delgado M, Munoz-Elias EJ, Gomariz RP, et al. (1999). VIP and PACAP inhibit IL-12 production in LPS-stimulated macrophages. Subsequent effect on IFNγ synthesis by T cells. J Neuroimmunol 96: 167–181.

Delgado M, Leceta J, Ganea D (2002). Vasoactive intestinal peptide and pituitary adenylate cyclase-activating polypeptide promote in vivo generation of memory Th2 cells. FASEB J 16: 1844–1846.

Delgado M, Gonzalez-Rey E, Ganea D (2004). VIP/PACAP preferentially attract Th2 effectors through differential regulation of chemokine production by dendritic cells. FASEB J 18: 1453–1455.

Dellisanti CD, Yao Y, Stroud JC, et al. (2007). Crystal structure of the extracellular domain of nAChR alpha1 bound to alpha-bungarotoxin at 1.94 A resolution. Nat Neurosci 10: 953–962.

Demaine A, Willcox N, Janer M, et al. (1992). Immunoglobulin heavy chain gene associations in myasthenia gravis: new evidence for disease heterogeneity. J Neurol 239: 53–56.

Deng C, Goluszko E, Tuzun E, et al. (2002). Resistance to experimental autoimmune myasthenia gravis in IL-6-deficient mice is associated with reduced germinal center formation and C3 production. J Immunol 169: 1077–1083.

Diaz-Manera J, Rojas-Garcia R, Gallardo E, et al. (2007). Antibodies to AChR, MuSK and VGKC in a patient with myasthenia gravis and Morvan's syndrome. Nat Clin Pract Neurol 3: 405–410.

Djabiri F, Caillat-Zucman S, Gajdos P, et al. (1997a). Association of the AChRα-subunit gene (CHRNA), DQA1*0101, and the DR3 haplotype in myasthenia gravis. Evidence for a three-gene disease model in a subgroup of patients. J Autoimmun 10: 407–413.

Djabiri F, Gajdos P, Eymard B, et al. (1997b). No evidence for an association of AChR β-subunit gene (CHRNB1) with myasthenia gravis. J Neuroimmunol 78: 86–89.

Dondi E, Gajdos P, Bach JF, et al. (1994). Association of Km3 allotype with increased serum levels of autoantibodies against muscle acetylcholine receptor in myasthenia gravis. J Neuroimmunol 51: 221–224.

Dönmez B, Ozakbas S, Oktem MA, et al. (2004). HLA genotypes in Turkish patients with myasthenia gravis: comparison with multiple sclerosis patients on the basis of clinical subtypes and demographic features. Hum Immunol 65: 752–757.

Dourov N (1986). Thymic atrophy and immune deficiency in malnutrition. Curr Top Pathol 75: 127–150.

Drachman DB, Adams RN, Josifek LF, et al. (1982). Functional acitivities of autoantibodies to acetylcholine receptors and the clinical severity of myasthenia gravis. N Engl J Med 307: 769–775.

Drenckhahn D, von Gaudecker B, Muller-Hermelink HK, et al. (1979). Myosin and actin containing cells in the human postnatal thymus. Ultrastructural and immunohistochemical findings in normal thymus and in myasthenia gravis. Virchows Arch B Cell Pathol Incl Mol Pathol 32: 33–45.

Duan RS, Wang HB, Yang JS, et al. (2002). Anti-TNF-α antibodies suppress the development of experimental autoimmune myasthenia gravis. J Autoimmun 19: 169–174.

Dumas P, Archambeaud-Mouveroux F, Vallat JM, et al. (1985). Myasthenia gravis associated with adrenocortical insufficiency. J Neurol 232: 354–356.

Dupont BL, Richman DP (1987). Complement activation by anti-acetylcholine receptor monoclonal antibody in vivo correlates with potency of EAMG response in vivo. Ann N Y Acad Sci 505: 725–727.

Dwyer DS, Bradley RJ, Urquhart CK, et al. (1983). Naturally occurring anti-idiotypic antibodies in myasthenia gravis patients. Nature 301: 611–614.

Eddy S, Wim R, Peter VE, et al. (1999). Myasthenia gravis. Another autoimmune disease associated with hepatitis C virus infection. Dig Dis Sci 44: 186–189.

Ehlers M, Ravetch JV (2007). Opposing effects of Toll-like receptor stimulation induce autoimmunity or tolerance. Trends Immunol 28: 74–79.

Engel AG (1961). Thyroid function and myasthenia gravis. Arch Neurol 4: 95–106.

Engel AG (1992). Myasthenia gravis and myasthenic syndromes. In: PJ Vinken, GW Bruyn, HL Klawans (Eds.), Handbook of Clinical Neurology. Myopathies. Elsevier, Amsterdam, London, New York, Tokyo, pp. 391–455.

Engel AG, Arahata K (1987). The membrane attack complex of complement at the endplate in myasthenia gravis. Ann N Y Acad Sci 505: 326–332.

Engel AG, Tsujihata M, Lambert EH, et al. (1976a). Experimental autoimmune myasthenia gravis: a sequential and quantitative study of the neuromuscular junction ultrastructure and electrophysiologic correlations. J Neuropathol Exp Neurol 35: 569–587.

Engel AG, Tsujihata M, Lindstrom JM, et al. (1976b). The motor endplate in myasthenia gravis and in experimental autoimmune myasthenia gravis: a quantitative ultrastructural study. Ann N Y Acad Sci 274: 60–79.

Engel AG, Lindstrom JM, Lambert EH, et al. (1977a). Ultrastructural localization of the acetylcholine receptor in myasthenia gravis and in its experimental autoimmune model. Neurology 27: 307–315.

Engel AG, Lambert EH, Howard FM (1977b). Immune complexes (IgG and C3) at the motor end-plate in myasthenia gravis: ultrastructural and light microscopic localization and electrophysiologic correlations. Mayo Clin Proc 52: 267–280.

Engel AG, Sahashi K, Fumagalli G (1981). The immunopathology of acquired myasthenia gravis. Ann N Y Acad Sci 377: 158–174.

Evoli A, Tonali PA, Padua L, et al. (2003). Clinical correlates with anti-musk antibodies in generalized seronegative myasthenia gravis. Brain 126: 2304–2311.

Farrugia ME, Kennett RP, Newsom-Davis J, et al. (2006a). Single-fiber electromyography in limb and facial muscles in muscle-specific kinase antibody and acetylcholine receptor antibody myasthenia gravis. Muscle Nerve 33: 568–570.

Farrugia ME, Robson MD, Clover L, et al. (2006b). MRI and clinical studies of facial and bulbar muscle involvement in musk antibody-associated myasthenia gravis. Brain 129: 1481–1492.

Fattorossi A, Battaglia A, Buzzonetti A, et al. (2005). Circulating and thymic CD4 CD25 T regulatory cells in myasthenia gravis: effect of immunosuppressive treatment. Immunology 116: 134–141.

Fazekas A, Komoly S, Bozsik B, et al. (1986). Myasthenia gravis: demonstration of membrane attack complex in muscle end-plates. Clin Neuropathol 5: 78–83.

Feferman T, Maiti PK, Berrih-Aknin S, et al. (2005). Overexpression of IFN-induced protein 10 and its receptor CXCR3 in myasthenia gravis. J Immunol 174: 5324–5331.

Felix NJ, Donermeyer DL, Horvath S, et al. (2007). Alloreactive T cells respond specifically to multiple distinct peptide–MHC complexes. Nat Immunol 8: 388–397.

Feltkamp TE, van den Berg-Loonen PM, Nijenhuis LE, et al. (1974). Myasthenia gravis, autoantibodies, and HL-A antigens. Br Med J 1: 131–133.

Fernandez-Mestre MT, Vargas V, Montagnani S, et al. (2004). HLA class II and class I polymorphism in Venezuelan patients with myasthenia gravis. Hum Immunol 65: 54–59.

Flores KG, Li J, Sempowski GD, et al. (1999). Analysis of the human thymic perivascular space during aging. J Clin Invest 104: 1031–1039.

Frese A, Bethke F, Ludemann P, et al. (2000). Development of myasthenia gravis in a patient with multiple sclerosis during treatment with glatiramer acetate. J Neurol 247: 713.

Fritze D, Herrman CJR, Naeim F, et al. (1974). HL-A antigens in myasthenia gravis. Lancet 1: 240–242.

Fujii Y, Monden Y, Nakahara K, et al. (1984). Antibody to acetylcholine receptor in myasthenia gravis: production by lymphocytes from thymus or thymoma. Neurology 34: 1182–1186.

Fukui Y, Ishimoto T, Utsuyama M, et al. (1997). Positive and negative CD4+ thymocyte selection by a single MHC class II/peptide ligand affected by its expression level in the thymus. Immunity 6: 401–410.

Fumagalli G, Engel AG, Lindstrom J (1982a). Estimation of acetylcholine receptor degradation rate by external gamma counting in vivo. Mayo Clin Proc 57: 758–764.

Fumagalli G, Engel AG, Lindstrom J (1982b). Ultrastructural aspects of acetylcholine receptor turnover at the normal end-plate and in autoimmune myasthenia gravis. J Neuropathol Exp Neurol 41: 567–579.

Garchon HJ (2003). Genetics of autoimmune myasthenia gravis, a model for antibody-mediated autoimmunity in man. J Autoimmun 21: 105–110.

Garcia-Ramos G, Tellez-Zenteno JF, Zapata-Zuniga M, et al. (2003). HLA class II genotypes in Mexican Mestizo patients with myasthenia gravis. Eur J Neurol 10: 707–710.

Gattenloehner S, Vincent A, Leuschner I, et al. (1998). The fetal form of the acetylcholine receptor distinguishes rhabdomyosarcomas from other childhood tumors. Am J Pathol 152: 437–444.

Gautel M, Lakey A, Barlow DP, et al. (1993). Titin antibodies in myasthenia gravis: identification of a major immunogenic region of titin. Neurology 43: 1581–1585.

Genkins G, Mendelow H, Sobel HJ, et al. (1961). Myasthenia gravis: analysis of thirty-one consecutive post-mortem examinations. In: HR Viets, GW Bruyn, HL Klawans (Eds.), Myasthenia Gravis. Proceedings of the Second International Symposium. Charles C Thomas, Springfield, pp. 519–530.

Geuder KI, Marx A, Witzemann V, et al. (1992). Pathogenetic significance of fetal-type acetylcholine receptors on thymic myoid cells in myasthenia gravis. Dev Immunol 2: 69–75.

Gilhus HB, Aarli JA, Skogen OR (1992). Fulminant myasthenia gravis and polymyositis after thymectomy for thymoma. Acta Neurol Scand 85: 63–65.

Gilhus NE, Pandey JP, Gaarder PI, et al. (1990). Immunoglobulin allotypes in myasthenia gravis patients with a thymoma. J Autoimmun 3: 299–305.

Giraud M, Beaurain G, Yamamoto AM, et al. (2001). Linkage of HLA to myasthenia gravis and genetic heterogeneity depending on anti-titin antibodies. Neurology 57: 1555–1560.

Giraud M, Beaurain G, Eymard B, et al. (2004a). Genetic control of autoantibody expression in autoimmune myasthenia gravis: role of the self-antigen and of HLA-linked loci. Genes Immun 5: 398–404.

Giraud M, Eymard B, Tranchant C, et al. (2004b). Association of the gene encoding the delta-subunit of the muscle acetylcholine receptor (CHRND) with acquired autoimmune myasthenia gravis. Genes Immun 5: 80–83.

Giraud M, Taubert R, Vandiedonck C, et al. (2007). An IRF8-binding promoter variant and AIRE control CHRNA1 promiscuous expression in thymus. Nature 448: 934–937.

Goluszko E, Deng C, Poussin MA, et al. (2002). Tumor necrosis factor receptor p55 and p75 deficiency protects mice from developing experimental autoimmune myasthenia gravis. J Neuroimmunol 122: 85–93.

Gonzalez-Rey E, Chorny A, Delgado M (2007). Regulation of immune tolerance by anti-inflammatory neuropeptides. Nat Rev Immunol 7: 52–63.

Grau JM, Casademont J, Monforte R, et al. (1990). Myasthenia gravis after allogenic bone marrow transplantation: report of a case and pathogenic considerations. Bone Marrow Transplant 5: 435–437.

Guyon T, Wakkach A, Poea S, et al. (1998). Regulation of acetylcholine receptor gene expression in human myasthenia gravis muscles. Evidence for a compensatory mechanism triggered by receptor loss. J Clin Invest 102: 249–263.

Hanisch F, Eger K, Zierz S (2006). Musk-antibody positive pure ocular myasthenia gravis. J Neurol 253: 659–660.

Harcourt GC, Sommer N, Rothbard J, et al. (1988). A juxtamembrane epitope on the human acetylcholine receptor recognized by T cells in myasthenia gravis. J Clin Invest 82: 1295–1300.

Hawke S, Matsuo H, Nicolle M, et al. (1996). Autoimmune T cells in myasthenia gravis: heterogeneity and potential for specific immunotargeting. Immunol Today 17: 307–311.

Hawkins BR, Ip MS, Lam KS, et al. (1986). HLA antigens and acetylcholine receptor antibody in the subclassification of myasthenia gravis in Hong Kong Chinese. J Neurol Neurosurg Psychiatry 49: 316–319.

Hawkins BR, Yu YL, Wong V, et al. (1989). Possible evidence for a variant of myasthenia gravis based on HLA and acetylcholine receptor antibody in Chinese patients. Q J Med 70: 235–241.

Hawn TR, Wu H, Grossman JM, et al. (2005). A stop codon polymorphism of Toll-like receptor 5 is associated with resistance to systemic lupus erythematosus. Proc Nat Acad Sci USA 102: 10593–10597.

Heidenreich FR, Vincent A (1998). Antibodies to ion-channel proteins in thymoma with myasthenia, neuromyotonia, and peripheral neuropathy. Neurology 50: 1483–1485.

Hemmer B, Vergelli M, Pinilla C, et al. (1998). Probing degeneracy in T-cell recognition using peptide combinatorial libraries. Immunol Today 19: 163–168.

Hemminki K, Li X, Sundquist K (2006). Familial risks for diseases of myoneural junction and muscle in siblings based on hospitalizations and deaths in Sweden. Twin Res Hum Genet 9: 573–579.

Hill M, Moss P, Wordsworth P, et al. (1999a). T cell responses to D-penicillamine in drug-induced myasthenia gravis: recognition of modified DR1: peptide complexes. J Neuroimmunol 97: 146–153.

Hill M, Beeson D, Moss P, et al. (1999b). Early-onset myasthenia gravis: a recurring t-cell epitope in the adult-specific acetylcholine receptor epsilon subunit presented by the susceptibility allele HLA-DR52a. Ann Neurol 45: 224–231.

Hirabayashi H, Ohta M, Okumura M, et al. (2002). Appearance of thymoma 15 years after extended thymectomy for myasthenia gravis without thymoma. Eur J Cardiothorac Surg 22: 479–481.

Hoch W, McConville J, Helms S, et al. (2001). Auto-antibodies to the receptor tyrosine kinase musk in patients with myasthenia gravis without acetylcholine receptor antibodies. Nat Med 7: 365–368.

Hoedemaekers A, Graus Y, Beijleveld L, et al. (1997). Macrophage infiltration at the neuromuscular junction does not contribute to AChR loss and age-related resistance to EAMG. J Neuroimmunol 75: 147–155.

Hoff JM, Daltveit AK, Gilhus NE (2006). Arthrogryposis multiplex congenita—a rare fetal condition caused by maternal myasthenia gravis. Acta Neurol Scand 113(S 183): 26–27.

Hoffacker V, Schultz A, Tiesinga JJ, et al. (2000). Thymomas alter the t-cell subset composition in the blood: a potential mechanism for thymoma-associated autoimmune disease. Blood 96: 3872–3879.

Hogquist KA, Jameson SC, Bevan MJ (1994). The ligand for positive selection of T lymphocytes in the thymus. Curr Opin Immunol 6: 273–278.

Hohlfeld R (1997). Biotechnological agents for the immunotherapy of multiple sclerosis. Principles, problems and perspectives. Brain 120: 865–916.

Hohlfeld R, Engel AG (1990). Induction of HLA-DR expression on human myoblasts with interferon-γ. Am J Pathol 136: 503–508.

Hohlfeld R, Wekerle H (1999). The immunopathogenesis of myasthenia gravis. In: AG Engel (Ed.), Myasthenia Gravis and Myasthenic Disorders. Oxford University Press, Oxford, pp. 87–110.

Hohlfeld R, Toyka KV, Heininger K, et al. (1984). Autoimmune human t lymphocytes specific for acetylcholine receptor. Nature 319: 244–246.

Hohlfeld R, Toyka KV, Besinger UA, et al. (1985). Myasthenia gravis: reactivation of clinical disease and of autoimmune factors after discontinuation of long-term azathioprine. Ann Neurol 17: 238–242.

Hohlfeld R, Kalies I, Kohleisen B, et al. (1986). Myasthenia gravis: stimulation of antireceptor autoantibodies by autoreactive T cell lines. Neurology 36: 618–621.

Hohlfeld R, Toyka KV, Tzartos SJ, et al. (1987). Human T-helper lymphocytes in myasthenia gravis recognize the nicotinic receptor alpha subunit. Proc Nat Acad Sci USA 84: 5379–5383.

Hohlfeld R, Toyka KV, Miner LL, et al. (1988). Amphipathic segment of the nicotinic receptor alpha subunit contains epitopes recognized by T lymphocytes in myasthenia gravis. J Clin Invest 81: 657–660.

Horton RM, Manfredi AA, Conti-Tronconi EM (1993). The "embryonic" gamma subunit of the nicotinic acetylcholine receptor is expressed in adult extraocular muscle. Neurology 43: 983.

Huang D, Liu L, Noren K, et al. (1998a). Genetic association of CTLA-4 to myasthenia gravis with thymoma. J Neuroimmunol 88: 192–198.

Huang D, Pirskanen R, Hjelmstrom P, et al. (1998b). Polymorphisms in IL-1beta and IL-1 receptor antagonist genes are associated with myasthenia gravis. J Neuroimmunol 81: 76–81.

Huang D, Xia S, Zhou Y, et al. (1998c). No evidence for interleukin-4 gene conferring susceptibility to myasthenia gravis. J Neuroimmunol 92: 208–211.

Huang DR, Zhou YH, Xia SQ, et al. (1999a). Markers in the promoter region of interleukin-10 (IL-10) gene in myasthenia gravis: implications of diverse effects of IL-10 in the pathogenesis of the disease. J Neuroimmunol 94: 82–87.

Huang D, Zheng C, Giscombe R, et al. (1999b). Polymorphisms at −174 and in the 3′ flanking region of interleukin-6 (IL-6) gene in patients with myasthenia gravis. J Neuroimmunol 101: 197–200.

Huang D, Giscombe R, Zhou Y, et al. (2000). Dinucleotide repeat expansion in the CTLA-4 gene leads to T cell hyper-reactivity via the CD28 pathway in myasthenia gravis. J Neuroimmunol 105: 69–77.

Hughes BW, Moro De Casillas ML, Kaminski HJ (2004). Pathophysiology of myasthenia gravis. Semin Neurol 24: 21–30.

Hughes BW, Kusner LL, Kaminski HJ (2006). Molecular architecture of the neuromuscular junction. Muscle Nerve 33: 445–461.

Hyttinen V, Kaprio J, Kinnunen L, et al. (2003). Genetic liability of type 1 diabetes and the onset age among 22,650 young Finnish twin pairs: a nationwide follow-up study. Diabetes 52: 1052–1055.

Im SH, Barchan D, Maiti PK, et al. (2001a). Blockade of CD40 ligand suppresses chronic experimental myasthenia gravis by down-regulation of Th1 differentiation and up-regulation of CTLA-4. J Immunol 166: 6893–6898.

Im SH, Barchan D, Maiti PK, et al. (2001b). Suppression of experimental myasthenia gravis, a B cell-mediated autoimmune disease, by blockade of IL-18. FASEB J 15: 2140–2148.

Inoue M, Marx A, Zettl A, et al. (2002). Chromosome 6 suffers frequent and multiple aberrations in thymoma. Am J Pathol 161: 1507–1513.

Inoue M, Starostik P, Zettl A, et al. (2003). Correlating genetic aberrations with World Health Organization-defined histology and stage across the spectrum of thymomas. Cancer Res 63: 3708–3715.

Ito Y, Kanda N, Mitsui H, et al. (1999). Cutaneous manifestations of Sjogren's syndrome associated with myasthenia gravis. Br J Dermatol 141: 362–363.

Izumi Y, Kinoshita I, Kita Y, et al. (2002). Myasthenia gravis with diffuse alopecia areata and pemphigus foliaceous. J Neurol 249: 1455–1456.

Jacobsen M, Schweer D, Ziegler A, et al. (2000). A point mutation in PTPRC is associated with the development of multiple sclerosis. Nat Genet 26: 495–499.

Jambou F, Cohen-Kaminsky S (2003). Immunoregulation by Vβ specific antibodies in myasthenia gravis: mining physiological T cell homeostasis for TCR specific therapy. Cell Mol Biol (Noisy-le-grand) 49: 181–192.

Jambou F, Zhang W, Menestrier M, et al. (2003). Circulating regulatory anti-T cell receptor antibodies in patients with myasthenia gravis. J Clin Invest 112: 265–274.

Janeway CA, Travers P, Walport M, et al. (2005). Immunobiology. 6th ed. Garland Science, New York, London.

Jermy A, Beeson D, Vincent A (1993). Pathogenic autoimmunity to affinity-purified mouse acetylcholine receptor induced without adjuvant in BALB/c mice. Eur J Immunol 23: 973–976.

Jerne NK (1985). The generative grammar of the immune system. EMBO J 4: 847–852.

Jha S, Xu K, Maruta T, et al. (2006). Myasthenia gravis induced in mice by immunization with the recombinant extracellular domain of rat muscle-specific kinase (MuSK). J Neuroimmunol 175: 107–117.

Jiang W, Anderson MS, Bronson R, et al. (2005). Modifier loci condition autoimmunity provoked by AIRE deficiency. J Exp Med 202: 805–815.

Kaminski HJ, Ruff RL (1997). Ocular muscle involvement by myasthenia gravis. Ann Neurol 41: 419–420.

Kaminski HJ, Kusner LL, Block CH (1996). Expression of acetylcholine receptor isoforms at extraocular muscle endplates. Invest Ophthalmol Vis Sci 37: 345–351.

Kao I, Drachman DB (1977). Thymic muscle cells bear acetylcholine receptors: possible relation to myasthenia gravis. Science 195: 74–75.

Kaul R, Shenoy M, Goluszko E, et al. (1994). Major histocompatibility complex class II gene disruption prevents experimental autoimmune myasthenia gravis. J Immunol 152: 3152–3157.

Kerzin-Storrar L, Metcalfe RA, Dyer PA, et al. (1988). Genetic factors in myasthenia gravis: a family study. Neurology 38: 38–42.

Kiechl S, Kohlendorfer U, Willeit J, et al. (1996). Myasthenia gravis and primary biliary cirrhosis. Acta Neurol Scand 93: 263–265.

Kimura K, Nezu A, Kimura S, et al. (1998). A case of myasthenia gravis in childhood associated with chronic inflammatory demyelinating polyradiculoneuropathy. Neuropediatrics 29: 108–112.

Kirchner T, Schalke B, Melms A, et al. (1986). Immunohistological patterns of non-neoplastic changes in the thymus in myasthenia gravis. Virchows Arch B Cell Pathol Incl Mol Pathol 52: 237–257.

Kirchner T, Hoppe F, Schalke B, et al. (1988). Microenvironment of thymic myoid cells in myasthenia gravis. Virchows Arch B Cell Pathol Incl Mol Pathol 54: 295–302.

Kirchner T, Schalke B, Buchwald J, et al. (1992). Well-differentiated thymic carcinoma. An organotypical low-grade carcinoma with relationship to cortical thymoma. Am J Surg Pathol 16: 1153–1169.

Köhler G, Milstein C (1975). Continuous cultures of fused cells secreting antibody of predefined specificity. Nature 256: 495–497.

Kohno T, Tsuji T, Hirayama K, et al. (2005). A novel immunomodulator, FTY720, prevents development of experimental autoimmune myasthenia gravis in C57BL/6 mice. Biol Pharm Bull 28: 736–739.

Kolte L, Dreves AM, Ersboll AK, et al. (2002). Association between larger thymic size and higher thymic output in human immunodeficiency virus-infected patients receiving highly active antiretroviral therapy. J Infect Dis 185: 1578–1585.

Komal Kumar RN, Patil SA, Taly AB, et al. (2004). Effect of D-penicillamine on neuromuscular junction in patients with Wilson disease. Neurology 63: 935–936.

Kornstein MJ, Asher O, Fuchs S (1995). Acetylcholine receptor α-subunit and myogenin mRNAs in thymus and thymomas. Am J Pathol 146: 1320–1324.

Krolick KA, Urso OE (1987). Analysis of helper-T-cell function by acetylcholine receptor–reactive cell lines of defined AChR-subunit specificity. Cell Immunol 105: 75–85.

Kuks JB, Skallebaek D (1998). Plasmapheresis in myasthenia gravis. A survey. Transfus Sci 19: 129–136.

Lambert EH, Lindstrom JM, Lennon VA (1976). End-plate potentials in experimental autoimmune myasthenia gravis. Ann N Y Acad Sci 274: 300–318.

Lanzavecchia A (1990). Receptor-mediated antigen uptake and its effects on antigen presentation to class II-restricted T lymphocytes. Ann Rev Immunol 8: 773–794.

Lanzavecchia A, Sallusto F (2007). Toll-like receptors and innate immunity in B-cell activation and antibody responses. Curr Opin Immunol 19: 268–274.

Laufer TM, Fan L, Glimcher LH (1999). Self-reactive T cells selected on thymic cortical epithelium are polyclonal and are pathogenic in vivo. J Immunol 162: 5078–5084.

Lefvert A (1982). Differences in the interaction of acetylcholine receptor antibodies with receptor from normal, denervated and myasthenic human muscle. J Neurol Neurosurg Psychiatry 45: 70–73.

Lefvert AK, Björkholm M (1987). Antibodies against the acetylcholine receptor in hematologic disorders: implications for the development of myasthenia gravis after bone marrow grafting. N Engl J Med 317: 170.

Lefvert A, Bergstrom K, Matell G, et al. (1978). Determination of acetylcholine receptor antibody in myasthenia gravis: clinical usefulness and pathogenic implications. J Neurol Neurosurg Psychiatry 41: 394–403.

Lennon VA (1982). Myasthenia gravis: diagnosis by assay of serum antibodies. Mayo Clin Proc 57: 723–724.

Lennon VA, Lindstrom JM, Seybold ME (1975). Experimental autoimmune myasthenia gravis in rats and guinea pigs. J Exp Med 141: 1365–1375.

Lennon VA, Lindstrom JM, Seybold M (1976). Experimental autoimmune myasthenia gravis: cellular and humoral immune responses. Ann N Y Acad Sci 274: 283–299.

Lennon VA, Seybold ME, Lindstrom JM, et al. (1978). Role of complement in the pathogenesis of experimental autoimmune myasthenia gravis. J Exp Med 147: 973–983.

Levy YA, Afek Y, Sherer Y, et al. (1998). Malignant thymoma associated with autoimmune diseases: a retrospective study and review of the literature. Semin Arthritis Rheum 28: 73–79.

Ligers A, Teleshova N, Masterman T, et al. (2001). CTLA-4 gene expression is influenced by promoter and exon 1 polymorphisms. Genes Immun 2: 145–152.

Limburg PC, The TH, Hummel-Tappel E, et al. (1983). Anti-acetylcholine receptor antibodies in myasthenia gravis. Part 1: relation to clinical parameters in 250 patients. J Neurol Sci 58: 357–370.

Lindstrom J (2004). Is "seronegative" MG explained by autoantibodies to MuSK? Neurology 62: 1920–1921.

Lindstrom J, Lambert EH (1978). Content of acetylcholine receptor and antibodies bound to receptor in myasthenia gravis, experimental autoimmune myasthenia gravis, and Eaton–Lambert syndrome. Neurology 28: 130–138.

Lindstrom JM, Seybold ME, Lennon VA, et al. (1976a). Antibody to acetylcholine receptor in myasthenia gravis. Prevalence, clinical correlates, and diagnostic value. Neurology 26: 1054–1059.

Lindstrom JM, Einarson BL, Lennon VA, et al. (1976b). Pathological mechanisms in experimental autoimmune myasthenia gravis. I. Immunogenicity of syngeneic muscle acetylcholine receptor and quantitative extraction of receptor and antibody–receptor complexes from muscles of rats with experimental autoimmune myasthenia gravis. J Exp Med 144: 726–738.

Lindstrom JM, Engel AG, Seybold ME, et al. (1976c). Pathological mechanisms in experimental autoimmune myasthenia gravis. II. Passive transfer of experimental autoimmune myasthenia gravis in rats with anti-acetylcholine receptor antibodies. J Exp Med 144: 739–753.

Liston A, Lesage S, Wilson J, et al. (2003). AIRE regulates negative selection of organ-specific T cells. Nat Immunol 4: 350–354.

Liu R, La Cava A, Bai XF, et al. (2005). Cooperation of invariant NKT cells and CD4+CD25+ T regulatory cells in the prevention of autoimmune myasthenia. J Immunol 175: 7898–7904.

Liu R, Van Kaer L, La Cava A, et al. (2006). Autoreactive T cells mediate NK cell degeneration in autoimmune disease. J Immunol 176: 5247–5254.

Liyanage Y, Hoch W, Beeson D, et al. (2002). The agrin/muscle-specific kinase pathway: new targets for autoimmune and genetic disorders at the neuromuscular junction. Muscle Nerve 25: 4–16.

Lodoen MB, Lanier LL (2006). Natural killer cells as an initial defense against pathogens. Curr Opin Immunol 18: 391–398.

Lohr J, Knoechel B, Wang JJ, et al. (2006). Role of IL-17 and regulatory T lymphocytes in a systemic autoimmune disease. J Exp Med 203: 2785–2791.

Losen M, Stassen MH, Martinez-Martinez P, et al. (2005). Increased expression of rapsyn in muscles prevents acetylcholine receptor loss in experimental autoimmune myasthenia gravis. Brain 128: 2327–2337.

Lossos A, River Y, Eliakim A, et al. (1995). Neurologic aspects of inflammatory bowel disease. Neurology 45: 416–421.

Luther C, Poeschel S, Varga M, et al. (2005). Decreased frequency of intrathymic regulatory T cells in patients with myasthenia-associated thymoma. J Neuroimmunol 164: 124–128.

Machens A, Loliger C, Pichlmeier U, et al. (1999). Correlation of thymic pathology with HLA in myasthenia gravis. Clin Immunol 91: 296–301.

Mackay F, Silveira PA, Brink R (2007). B cells and the BAFF/APRIL axis: fast-forward on autoimmunity and signaling. Curr Opin Immunol 19: 327–336.

MacLennan C, Beeson D, Buijs AM, et al. (1997). Acetylcholine receptor expression in human extraocular muscles and their susceptibility to myasthenia gravis. Ann Neurol 41: 423–431.

Maiti PK, Feferman T, Im SH, et al. (2004). Immunosuppression of rat myasthenia gravis by oral administration of a syngeneic acetylcholine receptor fragment. J Neuroimmunol 152: 112–120.

Manz RA, Hauser AE, Hiepe F, et al. (2005). Maintenance of serum antibody levels. Ann Rev Immunol 23: 367–386.

Markert ML, Alexieff MJ, Li J, et al. (2004). Postnatal thymus transplantation with immunosuppression as treatment for Digeorge syndrome. Blood 104: 2574–2581.

Marx A, Müller-Hermelink HK (1999). From basic immunobiology to the upcoming WHO-classification of tumors of the thymus. The Second Conference on Biological and Clinical Aspects of Thymic Epithelial Tumors and Related Recent Developments. Pathol Res Pract 195: 515–533.

Marx A, Kirchner T, Greiner A, et al. (1992). Neurofilament epitopes in thymoma and antiaxonal autoantibodies in myasthenia gravis. Lancet 339: 707–708.

Marx A, Schultz A, Wilisch A, et al. (1996). Myasthenia gravis. Verh Dtsch Ges Pathol 80: 116–126.

Marx A, Wilisch A, Schultz A, et al. (1997). Pathogenesis of myasthenia gravis. Virchows Arch 430: 355–364.

Marx A, Schultz A, Wilisch A, et al. (1998). Paraneoplastic autoimmunity in thymus tumors. Dev Immunol 6: 129–140.

Marx A, Müller-Hermelink HK, Ströbel P (2003). The role of thymomas in the development of myasthenia gravis. Ann N Y Acad Sci 998: 223–236.

Mason D (1998). A very high level of crossreactivity is an essential feature of the T-cell receptor. Immunol Today 19: 395–404.

Masters CL, Dawkins RL, Zilko PJ, et al. (1977). Penicillamine-associated myasthenia gravis, antiacetylcholine receptor and antistriational antibodies. Am J Med 63: 689–694.

Masunaga A, Arai T, Yoshitake T, et al. (1994). Reduced expression of apoptosis-related antigens in thymuses from patients with myasthenia gravis. Immunol Lett 39: 169–172.

Mathis D, Benoist C (2007). A decade of AIRE. Nat Rev Immunol 7: 645–650.

Matsuki K, Juji T, Tokunaga K, et al. (1990). HLA antigens in Japanese patients with myasthenia gravis. J Clin Invest 86: 392–399.

Matsumoto MY, Matsuo H, Oka T, et al. (2004). Thymic myoid cells as a myasthenogenic antigen and antigen-presenting cells. J Neuroimmunol 150: 80–87.

Matsumoto MY, Matsuo H, Sakuma H, et al. (2006). CDR3 spectratyping analysis of the TCR repertoire in myasthenia gravis. J Immunol 176: 5100–5107.

Matthews I, Sims G, Ledwidge S, et al. (2002). Antibodies to acetylcholine receptor in parous women with myasthenia: evidence for immunization by fetal antigen. Lab Invest 82: 1407–1417.

McConville J, Farrugia ME, Beeson D, et al. (2004). Detection and characterization of musk antibodies in seronegative myasthenia gravis. Ann Neurol 55: 580–584.

Meager A, Vincent A, Newsom-Davis J, et al. (1997). Spontaneous neutralising antibodies to interferon-α and interleukin-12 in thymoma-associated autoimmune disease. Lancet 350: 1596–1597.

Meager A, Wadhwa M, Dilger P, et al. (2003). Anti-cytokine autoantibodies in autoimmunity: preponderance of neutralizing autoantibodies against interferon-α, interferon-ω and interleukin-12 in patients with thymoma and/or myasthenia gravis. Clin Exp Immunol 132: 128–136.

Medzhitov R, Janeway CA (2000). Innate immunity. N Engl J Med 343: 338–344.

Meinl E, Klinkert WE, Wekerle H (1991). The thymus in myasthenia gravis. Changes typical for the human disease are absent in experimental autoimmune myasthenia gravis of the Lewis rat. Am J Pathol 139: 995–1008.

Melms A, Schalke BC, Kirchner T, et al. (1988). Thymus in myasthenia gravis. Isolation of T-lymphocyte lines specific for the nicotinic acetylcholine receptor from thymuses of myasthenic patients. J Clin Invest 81: 902–908.

Melms A, Malcherek G, Gern U, et al. (1992a). T cells from normal and myasthenic individuals recognize the human acetylcholine receptor: heterogeneity of antigenic sites on the α-subunit. Ann Neurol 31: 311–318.

Melms A, Faul C, Sommer N, et al. (1992b). Myasthenia gravis after BMT: identification of patients at risk? Bone Marrow Transplant 9: 78–79.

Mendelow H (1958). II. Pathology. In: KE Osserman (Ed.), Myasthenia Gravis. Grune and Stratton, New York, pp. 10–43.

Meraouna A, Cizeron-Clairac G, Panse RL, et al. (2006). The chemokine CXCL13 is a key molecule in autoimmune myasthenia gravis. Blood 108: 432–440.

Merlie JP, Heinemann S, Einarson B, et al. (1979). Degradation of acetylcholine receptor in diaphragms of rats with experimental autoimmune myasthenia gravis. J Biol Chem 254: 6328–6332.

Middleton G, Schoch EM (2000). The prevalence of human thymic lymphoid follicles is lower in suicides. Virchows Arch 436: 127–130.

Mier AK, Havard CW (1985). Diaphragmatic myasthenia in mother and child. Postgrad Med J 61: 725–727.

Milani M, Ostlie N, Wang W, et al. (2003). T cells and cytokines in the pathogenesis of acquired myasthenia gravis. Ann N Y Acad Sci 998: 284–307.

Milani M, Ostlie N, Wu H, et al. (2006). CD4+ T and B cells cooperate in the immunoregulation of experimental autoimmune myasthenia gravis. J Neuroimmunol 179: 152–162.

Miller JF (1961). Immunological function of the thymus. Lancet 2: 748–749.

Miller JF (2001). Ruby anniversary: forty years of thymus immunology research. Nat Immunol 2: 663–664.

Mishina M, Takai T, Imoto K, et al. (1986). Molecular distinction between fetal and adult forms of muscle acetylcholine receptor. Nature 321: 406–411.

Mittag T, Massa T, Kornfeld P (1981). Multiple forms of antiacetylcholine receptor antibody in myasthenia gravis. Muscle Nerve 4: 16–25.

Moiola L, Karachunski P, Protti MP, et al. (1994). Epitopes on the β subunit of human muscle acetylcholine receptor recognized by CD4+ cells of myasthenia gravis patients and healthy subjects. J Clin Invest 93: 1020–1028.

Moiola L, Galbiati F, Martino G, et al. (1998). IL-12 is involved in the induction of experimental autoimmune myasthenia gravis, an antibody-mediated disease. Eur J Immunol 28: 2487–2497.

Morgutti M, Conti-Tronconi BM, Sghirlanzoni A, et al. (1979). Cellular immune response to acetylcholine receptor in myasthenia gravis. II. Thymectomy and corticosteroids. Neurology 29: 734–738.

Mosmann TR, Coffman RL (1989). TH1 and TH2 cells: different patterns of lymphokine secretion lead to different functional properties. Ann Rev Immunol 7: 145–173.

Mossmann S, Vincent A, Newsom-Davis J (1986). Myasthenia gravis without acetylcholine-receptor antibody: a distinct disease entity. Lancet 1: 116–119.

Moulian N, Bidault J, Planche C, et al. (1998). Two signaling pathways can increase fas expression in human thymocytes. Blood 92: 1297–1307.

Müller-Hermelink HK, Marx A (1999). Pathological aspects of malignant and benign thymic disorders. Ann Med 31(S2): 5–14.

Müller-Hermelink HK, Marx A (2000). Thymoma. Curr Opin Oncol 12: 426–433.

Müller-Hermelink HK, Marx A, Marx KT (1996). Thymus. In: LJ Damjanov I (Ed.), Anderson's Pathology. Mosby, St. Louis, pp. 1218–1243.

Murakami M, Hosoi Y, Negishi T, et al. (1996). Thymic hyperplasia in patients with Graves' disease. Identification of thyrotropin receptors in human thymus. J Clin Invest 98: 2228–2234.

Murphy J, Murphy SF (1986). Myasthenia gravis in identical twins. Neurology 36: 78–80.

Nagane Y, Utsugisawa K, Akutsu H, et al. (2005). Perivascular infiltrate of memory lymphocytes and mature dendritic cells in MG thymomas. Neurology 65: 770–772.

Nagvekar N, Moody AM, Moss P, et al. (1998a). A pathogenetic role for the thymoma in myasthenia gravis. Autosensitization of IL-4-producing T cell clones recognizing extracellular acetylcholine receptor epitopes presented by minority class II isotypes. J Clin Invest 101: 2268–2277.

Nagvekar N, Jacobson LW, Willcox N, et al. (1998b). Epitopes expressed in myasthenia gravis (MG) thymomas are not recognized by patients' T cells or autoantibodies. Clin Exp Immunol 112: 17–20.

Nakano S, Engel AG (1993). Myasthenia gravis: quantitative immunocytochemical analysis of inflammatory cells and detection of complement membrane attack complex at the end-plate in 30 patients. Neurology 43: 1167–1172.

Nakao Y, Matsumoto H, Miyazaki T, et al. (1980). Gm allotypes in myasthenia gravis. Lancet 1: 677–680.

Namba T, Brunner NG, Brown SB, et al. (1971). Familial myasthenia gravis. Report of 27 patients in 12 families and review of 164 patients in 73 families. Arch Neurol 25: 49–60.

Namba T, Brunner NG, Grob D (1974). Idiopathic giant cell polymyositis. Archives of Neurology 31: 27–30.

Nath A, Kerman RH, Novak IS, et al. (1990). Immune studies in human immunodeficiency virus infection with myasthenia gravis: a case report. Neurology 40: 581–583.

Navaneetham D, Penn AS, Howard JF Jr, et al. (2001). Human thymuses express incomplete sets of muscle acetylcholine receptor subunit transcripts that seldom include the δ subunit. Muscle Nerve 24: 203–210.

Nenninger R, Schultz A, Hoffacker V, et al. (1998). Abnormal thymocyte development and generation of autoreactive T cells in mixed and cortical thymomas. Lab Invest 78: 743–753.

Neufert C, Becker C, Wirtz S, et al. (2007). IL-27 controls the development of inducible regulatory T cells and Th17 cells via differential effects on STAT1. Eur J Immunol 37: 1809–1816.

Newsom-Davis J, Willcox N, Schluep M, et al. (1987). Immunological heterogeneity and cellular mechanisms in myasthenia gravis. Ann N Y Acad Sci 505: 12–26.

Newsom-Davis J, Leys K, Vincent A, et al. (1991). Immunological evidence for the co-existence of the Lambert–Eaton myasthenic syndrome and myasthenia gravis in two patients. J Neurol Neurosurg Psychiatry 54: 452–453.

Newsom-Davis J, Buckley C, Clover L, et al. (2003). Autoimmune disorders of neuronal potassium channels. Ann N Y Acad Sci 998: 202–210.

Nicolle MW (1999). Pseudo-myasthenia gravis and thymic hyperplasia in Graves' disease. Can J Neurol Sci 26: 201–203.

Nieto IP, Robledo JP, Pajuelo MC, et al. (1999). Prognostic factors for myasthenia gravis treated by thymectomy: review of 61 cases. Ann Thorac Surg 67: 1568–1571.

Niks EH, Kuks JB, Roep BO, et al. (2006). Strong association of musk antibody-positive myasthenia gravis and hla-dr 14-dq5. Neurology 66: 1772–1774.

Niks EH, Kuks JBM, Verschuuren JJGM (2007). Epidemiology of myasthenia gravis with anti-musk antibodies in the Netherlands. J Neurol Neurosurg Psychiatry 78: 417–418.

Noda M, Takahashi H, Tanabe T, et al. (1983). Structural homology of Torpedo californica acetylcholine receptor subunits. Nature 302: 528–532.

Oda K, Goto I, Kuriowa Y, et al. (1980). Myasthenia gravis: antibodies to acetylcholine receptor with human and rat antigens. Neurology 30: 543–546.

Ohta K, Shigemoto K, Kubo S, et al. (2004). MuSK antibodies in AChR ab-seropositive MG vs. AChR ab-seronegative MG. Neurology 62: 2132–2133.

Olmos P, A'Hern R, Heaton DA, et al. (1988). The significance of the concordance rate for type 1 (insulin-dependent) diabetes in identical twins. Diabetologia 31: 747–750.

Onodera J, Nakamura S, Nagano I, et al. (1996). Upregulation of Bcl-2 protein in the myasthenic thymus. Ann Neurol 39: 521–528.

Oosterhuis HJGH, Limburg PC, Hummel-Tappel E, et al. (1983). Anti-acetylcholine receptor antibodies in myasthenia gravis. Part 2. Clinical and serological follow-up of individual patients. J Neurol Sci 58: 371–385.

Oshima M, Ashizawa T, Pollack MS, et al. (1990). Autoimmune T cell recognition of human acetylcholine receptor: the sites of T cell recognition in myasthenia gravis on the extracellular part of the alpha subunit. Eur J Immunol 20: 2563–2569.

Oshima M, Ohtani M, Deitiker PR, et al. (2005a). Suppression by mAbs against DQB1 peptides of in vitro proliferation of AChR-specific T cells from myasthenia gravis patients. Autoimmunity 38: 161–169.

Oshima M, Deitiker PR, Mosier DR, et al. (2005b). Responses in vitro of peripheral blood lymphocytes from patients with myasthenia gravis to stimulation with human acetylcholine receptor α-chain peptides: analysis in relation to age, thymic abnormality, and ethnicity. Hum Immunol 66: 32–42.

Oshima M, Maruta T, Ohtani M, et al. (2006). Vaccination with a MHC class II peptide in alum and inactive pertussis strongly ameliorates clinical MG in C57BL/6 mice. J Neuroimmunol 171: 8–16.

Osserman KE, Tsairis P, Weiner LB (1967). Myasthenia gravis and thyroid disease: clinical and immunological correlation. J Mt Sinai Hosp NY 34: 469–481.

Ostlie N, Milani M, Wang W, et al. (2003). Absence of IL-4 facilitates the development of chronic autoimmune myasthenia gravis in C57BL/6 mice. J Immunol 170: 604–612.

Pachner AR (1989). Anti-acetylcholine receptor antibodies block bungarotoxin binding to native human acetylcholine receptor on the surface of te671 cells. Neurology 39: 1057–1061.

Padua L, Tonali P, Aprile I, et al. (2006). Seronegative myasthenia gravis: comparison of neurophysiological picture in MuSK+ and MuSK– patients. Eur J Neurol 13: 273–276.

Palmieri G, Selleri C, Montella L, et al. (2006). Thymoma followed by paroxysmal nocturnal hemoglobinuria: a unique clinical association in the context of multiorgan autoimmunity with a potential role for CD8+ T lymphocytes. Am J Hematol 81: 774–778.

Parkin J, Cohen B (2001). An overview of the immune system. Lancet 357: 1777–1789.

Pasaoglu I, Dogan R, Topcu M, et al. (1994). Multicentric angiofollicular lymph node hyperplasia associated with myasthenia gravis. Thorac Cardiovasc Surg 42: 253–256.

Pascuzzi RM, Campa JF (1988). Lymphorrhage localized to the muscle end-plate in myasthenia gravis. Arch Pathol Lab Med 112: 934–937.

Pascuzzi RM, Roos KL, Phillips LH (1986). Granulomatous inflammatory myopathy associated with myasthenia gravis. A case report and review of the literature. Arch Neurol 43: 621–623.

Patrick J, Lindström J (1973). Autoimmune response to acetylcholine receptor. Science 25: 871–872.

Penn AS, Low BW, Jaffe IA, et al. (1998). Drug-induced autoimmune myasthenia gravis. Ann N Y Acad Sci 841: 433–449.

Phillips LH, Torner JC (1996). Epidemiologic evidence for a changing natural history of myasthenia gravis. Neurology 47: 1233–1238.

Piddlesden SJ, Jiang S, Levin JL, et al. (1996). Soluble complement receptor 1 (sCR1) protects against experimental autoimmune myasthenia gravis. J Neuroimmunol 71: 173–177.

Pinching AJ, Peters DK, Newsom-Davis J (1977). Plasma exchange in myasthenia gravis. Lancet 1: 428–429.

Pirskanen R (1976). Genetic associations between myasthenia gravis and the HL-A system. J Neurol Neurosurg Psychiatry 39: 23–33.

Pirskanen R (1977). Genetic aspects in myasthenia gravis. A family study of 264 Finnish patients. Acta Neurol Scand 56: 365–388.

Plested P, Tang T, Spreadbury I, et al. (2002). AChr phosphorylation and indirect inhibition of AChR function in seronegative MG. Neurology 59: 1682–1688.

Poea-Guyon S, Christadoss P, Le Panse R, et al. (2005). Effects of cytokines on acetylcholine receptor expression: implications for myasthenia gravis. J Immunol 174: 5941–5949.

Poussin MA, Goluszko E, Franco JU, et al. (2002). Role of IL-5 during primary and secondary immune response to acetylcholine receptor. J Neuroimmunol 125: 51–58.

Poussin MA, Tuzun E, Goluszko E, et al. (2003). B7–1 costimulatory molecule is critical for the development of experimental autoimmune myasthenia gravis. J Immunol 170: 4389–4396.

Price P, Witt C, Allcock R, et al. (1999). The genetic basis for the association of the 8.1 ancestral haplotype (A1, B8, DR3) with multiple immunopathological diseases. Immunol Rev 167: 257–274.

Protti MP, Manfredi AA, Howard JF Jr, et al. (1991). T cells in myasthenia gravis specific for embryonic acetylcholine receptor. Neurology 41: 1809–1814.

Provenzano C, Arancio O, Evoli A, et al. (1988). Familial autoimmune myasthenia gravis with different pathogenetic antibodies. J Neurol Neurosurg Psychiatry 51: 1228–1230.

Ragheb S, Mohamed M, Lisak RP (2005). Myasthenia gravis patients, but not healthy subjects, recognize epitopes that are unique to the ε-subunit of the acetylcholine receptor. J Neuroimmunol 159: 137–145.

Raju R, Spack EG, David CS (2001). Acetylcholine receptor peptide recognition in HLA DR3-transgenic mice: in vivo responses correlate with MHC–peptide binding. J Immunol 167: 1118–1124.

Rasheed AU, Rahn HP, Sallusto F, et al. (2006). Follicular B helper T cell activity is confined to CXCR5(hi)ICOS(hi) CD4 T cells and is independent of CD57 expression. Eur J Immunol 36: 1892–1903.

Riemersma S, Vincent A, Beeson D, et al. (1996). Association of arthrogryposis multiplex congenita with maternal antibodies inhibiting fetal acetylcholine receptor function. J Clin Invest 98: 2358–2363.

Robey E, Fowlkes BJ (1994). Selective events in t cell development. Ann Rev Immunol 12: 675–705.

Romagnani S (2006). Regulation of the T cell response. Clin Exp Allergy 36: 1357–1366.

Romi F, Skeie GO, Gilhus NE, et al. (2005). Striational antibodies in myasthenia gravis: reactivity and possible clinical significance. Arch Neurol 62: 442–446.

Rosai J (1999). Histological Typing of Tumours of the Thymus. Springer-Verlag, Berlin, Heidelberg.

Rostedt Punga A, Ahlqvist K, Bartoccioni E, et al. (2006a). Neurophysiological and mitochondrial abnormalities in musk antibody seropositive myasthenia gravis compared to other immunological subtypes. Clin Neurophysiol 117: 1434–1443.

Rostedt Punga A, Flink R, Askmark H, et al. (2006b). Cholinergic neuromuscular hyperactivity in patients with myasthenia gravis seropositive for musk antibody. Muscle Nerve 34: 111–115.

Rowen L, Koop BF, Hood L (1996). The complete 685-kilobase DNA sequence of the human β T cell receptor locus. Science 272: 1755–1762.

Rowland LP, Hoefer PF, Aranow H Jr, et al. (1956). Fatalities in myasthenia gravis. A review of 39 cases with 26 autopsy reports. Neurology 6: 307–326.

Roxanis I, Micklem K, McConville J, et al. (2002). Thymic myoid cells and germinal center formation in myasthenia gravis: possible roles in pathogenesis. J Neuroimmunol 125: 185–197.

Sahashi K, Engel AG, Lambert EH, et al. (1980). Ultrastructural localization of the terminal and lytic ninth complement component (c9) at the motor end-plate in myasthenia gravis. J Neuropathol Exp Neurol 39: 160–172.

Saito R, Onodera H, Tago H, et al. (2005). Altered expression of chemokine receptor CXCR5 on T cells of myasthenia gravis patients. J Neuroimmunol 170: 172–178.

Saka E, Topcuoglu MA, Akkaya B, et al. (2005). Thymus changes in anti-MuSK-positive and -negative myasthenia gravis. Neurology 65: 782–783.

Salmon AM, Bruand C, Cardona A, et al. (1998). An acetylcholine receptor alpha subunit promoter confers intrathymic expression in transgenic mice. Implications for tolerance of a transgenic self-antigen and for autoreactivity in myasthenia gravis. J Clin Invest 101: 2340–2350.

Salvetti M, Jung S, Chang SF, et al. (1991). Acetylcholine receptor-specific T-lymphocyte clones in the normal human immune repertoire: target epitopes, HLA restriction, and membrane phenotypes. Ann Neurol 29: 508–516.

Sato T, Tamaoki N (1989). Myoid cells in the human thymus and thymoma revealed by three different immunohistochemical markers for striated muscle. Acta Pathol Jpn 39: 509–519.

Scadding GK, Vincent A, Newsom-Davis J, et al. (1981). Acetylcholine receptor antibody synthesis by thymic lymphocytes: correlation with thymic histology. Neurology 31: 935–943.

Scarpino S, Di Napoli A, Stoppacciaro A, et al. (2007). Expression of autoimmune regulator gene (AIRE) and T regulatory cells in human thymomas. Clin Exp Immunol 149: 504–512.

Schluep M, Willcox N, Vincent A, et al. (1987). Acetylcholine receptors in human thymic myoid cells in situ: an immunohistological study. Ann Neurol 22: 212–222.

Schluep M, Willcox N, Ritter MA, et al. (1988). Myasthenia gravis thymus: clinical, histological and culture correlations. J Autoimmun 1: 445–467.

Schönbeck S, Padberg F, Hohlfeld R, et al. (1992). Transplantation of thymic autoimmune microenvironment to severe combined immunodeficiency mice. A new model of myasthenia gravis. J Clin Invest 90: 245–250.

Schultz A, Hoffacker V, Wilisch A, et al. (1999). Neurofilament is an autoantigenic determinant in myasthenia gravis. Ann Neurol 46: 167–175.

Schumacher E, Roth W (1912). Thymektomie bei einem fall von morbus basedowi mit myasthenie. Mitt Grenzgeb Med Chir 25: 746–765.

Schumm F, Fateh-Moghadam A, Dichgans J (1984). Correlation between serum-anti-acetylcholine receptor antibody levels and clinical state under immunosuppressive therapy in myasthenia gravis. Eur Arch Psychiatry Neurol Sci 234: 224–230.

Schumm F, Wiethölter H, Fateh-Moghadam A, et al. (1985). Thymectomy in myasthenia with pure ocular symptoms. J Neurol Neurosurg Psychiatry 48: 332–337.

Sciamanna MA, Griesmann GE, Williams CL, et al. (1997). Nicotinic acetylcholine receptors of muscle and neuronal (alpha7) types coexpressed in a small cell lung carcinoma. J Neurochem 69: 2302–2311.

Scott BG, Yang H, Tuzun E, et al. (2004). ICOS is essential for the development of experimental autoimmune myasthenia gravis. J Neuroimmunol 153: 16–25.

Seifert R, Christ B (1990). On the differentiation and origin of myoid cells in the avian thymus. Anat Embryol 181: 287–298.

Selcen D, Fukuda T, Shen XM, et al. (2004). Are MuSK antibodies the primary cause of myasthenic symptoms? Neurology 62: 1945–1950.

Sempowski GD, Hale LP, Sundy JS, et al. (2000). Leukemia inhibitory factor, oncostatin m, IL-6, and stem cell factor mRNA expression in human thymus increases with age and is associated with thymic atrophy. J Immunol 164: 2180–2187.

Seybold ME (1999). Diagnosis of myasthenia gravis. In: AG Engel (Ed.), Myasthenia Gravis and Myasthenic Disorders. Oxford University Press, New York, pp. 167–201.

Sheng JR, Li L, Ganesh BB, et al. (2006). Suppression of experimental autoimmune myasthenia gravis by granulocyte-macrophage colony-stimulating factor is associated with an expansion of FoxP3+ regulatory T cells. J Immunol 177: 5296–5306.

Shi FD, Wang HB, Li H, et al. (2000). Natural killer cells determine the outcome of B cell-mediated autoimmunity. Nat Immunol 1: 245–251.

Shimizu H, Kataoka H, Kawahara M, et al. (2007). Interferon causes no myasthenia in a seropositive patient with multiple sclerosis. Clin Neurol Neurosurg 109: 277–278.

Shinomiya N, Nomura Y, Segawa M (2004). A variant of childhood-onset myasthenia gravis: HLA typing and clinical characteristics in Japan. Clin Immunol 110: 154–158.

Shiono H, Roxanis I, Zhang W, et al. (2003). Scenarios for autoimmunization of T and B cells in myasthenia gravis. Ann N Y Acad Sci 998: 237–256.

Shiraishi H, Motomura M, Yoshimura T, et al. (2005). Acetylcholine receptors loss and postsynaptic damage in musk antibody-positive myasthenia gravis. Ann Neurol 57: 289–293.

Silman AJ, MacGregor AJ, Thomson W, et al. (1993). Twin concordance rates for rheumatoid arthritis: results from a nationwide study. British J Rheumatol 32: 903–907.

Simpson IA (1960). Myasthenia gravis: a new hypothesis. Scott Med J 5: 419–436.

Slater CR, Lyons PR, Walls TJ, et al. (1992). Structure and function of neuromuscular junctions in the vastus lateralis of man. Brain 115: 451–478.

Smith CI, Grubb R, Hammarstrom L, et al. (1983). Gm allotypes in Swedish myasthenia gravis patients. J Immunogenet 10: 1–9.

Smith CI, Grubb R, Hammarstrom L, et al. (1984). Gm allotypes in Finnish myasthenia gravis patients. Neurology 34: 1604–1605.

Smith KY, Valdez H, Landay A, et al. (2000). Thymic size and lymphocyte restoration in patients with human immunodeficiency virus infection after 48 weeks of Zidovudine, Lamivudine, and Ritonavir therapy. J Infect Dis 181: 141–147.

Somer H, Müller K, Kinnunen E (1989). Myasthenia gravis associated with multiple sclerosis. Epidemiological survey and immunological findings. J Neurol Sci 89: 37–48.

Sommer N, Willcox N, Harcourt GC, et al. (1990). Myasthenic thymus and thymoma are selectively enriched in acetylcholine receptor-reactive t cells. Ann Neurol 28: 312–319.

Sommer N, Harcourt GC, Willcox N, et al. (1991). Acetylcholine receptor-reactive T lymphocytes from healthy subjects and myasthenia gravis patients. Neurology 41: 1270–1276.

Sommer N, Melms A, Weller M, et al. (1993). Ocular myasthenia gravis. A critical review of clinical and pathophysiological aspects. Doc Ophthalmol 84: 309–333.

Somnier FE (1994). Exacerbation of myasthenia gravis after removal of thymomas. Acta Neurol Scand 90: 56–66.

Somnier FE (2005). Increasing incidence of late-onset anti-AChr antibody-seropositive myasthenia gravis. Neurology 65: 928–930.

Somnier FE, Engel PJ (2002). The occurrence of anti-titin antibodies and thymomas: a population survey of MG 1970–1999. Neurology 59: 92–98.

Spits H (2002). Development of ab T cells in the human thymus. Nat Rev Immunol 2: 760–772.

Spuler S, Marx A, Kirchner T, et al. (1994). Myogenesis in thymic transplants in the severe combined immunodeficient mouse model of myasthenia gravis. Differentiation of thymic myoid cells into striated muscle. Am J Pathol 145: 766–770.

Spuler S, Sarropoulos A, Marx A, et al. (1996). Thymoma-associated myasthenia gravis. Transplantation of thymoma and extrathymomal thymic tissue into SCID mice. Am J Pathol 148: 1359–1365.

Stanley FF, Drachman DB (1983). Rapid degradation of "new" acetylcholine receptors at neuromuscular junctions. Science 222: 67–69.

Stassen MH, Meng F, Melgert E, et al. (2003). Experimental autoimmune myasthenia gravis in mice expressing human immunoglobulin loci. J Neuroimmunol 135: 56–61.

Steinman L (2007). A brief history of T(H)17, the first major revision in the T(H)1/T(H)2 hypothesis of T cell-mediated tissue damage. Nat Med 13: 139–145.

Stickler DE, Massey JM, Sanders DB (2005). Musk-antibody positive myasthenia gravis: clinical and electrodiagnostic patterns. Clin Neurophysiol 116: 2065–2068.

Strauss AJ, Kemp PG Jr (1967). Serum autoantibodies in myasthenia gravis and thymoma: selective affinity for I-bands of striated muscle as a guide to identification of antigen(s). J Immunol 99: 945–953.

Strauss AJL, Seegal BC, Hsu KC, et al. (1960). Immunofluorescence demonstration of a muscle binding, complement-fixing serum globulin fraction in myasthenia gravis. Proc Soc Exp Biol Med 105: 184–191.

Ströbel P, Helmreich M, Kalbacher H, et al. (2001). Evidence for distinct mechanisms in the shaping of the CD4 T cell repertoire in histologically distinct myasthenia gravis-associated thymomas. Dev Immunol 8: 279–290.

Ströbel P, Rosenwald A, Beyersdorf N, et al. (2004). Selective loss of regulatory T cells in thymomas. Ann Neurol 56: 901–904.

Ströbel P, Murumagi A, Klein R, et al. (2007). Deficiency of the autoimmune regulator AIRE in thymomas is insufficient to elicit autoimmune polyendocrinopathy syndrome type 1 (APS-1). J Pathol 211: 563–571.

Suzuki Y, Onodera H, Tago H, et al. (2005). Altered populations of natural killer cell and natural killer T cell subclasses in myasthenia gravis. J Neuroimmunol 167: 186–189.

Suzuki Y, Onodera H, Tago H, et al. (2006). Altered expression of Th1-type chemokine receptor CXCR3 on CD4+ T cells in myasthenia gravis patients. J Neuroimmunol 172: 166–174.

Szobor A (1991). Familial myasthenia gravis: nine patients in two generations. Acta Med Hung 48: 145–149.

Tackenberg B, Hemmer B, Oertel WH, et al. (2001). Immunosuppressive treatment of ocular myasthenia gravis. BioDrugs 15: 369–378.

Tackenberg B, Nitschke M, Willcox N, et al. (2003). CD45 isoform expression in autoimmune myasthenia gravis. Autoimmunity 36: 117–121.

Tackenberg B, Kruth J, Bartholomaeus JE, et al. (2007). Clonal expansions of CD4+ B helper T cells in autoimmune myasthenia gravis. Eur J Immunol 37: 849–863.

Takahashi H, Amagai M, Tanikawa A, et al. (2007). T helper type 2-biased natural killer cell phenotype in patients with pemphigus vulgaris. J Invest Dermatol 127: 324–330.

Tami JA, Urso OE, Krolick KA (1987). T cell hybridomas reactive with the acetylcholine receptor and its subunits. J Immunol 138: 732–738.

Thangarajh M, Masterman T, Helgeland L, et al. (2006). The thymus is a source of B-cell-survival factors—APRIL and BAFF—in myasthenia gravis. J Neuroimmunol 178: 161–166.

Thorlacius S, Mollnes TE, Garred P, et al. (1988). Plasma exchange in myasthenia gravis: changes in serum complement and immunoglobulins. Acta Neurol Scand 78: 221–227.

Thorlacius S, Aarli JA, Riise T, et al. (1989). Associated disorders in myasthenia gravis: autoimmune diseases and their relation to thymectomy. Acta Neurol Scand 80: 290–295.

Tiller T, Tsuiji M, Yurasov S, et al. (2007). Autoreactivity in human IgG+ memory B cells. Immunity 26: 205–213.

Tindall R (1981). Humoral immunity in myasthenia gravis: biochemical characterization of acquired antireceptor antibodies and clinical correlations. Ann Neurol 10: 437–447.

Tindall RSA (1980). Humoral immunity in myasthenia gravis: effects of steroids and thymectomy. Neurology 30: 554–557.

Tindall RSA, Rollins JA, Phillips JT, et al. (1987). Preliminary results of a double-blind, randomized, placebo-controlled trial of cyclosporine in myasthenia gravis. N Engl J Med 316: 719–724.

Tonegawa S (1983). Somatic generation of antibody diversity. Nature 302: 575–581.

Toyka KV, Drachman DB, Griffin DE, et al. (1977). Myasthenia gravis. Study of humoral immune mechanisms by passive transfer to mice. N Engl J Med 296: 125–131.

Tsao CY, Mendell JR, Lo WD, et al. (2000). Myasthenia gravis associated with autoimmune diseases in children. J Child Neurol 15: 767–769.

Tsuchida M, Yamato Y, Souma T, et al. (1999). Efficacy and safety of extended thymectomy for elderly patients with myasthenia gravis. Ann Thorac Surg 67: 1563–1567.

Tuzun E, Li J, Saini SS, et al. (2007). Pros and cons of treating murine myasthenia gravis with anti-C1q antibody. J Neuroimmunol 182: 167–176.

Tzartos SJ, Lindstrom JM (1980). Monoclonal antibodies used to probe acetylcholine receptor structure: localization of the main immunogenic region and detection of similarities between subunits. Proc Natl Acad Sci U S A 77: 755–759.

Tzartos SJ, Seybold ME, Lindstrom J (1982). Specificities of antibodies to acetylcholine receptors in sera from myasthenia gravis patients measured by monoclonal antibodies. Proc Natl Acad Sci U S A 70: 188–192.

Tzartos SJ, Kokla A, Walgrave SL, et al. (1988a). Localization of the main immunogenic region of human acetylcholine receptor to residues 67–76 of the α-subunit. Proc Natl Acad Sci U S A 85: 2899–2903.

Tzartos SJ, Morel E, Efthimiadis A, et al. (1988b). Fine antigenic specificities of antibodies in sera from patients with D-penicillamine-induced myasthenia gravis. Clin Exp Immunol 73: 80–86.

Tzartos SJ, Barkas T, Cung MT, et al. (1998). Anatomy of the antigenic structure of a large membrane autoantigen, the muscle-type nicotinic acetylcholine receptor. Immunol Rev 163: 89–120.

van de Velde RL, Friedman NB (1970). Thymic myoid cells and myasthenia gravis. Am J Pathol 59: 347–368.

van de Warrenburg BP, Hengstman GJ, Vos PE, et al. (2002). Concomitant dermatomyositis and myasthenia gravis presenting with respiratory insufficiency. Muscle Nerve 25: 293–296.

van der Pol WL, Jansen MD, Kuks JB, et al. (2003). Association of the Fc gamma receptor IIA-R/R131 genotype with myasthenia gravis in Dutch patients. J Neuroimmunol 144: 143–147.

Vandiedonck C, Beaurain G, Giraud M, et al. (2004). Pleiotropic effects of the 8.1 HLA haplotype in patients with autoimmune myasthenia gravis and thymus hyperplasia. Proc Nat Acad Sci USA 101: 15464–15469.

Vandiedonck C, Giraud M, Garchon HJ (2005). Genetics of autoimmune myasthenia gravis: the multifaceted contribution of the HLA complex. J Autoimmun 25: 6–11.

Vandiedonck C, Capdevielle C, Giraud M, et al. (2006). Association of the PTPN22*R620W polymorphism with autoimmune myasthenia gravis. Ann Neurol 59: 404–407.

van Ewijk W, Shores EW, Singer A (1994). Crosstalk in the mouse thymus. Immunol Today 15: 214.

Vanhecke D, Leclercq G, Plum J, et al. (1995). Characterization of distinct stages during the differentiation of human CD69+CD3+ thymocytes and the identification of thymic emigrants. J Immunol 155: 1862–1872.

van Meerwijk JP, MacDonald HR (1999). In vivo T-lymphocyte tolerance in the absence of thymic clonal deletion mediated by hematopoietic cells. Blood 93: 3856–3862.

Vernet-der Garabedian B, Lacokova M, Eymard B, et al. (1994). Association of neonatal myasthenia gravis with antibodies against the fetal acetylcholine receptor. J Clin Invest 94: 555–559.

Vincent A (1994). Aetiological factors in development of myasthenia gravis. Adv Neuroimmunol 4: 355–371.

Vincent A (2002). Unravelling the pathogenesis of myasthenia gravis. Nat Rev Immunol 2: 797–804.

Vincent A, Newsom-Davis J (1982). Acetylcholine receptor antibody characteristics in myasthenia gravis. I. Patients with generalized myasthenia or disease restricted to ocular muscles. Clin Exp Immunol 49: 257–265.

Vincent A, Newsom-Davis J (1985). Acetylcholine receptor antibody as a diagnostic test for myasthenia gravis: results in 153 validated cases and 2967 diagnostic assays. J Neurol Neurosurg Psychiatry 48: 1246–1252.

Vincent A, Willcox N (1999). The role of T-cells in the initiation of autoantibody responses in thymoma patients. Pathol Res Pract 195: 535–540.

Vincent A, Newsom-Davis J, Newton P, et al. (1983). Acetylcholine receptor antibody and clinical response to thymectomy in myasthenia gravis. Neurology 33: 1276–1282.

Vincent A, Newland C, Brueton L, et al. (1995). Arthrogryposis multiplex congenita with maternal autoantibodies specific for a fetal antigen. Lancet 346: 24–25.

Vincent A, Willcox N, Hill M, et al. (1998). Determinant spreading and immune responses to acetylcholine receptors in myasthenia gravis. Immunol Rev 164: 157–168.

Vincent A, Clover L, Buckley C, et al. (2003). Evidence of underdiagnosis of myasthenia gravis in older people. J Neurol Neurosurg Psychiatry 74: 1105–1108.

Vincent AC, McConville J, Newsom-Davis J (2005). Is "seronegative" MG explained by autoantibodies to MuSK? Neurology 64: 399.

Vinuesa CG, Tangye SG, Moser B, et al. (2005). Follicular B helper T cells in antibody responses and autoimmunity. Nat Rev Immunol 5: 853–865.

Voltz R, Albrich W, Hohlfeld R, et al. (2003). Anti-titin antibodies are not associated with a specific thymoma histology. J Neurol Neurosurg Psychiatry 74: 282.

von Boehmer H (1993). Positive selection of lymphocytes. Cell 76: 219–228.

AChR function (Drachman et al., 1978; Stanley and Drachman, 1978).

6.2.4. Characteristics of AChR antibodies

The AChR antibodies, as measured by immunoprecipitation, are mostly, if not entirely, IgG, polyclonal (i.e. both κ and λ light chains can be present in any individual), very high affinity with Kd values $>10^{-10}$M, and mainly IgG1 and IgG3 subclasses (Bray and Drachman, 1982; Vincent and Newsom-Davis, 1982a,b; Rodgaard et al., 1987). The antibodies bind variably to muscle AChRs extracted from different species, but generally bind similarly to non-human primate and human AChRs. They bind much more effectively to the native AChR than to denatured AChR subunits (i.e. on Western blots that measure antibody binding to the separated, denatured AChR subunits). For this reason, it is difficult to determine the exact epitopes to which they bind, but they compete variably with monoclonal antibodies derived from mice immunized with purified AChR (see Vincent et al., 1987; Tzartos et al., 1998). Many, but not all, of these antibodies bind to the two "main immunogenic regions" on the α-subunits (Tzartos et al., 1998). However, since some of these monoclonal antibodies have been shown to bind to different subunits, the competition with the patients' antibodies implies that the human antibodies also bind to different subunits (Jacobson et al., 1999a). In addition, as mentioned above, it is clear that some MG sera bind preferentially to adult or fetal AChR.

6.2.5. Antibodies during immunosuppressive treatments

It has already been mentioned that AChR antibodies fall during plasma exchange and that their levels during and after this treatment reflect well the clinical changes in the patient. Thus there is little doubt that within a patient, over a short period of time, antibody levels correlate well with clinical status (Newsom-Davis et al., 1978). In longer term studies, by contrast, such as after thymectomy, the evidence is less good or incomplete. Nevertheless, there were some studies that showed reasonable correlations after steroid treatments or thymectomy (Vincent et al., 1983; Kuks et al., 1991). In fact, if each antibody level is carefully measured and expressed as a percentage of the pretreatment value, the mean values correlate well with clinical score. It is very important in such studies to store the sera from each patient and assay all samples on a single occasion, taking care to titrate the serum

adequately to ensure an accurate result. Lack of care over these technical details may be responsible for some of the less conclusive studies. On the other hand, any long term study will undoubtedly be confounded by other factors that may influence antibody levels or clinical state.

6.2.6. Antibodies in different forms of MG

MG is a heterogeneous disease and patients can be divided into several groups according to age at onset, thymic pathology and antibody status. Table 6.1 summarizes the main groups, and mentions the other autoantibodies that the patients may have. The HLA associations found suggest that there are different underlying causes that lead, by a final common pathway, to the AChR antibodies. Overall other autoimmune diseases including thyroid disease, rheumatoid arthritis and systemic lupus erythematosus (SLE), and the associated autoantibodies, are found in up to 30% of MG patients, mostly those with AChR antibodies and with early age at onset of generalized MG (Tellez-Zenteno et al., 2004; Sthoeger et al., 2006; Toth et al., 2006). Thymectomy did not appear to be more beneficial in patients with or without associated autoantibodies, and it is not clear whether the associated autoimmune diseases benefited from the surgery.

Interestingly, thymoma-MG patients often develop other diseases such as acquired neuromyotonia, aplastic anemia, neuropathies and even limbic encephalitis, rather than the more usual autoimmune conditions such as thyroiditis, rheumatoid arthritis and SLE. In addition, late-onset MG patients not only have other autoimmune diseases less frequently, but share with thymoma-MG cases antibodies to muscle antigens, ryanodine receptor, and titin (see Romi et al., 2000; Aarli et al., 2003; Skeie et al., 2006), and to two cytokines, interferon-α and interleukin-12 (Meager et al., 1999; Buckley et al., 2001). Interestingly, in thymoma patients studied over time, changes in any of these antibodies do not necessarily correlate within an individual, although rises in cytokine antibodies appear to predict thymoma recurrence (Buckley et al., 2001).

6.2.7. Epidemiological studies based on serological studies

MG is widely recognized throughout the world and AChR antibody positivity is high in all published reports. One of the advantages of having a serological diagnostic test is the fact that it can be used to confirm

Table 6.1

Subtypes of myasthenia gravis, defined by antibodies, age at onset, generalized symptoms and thymic pathology

	AChR antibody seropositive					AChR antibody seronegative	
	Generalized		Thymoma-associated MG	Ocular		Generalized	
	Early onset MG	Late onset MG		Seropositive ocular MG	Seronegative ocular MG	MuSK-MG	SNMG
						MuSK antibody associated	Non-MuSK antibody associated
Age range (years)	<40 by definition	>40 by definition	2–80+	2–100	2–80+	Mainly <60	2–80+
Male:female approximate ratio	1:3	3:2	1:1	Not clear	Not clear	1:4	2:3
HLA association (in Caucasians)	HLA B8 DR3	HLA B7 DR2 (males>females)	No clear association	None known	None known	DR14DQ5	None known
Thymic pathology	Hyperplasia	Atrophy	Thymoma	Not known	Not known	Often normal for age	May have hyperplasia
Other antibodies	Other organ-specific antibodies common	Titin, ryanodine receptor, IFNα, IL-12	Titin, ryanodine receptor, IFNα, IL-12	Not frequent	Not frequent	Distinction between MuSK-MG and SNMG not made in most studies	Distinction between MuSK-MG and SNMG not made in most studies

The information is summarized from clinical data of Professor J. Newsom-Davis, and from unpublished observations on seronegative MG (Vincent et al., 2003).

the diagnosis in patients from different populations, thus facilitating direct comparisons on disease incidence and prevalence. This is particularly relevant to the relative incidence of MG presenting at different ages. In western populations several studies have shown a higher annual rate of AChR positive MG patients over 50 years of age, peaking at around age 70 years or even higher (see Vincent et al., 2003). Particularly striking is the reported high incidence of MG in children in China, Taiwan and Japan compared with the very low incidence in western countries (Chiu et al., 1987; Zhang et al., 2007). Several studies of patients from these countries have shown that a high proportion of the diagnosed children have AChR antibodies, thus confirming the diagnosis of MG (Zhang et al., 2007). The relatively low levels of such antibodies can be explained mainly by the high incidence of ocular MG. Thus, the relative proportions of ocular to generalized MG also differ between Oriental and Caucasian populations. Whether this is genetically determined or environmentally determined may become clearer when Oriental populations living in western countries, such as the USA, are studied.

6.3. Fetal AChR antibodies in maternal sera

An exception to the general rule that antibodies to the α-BuTx binding sites do not predominate in MG sera is illustrated by antibodies in mothers of babies with arthrogryposis multiplex congenita (AMC) (Polizzi et al., 2002). In this condition, multiple joint contractures form in utero and are present at birth, sometimes severely compromising survival. Lung hypoplasia may result and can be lethal. AMC is a relatively common congenital condition (many cases are restricted to distal joints and relatively mild) and maternal antibodies to AChR are only present in 1–2% (Dalton et al., 2006), but in the few well studied cases, a high proportion of the AChR antibodies bind to the α-BuTx binding site at the interface of the γ- and α-subunits (Fig. 6.1A). In theory, therefore, one would not expect these antibodies to be detected by radioimmunoprecipitation where both ^{125}I–α–BuTx binding sites are fully occupied. However, in practice, these antibodies often displace ^{125}I–α–BuTx from the gamma-specific binding site, with the result that even at high serum concentrations ^{125}I–α–BuTx binding is inhibited by 50% (Fig. 6.3). That these antibodies are directly able to block fetal AChR function, and not adult AChR function, was shown by cellular studies demonstrating a rapid inhibition of ACh-induced currents through the fetal but not the adult form of the AChR, and by analogous experiments that monitored agonist induced sodium flux through AChRs (Vincent et al.,

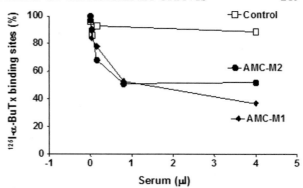

Fig. 6.3. Sera from two women whose babies were born with arthrogryposis multiplex congenita inhibit ^{125}I–α–BuTx binding to the fetal-specific AChR binding site by 50% (see Fig. 6.1A).

1995; Riemersma et al., 1997). The pathogenicity of the fetal-specific antibodies was strikingly confirmed by passive transfer of the maternal serum to pregnant mice that led to fetal joint contractures (Jacobson et al., 1999b).

6.4. Antibodies in seronegative MG

In the first comprehensive study of autoantibody status in MG patients, Lindstrom et al. (1976) noted that 12% were negative in the AChR-Ab assay and suggested that they might have antibodies to another protein, or have a different form of the disease. Interestingly, the proportion of such seronegative MG (SNMG) patients varies quite considerably (5–30%) between different studies (see Vincent et al., 2003) but it is difficult to know whether this is due to geographical or methodological differences. Some MG patients develop AChR antibodies over time, suggesting that these antibodies are present but undetectable by the radioimmunoprecipitation assay (Vincent and Newsom-Davis, 1985), and in addition, since AChR antibody assays have improved over time, with the introduction of both adult and fetal AChR isoforms, it is possible that some of the results of earlier studies were misleading.

6.4.1. Experimental evidence for antibodies in SNMG

The response to plasma exchange in SNMG (Mossman et al., 1986) and the transfer of SNMG from mother to child (Mier and Havard, 1985) clearly indicate that there is a circulating serum factor in SNMG, probably an IgG antibody. Moreover, early studies showed the transfer of disease to mice by injection of plasmas and immunoglobulin preparation from SNMG patients (Mossman et al., 1986; Burges et al., 1993; Evoli et al., 2003).

The mice did not show any obvious symptoms of MG, but in vivo or in vitro electrophysiological tests revealed defects in neuromuscular transmission in most animals. One possible explanation was that the plasmas did contain antibodies to the AChR, but at such low titers that they were undetectable in the immunoprecipitation assay. However, the AChRs extracted from the mouse muscles did not (except in one case) have human antibody attached (Mossman et al., 1986), in contrast to those in mice transferred with AChR antibody positive plasmas. Moreover, the number of AChRs at the mouse endplates was not substantially reduced, unlike in mice treated with AChR antibody positive plasmas (Mossman et al., 1986). Other passive transfer studies confirmed that the disease is transferable and, in one study, some presynaptic as well as postsynaptic electrophysiological abnormalities were found (Burges et al., 1993). The authors concluded that antibodies to non-AChR target(s) were likely to be involved.

There have been several attempts to demonstrate the presence of antibodies to neuromuscular junction proteins in SNMG. These included a search for antibodies to presynaptic membrane proteins (Lu et al., 1991), antibodies specific against fetal and adult AChR (Ohta et al., 2003), and filamin and vinculin, which are both postsynaptic cytoskeletal proteins (Yamamoto et al., 1987). However, most data supports the importance of antibodies that bind to the extracellular surface of the muscle fiber. These fall into two main categories and will be described in more detail.

6.4.2. IgG antibodies to MuSK

The first clear evidence that there were antibodies to another cell surface muscle protein in SNMG patients came from studies that demonstrated that IgG antibodies from about 50% of these sera bound to the TE671 muscle-like cells (Blaes et al., 1998). Somewhat similar results had been reported using a mouse muscle-like cell line (Brooks et al., 1990). However, the antibodies did not bind to human embryonic kidney cells that had been transformed to express human adult AChRs (Blaes et al., 1998). These results suggested that there were IgG antibodies specific for another muscle membrane protein.

A potential candidate was the muscle specific kinase (MuSK), which was identified as a neuromuscular-junction specific receptor tyrosine kinase in 1995 (Valenzuela et al., 1995). MuSK is a transmembrane receptor with three (or four) immunoglobulin-like domains and a cysteine-rich domain extracellularly, and an intracellular kinase domain. During development, it serves as the receptor for agrin released from the motor nerve. Agrin interacts with MuSK, MuSK dimerizes and the intracellular tyrosine kinase domain activates phosphorylation of other cytoplasmic proteins including the AChR-anchoring protein rapsyn. This then clusters AChRs on the postsynaptic muscle surface. Mice defective in MuSK, or rapsyn, do not cluster AChRs at the neuromuscular junction and cannot survive after birth (DeChiara et al., 1996). However, the role of MuSK at the adult neuromuscular junction is less clear.

MuSK antibodies were first detected in 70% of SNMG sera or plasmas by an ELISA assay and then by radioimmunoprecipitation (Hoch et al., 2001). The antibodies were only found in patients without AChR antibodies with generalized disease. They have been found only very infrequently in patients with purely ocular symptoms (McConville et al., 2004). The antibodies were also detected by Scuderi et al., (2003) using immunoprecipitation of biotinylated membrane proteins from TE671 cells. They found a 110 kDa biotinylated protein in the precipitate that they were subsequently able to identify as MuSK using Western blotting. Most of the patients studied initially (Hoch et al., 2001) had undergone plasma exchange because of severe symptoms, and this is likely to have influenced the proportion who were positive for MuSK antibodies, since it is now clear that patients with these antibodies tend to be more severe and more difficult to treat effectively with steroids alone. There appears to be a genetic predisposition to development of this form of MG since HLA DR14DQ5 is more common than in controls (Niks et al., 2006). Further studies on patients from around the world suggest that the proportion of SNMG patients with MuSK antibodies varies widely from 0 to 50% (Vincent et al., in preparation). It is particularly intriguing that the incidence of MuSK antibody positivity appears to be greatest at around the 40th parallel north of the equator and falls off further south and further north. These results suggest that there may be an environmental antigen that stimulates the formation of this antibody.

6.4.3. Characteristics and mechanisms of action of MuSK antibodies

MuSK antibodies are predominantly IgG and of high affinity (McConville et al., 2004). The antibodies affect the function of MuSK in in vitro assays, notably those using the C2C12 mouse cell line that forms myotubes when grown under conditions of serum depletion (Hoch et al., 2001; Farrugia et al., 2007). These cells express MuSK and AChRs, and the addition of agrin to the cultures for a few hours activates MuSK and induces clusters of AChRs that can be detected by fluorescent-labeled α-BuTx. MuSK antibodies, presumably by dimerizing and activating MuSK, can increase the number of spontaneous AChR clusters, but if added before or during the application of agrin, MuSK antibodies reduce the number of agrin-induced AChR clusters. However, in a recent study, the total number of AChRs was not reduced by the MuSK antibodies, even when clustering was reduced (Farrugia et al., 2007).

Another study, however, found a direct effect of MuSK antibodies on muscle cell proliferation. These authors used the cell line TE671, which expresses MuSK, and showed a reduction in cell numbers over a 3-day period of incubation in diluted serum (Boneva et al., 2006). There was a decrease in mRNA expression for AChR subunits and an increase in expression of MURF-1, a muscle atrophy-related gene. Although interesting there is no evidence that any of these changes relate to neuromuscular transmission defects in vivo.

It may be difficult to determine the role of MuSK antibodies using cell lines in vitro. It is likely that TE671 and C2C12 cells do not contain all of the intracellular machinery necessary to demonstrate a pathogenic effect of MuSK antibodies. For instance, a recently discovered molecule that binds intracellularly to MuSK is Dok-7. Since deletions in Dok-7 lead to a congenital myasthenic syndrome by an as yet unknown mechanism (Beeson et al., 2006; see Chapter 10), it is possible that reduced activity of the MuSK–Dok-7 interaction may alter downstream signals involved in the structure and maintenance of the AChR, or may affect intracellular signaling pathways that could reduce AChR function.

The alternative approach is to use the animal models to determine what happens in vivo. Initial suggestions were that MuSK antibodies would activate complement-dependent lysis of the neuromuscular junction, in a similar manner to the AChR antibodies (Hoch et al., 2001), but MuSK antibodies are IgG4

predominantly (McConville et al., 2004) and this IgG subclass does not activate complement effectively. Moreover, recent studies of biopsies from MuSK-MG patients show very little loss of AChRs or complement deposition, in contrast to results from both AChR-MG and patients with neither antibody (Selcen et al., 2004; Shiraishi et al., 2005; and H. Shiraishi and M. Motomura 2005, unpublished observations).

Various lines of evidence, however, are in favor of a direct role of the MuSK antibodies on neuromuscular transmission. First, in the passive transfer experiments of Mossman et al., (1985), there was clear evidence of a transmission defect despite the normal AChR numbers, and in a further study, miniature endplate potentials were reduced in amplitude (Burges et al., 1993). The majority of the patients whose serum or plasma preparations were studied in those two reports have been identified, retrospectively, as being MuSK antibody positive (A. Vincent 2001, unpublished). Secondly, there is a good correlation between MuSK antibody levels and clinical state, as shown in serial studies (e.g., Fig. 6.4). Thirdly, in vivo knock-down of MuSK in mature muscle by electroporation of mouse leg muscles with siRNA for MuSK produced a slow dispersal of AChRs from the neuromuscular junction, presumably leading to defective transmission, although this was not studied (Kong et al., 2004). Fourthly, immunization against MuSK in two reports has produced evidence of muscle weakness, electromyographic or electrophysiological evidence of neuromuscular transmission defect, and alterations to the morphology of the neuromuscular junctions (Jha et al., 2006; Shigemoto et al., 2006). These experimental observations indicate that MuSK antibodies can be pathogenic in vivo, although none of these studies used accurate measurements of AChRs, or extensive in vitro electrophysiology, or ultrastructural studies, to demonstrate that their

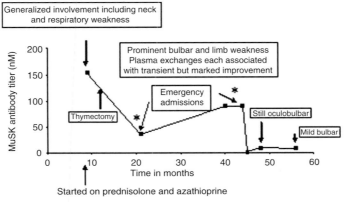

Fig. 6.4. Serial MuSK antibody titers in a young female patient with typical MuSK-MG showing the prolonged course and emergency admissions. (Some MuSK antibody measurements were taken after, rather than before, plasma exchange, e.g., *, explaining why the antibody levels are not as high as might be expected.) MuSK antibody data courtesy of Dr. J. McConville.

findings were analogous to those in patients' muscle biopsies. Therefore, the pathogenic role of MuSK antibodies, although highly probable, is still undetermined.

6.4.4. MuSK antibodies and muscle wasting

One observation that needs to be explained is the distribution of muscle weakness in patients with MuSK antibodies. These patients tend to have ocular weakness, like many MG patients, and often with relatively mild limb weakness but marked involvement of bulbar, neck and respiratory muscles (e.g., Sanders et al., 2003). They often respond less well to conventional immunosuppressive treatment with prednisolone and/or azathioprine (see Chapter 9). Ocular and bulbar muscles may show electromyographic (SFEMG) evidence of neuromuscular transmission defects when limb muscles are normal (Nemoto et al., 2005; Oh et al., 2005; Farrugia et al., 2006a). Fairly frequently they are left with severe bulbar symptoms and muscle wasting (Evoli et al., 2004; Farrugia et al., 2006b). The latter study quantified muscle bulk in MuSK-MG patients comparing with an AChR-MG group who were closely matched for age at onset, sex, disease duration and severity. Muscle dimensions were significantly less in the MuSK-MG patients, and there was more evidence of fatty replacement as indicated by a high signal on MRI (Farrugia et al., 2006b). Moreover, as mentioned above, and found also in C2C12 cells, MuSK antibodies can upregulate expression of muscle atrophy-related genes (Benveniste et al., 2005; Boneva et al., 2006), suggesting that they directly induce some of the changes found in muscle atrophy.

6.4.5. Evidence for serum antibodies in SNMG

The patients who are persistently negative for antibodies to AChR or to MuSK are called seronegative MG. An effect of purified IgG from MG patients on mouse muscle AChR ion channels was shown by Bufler et al., (1998) in both AChR antibody positive and negative patients. The reduction in AChR currents that they saw was reversible with washing, suggesting that there may be low affinity, reversible IgG antibodies that directly block AChR function. Such antibodies would not be expected to be detected in the ^{125}I-α–BuTx–AChR radioimmunoprecipitation assay because their reversibility would make detection in solution, where the AChR is not at a high concentration, very unlikely.

In a somewhat similar manner, sera or plasmas from SNMG patients were found to reduce the function of the muscle AChR in a cell line, TE671, originally derived from a rhabdomyosarcoma. In this case, AChR function was measured by carbachol-induced $\{\Sigma Y\}22$ $\{\Sigma Y\}$Na influx (carbachol is a non-hydrolysable ACh homolog) and measured over a 1 min time course. Inhibition occurred rapidly but was mostly studied after a 2 h incubation or overnight (Yamamoto et al., 1991). The effects were partially reversible (Plested et al., 2002) and the active plasma ingredient appeared to be in the non-IgG fraction. A similar partially reversible effect on AChR function was found after incubation in drugs that activated cAMP kinase or lectins that also affect membrane receptors (Li et al., 1996), and it was proposed that the antibodies might be acting indirectly via a second messenger system rather than by direct blocking of AChR function. This was supported by evidence that application of the serum or non-IgG fractions increased incorporation of ^{32}P into AChRs (Plested et al., 2002). Phosphorylation of AChRs is known to accompany receptor desensitization; thus these results were consistent with the idea that the antibodies acted indirectly and led to receptor desensitization and reduced function.

A more recent study, however, has produced evidence indicating that there are some antibodies binding directly to the AChR. Short pulses of sera or non-IgG preparations were applied to the CN21 cell line (TE671 cells permanently transformed to express excess adult AChR) between pulses of nicotine as an agonist (Spreadbury et al., 2005). The nicotine-induced AChR currents were reduced in amplitude within one minute of application of the antibodies. Intriguingly the inhibition varied between different individual CN21 cells, as also noted in another study (Plested et al., 2003), and correlated strongly with the desensitization that occurred in the presence of longer pulses of nicotine. These results were in line with those reported above. However, the same results were obtained when the antibody preparations were applied to human embryonic kidney cells expressing the AChR (and not muscle antigens), and the degree of inhibition of the antibodies correlated with that obtained with a monoclonal antibody, C7, that is known to bind to the AChR δ-subunit. Altogether therefore these results are more consistent with a direct effect of antibodies binding directly to the AChR and increasing its tendency to desensitize in the presence of agonist (Spreadbury et al., 2005).

6.4.6. Antibodies to AChRs in SNMG

Following these observations, my coworkers and I began to look more carefully at SNMG patients and their serum. First, it appears that SNMG is much more similar to AChR antibody positive MG in its clinical features, in electrophysiological defects, and in thymic pathology (Table 6.1). The thymus in SNMG patients frequently contains germinal centers with T and B cell domains, very similar to those found in typical AChR-MG (Lauriola et al., 2005; Leite et al., 2005; 2007). These results contrast with those in MuSK-MG where the thymic changes are unremarkable in most cases.

Based on these observations, and those described above that suggested antibodies bind to AChR with low affinity, we have attempted to detect antibodies to AChR using cell lines expressing adult AChRs that have been clustered by co-transfection with rapsyn. With this approach we have found IgG antibodies to AChR in over 50% of sera from patients previously negative by radioimmunoprecipitation assays (Leite et al., in preparation).

6.5. Antibodies in the Lambert–Eaton myasthenic syndrome

The criteria that helped to define MG as an autoimmune disease also applied to the Lambert–Eaton myasthenic syndrome (LEMS; see Chapter 9) but the sequence of events was somewhat different. It had been shown in the 1950s and 1960s that the defect was presynaptic and led to marked reductions in the quantal content of the endplate potential (number of ACh packets released per nerve impulse) probably involving a reduction in calcium-evoked release of ACh from the motor nerve terminal (Elmqvist and Lambert, 1968; Lambert and Elmqvist, 1971). Later freeze-fracture studies showed that the active zone particles on the presynaptic membrane, which are thought to be the voltage-gated calcium channels (VGCCs), were reduced in number (Fukunaga et al., 1983). Some of the patients had other autoimmune diseases, and plasma exchange produced a slow but marked improvement (Lang et al., 1981). Moreover, the disease could be passively transferred to mice by daily injections of LEMS IgG (Lang et al., 1987). This led to changes in the number and distribution of active zone particles (Fukuoka et al., 1987a,b), and reduced ACh release from the motor nerve terminals (Lang et al., 1987). These observations clearly implicated VGCCs as a target antigen in the disease.

VGCCs are a family of channels composed of an $\alpha 1$ subunit that contains the calcium pore and determines the functional subtype and sensitivity to various neurotoxins. Using different neurotoxins that bind to different subtypes of VGCC, it was possible to demonstrate antibodies in patients with LEMS (using the radioimmunoprecipitation technique similar to that illustrated in Fig. 6.1B). Antibodies were first detected in around 50% of patients using a snail toxin called ^{125}I-conotoxin GVIA (^{125}I-CgTx) (Sher et al., 1989) to label N-type VGCCs extracted from human brain tissue. Subsequently, however, using a different cone snail, ^{125}I-conotoxin MVIIC (^{125}I-CmTx), antibodies to P/Q-type VGCC antibodies were demonstrated in >85% of clinically definite LEMS patients (Lennon et al., 1995; Motomura et al., 1995).

About 50% of patients with LEMS have small cell lung cancer (SCLC) and these tumors express VGCC on their surface, and presumably it is the immune response to the tumor that leads to these antibodies. In fact LEMS is considered to be one of the most typical paraneoplastic diseases. The VGCC antibodies in the remaining 50% of patients appear to be the result of a spontaneous autoimmune disease, similar to early onset MG.

The pathogenicity of the VGCC antibodies is clear from passive transfer and cell culture studies (e.g., Roberts et al., 1985). However, VGCC antibodies can also be found at low levels in some patients with lung cancer without neurological dysfunction, including SCLC-associated cerebellar ataxia (Graus et al., 2003). In these cases the antibodies are probably acting as markers for the presence of the tumor rather than playing a pathogenic role, since the patients do not generally improve with immunosuppressive therapies.

It is not certain where on the VGCC α-subunit the antibodies bind. Some attempts to define the binding of antibodies to different peptides representing the VGCC sequence have suggested binding to an extracellular region (Takamori et al., 1998), but it is not clear what proportion of the patients' antibodies bind to this site. Some patients' sera also bind to synaptotagmin, and immunization against VGCC and synaptotagmin, peptides has induced the electrophysiological changes of LEMS (Takamori et al., 1998; Komai et al., 1999; Iwasa et al., 2000).

The antibodies reduce VGCC channel function in cell lines (Roberts et al., 1986; Meriney et al., 1996; Pinto et al., 1998) and most evidence suggests that this is by cross-linking the channels and leading to their internalization. This is partly because the effects take time to develop, as in similar studies in MG (see above), and are dependent on cross-linking by divalent antibody and independent of complement (Peers et al., 1990). Interestingly, when sera are applied to cultured cell lines overnight, there is often a compensatory upregulation of other VGCCs (e.g., N and R type), as if to compensate for the loss of P/Q-type VGCC (Pinto et al., 1998).

References

Aarli JA, Romi F, Skeie GO, et al. (2003). Myasthenia gravis in individuals over 40. Ann N Y Acad Sci 998: 424–431.

Almon RR, Andrew CG, Appel SH (1974). Serum globulin in myasthenia gravis: inhibition of α-bungarotoxin binding to acetylcholine receptors. Science 186: 55–57.

Beeson D, Jacobson L, Newsom-Davis J, et al. (1996). A transfected human muscle cell line expressing the adult subtype of the human muscle acetylcholine receptor for diagnostic assays in myasthenia gravis. Neurology 47: 1552–1555.

Beeson D, Higuchi O, Palace J, et al. (2006). Dok-7 mutations underlie a neuromuscular junction synaptopathy. Science 313: 1975–1978.

Bender AN, Ringel SP, Engel WK, et al. (1976). Immunoperoxidase localization of α-bungarotoxin: a new approach to myasthenia gravis. Ann N Y Acad Sci 274: 20–30.

Benveniste O, Jacobson L, Farrugia ME, et al. (2005). MuSK antibody positive myasthenia gravis plasma modifies MURF-1 expression in C2C12 cultures and mouse muscle in vivo. J Neuroimmunol 170: 41–48.

Blaes F, Beeson D, Plested P, et al. (2000). IgG from "seronegative" myasthenia gravis patients binds to a muscle cell line, TE671, but not to human acetylcholine receptor. Ann Neurol 47: 504–510.

Boneva N, Frenkian-Cuvelier M, Bidault J, et al. (2006). Major pathogenic effects of anti-MuSK antibodies in myasthenia gravis. J Neuroimmunol 177: 119–131.

Bray JJ, Drachman DB (1982). Binding affinities of anti-acetylcholine receptor autoantibodies in myasthenia gravis. J Immunol 128: 105–110.

Brooks EB, Pachner AR, Drachman DB, et al. (1990). A sensitive rosetting assay for detection of acetylcholine receptor antibodies using BC3H-1 cells: positive results in "antibody-negative" myasthenia gravis. J Neuroimmunol 28: 83–93.

Buckley C, Newsom-Davis J, Willcox N, et al. (2001). Do titin and cytokine antibodies in MG patients predict thymoma or thymoma recurrence? Neurology 57: 1579–1582.

Bufler J, Pitz R, Czep M, et al. (1998). Purified IgG from seropositive and seronegative patients with mysasthenia gravis reversibly blocks currents through nicotinic acetylcholine receptor channels. Ann Neurol 43: 458–464.

Burges J, Vincent A, Molenaar PC, et al. (1994). Passive transfer of seronegative myasthenia gravis to mice. Muscle Nerve 17: 1393–1400.

Chiu HC, Vincent A, Newsom-Davis J, et al. (1987). Myasthenia gravis: population differences in disease expression and acetylcholine receptor antibody titers between Chinese and Caucasians. Neurology 37: 1854–1857.

Dalton P, Clover L, Wallerstein R, et al. (2006). Fetal arthrogryposis and maternal serum antibodies. Neuromuscul Disord 16: 481–491.

DeChiara TM, Bowen DC, Valenzuela DM, et al. (1996). The receptor tyrosine kinase MuSK is required for neuromuscular junction formation in vivo. Cell 85: 501–512.

Drachman DB, Angus CW, Adams RN, et al. (1978). Myasthenic antibodies cross-link acetylcholine receptors to accelerate degradation. N Engl J Med 298: 1116–1122.

Elmqvist D, Lambert EH (1968). Detailed analysis of neuromuscular transmission in a patient with the myasthenic syndrome sometimes associated with bronchogenic carcinoma. Mayo Clin Proc 43: 689–713.

Engel AG (1984). Myasthenia gravis and myasthenic syndromes. Ann Neurol 16: 519–534.

Engel AG, Lambert EH, Howard FM (1977). Immune complexes (IgG and C3) at the motor end-plate in myasthenia gravis: ultrastructural and light microscopic localization and electrophysiologic correlations. Mayo Clin Proc 52: 267–280.

Evoli A, Tonali PA, Padua L, et al. (2003). Clinical correlates with anti-MuSK antibodies in generalized seronegative myasthenia gravis. Brain 126: 2304–2311.

Fambrough DM, Drachman DB, Satyamurti S (1973). Neuromuscular junction in myasthenia gravis: decreased acetylcholine receptors. Science 182: 293–295.

Farrugia ME, Kennett RP, Newsom-Davis J, et al. (2006a). Single-fiber electromyography in limb and facial muscles in muscle-specific kinase antibody and acetylcholine receptor antibody myasthenia gravis. Muscle Nerve 33: 568–570.

Farrugia ME, Robson MD, Clover L, et al. (2006b). MRI and clinical studies of facial and bulbar muscle involvement in MuSK antibody-associated myasthenia gravis. Brain 129: 1481–1492.

Farrugia ME, Kennett RP, Hilton-Jones D, et al. (2007). Quantitative EMG of facial muscles in myasthenia patients with MuSK antibodies. Clin Neurophysiol 118: 269–277.

Fukunaga H, Engel AG, Lang B, et al. (1983). Passive transfer of Lambert–Eaton myasthenic syndrome with IgG from man to mouse depletes the presynaptic membrane active zones. Proc Natl Acad Sci U S A 80: 7636–7640.

Fukuoka T, Engel AG, Lang B, et al. (1987a). Lambert–Eaton myasthenic syndrome: I. Early morphological effects of IgG on the presynaptic membrane active zones. Ann Neurol 22: 193–199.

Fukuoka T, Engel AG, Lang B, et al. (1987b). Lambert–Eaton myasthenic syndrome: II. Immunoelectron microscopy localization of IgG at the mouse motor end-plate. Ann Neurol 22: 200–211.

Gattenlohner S, Schneider C, Thamer C, et al. (2002). Expression of foetal type acetylcholine receptor is restricted to type 1 muscle fibres in human neuromuscular disorders. Brain 125: 1309–1319.

Gotti C, Balestra B, Mantegazza R, et al. (1997). Detection of antibody classes and subpopulations in myasthenia gravis patients using a new nonradioactive enzyme immunoassay. Muscle Nerve 20: 800–808.

Graus F, Lang B, Pozo-Rosich P, et al. (2002). P/Q type calcium-channel antibodies in paraneoplastic cerebellar degeneration with lung cancer. Neurology 59: 764–766.

Hewer R, Matthews I, Chen S, et al. (2006). A sensitive non-isotopic assay for acetylcholine receptor autoantibodies. Clin Chim Acta 364: 159–166.

Hoch W, McConville J, Helms S, et al. (2001). Auto-antibodies to the receptor tyrosine kinase MuSK in patients with myasthenia gravis without acetylcholine receptor antibodies. Nat Med 7: 365–368.

Howard FM Jr., Lennon VA, Finley J, et al. (1987). Clinical correlations of antibodies that bind, block, or modulate human acetylcholine receptors in myasthenia gravis. Ann N Y Acad Sci 505: 526–538.

Iwasa K, Takamori M, Komai K, et al. (2000). Recombinant calcium channel is recognized by Lambert–Eaton myasthenic syndrome antibodies. Neurology 54: 757–759.

Jacobson L, Beeson D, Tzartos S, et al. (1999a). Monoclonal antibodies raised against human acetylcholine receptor bind to all five subunits of the fetal isoform. J Neuroimmunol 98: 112–120.

Jacobson L, Polizzi A, Morriss-Kay G, et al. (1999b). Plasma from human mothers of fetuses with severe arthrogryposis multiplex congenita causes deformities in mice. J Clin Invest 103: 1031–1038.

Jha S, Xu K, Maruta T, et al. (2006). Myasthenia gravis induced in mice by immunization with the recombinant extracellular domain of rat muscle-specific kinase (MuSK). J Neuroimmunol 175: 107–117.

Komai K, Iwasa K, Takamori M (1999). Calcium channel peptide can cause an autoimmune-mediated model of Lambert–Eaton myasthenic syndrome in rats. J Neurol Sci 166: 126–130.

Kong XC, Barzaghi P, Ruegg MA (2004). Inhibition of synapse assembly in mammalian muscle in vivo by RNA interference. EMBO Rep 5: 183–188.

Kuks JB, Oosterhuis HJ, Limburg PC, et al. (1991). Anti-acetylcholine receptor antibodies decrease after thymectomy in patients with myasthenia gravis. Clinical correlations. J Autoimmun 4: 197–211.

Lambert EH, Elmqvist D (1971). Quantal components of end-plate potentials in the myasthenic syndrome. Ann N Y Acad Sci 183: 183–199.

Lang B, Newsom-Davis J, Peers C, et al. (1987). The effect of myasthenic syndrome antibody on presynaptic calcium channels in the mouse. J Physiol 390: 257–270.

Lang B, Richardson G, Rees J, et al. (1988). Plasma from myasthenia gravis patients reduces acetylcholine receptor agonist-induced Na+ flux into TE671 cell line. J Neuroimmunol 19: 141–148.

Lauriola L, Ranelletti F, Maggiano N, et al. (2005). Thymus changes in anti-MuSK-positive and -negative myasthenia gravis. Neurology 64: 536–538.

Leite MI, Strobel P, Jones M, et al. (2005). Fewer thymic changes in MuSK antibody-positive than in MuSK antibody-negative MG. Ann Neurol 57: 444–448.

Leite MI, et al. (2007). Myasthenia gravis thymus: complement vulnerability of epithelial and myoid cells, complement attack on them, and correlations with autoantibody status. Am J Pathol 171: 893–905.

Leite MI, Jacob S, Viegas S, et al. (2007). IgG1 antibodies to acetylcholine receptors in "seronegative" MG. (submitted)

Lennon VA, Kryzer TJ, Griesmann GE, et al. (1995). Calcium-channel antibodies in the Lambert–Eaton syndrome and other paraneoplastic syndromes. N Engl J Med 332: 1467–1474.

Li Z, Forester N, Vincent A (1996). Modulation of acetylcholine receptor function in TE671 (rhabdomyosarcoma) cells by non-AChR ligands: possible relevance to seronegative myasthenia gravis. J Neuroimmunol 64: 179–183.

Lindstrom JM, Seybold ME, Lennon VA, et al. (1976). Antibody to acetylcholine receptor in myasthenia gravis. Prevalence, clinical correlates, and diagnostic value. Neurology 26: 1054–1059.

Lu CZ, Link H, Mo XA, et al. (1991). Anti-presynaptic membrane receptor antibodies in myasthenia gravis. J Neurol Sci 102: 39–45.

McConville J, Farrugia ME, Beeson D, et al. (2004). Detection and characterization of MuSK antibodies in seronegative myasthenia gravis. Ann Neurol 55: 580–584.

Meager A, Wadhwa M, Bird C, et al. (1999). Spontaneously occurring neutralizing antibodies against granulocyte-macrophage colony-stimulating factor in patients with autoimmune disease. Immunology 97: 526–532.

Meriney SD, Hulsizer SC, Lennon VA, et al. (1996). Lambert–Eaton myasthenic syndrome immunoglobulins react with multiple types of calcium channels in small-cell lung carcinoma. Ann Neurol 40: 739–749.

Mier AK, Havard CW (1985). Diaphragmatic myasthenia in mother and child. Postgrad Med J 61: 725–727.

Mossman S, Vincent A, Newsom-Davis J (1986). Myasthenia gravis without acetylcholine-receptor antibody: a distinct disease entity. Lancet 1: 116–119.

Motomura M, Johnston I, Lang B, et al. (1995). An improved diagnostic assay for Lambert–Eaton myasthenic syndrome. J Neurol Neurosurg Psychiatry 58: 85–87.

Nastuk WL, Strauss AJ, Osserman KE (1959). Search for a neuromuscular blocking agent in the blood of patients with myasthenia gravis. Am J Med 26: 394–409.

Nastuk WL, Plescia OJ, Osserman KE (1960). Changes in serum complement activity in patients with myasthenia gravis. Proc Soc Exp Biol Med 105: 177–184.

Nemoto Y, Kuwabara S, Misawa S, et al. (2005). Patterns and severity of neuromuscular transmission failure in seronegative myasthenia gravis. J Neurol Neurosurg Psychiatry 76: 714–718.

Newsom-Davis J, Pinching AJ, Vincent A, et al. (1978). Function of circulating antibody to acetylcholine receptor in myasthenia gravis: investigation by plasma exchange. Neurology 28: 266–272.

Niks EH, Kuks JB, Roep BO, et al. (2006). Strong association of MuSK antibody-positive myasthenia gravis and HLA-DR14-DQ5. Neurology 66: 1772–1774.

Oh SJ, Hatanaka Y, Hemmi S, et al. (2006). Repetitive nerve stimulation of facial muscles in MuSK antibody-positive myasthenia gravis. Muscle Nerve 33: 500–504.

Ohta K, Fujinami A, Saida T, et al. (2003). Frequency of anti-AChR ε subunit-specific antibodies in MG. Autoimmunity 36: 151–154.

Patrick J, Lindstrom J (1973). Autoimmune response to acetylcholine receptor. Science 180: 871–872.

Peers C, Johnston I, Lang B, et al. (1993). Cross-linking of presynaptic calcium channels: a mechanism of action for

Lambert–Eaton myasthenic syndrome antibodies at the mouse neuromuscular junction. Neurosci Lett 153: 45–48.

Pinching AJ, Peters DK (1976). Remission of myasthenia gravis following plasma-exchange. Lancet 2: 1373–1376.

Pinto A, Gillard S, Moss F, et al. (1998). Human autoantibodies specific for the alpha1A calcium channel subunit reduce both P-type and Q-type calcium currents in cerebellar neurons. Proc Natl Acad Sci U S A 95: 8328–8333.

Plested CP, Tang T, Spreadbury I, et al. (2002). AChR phosphorylation and indirect inhibition of AChR function in seronegative MG. Neurology 59: 1682–1688.

Polizzi A, Huson SM, Vincent A (2000). Teratogen update: maternal myasthenia gravis as a cause of congenital arthrogryposis. Teratology 62: 332–341.

Riemersma S, Vincent A, Beeson D, et al. (1996). Association of arthrogryposis multiplex congenita with maternal antibodies inhibiting fetal acetylcholine receptor function. J Clin Invest 98: 2358–2363.

Roberts A, Perera S, Lang B, et al. (1985). Paraneoplastic myasthenic syndrome IgG inhibits $45Ca^{2+}$ flux in a human small cell carcinoma line. Nature 317: 737–739.

Rodgaard A, Nielsen FC, Djurup R, et al. (1987). Acetylcholine receptor antibody in myasthenia gravis: predominance of IgG subclasses 1 and 3. Clin Exp Immunol 67: 82–88.

Romi F, Skeie GO, Aarli JA, et al. (2000). Muscle autoantibodies in subgroups of myasthenia gravis patients. J Neurol 247: 369–375.

Sahashi K, Engel AG, Linstrom JM, et al. (1978). Ultrastructural localization of immune complexes (IgG and C3) at the end-plate in experimental autoimmune myasthenia gravis. J Neuropathol Exp Neurol 37: 212–223.

Sanders DB, El-Salem K, Massey JM, et al. (2003). Clinical aspects of MuSK antibody positive seronegative MG. Neurology 60: 1978–1980.

Scuderi F, Marino M, Colonna L, et al. (2002). Anti-p110 autoantibodies identify a subtype of "seronegative" myasthenia gravis with prominent oculobulbar involvement. Lab Invest 82: 1139–1146.

Selcen D, Fukuda T, Shen XM, et al. (2004). Are MuSK antibodies the primary cause of myasthenic symptoms? Neurology 62: 1945–1950.

Sher E, Gotti C, Canal N, et al. (1989). Specificity of calcium channel autoantibodies in Lambert–Eaton myasthenic syndrome. Lancet 2: 640–643.

Shigemoto K, Kubo S, Maruyama N, et al. (2006). Induction of myasthenia by immunization against muscle-specific kinase. J Clin Invest 116: 1016–1024.

Shiraishi H, Motomura M, Yoshimura T, et al. (2005). Acetylcholine receptors loss and postsynaptic damage in MuSK antibody-positive myasthenia gravis. Ann Neurol 57: 289–293.

Simpson JA (1960). Myasthenia gravis, a new hypothesis. Scott Med J 5: 419–436.

Skeie GO, Aarli JA, Gilhus NE (2006). Titin and ryanodine receptor antibodies in myasthenia gravis. Acta Neurol Scand Suppl 183: 19–23.

Spreadbury I, Kishore U, Beeson D, et al. (2005). Inhibition of acetylcholine receptor function by seronegative myasthenia gravis non-IgG factor correlates with desensitisation. J Neuroimmunol 162: 149–156.

Stanley EF, Drachman DB (1978). Effect of myasthenic immunoglobulin on acetylcholine receptors of intact mammalian neuromuscular junctions. Science 200: 1285–1287.

Sthoeger Z, Neiman A, Elbirt D, et al. (2006). High prevalence of systemic lupus erythematosus in 78 myasthenia gravis patients: a clinical and serologic study. Am J Med Sci 331: 4–9.

Takamori M, Hamada T, Komai K, et al. (1994). Synaptotagmin can cause an immune-mediated model of Lambert–Eaton myasthenic syndrome in rats. Ann Neurol 35: 74–80.

Takamori M, Iwasa K, Komai K (1997). Antibodies to synthetic peptides of the $\alpha 1A$ subunit of the voltage-gated calcium channel in Lambert–Eaton myasthenic syndrome. Neurology 48: 1261–1265.

Takamori M, Iwasa K, Komai K (1998). Antigenic sites of the voltage-gated calcium channel in Lambert–Eaton myasthenic syndrome. Ann N Y Acad Sci 841: 625–635.

Tellez-Zenteno JF, Cardenas G, Estanol B, et al. (2004). Associated conditions in myasthenia gravis: response to thymectomy. Eur J Neurol 11: 767–773.

Toth C, McDonald D, Oger J, et al. (2006). Acetylcholine receptor antibodies in myasthenia gravis are associated with greater risk of diabetes and thyroid disease. Acta Neurol Scand 114: 124–132.

Toyka KV, Brachman DB, Pestronk A, et al. (1975). Myasthenia gravis: passive transfer from man to mouse. Science 190: 397–399.

Tzartos SJ, Barkas T, Cung MT, et al. (1998). Anatomy of the antigenic structure of a large membrane autoantigen, the muscle-type nicotinic acetylcholine receptor. Immunol Rev 163: 89–120.

Valenzuela DM, Stitt TN, DiStefano PS, et al. (1995). Receptor tyrosine kinase specific for the skeletal muscle lineage: expression in embryonic muscle, at the neuromuscular junction, and after injury. Neuron 15: 573–584.

Vincent A (2002). Unravelling the pathogenesis of myasthenia gravis. Nat Rev Immunol 2: 797–804.

Vincent A, Newsom-Davis J (1982a). Acetylcholine receptor antibody characteristics in myasthenia gravis. I. Patients with generalized myasthenia or disease restricted to ocular muscles. Clin Exp Immunol 49: 257–265.

Vincent A, Newsom-Davis J (1982b). Acetylcholine receptor antibody characteristics in myasthenia gravis. II. Patients with penicillamine-induced myasthenia or idiopathic myasthenia of recent onset. Clin Exp Immunol 49: 266–272.

Vincent A, Newsom-Davis J, Newton P, et al. (1983). Acetylcholine receptor antibody and clinical response to thymectomy in myasthenia gravis. Neurology 33: 1276–1282.

Vincent A, Newsom-Davis J (1985). Acetylcholine receptor antibody as a diagnostic test for myasthenia gravis: results in 153 validated cases and 2967 diagnostic assays. J Neurol Neurosurg Psychiatry 48: 1246–1252.

Vincent A, Whiting PJ, Schluep M, et al. (1987). Antibody heterogeneity and specificity in myasthenia gravis. Ann N Y Acad Sci 505: 106–120.

Vincent A, Newland C, Brueton L, et al. (1995). Arthrogryposis multiplex congenita with maternal autoantibodies specific for a fetal antigen. Lancet 346: 24–25.

Vincent A, Bowen J, Newsom-Davis J, et al. (2003). Seronegative generalised myasthenia gravis: clinical features, antibodies, and their targets. Lancet Neurol 2: 99–106.

Vincent A, Clover L, Buckley C, et al. (2003). Evidence of underdiagnosis of myasthenia gravis in older people. J Neurol Neurosurg Psychiatry 74: 1105–1108.

Whiting PJ, Vincent A, Newsom-Davis J (1983). Acetylcholine receptor antibody characteristics in myasthenia gravis. Fractionation of α-bungarotoxin binding site antibodies and their relationship to IgG subclass. J Neuroimmunol 5: 1–9.

Yamamoto T, Sato T, Sugita H (1987). Antifilamin, antivinculin, and antitropomyosin antibodies in myasthenia gravis. Neurology 37: 1329–1333.

Yamamoto T, Vincent A, Ciulla TA, et al. (1991). Seronegative myasthenia gravis: a plasma factor inhibiting agonist-induced acetylcholine receptor function copurifies with IgM. Ann Neurol 30: 550–557.

Zhang X, Yang M, Xu J, et al. (2007). Clinical and serological study of myasthenia gravis in HuBei province, China. J Neurol Neurosurg Psychiatry 78: 386–390.

Handbook of Clinical Neurology, Vol. 91 (3rd series)
Neuromuscular junction disorders
A.G. Engel, Editor

Chapter 7

Clinical features of myasthenia gravis

DONALD B. SANDERS* AND JANICE M. MASSEY

Duke University Medical School, Durham, NC, USA

7.1. Introduction

In few diseases of the nervous system is the early diagnosis and treatment more critical and more gratifying than in myasthenia gravis (MG). To assure early diagnosis, it is essential that the typical clinical features be recognized so that appropriate treatment can be instituted.

7.2. Clinical presentations of MG

Almost all patients with MG seek medical attention because of dysfunction referable to specific muscles. Although they may also complain of generalized fatigue, this is rarely the major or presenting complaint.

7.2.1. Symptoms

"With one auspicious and one dropping eye."
As You Like It
"Methinks I see these things with parted eye, when every thing seems double." A Midsummer Night's Dream

Blurred vision, frank diplopia or eyelid ptosis is the initial symptom in about 60% of patients with MG (Grob et al., 1981; Kuks and Oosterhuis, 2004), and most of the others have these symptoms within 2 years of onset (Table 7.1). Lid ptosis typically begins unilaterally, but the other lid may become worse later—such alternating lid ptosis is virtually diagnostic of MG. Symptoms of oropharyngeal ("bulbar") muscle weakness—difficulty chewing, swallowing, or talking—are present at onset in about 20% of patients (Grob et al., 1981; Kuks and Oosterhuis, 2004) (Table 7.1). About 20% of patients begin with weakness of single

muscle groups, such as neck or finger extensors, hip flexors or ankle dorsiflexors (Grob et al., 1981; Kuks and Oosterhuis, 2004) (Table 7.1). Respiratory dysfunction is rarely the first symptom of MG with the exception of some patients with MuSK antibody positive MG (see below). Isolated dysphagia is rarely the initial symptom in MG (Llabres et al., 2005).

A careful history often uncovers symptoms of previously unappreciated myasthenic weakness, such as: frequent purchases of new eyeglasses to correct blurred vision; avoidance of foods that have become difficult to chew or swallow; or cessation of activities that require prolonged use of affected muscles, such as singing or public speaking. Friends or family members may have observed a sleepy or sad facial appearance due to lid ptosis or facial weakness. Many patients do not appreciate how long they have had MG until treatment has relieved their symptoms.

Exaggerated fatigability is the hallmark of abnormal neuromuscular transmission—symptoms typically are less in the morning or after rest, and become more pronounced as the day goes on or after prolonged use of the affected muscles. Ocular symptoms become worse after reading or watching television or in bright light—many patients use dark glasses to reduce diplopia and hide drooping eyelids. Speech becomes nasal or slurred after prolonged talking—patients with these symptoms are frequently accused of being intoxicated. Difficulty swallowing may be worse with liquids, which may regurgitate through the nose. Food may stick in the back of the throat, or worse, be aspirated. Frequent coughing while eating is a worrisome sign of aspiration. Chewing may worsen during meals, particularly with meat, and patients may have to use a hand to assist in closing the jaw while eating. Difficulty eating may lead to otherwise unexplained weight loss.

*Correspondence to: Donald B. Sanders, MD, Professor of Medicine (Neurology), Duke University Medical School, Box 3403, Duke University Medical Center, Durham, NC 27710, USA. E-mail: Donald.Sanders@Duke.edu, Tel: 1-919-684-6078, Fax: 1-919-660-3853.

Table 7.1

Initial symptoms as recorded from 919 patients in the Duke MG Clinic

Ocular (ptosis, diplopia)	643 (70%)
Bulbar (dysarthria, dysphagia, difficulty chewing)	200 (22%)
Isolated limb or axial muscle weakness	50 (5.4%)

7.2.2. Physical findings

The examination of patients with suspected MG is performed to detect variable weakness in certain muscle groups. Strength should be assessed repetitively during maximum effort and again after a brief rest. Fluctuating strength is best shown by examining ocular and oropharyngeal muscle functions as these are less likely to be affected by effort, pain or other factors.

7.2.2.1. Mental status

The mental status is normal unless there is oxygen deprivation due to respiratory compromise. Patients with air hunger have frequent yawning and sighing.

7.2.2.2. Ocular muscle examination

Ocular muscles are usually involved in MG and are uniquely suited for direct observation of weakness. Asymmetrical weakness of several muscles in both eyes is typical. The pattern of weakness does not usually fit that of lesions affecting one or more individual nerves and pupillary reactions are normal.

Eyelid ptosis is easily observed during the interview and examination. Ptosis is usually asymmetric and varies during sustained activity. When ptosis is mild or subtle, frontalis muscle contraction may be a clue that eyelid elevation is not normal (Figs. 7.1A, 7.2). Several maneuvers have been described to demonstrate or exacerbate lid ptosis in MG: prolonged gaze up or to the side, passive elevation of the opposite lid (Cogan, 1965) (Fig. 7.3), even forced or repeated eye closure (Osserman, 1958). The salient feature is variability of ptosis, which is manifest as worsening after these maneuvers and rapid recovery after rest. Other observations that support a diagnosis of MG include the "lid twitch sign" (characterized by one or more twitches of the upper eyelid when the eyes are directed downwards and then returned to the primary position), quick lid retraction after refixation to the primary position from sustained downgaze (Cogan, 1965) and improvement of ptosis in response to eyelid cooling—the "ice pack test" (Sethi et al., 1987). Unsustained nystagmus, exophthalmos, and amblyopia are rare manifestations

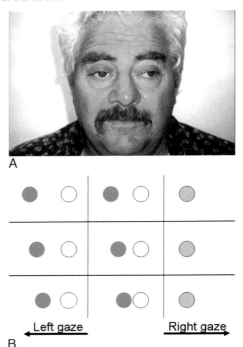

A

B

Left gaze ←   Right gaze →

Fig. 7.1. (A) MG. Bilateral lid ptosis, which is partially corrected by contraction of the frontalis muscle bilaterally. The right eye does not move medially beyond the mid-position as he looks to his left. (B) The images as the patient sees them in the cardinal fields of gaze with a red lens over the right eye; there is horizontal diplopia that increases on looking to his left and up.

of ocular muscle weakness in MG (Walsh and Hoyt, 1969; Ellenhorn et al., 1986; Mullaney et al., 2000).

Particular attention should be paid to diplopia or visible divergence of the eyes. The second image may be suppressed if acuity is poor or divergence is extreme or has been present for many years. The medial rectus is the most frequently involved ocular muscle, producing horizontal diplopia when looking to the opposite side. When moderate or severe, limited medial movement of the affected eye can be directly

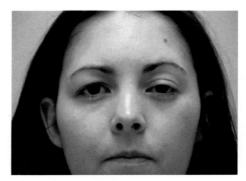

Fig. 7.2. MG. Mild left lid ptosis, which is partially compensated by asymmetric contraction of the left frontalis, which elevates the left eyebrow.

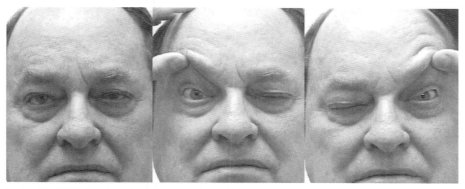

Fig. 7.3. "Curtain sign" in MG. Passive elevation of each eyelid in turn unmasks or exaggerates ptosis in the contralateral lid.

observed and is typically worse after prolonged gaze. More subtle weakness of the medial rectus can be brought out by covering the adducting eye for several seconds, then observing the position and movement of that eye immediately after uncovering it. When covered, the eye drifts toward the midline, then jerks back in the direction of gaze when uncovered. Sustained activation of any paretic ocular muscle may produce nystagmoid movements in the direction of gaze as the paretic muscle fatigues. Concomitant weakness of the medial rectus and the contralateral lateral rectus can produce a "pseudo-internuclear ophthalmoplegia," a common finding in MG that may be mistakenly attributed to multiple sclerosis (Glaser, 1966). During upgaze the medial rectus normally holds the eyes in conjugate gaze against the lateral pull of the superior rectus. When the medial rectus is weak, as in MG, the eyes tend to diverge with upgaze, and this is exaggerated if one eye is covered. After the medial rectus, the superior rectus is the next most frequently involved muscle, producing vertical diplopia that is worse or present only during upgaze. When several ocular muscles are weak, as is usually the case, more complex patterns of diplopia are seen. With red lens testing the relative positions of the images from each eye can be diagrammed (Fig. 7.1B), thus identifying the weak muscles and quantifying the diplopia. These findings may fluctuate over a short period of time.

7.2.2.3. Oropharyngeal and facial muscle examination

Weakness of the oropharyngeal muscles causes changes in the voice, difficulty chewing and swallowing and inadequate protection of the upper airway. Nasal speech is common, especially after prolonged talking, and liquids may escape through the nose when swallowing because of palatal muscle weakness. Weakness of the laryngeal muscles causes hoarseness and difficulty making a high-pitched "eeeee" sound.

Difficulty swallowing is detected from a history of frequent choking or throat clearing or coughing after eating.

Weakness of facial muscles produces a characteristic facial appearance—at rest, the corners of the mouth droop downward, making the patient appear depressed. Attempts to smile often produce contraction of the medial portion of the upper lip and a horizontal contraction of the corners of the mouth without the natural upward curling, which gives the appearance of a sneer (Fig. 7.4).

Jaw weakness can be shown by having the patient bite on a tongue blade, or by manually opening the jaw against resistance, which is not normally possible. The patient may support a weak jaw with the thumb under the chin, the middle finger curled under the nose or lower lip and the index finger extended up the cheek, producing a studious or attentive appearance.

Eyelid closure is almost always weak in MG, even when strength is normal in all other facial muscles, and may be the only residual weakness in those with otherwise complete remission. This is usually asymptomatic unless it is severe enough to allow soap or water in the eyes during bathing. With moderate

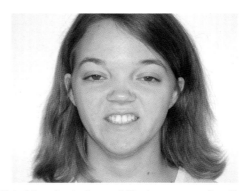

Fig. 7.4. Myasthenic "sneer." During attempted smile, there is contraction of the medial portion of the upper lip and horizontal contraction of the corners of the mouth without the natural upward curling.

weakness of these muscles, the patient does not "bury" the eyelashes during forced eye closure. Fatigue in eye closure as the patient tries to keep the eyes gently closed may result in slight involuntary opening of the eyes, the so-called "peek" sign (Fig. 7.5) (Osher and Griggs, 1979).

Tongue weakness produces slurred speech and can be assessed by having the patient push the tongue against the inside of the cheek while the examiner presses against the cheek. Chronic, untreated weakness of the tongue may result in severe lingual atrophy (De Assis et al., 1994), which classically has a "triple furrowed" appearance.

Patients with respiratory insufficiency may frequently yawn or sigh deeply. Vital capacity can be estimated by having the patient count out loud as far as possible on a single breath—counts more than 30 usually indicate adequate breathing capacity. Producing a vigorous cough assesses both diaphragm and laryngeal muscle function. Producing a sharp sniff assesses negative inspiratory function. Formal pulmonary function tests (e.g., spirometry) quantify respiratory effort and pulse oximetry quantifies oxygen saturation. However, it should be kept in mind that these tests measure function only at one point in time and the weakness in MG characteristically fluctuates. It is important to look for trends in these functions that may indicate deterioration.

7.2.2.4. Limb muscle examination

Any trunk or limb muscle can be weak in MG but some are more often affected than others. Neck flexors are usually weaker than neck extensors and the deltoids, triceps, extensors of the wrist and fingers and dorsiflexors of the ankle are frequently weaker than other limb muscles. In 5–10% of patients, symptomatic weakness begins in one or more of these limb muscles, producing a clinical pattern more suggestive of a neuropathy or focal myopathy. Unless weakness

has been untreated for a long time, muscles are not usually atrophic, which helps distinguish nerve disease. Muscle stretch reflexes are not reduced.

Pain is not a prominent feature of MG, though severe weakness of neck extensors may be accompanied by local pain.

7.2.3. Course

MG follows a variable course but usually progresses in severity and distribution of weakness during the first 1–2 years. Early on, spontaneous improvement is common, even for long periods, but these "remissions" are rarely permanent.

Weakness remains restricted to the ocular muscles in 10–16% of cases (Grob et al., 1981; Kuks and Oosterhuis, 2004) (see Section 7.8.1). Most patients develop oropharyngeal or limb muscle weakness, which reaches maximum severity during the first year in two-thirds of patients. Without treatment, weakness may become fixed and severely involved muscles may atrophy, but this is rarely seen today except in patients with MuSK antibody-positive myasthenia (see 7.8.3.1).

Many factors may worsen myasthenic symptoms—systemic illness (especially viral respiratory infections with fever), hypothyroidism or hyperthyroidism, pregnancy, the menstrual cycle, drugs that affect neuromuscular transmission, increased body temperature, and emotional upset. Vaccinations and insect bites may precipitate onset or exaggerate symptoms. Neuromuscular blocking agents used during surgery have heightened and prolonged effects in MG and the disease may be revealed when a patient requires prolonged ventilatory support after receiving these during surgery. Some antibiotics, antiarrhythmics (quinine, quinidine and procainamide), and β-adrenergic blocking drugs that compromise neuromuscular transmission may increase weakness in MG (see Chapter 12).

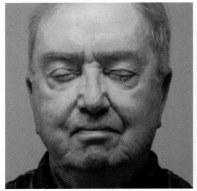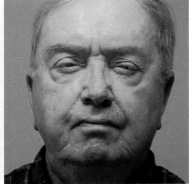

Fig. 7.5. "Peek" sign in MG. During sustained forced eyelid closure he is unable to bury his eyelashes (left) and, after 30 s, he is unable to keep the lids fully closed (right).

7.2.4. Associated diseases

MG often occurs in association with other immune-mediated diseases, especially hyperthyroidism and rheumatoid arthritis (Christensen et al., 1995). The incidence of autoimmune disorders is increased in MG patients with thymic hyperplasia but not in those with thymoma (Aarli et al., 1992); autoimmune diseases have been reported to be equally frequent in seropositive and seronegative MG (Vujic et al., 2004) and are also common among family members of MG patients (Kerzin-Storrar et al., 1988).

Systemic lupus erythematosus (Thorlacius et al., 1989) and multiple sclerosis (Isbister et al., 2003) have been reported to occur more often in MG than by chance alone. Seizures have been reported to occur with increased frequency in children with MG (see Section 7.8.2).

Patients with thymoma, with and without MG, have a higher incidence of extrathymic malignancy (Evoli et al., 2004); this higher incidence has not been found in non-thymomatous MG (Monden et al., 1991; Evoli et al., 1998b).

Psychiatric disturbance occurs often in MG, in particular adjustment disorders with depressed mood and mixed emotional features, affective disorders and personality disorders (Magni et al., 1988).

A small number of patients have been described with onset of MG during the course of HIV infection (Wessel and Zitelli, 1987; Nath et al., 1990; Martini et al., 1991; Tiab et al., 1993; Wullenweber et al., 1993; Authier et al., 1995). Of seven reported patients, four had acetylcholine receptor (AChR) antibodies and five had marked improvement or remission as CD4 counts dropped with progression of AIDS. This rare occurrence of MG with HIV infection is likely coincidental. Immune mechanisms producing MG in these patients have been proposed based on the affinity of HIV for the thymus (Derossi et al., 1990). MG occurred early in the course of HIV infection in these patients, suggesting that it may have been the initial manifestation of AIDS seroconversion, as has also been reported with HIV inflammatory demyelinating polyneuropathy and HIV inflammatory myopathy (Gherardi et al., 1995).

7.3. Pathophysiology of MG

In most patients with MG, weakness results from the effects of circulating anti-AChR antibodies. Binding to AChR is on the terminal expansions of the junctional folds (Fig. 7.6). These antibodies cause complement-mediated destruction of the folds, accelerated internalization and destruction of AChR by antigenic

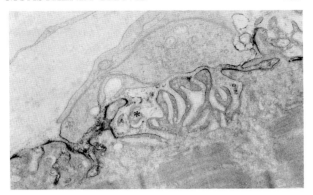

Fig. 7.6. Localization of IgG at a neuromuscular junction in MG. The immune deposits appear on short segments of some junctional folds and on degenerate material in the synaptic space. (From Engel et al., 1977a, with permission.)

modulation, and, in some cases, blocking of the binding of acetylcholine (ACh) to AChR. Destruction of the junctional folds results in distortion and simplification of the postsynaptic region (Fig. 7.6) (see Chapter 5). Approximately 10% of patients carry circulating antibodies to muscle specific tyrosine kinase (MuSK) instead of antibodies directed against AChR. The pathophysiological role of the anti-MuSK antibodies is yet to be determined. No specific antibodies have been identified in the remaining seronegative patients.

7.4. Epidemiology, age and gender

The incidence of MG estimated from a 1992 study in Virginia was 9 to 10 new cases per million population per year, and the estimated prevalence was 14.2 per 100 000 (Phillips et al., 1992). Later studies reported prevalence rates as high as 20.4 per 100 000, in British Columbia (Isbister et al., 2002). Based on these numbers, it is estimated that there are from 26 000 to 56 000 MG patients in the US (Phillips, 2003). The incidence of MG has increased progressively over the past 50 years, due in part to better diagnostic techniques and treatments.

The demographics of MG differ among different reports and are affected by referral patterns and other factors that determine patient recognition. In our clinic, the distribution of onset age among the 869 patients without thymoma follows the classic pattern, most women having symptom onset in the third decade, and men in the seventh (Fig. 7.7). However, when these data are adjusted for the number of patients at risk in the population, the age- and gender-specific incidence for all patients is greatest from age 60 to 80 and the incidence in males at that age is more than twice that of females (Sanders et al., 1997; Lavrnic

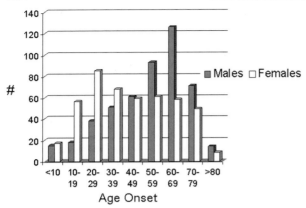

Fig. 7.7. Age onset of MG symptoms in 869 patients without thymoma in the Duke MG Clinic. For males, the number of patients increases progressively until the seventh decade, after which there is a sharp decrease. For females, the numbers peak in the third decade, with a blunted peak after age 40.

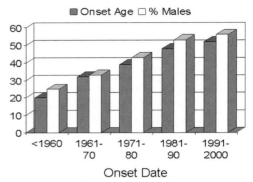

Fig. 7.9. Trends in the age of onset and gender distribution among 860 patients in the Duke MG Clinic whose symptoms began before 2001. As the population has aged, the age of disease onset and the proportion of males have increased. Most new onset MG patients now are male and over age 50.

et al., 1999; Vincent et al., 2003) (Fig. 7.8). As the population has aged, more patients now develop MG in their later years. Whereas women were more often affected by MG in the past, now males are more often affected and the average age at onset is over 50 (Phillips, 2003) (Fig. 7.9).

7.5. Diagnosis

Early and accurate diagnosis of MG is critical in determining and effecting the most appropriate treatment. A high level of suspicion is important in arriving at the correct diagnosis, which can be especially challenging if there is little weakness at the time of examination or there is no obvious ocular muscle involvement. If antibodies to the AChR or MuSK are found in a patient with weakness, the diagnosis is secure (see

Chapter 9). If no antibodies are found, the diagnosis is made by demonstrating weakness and abnormal neuromuscular transmission (NMT), and excluding other nerve or muscle disease. Abnormal NMT can be confirmed by observing unequivocal changes in strength or muscle function during voluntary activity or in response to anticholinesterase medications, or with electrodiagnostic testing.

Fewer than 70% of MG patients are correctly diagnosed within the first year after symptom onset (Beghi et al., 1991; Kalb et al., 2002). MG was the initial diagnosis given to only 49% of the MG patients in our clinic (Table 7.2); their myasthenic symptoms had variously been attributed to a number of conditions, the most common of which were ocular neuropathy or pathology (14%), cerebrovascular disease (10%), a psychological problem (4%), and myopathy (3%).

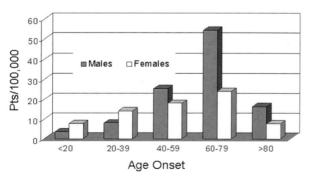

Fig. 7.8. The age-specific incidence of symptom onset among men and women with MG who were evaluated in the Duke MG Clinic within 2 years of onset, adjusted for gender and age by the North Carolina population in 1990 (Sanders et al., 1997).

Table 7.2

Initial diagnosis in 436 patients in the Duke MG Clinic

MG	212 (49%)
Eye disease	62 (14%)
CVA	44 (10%)
Psychological	18 (4%)
Myopathy	12 (3%)
Brain lesion	5 (1%)
Bell palsy	5 (1%)
Multiple sclerosis	4 (0.9%)
Allergy	4 (0.9%)
Blepharospasm	2 (0.4%)
Other	68 (16%)

7.5.1. Diagnostic tests

7.5.1.1. Edrophonium (Tensilon©) test

Edrophonium and other cholinesterase inhibitors impede the breakdown of acetylcholine by inhibiting the action of acetylcholinesterase, thus allowing ACh to diffuse more widely throughout the synaptic cleft and to have a more prolonged interaction with ACh receptors on the postsynaptic muscle membrane. This facilitates repeated interaction of ACh with the reduced number of AChRs and results in a larger endplate potential (Katz and Miledi, 1973). Weakness from abnormal neuromuscular transmission characteristically improves after administration of cholinesterase inhibitors, and this is the basis of the diagnostic edrophonium test.

Assessing the effect of edrophonium on most muscles depends on the patient exerting maximum effort before and after drug administration. For ocular and pharyngeal muscle function the observer can see changes in the position of the eyelid or ocular deviation (Fig. 7.10) or hear changes in speech. The edrophonium test is most reliable when it produces dramatic improvement in eyelid ptosis, ocular muscle weakness or dysarthria. Resolution of eyelid ptosis and unequivocal improvement in function of a single paretic extraocular muscle are the best endpoints, because observed function in these muscles is largely independent of voluntary effort. Changes in strength of other muscles after edrophonium must be interpreted cautiously, especially in a suggestible patient. Double-blinded administration of edrophonium adds a measure of objectivity to strength testing in limb muscles but even this should not be used as the only objective confirmation of the diagnosis.

The edrophonium test is reported to be positive in 60–95% of patients with ocular myasthenia and in 72–95% with generalized MG (Pascuzzi, 2003). However, improvement after edrophonium is not unique to MG and may also be seen in congenital myasthenic syndromes (CMSs) (see Chapter 10), the Lambert–Eaton myasthenic syndrome (LEMS) (Dell'Osso et al., 1983; Oh and Cho, 1990), motor neuron disease (Mulder et al., 1959; Trojan et al., 1993), intracranial aneurysms (Mindel and Charney, 1989), brainstem lesions (Dirr et al., 1989; Gupta et al., 2003; Rodolico et al., 2003), cavernous sinus tumors (personal observations), end-stage renal disease (Khan and Bank, 1995) and in muscle disease affecting the ocular muscles (Okamoto et al., 1996).

The optimal dose of edrophonium varies among patients and cannot be predetermined. In a study of ocular myasthenia, the mean dose of edrophonium that gave a positive response was 3.3 mg for ptosis and 2.6 mg for ocular motor dysfunction (Kupersmith et al., 2003). The lowest effective dose can be determined by injecting small incremental doses up to a maximum total of 10 mg. Most commonly, a test dose of 2 mg is injected initially and the response is monitored for 60 s. Subsequent injections of 3 mg and 5 mg may then be given, but if clear improvement is seen within 60 s after any dose, no further injections are necessary. If weakness develops or worsens after injections of <10 mg edrophonium this also indicates a neuromuscular transmission defect, as this dose will not weaken normal muscle.

Some patients who do not respond to intravenous edrophonium may respond to parenteral neostigmine methylsulfate, 0.5 mg I.M. (intramuscular) or S.C. (subcutaneous), which has a longer duration of action. Onset of action after I.M. injection of neostigmine is 5–15 min. The longer duration of action compared to edrophonium is particularly useful in children. A therapeutic trial of oral pyridostigmine or neostigmine for several days may produce improvement that cannot be appreciated after a single dose of edrophonium or

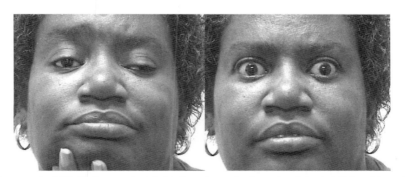

Fig. 7.10. Edrophonium test in MG. Before testing (left) there is marked ptosis of the left lid and lateral deviation of the left eye, and the jaw must be supported. Within 5 s after injection of 0.1 mg edrophonium (right), function of both lids and left medial rectus are improved.

neostigmine. Results should be interpreted with caution if the patient's subjective reports are the main measure of response.

Common side effects of edrophonium are increased salivation and sweating, nausea, stomach cramps, and fasciculations. Hypotension and bradycardia occur infrequently and generally resolve with rest in the supine position. Atropine (0.4–2 mg) should be available for I.V. injection in the event that bradycardia is severe. Serious complications (bradyarrythmia or syncope) have been reported in only 0.16% of edrophonium tests (Ing et al., 2005). The risk of these rare complications must be weighed against the potential diagnostic information that the edrophonium test may uniquely provide.

Many patients with MuSK antibody-positive MG (see Section 7.8.3.1) do not improve or even become worse with edrophonium or pyridostigmine, which often produces profuse fasciculations in these patients (Hatanaka et al., 2005).

7.5.1.2. Ocular cooling

Myasthenic weakness typically improves with muscle cooling. This is the basis of the "ice pack" test, in which cooling of a ptotic lid improves lid elevation (Saavedra et al., 1979; Sethi et al., 1987; Ertas et al., 1994; Golnik et al., 1999; Czaplinski et al., 2003). An ice pack is placed over the ptotic eyelid, usually for 2 min, and improvement in ptosis is assessed. Positive responses have been reported even when edrophonium tests are negative (Sethi et al., 1987). A meta analysis of six studies showed this test to have a sensitivity of 89% and a specificity of 100% in MG, suggesting that it may be useful in patients with lid ptosis, particularly if the edrophonium test is negative or contraindicated (Larner, 2004).

7.5.1.3. Autoantibodies in MG

7.5.1.3.1. Acetylcholine receptor antibodies

Assay for acetylcholine receptor antibodies (AChR-Abs) is an essential diagnostic test for MG (see Chapter 6 and Section 7.8.3). The most commonly performed assay measures binding to purified AChR from human skeletal muscle that is labeled with radioiodinated α-bungarotoxin. The reported sensitivity of this binding assay ranges from 70% to 95% for generalized MG, and 50% to 75% for ocular myasthenia (Lindstrom et al., 1976; Lindstrom, 1977; Vincent and Newsom-Davis, 1985). In a comparison of diagnostic tests performed in 550 untreated MG patients, we found elevated binding antibodies in 80% of patients with generalized MG and 55% of those with purely ocular weakness (Fig. 7.11).

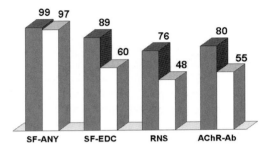

Fig. 7.11. The results of diagnostic tests performed in 550 patients with untreated generalized or ocular myasthenia. The percentage of tests with abnormal results is shown for each. SF-ANY—jitter measurements in any tested muscle; SF-EDC—jitter measurements in the extensor digitorum communis; RNS—repetitive nerve stimulation in a hand and a shoulder muscle; AChR-Ab—acetylcholine receptor antibody assay. (D.B. Sanders, J.M. Massey and J.F. Howard, Jr., unpublished observations.)

Another assay for AChR antibodies measures inhibition of binding of radiolabeled α-bungarotoxin to the AChR (Howard et al., 1987). Antibodies measured by this technique are directed against the ACh binding site on the α-subunit of the AChR. In most patients, relatively few of the circulating antibodies recognize this site, resulting in a lower sensitivity for this assay. These blocking antibodies are found in less than 1% of MG patients who do not have measurable binding antibodies and thus have little diagnostic value.

AChR antibodies cross-link the AChR in the membrane and increase their rate of degradation. The AChR modulating antibody assay measures the rate of loss of labeled AChR from cultured human myotubes (Drachman et al., 1982). AChR modulating antibodies are found in about 10% of MG patients who do not have elevated binding antibodies. This test may give false positive results if the blood sample is hemolyzed, contaminated, or exposed to ambient heat (Lennon, 1997). MG patients with thymoma often have high levels of anti-AChR modulating antibodies but we have not found this to be different from patients without thymoma (Husain et al., 1998).

Finding elevated AChR antibodies in a patient with compatible clinical features essentially confirms the diagnosis of MG but normal antibody measurements do not exclude the disease. False positive AChR antibody tests are rare, but have been reported in autoimmune liver disease, systemic lupus, inflammatory neuropathies, amyotrophic lateral sclerosis, patients with rheumatoid arthritis receiving penicillamine, patients with thymoma without MG, and in first degree relatives of patients with acquired autoimmune MG (Lennon, 1994).

AChR antibody levels tend to be lower in patients with ocular or mild generalized MG but the serum antibody concentration varies widely among patients with similar degrees of weakness, and does not reliably predict the severity of disease in individual patients. AChR antibodies are found in virtually all patients with thymoma. Antibody levels fall in most MG patients after immunosuppressive treatment, but only rarely become normal, and may actually rise in some patients in clinical remission. The AChR antibody level is thus not an accurate marker of response to therapy.

7.5.1.3.2. Anti-striated muscle antibodies

Antibodies to the striated elements in the contractile apparatus of skeletal muscle (StrAbs) were the first autoantibodies discovered in MG (Strauss et al., 1960). These antibodies are not pathogenic and are not specific for MG—they are also found in autoimmune liver disease and infrequently in LEMS and in patients with primary lung cancer. They are found in more than 90% of MG with thymoma and in one-third of patients with thymoma who do not have MG. One-third of MG patients without thymoma also have StrAbs; they are more frequent in older patients and in those with more severe disease.

StrAbs are rarely, if ever, elevated in MG in the absence of AChR antibodies and are therefore of little value in confirming the diagnosis. They have some clinical value in predicting thymomas—60% of patients with MG beginning before age 50 who have these antibodies have a thymoma. Although changes in the StrAb level have been associated with tumor recurrence, they may disappear in patients with persistent thymoma and may reappear after thymothymectomy in the absence of tumor recurrence (Husain et al., 1998). Thus, they do not consistently indicate the persistence or recurrence of tumor.

7.5.1.3.3. Anti-MuSK antibodies

Antibodies to muscle-specific receptor tyrosine kinase (MuSK), a surface membrane component essential in the development of the neuromuscular junction, have recently been described in patients with MG who are seronegative for AChR antibodies (see Section 7.8.3.1).

7.5.1.3.4. Other autoantibodies

Autoantibodies directed against several muscle antigens other than the AChR are found in the serum of many MG patients, mainly those with thymoma or late-onset MG. Although these antibodies are not pathogenic, they are found more often in patients with more severe disease, suggesting that disease severity is related to a more vigorous humoral response against these non-AChR antigens (Romi et al., 2000b).

Titin is a large muscle antigen and is at least partially responsible for the binding of StrAbs (Aarli et al., 1990). Anti-titin antibodies are found in patients with late-onset disease or thymoma (Gautel et al., 1993; Buckley et al., 2001; Somnier and Engel, 2002) and thus are a marker for thymoma in young MG patients.

The ryanodine receptor (RyR) is a calcium release channel in the sarcoplasmic reticulum of skeletal muscle. Anti-RyR antibodies are found in 75% of MG patients with thymoma, and in approximately 10–20% of late-onset MG without thymoma (Romi et al., 2000b; Skeie et al., 2001). RyR antibody testing has been reported to have 70% sensitivity and specificity for thymoma in patients with MG (Romi et al., 2000a).

7.5.1.4. Electrodiagnostic tests (see Chapter 4)

7.5.1.4.1. Repetitive nerve stimulation

Repetitive nerve stimulation (RNS) is the most frequently used electrodiagnostic test to demonstrate abnormal neuromuscular transmission. In a direct comparison study, we found an abnormal decrement in a hand or shoulder muscle in 75% of patients with generalized MG, and in less than 50% of those with ocular myasthenia (Fig. 7.11). The major limitation to RNS testing in MG is its relative insensitivity, especially when weakness is mild or limited to ocular muscles. A positive RNS test confirms that neuromuscular transmission is abnormal, but a normal test does not exclude the diagnosis.

7.5.1.4.2. Single-fiber EMG

Single-fiber EMG (SFEMG) is the most sensitive clinical test of neuromuscular transmission and shows increased jitter with normal fiber density in some muscles in almost all patients with MG (Sanders and Howard, Jr., 1986). The jitter measured by SFEMG is greatest in weak muscles but is usually abnormal even in muscles with normal strength. In most patients with MG, the jitter is greater and more often abnormal in facial muscles than in limbs. This distribution pattern is not invariable, however, especially in patients with MuSK antibody-positive MG (see Section 7.8.3.1).

In ocular myasthenia, jitter is abnormal in a limb muscle in 60% of patients and in a facial muscle in 97% (Fig. 7.11). When there is any degree of non-ocular muscle weakness, jitter is increased in the forearm extensor digitorum communis in almost 90% of examinations. In the rare patient who has weakness in only a few limb muscles, abnormal jitter may be demonstrated only if a weak muscle is examined.

This is particularly true in some patients with MuSK antibody-positive MG (Stickler et al., 2005) (see Section 7.8.3.1).

7.5.1.4.3. Histopathology

Conventional light microscopic studies are usually unrevealing in MG, and thus are used mainly to exclude other diseases of nerve or muscle. Small accumulations of lymphoid cells ("lymphorrhages") are occasionally seen in peripheral muscle, but are not specific for MG. Ultrastructural studies demonstrate reduction in the nerve terminal area and simplification of the postsynaptic membrane (Engel and Santa, 1971) (Fig. 7.12). Special studies of AChR concentration demonstrate that the number of receptors is decreased at the neuromuscular junction in acquired MG (Fambrough et al., 1973). IgG deposits are found on the postsynaptic membrane (Engel and Santa, 1971), as are complement deposits, which are also found in the synaptic clefts (Engel et al., 1979). Studies such as these are important in advancing our understanding of the disease, but because of their limited availability are not used in the clinical diagnosis of MG.

7.5.1.5. Chest imaging

Imaging studies of the chest are performed in newly-diagnosed MG to detect a thymoma, which occurs in 10–15% of MG (see below). Chest CT, which is usually the imaging study of choice, accurately identifies

thymoma in 81% of patients, but is only 91% correct in predicting the absence of a tumor (Seybold, 1999). Small tumors that may elude detection by CT scan would be found if the patient undergoes thymectomy with wide exploration; however, less extensive surgery is less likely to detect tumors (Austin et al., 1983). Identification of a tumor by imaging is thus particularly critical when thymectomy might not otherwise be performed, for example in elderly patients or those with ocular myasthenia, or if thymectomy is to be performed by a less extensive procedure.

In all our MG patients with thymoma, the tumor was identified during the initial evaluation or at subsequent sternal-splitting thymectomy. Thus, we do not routinely perform imaging studies in search for thymoma after the initial evaluation if the patient has had a sternal-splitting thymectomy. In patients who have had thymoma or in whom thymectomy was performed with a less extensive exploration, periodic assessment for thymoma is indicated, particularly when AChR antibodies are elevated.

7.5.1.6. Other

Thyroid function tests should be performed as part of the initial evaluation and periodically thereafter to detect coincidental hyper- or hypo-thyroidism, which may induce exacerbation of MG. A skin test for tuberculosis should be performed before beginning any form of immunosuppression.

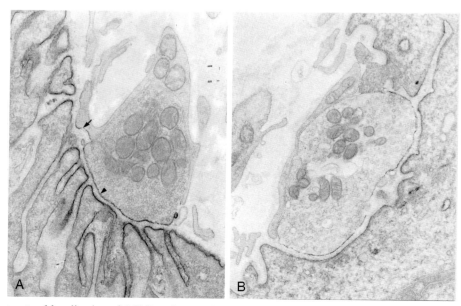

Fig. 7.12. Ultrastructural localization of AChR at the muscle endplate in a control subject (A) and in a patient with generalized MG (B). The AChR staining seen in A is virtually absent in B, in which only short segments of simplified postsynaptic membrane react. (From Engel et al., 1977b, with permission.)

7.5.1.7. Comparison of diagnostic tests

The edrophonium test is often diagnostic in patients with ptosis or ophthalmoparesis but is less useful in other muscles. The results are not entirely objective or specific and a positive test should be supported by other information, such as RNS, SFEMG, antibody levels or response to treatment. Abnormal results from AChR or anti-MuSK antibody assay virtually ensure the diagnosis of MG, but a normal result does not exclude it. AChR antibodies are found in virtually all patients with thymoma. RNS confirms impaired neuromuscular transmission but is not specific to MG, and is frequently normal in patients with mild or purely ocular disease. SFEMG demonstrates abnormal jitter in almost all patients with MG but abnormal jitter is also seen in other motor unit disorders. However, normal jitter in a weak muscle excludes MG as the cause of the weakness. The sensitivity of various diagnostic tests in MG is shown in Fig. 7.11.

7.5.2. Differential diagnosis of MG

The differential diagnosis of muscle weakness or oculomotor symptoms is broad, but in typical MG, the correct diagnosis is usually apparent to the careful observer. This is particularly true if eyelid ptosis clearly fluctuates or alternates from side to side. In patients with less typical manifestations, the differential diagnosis includes motor neuron disease, some primary muscle diseases, lesions affecting the brainstem nuclei including aneurysms (Ajtai et al., 2004; Akkaya et al., 2005), cavernous sinus thrombosis, various toxins, botulism including iatrogenically administered botulinum toxin (Sunness and Kelman, 2004), and diphtheritic neuropathies. The differential diagnosis can be reduced by attention to the clinical findings. Mitochondrial myopathies produce lid ptosis and ocular muscle paresis, but the course of these conditions is inexorably progressive, without fluctuations, and weakness is symmetric. The ocular muscle and lid weakness of myotonic dystrophy is accompanied by temporalis atrophy and myotonia in limb or facial muscles. The intermittent forced eye closure of blepharospasm is frequently mistaken for intermittent lid ptosis, though the distinction is obvious if the sudden fluctuations and simultaneous contraction of upper and lower lids that mark this condition are recognized. When MG produces severe oropharyngeal and tongue weakness, amyotrophic lateral sclerosis or a brainstem lesion may be considered, especially if the tongue is atrophic. Attention to the stretch reflexes usually distinguishes these from MG.

Application of appropriate diagnostic procedures will also greatly narrow the differential. Patients with MuSK antibody-positive MG may present with findings more suggestive of motor neuron disease or myopathy (see Section 7.8.3.1). Electrodiagnostic studies of weak muscles give the most convincing evidence of MG in these patients.

Although the clinical presentations of MG and LEMS are usually quite distinct (Wirtz et al., 2002), the clinical and electrodiagnostic findings may be similar in some patients, in which case making the correct diagnosis may be challenging (see Chapter 9). Features that strongly suggest MG are prominent ocular muscle weakness, limb weakness that predominates in the arms, and normal muscle stretch reflexes (Wirtz et al., 2002). Features that favor LEMS include weakness that predominates in the hip girdle muscles, hypoactive or absent reflexes, and autonomic symptoms, especially dry mouth.

There are many reports of patients with various overlapping features of MG and LEMS. These include clinical features of one condition but facilitation on manual muscle testing or high-frequency nerve stimulation, or lack thereof, typical of the other; clinical and electrodiagnostic patterns typical of one condition initially, but changing to the other later; or electrodiagnostic patterns typical of MG in one muscle, and of LEMS in another. Six patients have been reported who appear to have a true MG/LEMS overlap syndrome, with antibodies to both the AChR and VGCC (Newsom-Davis et al., 1991; Katz et al., 1998; Kanzato et al., 1999; Oh and Sher, 2005). The ultimate diagnosis in patients with mixed features of MG and LEMS may be moot because many treatments are the same for both conditions. Exceptions are that we do not search for cancer other than thymoma in MG, and thymectomy would not be considered as potential treatment in LEMS.

7.6. Genetics of MG

Autoimmune MG per se is not a hereditary disease, but, like other autoimmune conditions, occurs more often in family members than by chance alone. First-degree relatives of MG patients are approximately 1000 times more likely to develop the disease than is the general population and familial cases have been reported in up to 7% of MG families (Pirskanen, 1977). The severity, pattern of involvement and response to treatment may vary among affected family members. Either one or two generations can be affected and no association with a single human leukocyte antigen (HLA) haplotype has been found (Evoli et al., 1995). Among 949 MG patients in our clinic, MG has affected first-degree relatives in 18 families, including both members of three sets of monozygotic twins. These observations suggest that there is a genetically determined predisposition to develop MG.

The HLA complex occupies a large region of chromosome 6p21 and is divided into three regions, or classes: Classes I and II contain genes that encode membrane-bound molecules that present antigenic epitopes to lymphoid cells. The HLA-A1 and HLA-B8 genes from Class I and DRB3 from Class II are closely associated and form the most highly conserved HLA haplotype in Caucasians. This combination of genes has been associated with a large number of autoimmune and immune-related diseases. Because of its size, however, it is associated with a large number of alleles that may have no relationship to a disease with which it is associated.

The demonstrated association of certain HLA antigens with MG provides further evidence for a genetic factor. Among Caucasians, MG has a moderate association with HLA-B8 and DRw3 (Naeim et al., 1978; Drachman, 1994). In American blacks with MG, there is a significant increase in both HLA-A1 and B8 but there was an increase in DR5 rather than DR3 (Christiansen et al., 1984). Among Japanese, DR9 and DRw13 are significantly increased in patients who develop MG before 3 years of age but not in those with adult-onset MG (Matsuki et al., 1990). MG with thymus hyperplasia has been associated with, but not genetically linked to, the HLA-DR3 haplotype. Other HLA antigens are found with increased frequency in MG associated with thymoma, though the specific antigens differ among different ethnic groups (Machens et al., 1999; Garcia-Ramos et al., 2003). Yet other HLA antigens have been associated to MG with thymic atrophy, though this also varies among different ethnic groups (Garcia-Ramos et al., 2003). Other studies have shown that ocular myasthenia is associated with different HLA antigens than is generalized MG (Kida et al., 1987). These findings suggest that ocular, generalized and thymoma-associated MG might have different immunogenetic bases.

7.7. The thymus in MG (see Chapter 5)

The thymus gland plays a role in the induction of tolerance to self-antigens, which appears to be the primary abnormality in MG. The thymus contains all the necessary elements for the pathogenesis of most MG: myoid cells that express the AChR antigen, antigen-presenting cells, and immunocompetent T-cells. Cultured thymic myoid cells express transcripts that encode for AChR subunits. Expression of these subunits may serve as an antigen for the autosensitization of the patient against AChR. Thymic abnormalities are found in more than 80% of MG patients: 10–15% have a thymic tumor, and 70% have hyperplastic changes (germinal centers) that indicate an active immune response. Surgical removal of the thymus seems to improve the clinical course in many patients (Gronseth and Barohn, 2000).

7.7.1. Thymoma

Thymic tumors are found in 10–15% of patients with MG (Osserman and Genkins, 1971; Sorensen and Holm, 1989) and approximately 35% of patients with thymoma are reported to have MG (Rosenow and Hurley, 1984). Inasmuch as patients with thymoma who have no symptoms of MG may have evidence of subclinical neuromuscular dysfunction (Sanders and Howard, Jr., 1988) and symptoms of MG may begin even years after removal of thymoma (Madonick et al., 1957; Rowland et al., 1957; Namba et al., 1978), the frequency of MG in thymoma is probably underestimated.

Almost 10% of our patients with MG whose symptoms began between the ages of 30 and 60 years had thymoma; the frequency of thymoma was much lower when symptoms began before the age of 20 and after the age of 60 years (Table 7.3) (Fig. 7.13). In thymoma-associated MG, symptoms are on average more severe than in non-thymomatous MG (Grob et al., 1987; Oosterhuis and Kuks, 1997; Evoli et al., 2003a) and fewer patients have ocular myasthenia (D.B. Sanders, J.M. Massey, unpublished observations). Almost all thymoma-associated MG patients are seropositive.

Thymoma is the most common neoplasm of the mediastinum and accounts for 50% of anterior mediastinal masses. Most MG-associated thymic tumors are benign, well-differentiated, and encapsulated and can be removed completely at surgery. There is no clear histologic distinction between benign and most malignant thymomas other than by their invasiveness. Approximately 5% of malignant thymomas are associated with paraneoplastic syndromes other than MG, particularly red cell aplasia (Muller-Hermelink and Marx, 2000). In these patients, the associated neoplasm represents the most severe threat to life and determines the prognosis. Non-thymic malignancies have been reported in up to 21% of patients with thymoma (Souadijian et al., 1968), and may occur less often in those with MG (Evoli et al., 2004). Thymoma also has a better prognosis with than without associated MG (Monden et al., 1988; Budde et al., 2001; Moore et al., 2001).

Table 7.3

Age onset of acquired MG in 949 patients in the Duke MG Clinic

Age onset	Males				Females			
	Thymoma	African-American	Ocular MG	Total	Thymoma	African-American	Ocular MG	Total
<10	0	6	1	15	0	10	2	17
10–19	0	7	2	18	1	14	1	56
20–29	6	13	5	38	4	28	3	85
30–39	6	14	9	51	6	25	5	68
40–49	8	18	13	61	11	12	11	59
50–59	6	11	13	93	9	9	9	61
60–69	3	8	15	126	6	5	3	59
70–79	3	1	9	71	1	1	1	48
≥80	0	0	3	14	0	0	1	8
All	42	78	70	487	38	104	36	462

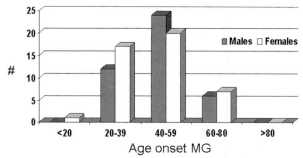

Fig. 7.13. Age onset of MG symptoms among 80 patients with thymoma seen in the Duke MG Clinic.

7.8. Special situations

7.8.1. Ocular myasthenia

Ocular myasthenia is defined as weakness that begins in and remains limited to the eyelids and muscles of ocular movement. Approximately two-thirds of MG patients have purely ocular symptoms at disease onset (Grob et al., 1981; Bever et al., 1983). The proportion of patients who subsequently develop generalized MG varies among different reports, possibly because of differences in the rigor with which weakness of non-ocular muscles is assessed. The majority of patients who develop generalized MG do so within the first year (Grob et al., 1981) and 80–90% do so within 2 years of symptom onset (Bever et al., 1983; Oosterhuis, 1989; Grob, 1999). Sixty-one percent of our patients had only ocular symptoms at onset but

weakness remained confined to the ocular muscles in only 11% (Table 7.3). Patients with ocular myasthenia are often seronegative—this was true in 52% of the ocular myasthenia patients in our clinic. Males with ocular myasthenia outnumbered females almost 2:1 in our clinic, and the male predominance was more marked in patients with late-onset disease (Fig. 7.14).

It is unclear whether ocular myasthenia is a different disease than generalized MG or merely one end of a spectrum of disease severity. The observation that abnormal neuromuscular transmission can be demonstrated in limb muscles by SFEMG in at least half the patients with ocular myasthenia favors the unitary hypothesis (Sanders and Howard, Jr., 1986). However, differences in the distribution of HLA subtypes suggests that ocular and generalized myasthenia might have different immunogenetic bases (Kida et al., 1987).

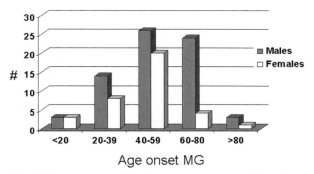

Fig. 7.14. Age onset of MG symptoms among 106 patients with ocular myasthenia seen in the Duke MG Clinic.

It has been hypothesized that the predominant involvement of ocular muscles in MG is due to antibodies specific for the γ-subunit of the AChR, which is found in adult extraocular muscle. However, AChR in the levator palpebrae harbors the epsilon and not the γ-subunit, yet this muscle is frequently involved in ocular myasthenia. Moreover, γ-subunits are present in some AChRs, even in normal limb muscle.

7.8.1.1. Predicting generalization

Eighty percent of patients who progress from ocular to generalized myasthenia do so within 1 year after onset of symptoms, and only 6% do so after 3 years (Grob et al., 1987). The longer a patient continues to have only ocular muscle weakness, the less likely it is that generalized weakness will occur. No clinical, laboratory, or electrophysiological features have been identified that predict which patients will develop generalized MG (Bever, Jr. et al., 1983; Weinberg et al., 1999; Rostedt et al., 2000; Kupersmith et al., 2003), though a later age at onset seems to predict early generalization (Thomas et al., 1993) and the risk of generalization is greater in patients with higher titers of AChR antibody (Kupersmith et al., 2003).

7.8.2. Childhood myasthenia gravis

Autoimmune MG beginning before age 20 is called juvenile MG (JMG). JMG is uncommon and only rarely develops before 1 year of age (Geh and Bradbury, 1998). JMG accounts for about 10–15% of all MG in North America, an annual incidence of 1.1 per million

(Phillips et al., 1992). Among Chinese, JMG accounts for 43% of all MG (Chiu et al., 1987) and a similar high frequency of early onset disease is reported in Japan, where there is a peculiar peak incidence at about 2 or 3 years of age (Uono, 1980).

In Caucasian patients with prepubertal onset, the sex ratio is equal, whereas females increasingly predominate during and after puberty (Batocchi et al., 1990; Andrews et al., 1994; Evoli et al., 1998a). In African-Americans, the incidence of JMG is greater than in Caucasians, and females are more commonly affected than males in early childhood and adolescence (Phillips et al., 1992; Andrews et al., 1994).

Although the clinical manifestations of MG in children are similar to those in adults, symptoms are harder to detect in infants and early childhood, and accurate assessment of strength and fatigability is difficult. As in adults, onset and exacerbation of symptoms of JMG often follow febrile illnesses. A transient form of MG preceded by viral illness has been reported in children (Felice et al., 2005).

In our clinic, 74% of children with JMG had ocular symptoms at onset and these were the only symptoms in 55%. Children often do not complain of ocular symptoms, but may tilt their head back to look beneath droopy lids (Fig. 7.15), or hold one eye closed to minimize diplopia.

The frequency with which JMG remains limited to ocular muscles is 10–15% in some reports (Evoli et al., 1998a; Linder et al., 1997; Rodriguez et al., 1983), and from 50% to 93% in others (Brodsky et al., 1996; Anlar et al., 2005). Weakness remains limited to ocular muscles in a higher percentage of Japanese (Fukuyama et al., 1970) and Chinese patients (Wong et al., 1992),

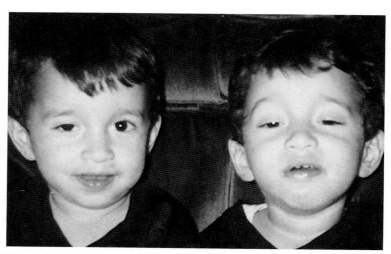

Fig. 7.15. Twins, aged 26 months, with SP-MG. One has asymmetric lid ptosis, the other (right) holds his head back to see beneath bilaterally ptotic lids.

and in children with prepubertal onset (Andrews et al., 1994; Evoli et al., 1998a).

Oropharyngeal weakness in children produces slow chewing and swallowing, drooling, weak or nasal voice, or poor pronunciation. Weakness and fatigability may be demonstrated by observing how well and how much the child can drink through a straw, or by listening for progressive dysarthria during a long count. As in adults, facial weakness may produce a characteristic flattened or horizontal smile, or diminished facial expression. Weakness in limb muscles is most obvious as fatigability and inability to run, climb stairs, or keep up with peers. Respiratory function can be assessed by seeing how far the patient can count with one breath, listening to a strong cough or sniff, and by measurements of peak flow, vital capacity, and maximum inspiratory and expiratory flow. The combination of bulbar weakness and weakness of respiratory musculature is of particular concern, and requires early recognition and aggressive treatment.

Spontaneous remissions have been reported within 3 years of disease onset in 7.6% of JMG patients, and in 30.1% within 15 years (Rodriguez et al., 1983). Spontaneous remissions are more common in younger, prepubertal patients (Rodriguez et al., 1983; Andrews et al., 1994) and are less frequent among African-American than Caucasian patients (Andrews et al., 1994). Unfortunately, these remissions are often only transient.

Thymomas are rare in JMG (Table 7.3). Among 119 JMG patients in our clinic, only two had thymoma and, in another series, four of 133 had thymoma (Evoli et al., 1998a); all six of these patients were older than 14 years at symptom onset.

The most common coincidental autoimmune diseases in JMG are juvenile diabetes mellitus, thyroid disease, and juvenile rheumatoid arthritis. Seizures have been reported to occur more frequently in JMG than in a non-myasthenic population (Snead et al., 1980; Rodriguez et al., 1983; Andrews et al., 1994; Evoli et al., 1998a).

7.8.2.1. Diagnostic testing in childhood myasthenia

Demonstration of weakness and fatigability in characteristically involved muscles often leads to a confident clinical diagnosis. If antibodies to AChR or MuSK are elevated, the diagnosis is virtually assured, and no further testing may be necessary. Other diagnostic testing represents a particular challenge in children and infants; those over age 12–14 can usually cooperate with the same testing procedures as adults.

In children the dose of edrophonium is 0.1 mg/kg intravenously, preceded by an intravenous test dose of 0.01 mg/kg. The maximum dose of 10 mg is rarely indicated in children. Edrophonium side-effects can make interpretation of the test difficult. Atropine should be available for resuscitation, especially in children with respiratory distress in whom edrophonium-induced bronchorrhea may be dangerous. Intramuscular or subcutaneous injection of edrophonium (0.15 mg/kg) may prolong the beneficial effect, facilitating observation of the response (Fenichel, 1989; Papazian, 1992).

Most children older than eight can usually cooperate well enough with EMG testing, but conscious sedation may be necessary for adequate testing in younger children. Several rare congenital myasthenic syndromes can be identified by characteristic findings on RNS and particular care should be taken to look for these (see Chapter 10). Because these procedures require considerable expertise and are painful, they have a lesser role in diagnosis and management in children than in adults with MG.

7.8.2.2. Differential diagnosis of childhood myasthenia

Once the diagnosis of myasthenia has been determined in an infant or child, it is essential to distinguish between autoimmune MG and a congenital myasthenic syndrome in order to offer potentially effective immunotherapies to the former and to avoid ineffective, potentially dangerous treatments in the latter group (see Chapter 10). Thirty six percent to 50% of prepubertal patients are seronegative, as are 18–32% of peripubertal patients and less than 9% of postpubertal adolescents with acquired MG (Snead et al., 1980; Andrews et al., 1993, 1994; Evoli et al., 1998a). The frequency of seronegative MG in young children creates special problems. These are the very patients in whom discrimination between seronegative autoimmune MG and CMS is most difficult. Repeated AChR antibody measurements may demonstrate conversion from seronegative to seropositive, confirming autoimmune MG (Anlar et al., 2005).

Careful questioning to identify the earliest symptoms is crucial in distinguishing CMS from autoimmune MG inasmuch as most CMS present at birth and autoimmune MG rarely begins before 18 months. However, some CMS patients, namely those suffering from the slow-channel syndrome, choline acetyltransferase deficiency, limb-girdle myasthenia, and a few with rapsyn deficiency, can present later in childhood or adolescence (see Chapter 10). Other, very rare neuromuscular transmission disorders of childhood include botulism, some venoms and toxins, including tick paralysis, and LEMS (see Chapter 9).

In young, seronegative children with suspected autoimmune MG and moderate to severe weakness that is not adequately controlled by cholinesterase inhibitors, a trial of plasmapheresis or IVIg may provide critical diagnostic information. Definite improvement after either of these procedures confirms that the disease has an autoimmune etiology. For mildly affected young children, the benefit of making an accurate diagnosis must be weighed against the invasiveness and logistical demands of muscle biopsy and microphysiologic studies to demonstrate the characteristic findings of CMS (Engel et al., 1999).

The differential diagnosis of JMG also includes myopathies, especially those with ptosis and extraocular muscle weakness. Mitochondrial myopathies often manifest in childhood after a normal neonatal period, commonly with ptosis and ocular and generalized muscle weakness; however, these findings are typically static and not fatigable. Also in the differential are congenital myopathies with prominent ptosis; brainstem tumors; brainstem encephalitis; Guillain-Barré syndrome (especially the Miller–Fisher variant); mass lesions near the orbit, cavernous sinus, or sella turcica; diphtheria; and Fazio–Londe disease (progressive bulbar paralysis of childhood). The remote paraneoplastic effects of neuroblastoma also should be considered (Hassan, 1977). Fatigability is an important aid in differentiating MG from these conditions.

7.8.2.3. Transient neonatal myasthenia gravis

Ten percent to 20% of infants born to mothers with MG develop transient neonatal MG (TNMG), which typically presents with hypotonia, poor suck, weak cry, respiratory weakness and intermittent cyanosis, especially during feeds. Ptosis and external ophthalmoplegia also occur. These symptoms usually develop a few hours after birth, but may not be seen for up to 3 days. TNMG typically lasts about 3 weeks, but may last for up to 3 months (Desmedt and Borenstein, 1977). MG does not reappear later, although there is one report that a patient with TNMG later developed JMG (Teng and Osserman, 1956).

TNMG was one of the observations that led to early hypotheses that MG is an autoimmune disease (Simpson, 1960) and this natural experiment underscores many aspects of the immunopathology of MG. Similar transient, neonatal disorders are seen in other antibody-mediated disorders, such as autoimmune thyroid disease and systemic lupus erythematosus. During pregnancy, circulating maternal IgG antibodies normally cross the placenta to enter the fetal circulation, especially during the second half of gestation. In mothers with autoimmune MG pathogenic autoantibodies cross the placenta and interfere with the normal AChR function of the fetus. Clearance of these autoantibodies from the neonate may take up to 5 months after birth.

Although almost all infants of seropositive mothers have elevated circulating AChR antibodies, only about 20% have symptoms of TNMG (Namba et al., 1970; Papazian, 1992; Volpe, 1995). Once an affected mother delivers an infant with TNMG, it is likely that her subsequent infants will be similarly affected (Morel et al., 1988; Papazian, 1992). There is no correlation between disease severity in mothers and their infants with TNMG (Hoff et al., 2004) and maternal AChR antibody levels correlate poorly with disease severity in the infants. However, falling AChR antibody levels in the infant correlate with clinical improvement. Mothers with high levels of antibodies directed against fetal AChR are more likely to deliver infants with TNMG (Vernet-der Garabedian et al., 1994; Gardnerova et al., 1997). Maternal antibodies directed against fetal AChR are also associated with weakness of the developing fetus and arthrogryposis (Stoll et al., 1991; Dinger and Prager, 1993; Vincent et al., 1995; Riemersma et al., 1996). Some mothers with antibodies directed specifically against fetal AChR may themselves be asymptomatic, which makes diagnosis more difficult (Vincent et al., 1995).

All infants born of myasthenic mothers should be examined carefully at birth for any weakness. Detection of AChR antibodies in the child provides strong evidence for the diagnosis, although seronegative mothers have delivered affected seronegative infants (Mier and Havard, 1985; Sisman et al., 2004). Improvement following injection of 0.1 mg/ kg of edrophonium supports the diagnosis of TNMG but it may be hard to assess the response to edrophonium in an intubated and ventilated neonate. Improvement after edrophonium does not distinguish TNMG from some congenital myasthenic syndromes. A decremental response to RNS confirms abnormal neuromuscular transmission, but also does not distinguish TNMG from many congenital myasthenic syndromes.

7.8.3. "Seronegative" MG

Twenty percent to 25% of patients with generalized MG do not have detectable AChR antibodies (Sanders et al., 1997), and have been called "seronegative" (SN-MG). Seropositive (SP-MG) and seronegative patients have similar clinical features except that SN-MG patients (particularly males) tend to have milder disease. Seroconversion is not rare, especially within the first 6 months of disease, after which time antibodies may be found in some patients who were initially seronegative. Age-adjusted incidence patterns are different in SN and SP-MG (Sanders et al., 1997): advanced age and levels of endogenous female sex hormones parallel the incidence of SP-MG, but not SN-MG. This may be a clue to disease pathogenesis.

7.8.3.1. MuSK antibody-positive MG

Muscle specific receptor tyrosine kinase is a transmembrane polypeptide, specific for skeletal muscle. It is expressed in low levels in myoblasts, and is then induced during muscle differentiation. MuSK is down-regulated in mature muscle, where it remains prominent only at the endplate. It can be induced in mature muscle by denervation or block of electrical activity. In the developing muscle, MuSK, which is activated by motor nerve-derived agrin, is essential in aggregation of the AChR at the developing neuromuscular junction. Knock-out mice who lack MuSK develop normally in utero, but AChR does not cluster normally at the endplate and these animals die perinatally from muscle weakness (DeChiari et al., 1996). The role of MuSK in adult muscle is still uncertain.

One family has been reported in which two siblings with dual mutations of the gene encoding MuSK had a congenital myasthenic syndrome, with neonatal respiratory insufficiency, which improved with age in the one who survived infancy (Chevessier et al., 2004). The father had a frame shift deletion of the MuSK gene, the mother had a missense mutation of the same gene, and the surviving daughter had both.

Antibodies to MuSK have been reported in 40–50% of patients with generalized SN-MG (Evoli et al., 2003b; Sanders et al., 2003; McConville et al., 2004; Vincent et al., 2004), and more recently, in ocular myasthenia as well (Caress et al., 2005). MuSK antibody-positive MG (MMG) predominantly affects females and begins from childhood through middle age. Several clinical patterns have been reported. The clinical picture may be indistinguishable from MuSK-negative MG, with fluctuating ocular, bulbar and limb weakness. However, many patients have predominant weakness in cranial and bulbar muscles, frequently with marked atrophy of these muscles (Evoli et al., 2003b) (Fig. 7.16). Others have prominent neck, shoulder and respiratory weakness, with little or no involvement of ocular or bulbar muscles (Sanders et al., 2003).

Many MMG patients do not improve with cholinesterase inhibitors—some actually become worse, and many have profuse fasciculations with these medications (Hatanaka et al., 2005). Most improve dramatically with plasma exchange or corticosteroids, but the response to other immunosuppressive agents varies. Thymic changes are absent or minimal compared to those in SP-MG (Lauriola et al., 2005; Leite et al., 2005) and the role of thymectomy in MMG is not yet clear (Sanders et al., 2003; Lavrnic et al., 2005).

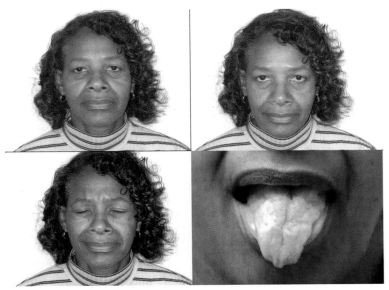

Fig. 7.16. MuSK antibody-positive MG with marked upper facial muscle weakness and atrophy. At rest (upper left), there is slight bilateral lid ptosis. There is no visible (or palpable) contraction of the frontalis muscle on attempted elevation of the eyebrows (upper right) and she does not bury the eyelashes during forced eyelid closure (lower left). The tongue is markedly wasted (lower right).

Muscle atrophy, particularly in facial and oropharyngeal muscles, is a prominent finding in many MMG patients and muscle biopsy changes (muscle fiber atrophy and variable diameter and focal necrosis) have suggested a myopathic process (Evoli et al., 2003b; Sanders et al., 2003).

The diagnosis of MMG may be elusive when the clinical features, electrodiagnostic findings and response to cholinesterase inhibitors differ from typical MG. Electrodiagnostic abnormalities may not be found as diffusely as in other forms of MG and it may be necessary to examine different muscles to demonstrate abnormal neuromuscular transmission (Stickler et al., 2005). The potentially more limited distribution of physiologic abnormalities also may limit the interpretation of microphysiologic and histologic studies in MMG, inasmuch as abnormalities might not be seen in the muscles that are usually biopsied for these studies.

7.8.4. Crisis

The term crisis in myasthenic patients denotes a medical emergency due to rapidly increasing weakness affecting the oropharyngeal and respiratory muscles. "Myasthenic crisis" is attributed to factors that exacerbate MG weakness, such as infection, and is generally defined as weakness that is severe enough to necessitate intubation for ventilatory support or airway protection. Myasthenic crisis occurs most often early in the illness, before effective treatment has begun. Crises are usually heralded by a period of deteriorating ocular and bulbar muscle function. In one report, the time between the start of deterioration and crisis was 1–3 days in 68%, 4–7 days in 22%, and 14–21 days in 10% of patients (Berrouschot et al., 1997). During this period of deterioration it is often possible to identify factors that trigger the exacerbation.

Infections are associated with 30–40% of crises, the most common being viral upper respiratory infection, bronchitis and bacterial pneumonia. Pneumonitis from aspiration is associated with 10% of crises. Physical stress (such as trauma or surgery, including thymectomy) and changes in medications (including recent initiation or discontinuation of corticosteroids or change in anticholinesterase dose) are also implicated. No obvious trigger is identified in 30–40% of crises.

"Cholinergic crisis" results from excess anticholinesterase medications. It was more common before the introduction of immunosuppressive therapy, when very large doses of anticholinesterase medications were used. In theory, it should be easy to determine if a patient is weak because of too little or too much anticholinesterase, but in practice this is often difficult. Administration of edrophonium should distinguish

overdose from underdose, but its use in crisis is dangerous unless the patient is intubated and ventilated. Also, an apprehensive patient in crisis frequently cannot cooperate with the test. Further, edrophonium frequently makes some muscles stronger and others weaker.

Cardiac arrhythmia has been reported in 11–14% of hospitalizations for crisis, usually in patients with underlying heart disease or receiving intravenous pyridostigmine (Thomas et al., 1997). These ranged from relatively benign arrhythmias, such as atrial fibrillation, to fatal episodes of ventricular fibrillation and asystole.

7.8.5. Pregnancy in MG

Women in their childbearing years represent a prominent group of patients with MG. Pregnancy or the postpartum state can trigger exacerbation or onset of MG. Severe generalized weakness, and in particular respiratory insufficiency, may endanger both mother and fetus. A pregnant woman with MG presents many challenging therapeutic decisions, which must consider the mother, the fetus and the integrity of the pregnancy.

Myasthenia may improve, worsen, or remain unchanged during pregnancy. First-trimester worsening is more common in first pregnancies, whereas third-trimester worsening and postpartum exacerbations are more common in subsequent pregnancies. It is not uncommon for the first symptoms of MG to begin during pregnancy or postpartum. The clinical state at onset of pregnancy does not reliably predict the course during pregnancy. In older reports, maternal death from myasthenic crisis occurred only rarely. There is an inverse correlation between disease duration and maternal mortality risk, which is greatest in the first year after onset of disease and minimal after seven years (Scott, 1997). In our experience, exacerbation is minimal in patients who are treated successfully prior to pregnancy, even when immunosuppression must be discontinued during pregnancy. Worsening occurs in 30–40% of pregnancies (Osserman, 1955; Plauche, 1991). This may occur at any time, but is more likely in the first trimester or postpartum (Batocchi et al., 1999). In some patients, worsening occurs during the first trimester and is followed by an improvement in the last two trimesters. Complete remission may occur late in pregnancy. All women with puerperal infections developed exacerbation (Djelmis et al., 2002).

7.8.5.1. Obstetric complications

Therapeutic abortion is rarely, if ever, needed because of MG, and the frequency of spontaneous abortion is not increased (Abel, 2002). Preterm delivery due to premature rupture of membranes has been reported in myasthenic mothers taking corticosteroids. Labor and delivery are usually normal, and cesarean section is needed only for obstetrical indications. MG does not affect uterine smooth muscle and therefore the first stage of labor is not compromised. In the second stage of labor, striated muscles are at risk for easy fatigue and therefore outlet forceps or vacuum extraction may be needed.

Inasmuch as myasthenic patients are very sensitive to many anesthetic agents, epidural anesthesia is preferred for both vaginal and operative delivery. Non-depolarizing muscle relaxants may induce an exaggerated or prolonged response and should be avoided if possible. Magnesium sulfate should not be used to manage pre-eclampsia because of its neuromuscular blocking effects. In our experience, breast-feeding is not a problem, despite the theoretical risk of passing maternal AChR antibodies to the newborn.

Weakness due to transplacental passage of maternal pathogenic autoantibodies may be manifest by the fetus in utero as arthrogryposis, weak fetal movements, polyhydramnios (due to poor fetal swallowing), pulmonary hypoplasia (due to reduced fetal respiratory movements), hydrops fetalis and stillbirth. Lack of fetal movements is probably the factor responsible for this complex phenotype, also known as the fetal akinesia deformation sequence. There is no evident correlation between maternal disease severity and fetal condition (Polizzi et al., 2000). The explanation probably lies in the very high levels of antibodies specific for the fetal isoform of AChR, which can cross the placenta and paralyze the fetus in utero (Vincent et al., 1995; Riemersma et al., 1996). Complications of pregnancy in MG may also result from coincidental autoimmune disease or underlying immunological dysfunction (Hoff et al., 2004).

7.8.6. MG in the elderly

Some reports have suggested that patients with late-onset MG have more severe disease and are more likely to have thymoma or to be seronegative, but this has not been our experience. In our clinic population, patients developing MG before or after age 60 have the same mean disease severity and percentage of ocular myasthenia, thymoma and seronegative disease (Figs. 7.13, 7.14; Table 7.3). One study found a high prevalence of previously unrecognized positive AChR antibodies in randomly selected subjects over 75 years old, suggesting that MG may be substantially under-diagnosed in older people (Vincent et al., 2003). In this age group particularly the symptoms of MG may be initially attributed to cerebrovascular or neuro-degenerative diseases. As the population continues to age, we can expect to see even more patients with

MG, who will live longer with their disease, be progressively older, and require treatment for longer periods.

7.8.7. Induced MG

7.8.7.1. D-Penicillamine-induced MG

D-Penicillamine (D-P) is used to treat Wilson's disease, cystinuria, rheumatoid arthritis, scleroderma and other inflammatory conditions. Patients treated with D-P for several months may develop any of a number of autoimmune conditions, including a myasthenic syndrome that disappears when the drug is stopped (Albers et al., 1980; Penn et al., 1998). D-P-induced MG is usually mild and often restricted to the ocular muscles but is otherwise indistinguishable from acquired MG. Weakness may not be recognized when there is severe arthritis. The diagnosis is established by the response to anticholinesterase medications, characteristic electrodiagnostic findings, and serum AChR antibodies. D-P has a reactive sulfhydryl group that is capable of modifying self-antigens and may directly couple to distinctive peptides in surface DR1 molecules on circulating macrophages or dendritic cells (Hill et al., 1999). It is likely that D-P stimulates or enhances an immunological reaction against the neuromuscular junction in susceptible patients. The myasthenia induced by D-P usually remits within 6–12 months after the drug is stopped. If myasthenic symptoms persist thereafter, the patient likely has coincidental MG.

7.8.7.2. MG following bone marrow transplantation

MG with elevated AChR antibodies is a rare complication of allogeneic bone marrow transplantation (BMT) (Mackey et al., 1997). In all reported cases MG occurred when decreasing immunosuppression was followed by graft-vs-host disease (GVHD), and usually improved when immunosuppression was reinstituted. Other autoimmune diseases have also been reported in post-BMT patients, the most common of which are hypothyroidism, hyperthyroidism, and immune cytopenias. Most patients with MG and GVHD have had aplastic anemia, which appears to be an important host factor in the development of all the autoimmune disorders seen with chronic GVHD (Nelson and McQuillen, 1988).

7.8.7.3. Interferon-induced MG

Patients treated with interferon-α develop several autoantibodies and autoimmune diseases, including MG. MG has been reported in patients receiving interferon-α-2b for malignancy and chronic active hepatitis C (Batocchi et al., 1995; Mase et al., 1996). Expression of interferon-γ at motor endplates of transgenic mice results in generalized weakness and abnormal NMJ function, which improve with cholinesterase inhibitors, suggesting that this expression of interferon provokes an autoimmune humoral response to the AChR (Gu et al., 1995).

References

Aarli JA, Stefansson K, Marton LSG, et al. (1990). Patients with myasthenia gravis and thymoma have human leukocyte antigen in their sera Igg autoantibodies against titin. Clin Exp Immunol 82: 284–288.

Aarli JA, Gilhus NE, Matre R (1992). Myasthenia gravis with thymoma is not associated with an increased incidence of non-muscle autoimmune disorders. Autoimmunity 11: 159–162.

Ajtai B, Fine EJ, Lincoff N (2004). Pupil-sparing, painless compression of the oculomotor nerve by expanding basilar artery aneurysm: a case of pseudomyasthenia. Arch Neurol 61: 1448–1450.

Akkaya OF, Sahin HA, Senel A, et al. (2005). Brain stem lesion mimicking myasthenia gravis. Clin Neurol Neurosurg 107: 246–248.

Albers JW, Hodach RJ, Kimmel DW, et al. (1980). Penicillamine-induced myasthenia gravis. Neurology 30: 1246–1250.

Andrews PI, Massey JM, Sanders DB (1993). Acetylcholine receptor antibodies in juvenile myasthenia gravis. Neurology 43: 977–982.

Andrews PI, Massey JM, Howard JF Jr., et al. (1994). Race, sex, and puberty influence onset, severity, and outcome in juvenile myasthenia gravis. Neurology 44: 1208–1214.

Anlar B, Senbil N, Kose G, et al. (2005). Serological followup in juvenile myasthenia: clinical and acetylcholine receptor antibody status of patients followed for at least 2 years. Neuromuscul Dis 15: 355–357.

Austin EH, Olanow W, Wechsler AS (1983). Thymoma following transcervical thymectomy for myasthenia gravis. Ann Thorac Surg 35: 548–550.

Authier FJ, De Grissac N, Degos JD, et al. (1995). Transient myasthenia gravis during HIV infection. Muscle Nerve 18: 914–916.

Batocchi AP, Evoli A, Palmisani MT, et al. (1990). Early-onset myasthenia gravis: clinical characteristics and response to therapy. Eur J Pediatr 150: 66–68.

Batocchi AP, Evoli A, Servidei S, et al. (1995). Myasthenia gravis during interferon alfa therapy. Neurology 45: 382–383.

Batocchi AP, Majolini L, Evoli A, et al. (1999). Course and treatment of myasthenia gravis during pregnancy. Neurology 52: 447–452.

Beghi E, Antozzi C, Batocchi AP, et al. (1991). Prognosis of myasthenia gravis: a multicenter follow-up study of 844 patients. J Neurol Sci 106: 213–220.

Berrouschot J, Baumann I, Kalischewski P, et al. (1997). Therapy of myasthenic crisis. Crit Care Med 25: 1228–1235.

Bever CT, Aquino AV, Penn AS, et al. (1983). Prognosis of ocular myasthenia. Ann Neurol 14: 516–519.

Brodsky MC, Baker RS, Hamed LM (1996). Pediatric Neuro-Ophthalmology. Springer, New York.

Buckley C, Newsom-Davis J, Willcox N, et al. (2001). Do titin and cytokine antibodies in MG patients predict thymoma or thymoma recurrence? Neurology 57: 1579–1582.

Budde JM, Morris CD, Gal AA, et al. (2001). Predictors of outcome in thymectomy for myasthenia gravis. Ann Thorac Surg 72: 197–202.

Caress JB, Hunt CH, Batish SD (2005). Anti-MuSK myasthenia gravis presenting with purely ocular findings. Arch Neurol 62: 1002–1003.

Chevessier F, Faraut B, Ravel-Chapuis A, et al. (2004). MuSK, a new target for mutations causing congenital myasthenic syndrome. Hum Mole Gen 13: 3229–3240.

Chiu HC, Newsom-Davis J, Hsieh KH, et al. (1987). Myasthenia gravis: population differences in disease expression and acetylcholine receptor antibody titers between Chinese and Caucasians. Neurology 37: 1854–1857.

Christensen PB, Jensen TS, Tsiropoulos I, et al. (1995). Associated autoimmune diseases in myasthenia gravis. A population-based study. Acta Neurol Scand 91: 192–195.

Christiansen FT, Pollack MS, Garlepp MJ, et al. (1984). Myasthenia gravis and HLA antigens in American blacks and other races. J Neuroimmunol 7: 121–129.

Cogan DG (1965). Myasthenia gravis. A review of the disease and a description of lid twitch as a characteristic sign. Arch Ophthalmol 62: 156–162.

Czaplinski A, Steck AJ, Fuhr P (2003). Ice pack test for myasthenia gravis. A simple, noninvasive and safe diagnostic method. J Neurol 250: 883–884.

De Assis JL, Marchiori PE, Scaff M (1994). Atrophy of the tongue with persistent articulation disorder in myasthenia gravis: report of 10 patients. Auris Nasus Larynx 21: 215–218.

DeChiari TM, Bowen DC, Valensuela DM, et al. (1996). The receptor tyrosine kinase MuSK is required for neuromuscular junction formation in vivo. Cell 85: 501–512.

Dell'Osso LF, Ayyar DR, Daroff RB, et al. (1983). Edrophonium test in Eaton–Lambert syndrome: quantitative oculography. Neurology 33: 1157–1163.

Derossi A, Calabro ML, Panozzo M, et al. (1990). In vitro studies of Hiv-1 infection in thymic lymphocytes—a putative role of the thymus in Aids pathogenesis. Aids Res Hum Retroviruses 6: 287–298.

Desmedt JE, Borenstein S (1977). Time course of neonatal myasthenia gravis and unsuspectedly long duration of neuromuscular block in distal muscles. N Engl J Med 296: 633.

Dinger J, Prager B (1993). Arthrogryposis multiplex in a newborn of a myasthenic mother—case report and literature. Neuromuscul Dis 3: 335–339.

Dirr LY, Donofrio PD, Patton JF, et al. (1989). A false-positive edrophonium test in a patient with a brainstem glioma. Neurology 39: 865–867.

Djelmis J, Sostarko M, Mayer D, et al. (2002). Myasthenia gravis in pregnancy: report on 69 cases. Eur J Ob Gyn Repro Biol 104: 21–25.

Drachman DB (1994). Medical progress: myasthenia gravis. N Engl J Med 330: 1797–1810.

Drachman DB, Adams RN, Josifek LF, et al. (1982). Functional activities of autoantibodies to acetylcholine receptors and the clinical severity of myasthenia gravis. N Engl J Med 307: 769–775.

Ellenhorn N, Lucchese N, Greenwald M (1986). Juvenile myasthenia gravis and amblyopia. Am J Ophthal 101: 214–217.

Engel AG, Santa T (1971). Histometric analysis of the ultrastucture of the neuromuscular junction in myasthenia gravis and in the myasthenic syndrome. Ann N Y Acad Sci 183: 46–63.

Engel AG, Sahashi K, Lambert EH, et al. (1979). The ultrastructural localization of the acetylcholine receptor, immunoglobulin G and the third and ninth complement components at the motor end-plate and their implications for the pathogenesis of myasthenia gravis. In: AJ Aguayo, G. Karpati (Eds.), Current Topics in Nerve and Muscle Research. Exc Med, Amsterdam, pp. 111–122.

Engel AG, Ohno K, Sine SM (1999). Congenital myasthenic syndromes. In: AG Engel (Ed.), Myasthenia Gravis and Myasthenic Disorders. Oxford University Press, New York, pp. 251–297.

Ertas M, Arac N, Kumral K, et al. (1994). Ice test as a simple diagnostic aid for myasthenia gravis. Acta Neurol Scand 89: 227–229.

Evoli A, Batocchi AP, Zelano G, et al. (1995). Familial autoimmune myasthenia gravis: report of four families. J Neurol Neurosurg Psychiatry 58: 729–731.

Evoli A, Batocchi AP, Bartoccioni E, et al. (1998a). Juvenile myasthenia gravis with prepubertal onset. Neuromuscul Dis 8: 561–567.

Evoli A, Batocchi AP, Tonali P, et al. (1998b). Risk of cancer in patients with myasthenia gravis. Ann N Y Acad Sci 841: 742–745.

Evoli A, Minisci C, Di Schino C, et al. (2003a). Thymoma in patients with MG. Neurology 59: 1844–1850.

Evoli A, Tonali PA, Padua L, et al. (2003b). Clinical correlates with anti-MuSK antibodies in generalized seronegative myasthenia gravis. Brain 126: 2304–2311.

Evoli A, Punzi C, Marsili F, et al. (2004). Extrathymic malignancies in patients with thymoma. Ann Oncol 15: 692–693.

Fambrough DM, Drachman DB, Satyamurti S (1973). Neuromuscular junction in myasthenia gravis: decreased acetylcholine receptors. Science 182: 293–295.

Felice KJ, DiMario FJ, Conway SR (2005). Postinfectious myasthenia gravis: report of two children. J Child Neurol 20: 441–444.

Fenichel GM (1989). Myasthenia gravis in children. Int Pediatr 4: 151–154.

Fukuyama Y, Suzuki M, Segawa M (1970). Studies on myasthenia gravis in childhood. Paediatr Univ Tokyo 18: 57–68.

Garcia-Ramos G, Tellez-Zenteno JF, Zapata-Zuniga M, et al. (2003). HLA class II genotypes in Mexican Mestizo patients with myasthenia gravis. Eur J Neurol 10: 707–710.

Gardnerova M, Eymard B, Morel E, et al. (1997). The fetal/adult acetylcholine receptor antibody ratio in mothers with myasthenia gravis as a marker for the transfer of the disease to the newborn. Neurology 48: 50–54.

Gautel M, Lakey A, Barlow DP, et al. (1993). Titin antibodies in myasthenia gravis: identification of a major immunogenic region of titin. Neurology 43: 1581–1585.

Geh VS, Bradbury JA (1998). Ocular myasthenia presenting in an 11-month-old boy. Eye 12: 319–320.

Gherardi R, Chariot P, Authier FJ (1995). Muscular involvement in HIV infection. Rev Neurol (Paris) 151: 603–607.

Glaser JS (1966). Myasthenic pseudo-internuclear ophthalmoplegia. Arch Ophthalmol 75: 363–366.

Golnik KC, Pena R, Lee AG, et al. (1999). An ice test for the diagnosis of myasthenia gravis. Ophthalmol 106: 1282–1286.

Grob D (1999). Natural history of myasthenia gravis. In: AG Engel (Ed.), Myasthenia Gravis and Myasthenic Disorders. Oxford University Press, New York, pp. 131–145.

Grob D, Brunner NG, Namba T (1981). The natural course of myasthenia gravis and effect of therapeutic measures. Ann N Y Acad Sci 377: 652–669.

Grob D, Arsura EL, Brunner NG, et al. (1987). The course of myasthenia gravis and therapies affecting outcome. Ann N Y Acad Sci 505: 472–499.

Gronseth GS, Barohn RJ (2000). Practice parameter: thymectomy for autoimmune myasthenia gravis (an evidence-based review). Neurology 55: 5–15.

Gu D, Wogensen L, Calcutt NA, et al. (1995). Myasthenia gravis-like syndrome induced by expression of interferon gamma in the neuromuscular junction. J Exp Med 181: 547–557.

Gupta M, Davis H, Rennie IG (2003). Positive tensilon test and intracranial tumor: a case report. Eur J Ophthalmol 13: 590–592.

Hassan MM (1977). Ganglioneuroblastoma presenting as myasthenia gravis. Childs Brain 3: 65–68.

Hatanaka Y, Claussen GC, Oh SJ (2005). Anticholinesterase hypersensitivity or intolerance is common in MuSK antibody positive myasthenia gravis. Neurology 64: A79.

Hill M, Moss P, Wordsworth P, et al. (1999). T cell responses to D-penicillamine in drug-induced myasthenia gravis: recognition of modified DR1:peptide complexes. J Neuroimmunol 97: 146–153.

Hoff JM, Daltveit AK, Gilhus NE (2004). Asymptomatic myasthenia gravis influences pregnancy and birth. Eur J Neurol 11: 559–562.

Howard FM, Lennon VA, Finley J, et al. (1987). Clinical correlations of antibodies that bind, block, or modulate human acetylcholine receptors in myasthenia gravis. Ann N Y Acad Sci 505: 526–538.

Husain AM, Massey JM, Howard JF, et al. (1998). Acetylcholine receptor antibody measurements in acquired myasthenia gravis. Diagnostic sensitivity and predictive value for thymoma. Ann N Y Acad Sci 841: 471–474.

Ing EB, Ing SY, Ing T, et al. (2005). The complication rate of edrophonium testing for suspected myasthenia gravis. Can J Ophthalmol 35: 141–144.

Isbister CM, Mackenzie PJ, Anderson D, et al. (2002). Co-occurrence of multiple sclerosis and myasthenia gravis in British Columbia: a population-based study. Neurology 58: A165–A186.

Isbister CM, Mackenzie PJ, Anderson D, et al. (2003). Co-occurrence of multiple sclerosis and myasthenia gravis in British Columbia. Multiple Sclerosis 9: 550–553.

Kalb B, Matell G, Pirskanen R, et al. (2002). Epidemiology of myasthenia gravis: a population-based study in Stockholm, Sweden. Neuroepidemiol 21: 221–225.

Kanzato N, Motomura M, Suehara M, et al. (1999). Lambert–Eaton myasthenic syndrome with ophthalmoparesis and pseudoblepharospasm. Muscle Nerve 22: 1727–1730.

Katz B, Miledi R (1973). The binding of acetylcholine to receptors and its removal from the synaptic cleft. J Physiol 231: 549–574.

Katz JS, Wolfe GI, Bryan WW, et al. (1998). Acetylcholine receptor antibodies in the Lambert–Eaton myasthenic syndrome. Neurology 50: 470–475.

Kerzin-Storrar L, Metcalfe RA, Dyer PA, et al. (1988). Genetic factors in myasthenia gravis: a family study. Neurology 38: 38–42.

Khan GA, Bank N (1995). Interpretation of positive edrophonium (Tensilon) testing in patients with end-stage renal disease. Ren Fail 17: 65–71.

Kida K, Hayashi M, Yamada I, et al. (1987). Heterogeneity in myasthenia gravis: HLA phenotypes and autoantibody responses in ocular and generalized types. Ann Neurol 21: 274–278.

Kuks JBM, Oosterhuis HJGH (2004). Clinical presentation and epidemiology of myasthenia gravis. In: HJ Kaminski (Ed.), Current Clinical Neurology: Myasthenia Gravis and Related Disorders. Humana Press, Totowa, NJ, pp. 93–113.

Kupersmith MJ, Latkany R, Homel P (2003). Development of generalized disease at 2 years in patients with ocular myasthenia gravis. Arch Neurol 60: 243–248.

Larner AJ (2004). The place of the ice pack test in the diagnosis of myasthenia gravis. Int J Clin Pract 58: 887–888.

Lauriola L, Ranelletti F, Maggiano N, et al. (2005). Thymus changes in anti-MuSK-positive and -negative myasthenia gravis. Neurology 64: 536–538.

Lavrnic D, Jarebinski M, Rakocevic-Stojanovic V, et al. (1999). Epidemiological and clinical characteristics of myasthenia gravis in Belgrade, Yugoslavia (1983–1992). Acta Neurol Scand 100: 168–174.

Lavrnic D, Losen M, de Baets M, et al. (2005). The features of myasthenia gravis with autoantibodies to MuSK. J Neurol Neurosurg Psychiatry 76: 1099–1102.

Leite MI, Strobel P, Jones M, et al. (2005). Fewer thymic changes in MuSK antibody-positive than in MuSK antibody-negative MG. Ann Neurol 57: 444–448.

Lennon VA (1994). Serological diagnosis of myasthenia gravis and the Lambert–Eaton myasthenic syndrome. In: RP Lisak (Ed.), Handbook of Myasthenia Gravis and Myasthenic Syndromes. Marcel Dekker, New York, pp. 149–164.

Lennon VA (1997). Serological profile of myasthenia gravis and distinction from the Lambert–Eaton myasthenic syndrome. Neurology 48: S23–S27.

Linder A, Schalke B, Toyka KV (1997). Outcome in juvenile-onset myasthenia gravis: a retrospective study with long-term follow-up of 79 patients. J Neurol 244: 515–520.

Lindstrom J (1977). An assay for antibodies to human acetylcholine receptor in serum from patients with myasthenia gravis. Clin Immunol Immunopathol 7: 36–43.

Lindstrom JM, Seybold ME, Lennon VA, et al. (1976). Antibody to acetylcholine receptor in myasthenia gravis. Neurology 26: 1054–1059.

Llabres M, Molina-Martinez FJ, Miralles F (2005). Dysphagia as the sole manifestation of myasthenia gravis. J Neurol Neurosurg Psychiatry 76: 1297–1300.

Machens A, Loliger C, Pichlmeier U, et al. (1999). Correlation of thymic pathology with HLA in myasthenia gravis. Clin Immunol 91: 296–301.

Mackey JR, Desai S, Larratt L, et al. (1997). Myasthenia gravis in association with allogeneic bone marrow transplantation. Bone Marrow Transplant 19: 939–942.

Madonick MJ, Rubin M, Levine LH, et al. (1957). Myasthenia gravis developing fifteen months after removal of thymoma. Arch Intern Med 99: 151–155.

Magni G, Micaglio GF, Lalli R, et al. (1988). Psychiatric disturbances associated with myasthenia gravis. Acta Psychiatr Scand 77: 443–445.

Martini L, Vion P, Le Gangneux E, et al. (1991). AIDS and myasthenia: an uncommon association. Rev Neurol (Paris) 147: 395–397.

Mase G, Zorzon M, Biasutti E, et al. (1996). Development of myasthenia gravis during interferon-α treatment for anti-HCV positive chronic hepatitis. J Neurol Neurosurg Psychiatry 60: 348–349.

Matsuki K, Juji T, Tokunaga K, et al. (1990). HLA antigens in Japanese patients with myasthenia gravis. J Clin Invest 86: 392–399.

McConville J, Farrugia ME, Beeson D, et al. (2004). Detection and characterization of MuSK antibodies in seronegative myasthenia gravis. Ann Neurol 55: 580–584.

Mier AK, Havard CW (1985). Diaphragmatic myasthenia in mother and child. Postgrad Med J 61: 725–727.

Mindel JS, Charney JZ (1989). Bilateral intracavernous carotid aneurysms presenting as pseudoocular myasthenia gravis. Trans Am Ophthalmol Soc 87: 445–457.

Monden Y, Uyama T, Taniki T, et al. (1988). The characteristics of thymoma with myasthenia gravis: a 28-year experience. J Surg Oncol 38: 151–154.

Monden Y, Uyama T, Kimura S, et al. (1991). Extrathymic malignancy in patients with myasthenia gravis. Eur J Cancer 27: 745–747.

Moore HK, Kenzie PR, Kennedy CW, et al. (2001). Thymoma: trends over time. Ann Thorac Surg 72: 203–207.

Morel E, Eymard B, Vernet-der Garabedian B, et al. (1988). Neonatal myasthenia gravis: a new clinical and immunologic appraisal on 30 cases. Neurology 38: 138–142.

Mulder DW, Lambert EH, Eaton LM (1959). Myasthenic syndrome in patients with amyotrophic lateral sclerosis. Neurology 9: 627–631.

Mullaney P, Vajsar J, Smith R, et al. (2000). The natural history and ophthalmic involvement in childhood myasthenia gravis at the hospital for sick children. Ophthalmol 107: 504–510.

Muller-Hermelink HK, Marx A (2000). Thymoma. Curr Opin Oncol 12: 426–433.

Naeim F, Keesey JC, Herrmann C, et al. (1978). Association of HLA-B8, DRw3, and anti-acetylcholine receptor antibodies in myasthenia gravis. Tissue Antigens 12: 381–386.

Namba T, Brown SB, Grob D (1970). Neonatal myasthenia gravis: a report of two cases and review of the literature. Pediatrics 45: 488–504.

Namba T, Brunner NG, Grob D (1978). Myasthenia gravis in patients with thymoma, with particular reference to onset after thymectomy. Medicine 57: 411–433.

Nath A, Kerman RH, Novak IS, et al. (1990). Immune studies in human-immunodeficiency-virus infection with myasthenia gravis—a case report. Neurology 40: 581–583.

Nelson KR, McQuillen MP (1988). Neurologic complications of graft-versus-host disease. Neurol Clin N Am 6: 389–403.

Newsom-Davis J, Leys K, Vincent A, et al. (1991). Immunological evidence for the co-existence of the Lambert–Eaton myasthenic syndrome and myasthenia gravis in two patients. J Neurol Neurosurg Psychiatry 54: 452–453.

Oh SJ, Cho HK (1990). Edrophonium responsiveness not necessarily diagnostic of myasthenia gravis. Muscle Nerve 13: 187–191.

Oh SJ, Sher E (2005). MG and LEMS overlap syndrome: case report with electrophysiological and immunological evidence. Clin Neurophysiol 116: 1167–1171.

Okamoto K, Ito J, Tokiguchi S, et al. (1996). Atrophy of bilateral extraocular muscles—CT and clinical features of seven patients. J Neuroophthalmol 16: 286–288.

Oosterhuis HJGH (1989). The natural course of myasthenia gravis: a long term follow-up study. J Neurol Neurosurg Psychiatry 52: 1121–1127.

Oosterhuis HJGH, Kuks JBM (1997). Myasthenia gravis with thymoma. In: A Marx, HK Muller-Hermelink (Eds.), Epithelial Tumors of the Thymus. Pathology, Biology, Treatment. Plenum Press, New York, pp. 271–280.

Osher RH, Griggs RC (1979). Orbicularis fatigue. Arch Ophthalmol 97: 677–679.

Osserman KE (1955). Pregnancy in myasthenia gravis and neonatal myasthenia gravis. Am J Med 19: 718–721.

Osserman KE (1958). Myasthenia Gravis. Grune & Stratton, New York.

Osserman KE, Genkins G (1971). Studies in myasthenia gravis: review of a 20-year experience in over 1200 patients. Mt Sinai J Med 38: 497–537.

Papazian O (1992). Transient neonatal myasthenia gravis. J Child Neurol 7: 135–141.

Pascuzzi RM (2003). The edrophonium test. Semin Neurol 23: 83–88.

Penn AS, Low BW, Jaffe IA, et al. (1998). Drug-induced autoimmune myasthenia gravis. Ann N Y Acad Sci 841: 433–449.

Phillips LH (2003). The epidemiology of myasthenia gravis. A United States perspective. Ann N Y Acad Sci 998: 407–412.

Phillips LH, Torner JC, Anderson MS, et al. (1992). The epidemiology of myasthenia gravis in central and western Virginia. Neurology 42: 1888–1893.

Pirskanen R (1977). Genetic aspects in myasthenia gravis. A family study of 264 Finnish patients. Acta Neurol Scand 56: 365–388.

Plauche WC (1991). Myasthenia gravis in mothers and their newborns. Clin Obstet Gynecol 34: 82–99.

Polizzi A, Huson SM, Vincent A (2000). Teratogen update: maternal myasthenia gravis as a cause of congenital arthrogryposis. Teratology 62: 332–341.

Riemersma S, Vincent A, Beeson D, et al. (1996). Association of arthrogryposis multiplex congenita with maternal antibodies inhibiting fetal acetylcholine receptor function. J Clin Invest 98: 2358–2363.

Rodolico C, Girlanda P, Nicolosi C, et al. (2003). Chiari I malformation mimicking myasthenia gravis. J Neurol Neurosurg Psychiatry 74: 388–394.

Rodriguez M, Gomez MR, Howard FM, Jr., et al. (1983). Myasthenia gravis in children: long-term follow-up. Ann Neurol 13: 504–510.

Romi F, Skeie GO, Aarli JA, et al. (2000a). Muscle auto-antibodies in subgroups of myasthenia gravis patients. J Neurol 247: 369–375.

Romi F, Skeie GO, Aarli JA, et al. (2000b). The severity of myasthenia gravis correlates with the serum concentration of titin and ryanodine receptor antibodies. Arch Neurol 57: 1596–1600.

Rosenow EC, Hurley BT (1984). Disorders of the thymus. Arch Intern Med 144: 763–770.

Rostedt A, Sanders LL, Edwards LJ, et al. (2000). Predictive value of single-fiber electromyography in the extensor digitorum communis muscle in patients with ocular myasthenia gravis: a retrospective study. J Clin Neuromusc Dis 2: 6–9.

Rowland LP, Aranow H, Hoefer PFA (1957). Myasthenia gravis appearing after the removal of thymoma. Neurology 7: 584–588.

Saavedra J, Femminini R, Kochen S, et al. (1979). A cold test for myasthenia gravis. Neurology 29: 1075.

Sanders DB, Howard JF, Jr. (1986). Single-fiber electromyography in myasthenia gravis. Muscle Nerve 9: 809–819.

Sanders DB, Howard JF, Jr. (1988). Thymoma without myasthenia gravis: electrophysiological study after thymectomy. J Neurol Neurosurg Psychiatry 51: 160–161.

Sanders DB, Andrews PI, Howard JF, Jr., et al. (1997). Seronegative myasthenia gravis. Neurology 48(Suppl 5): S40–S51.

Sanders DB, El Salem K, Massey JM, et al. (2003). Clinical aspects of MuSK antibody positive seronegative MG. Neurology 60: 1978–1980.

Scott JS (1997). Immunologic diseases in pregnancy. Prog Allergy 23: 371–375.

Sethi KD, Rivner MH, Swift TR (1987). Ice pack test for myasthenia gravis. Neurology 37: 1383–1385.

Seybold ME (1999). Diagnosis of myasthenia gravis. In: AG Engel (Ed.), Myasthenia Gravis and Myasthenic Disorders. Oxford University Press, New York, pp. 146–166.

Simpson JA (1960). Myasthenia gravis: a new hypothesis. Scot Med J 5: 419–436.

Sisman J, Ceri A, Nafday SM (2004). Seronegative neonatal myasthenia gravis in one of two twins. Indian Pediatr 41: 938–940.

Skeie GO, Lunde PK, Sejersted OM, et al. (2001). Autoimmunity against the ryanodine receptor in myasthenia gravis. Acta Physiol Scand 171: 379–384.

Snead OC, Benton JW, Dwyer D, et al. (1980). Juvenile myasthenia gravis. Neurology 30: 732–739.

Somnier FE, Engel PJH (2002). The occurrence of anti-titin antibodies and thymomas. Neurology 59: 92–98.

Sorensen TT, Holm E-B (1989). Myasthenia gravis in the county of Viborg, Denmark. Eur Neurol 29: 177–179.

Souadijian JV, Silverstein MN, Titus JL (1968). Thymoma and cancer. Cancer 22: 1221–1225.

Stickler DE, Massey JM, Sanders DB (2005). MuSK-antibody positive myasthenia gravis: clinical and electro-diagnostic patterns. Clin Neurophysiol 116: 2065–2068.

Stoll C, Ehret-Mentre MC, Treisser A, et al. (1991). Prenatal diagnosis of congenital myasthenia with arthrogryposis in a myasthenic mother. Prenat Diagn 11: 17–22.

Strauss AJL, Seegal BC, Hsu KC, et al. (1960). Immuno-fluorescence demonstration of a muscle-binding complement-fixing serum globulin fraction in myasthenia gravis. Proc Soc Exp Biol Med 105: 184–191.

Sunness JS, Kelman S (2004). Cosmetic botox injection mimicking myasthenia gravis. Plast Reconstruct Surg 113: 1515.

Teng P, Osserman KE (1956). Studies in myasthenia gravis: neonatal and juvenile types. J Mt Sinai Hosp 23: 711–727.

Thomas CE, Mayer SA, Gungor Y, et al. (1997). Myasthenic crisis: clinical features, mortality, complications, and risk factors for prolonged intubation. Neurology 48: 1253–1260.

Thomas M, Ahuja GK, Behari M, et al. (1993). Ocular myasthenia—factors predictive for generalisation. J Assoc Physicians India 41: 28–29.

Thorlacius S, Aarli JA, Riise T, et al. (1989). Associated disorders in myasthenia gravis: autoimmune diseases and their relation to thymectomy. Acta Neurol Scand 80: 290–295.

Tiab M, Letortorec S, Michelet C, et al. (1993). Occurrence of myasthenia in HIV infection. 2 cases. Ann Med Int 144: 456–462.

Trojan DA, Gendron D, Cashman NR (1993). Anti-choline-sterase-responsive neuromuscular junction transmission defects in post-poliomyelitis fatigue. J Neurol Sci 114: 170–177.

Uono M (1980). Clinical statistics of myasthenia gravis in Japan. Internat J Neurol 14: 87–99.

Vernet-der Garabedian B, Lacokova M, Eymard B, et al. (1994). Association of neonatal myasthenia gravis with antibodies against the fetal acetylcholine receptor. J Clin Invest 94: 555–559.

Vincent A, Newsom-Davis J (1985). Acetylcholine receptor antibody as a diagnostic test for myasthenia gravis: results in 153 validated cases and 2967 diagnostic assays. J Neurol Neurosurg Psychiatry 48: 1246–1252.

Vincent A, Newland C, Brueton L, et al. (1995). Arthrogry-posis multiplex congenita with maternal autoantibodies specific for a fetal antigen. Lancet 346: 24–25.

Vincent A, Clover L, Buckley C, et al. (2003). Evidence of underdiagnosis of myasthenia gravis in older people. J Neurol Neurosurg Psychiatry 74: 1105–1108.

Vincent A, Sanders DB, Drachman DB, et al. (2004). Multi-center study of clinical, geographical, and ethnic features of MuSK-antibody-associated myasthenia gravis. Ann Neurol 56(Suppl 8): S63.

Volpe JJ (1995). Neuromuscular disorders: levels above the lower motor neuron to the neuromuscular junction. In: JJ Volpe (Ed.), Neurology of the Newborn. 3rd edn. Saunders, Philadelphia, pp. 606–633.

Vujic A, Lavrnic D, Stojanovic V, et al. (2004). Myasthenia gravis and associated diseases. Eur J Neurol 11(Suppl 2): 272.

Walsh FB, Hoyt WF (1969). Chapter 9: Disorders of muscle. Clinical Ophthalmology 2. Baltimore, Williams & Wilkins, pp. 1242–1311.

Weinberg DH, Rizzo JF, Hayes MT, et al. (1999). Ocular myasthenia gravis: predictive value of single-fiber electro-myography. Muscle Nerve 22: 1222–1227.

Wessel HB, Zitelli BJ (1987). Myasthenia gravis associated with human T-cell lymphotropic virus type III infection. Pediatr Neurol 3: 238–239.

Wirtz PW, Sotodeh M, Nijnuis M, et al. (2002). Difference in distribution of muscle weakness between myasthenia gravis and the Lambert–Eaton myasthenic syndrome. J Neurol Neurosurg Psychiatry 73: 766–768.

Wong V, Hawkins BR, Yu YL (1992). Myasthenia gravis in Hong Kong Chinese. 2. Paediatric disease. Acta Neurol Scand 86: 68–72.

Wullenweber M, Schneider U, Hagenah R (1993). Myasthenia gravis in AIDS and neurosyphilis. Nervenarzt 64: 273–277.

Handbook of Clinical Neurology, Vol. 91 (3rd series)
Neuromuscular junction disorders
A.G. Engel, Editor

Chapter 8

Therapy of myasthenia gravis

DANIEL B. DRACHMAN*

Johns Hopkins School of Medicine, Baltimore, MD, USA

8.1. Introduction

Although the term "Myasthenia Gravis Pseudoparaly-tica," coined by Jolly in 1895 (Jolly, 1895), implied a grave prognosis, the outlook for myasthenic patients has improved dramatically in recent years as a result of important advances in treatment. At present, with optimal treatment, the mortality rate is essentially zero, and nearly all myasthenic patients can be returned to full productive lives (Grob et al., 1987). Myasthenia gravis (MG) is now the best understood human autoimmune disease, and is certainly the most treatable neuromuscular disease. Therapy of MG is based directly on concepts of the pathophysiology and immunology of MG. Therefore, successful practical treatment requires a clear understanding of both the physiological abnormalities at the neuromuscular junction (NMJ), and the immunological basis of the autoimmune attack, briefly reviewed below.

8.1.1. The neuromuscular junction in MG

The changes at the myasthenic NMJ—a reduction in the number of available acetylcholine receptors (AChRs) and alteration of postsynaptic membrane structure—account fully for the clinical and electro-physiological features of MG. Normal neuromuscular transmission depends on the release of acetylcholine (ACh) from the motor nerve terminal and its inter-action with AChRs at the postsynaptic membrane. ACh is stored in the presynaptic nerve terminal in packets or "quanta," estimated to contain approxi-mately 10 000 molecules (Miledi et al., 1983). ACh release occurs by exocytosis from the vesicles, which fuse with the nerve terminal membrane at "preferred" release sites. Vesicle release sites are situated directly

opposite the areas of highest concentration of AChRs, which are at the tops of the folds of the postsynaptic membrane. Normally, quantal release of ACh occurs both spontaneously and in response to nerve impulses. Spontaneous release of ACh involves single vesicles, and gives rise to local low-amplitude depolarizations of the muscle membrane, or "miniature end-plate poten-tials" (mepps). When a motor nerve impulse invades the nerve terminal, many quanta (50–300) are released (Ruff, 1998). The released ACh binds to the post-synaptic AChRs, producing transient opening of the receptors' ion channels. The rapid entry of cations results in a localized depolarization (the endplate potential). If the amplitude of the endplate potential is sufficient, it generates an action potential that spreads along the length of the muscle fiber, triggering the release of Ca^{2+} from internal stores, and leading to muscle contraction. At normal neuromuscular junc-tions, the endplate potential is more than sufficient to generate muscle action potentials without failures. The excess above threshold has been termed the "safety margin" of neuromuscular transmission (Waud, 1971).

In MG, the reduction in the numbers of AChRs results in a corresponding decrease of the amplitude of endplate potentials, and a reduction of the safety margin. This results in failure of transmission at some junctions (Stalberg et al., 1976). When transmission fails at many junctions, the power of the whole muscle is reduced, which is clinically manifested as weakness. If the safety margin is borderline, repeated stimulation may result in progressive decline in muscle power, or "neuromuscular fatigue," which is a typical clinical feature of MG. Fatigue occurs as a consequence of the reduced safety margin, in combination with the normal phenomenon of ACh "rundown." During repeated stimulation the amount of ACh released per

*Correspondence to: Daniel B. Drachman, MD, Professor of Neurology & Neuroscience, WW Smith Foundation Professor of Neuroimmunology, 5-119 Meyer Building, Johns Hopkins School of Medicine, 600 N. Wolfe St., Baltimore, MD 21287-7519, USA. E-mail: dandrac@aol.com, Tel: 1-410-955-5406, Fax: 1-410-955-1961.

impulse normally declines (runs down) after the first few impulses, since the nerve terminal is not able to sustain its initial rate of release (Stalberg et al., 1976). As the number of ACh–AChR interactions decreases, the endplate potential falls below threshold, resulting in progressive failure of contraction at more and more muscle fibers, or "fatigue." It is also manifested by a *decremental electrical response* on repetitive nerve stimulation. In healthy individuals, the safety margin is sufficient so that transmission failure and fatigue do not occur except at very rapid rates of nerve stimulation, above 40 Hz or 50 Hz.

The basic neuromuscular abnormality in MG—a reduction in the number of available AChRs at neuromuscular junctions—was first demonstrated quantitatively using radioactively labeled α-BuTx (Fambrough et al., 1973; Ito et al., 1978; Pestronk et al., 1985), and shown ultrastructurally, with peroxidase-labeled α-BuTx (Engel, 1992). In general, the degree of reduction of AChRs correlates with the clinical severity of MG. However, even patients with weakness restricted to the extraocular muscles may have reduced numbers of AChRs in clinically strong limb muscles (Pestronk et al., 1985). Additional morphological changes have been demonstrated at myasthenic NMJs, and contribute to impairment of transmission. "Simplification" of the normally complex folds of the postsynaptic membrane, increased distance between the motor nerve terminal and the postsynaptic membrane, and debris within the synaptic cleft are typical of the myasthenic junction (Engel et al., 1976).

8.1.2. The acetylcholine receptor

The molecular biology of the AChR is described in detail in Chapter 3. We will briefly summarize those features that are relevant to the immunology of MG. The AChR is a glycoprotein with a molecular weight of approximately 250 000, which projects through the muscle membrane. It is made up of 5 subunits, with 2 α-subunits, 1 β-subunit, either a γ- or an ε-subunit, and a δ-subunit, arranged around the circumference of a central ion channel (Kistler et al., 1982; Changeux, 1990; Unwin, 1995). There are two isoforms, a fetal isoform, which has a γ-subunit, and an adult isoform, in which the ε-subunit replaces the γ-subunit. The fetal isoform is present during embryonic life, and reappears in muscle that has been denervated. Each of the subunits has an extracellular domain of approximately 210 amino acids, and four transmembrane domains with a large cytoplasmic loop between M3 and M4. Each α-subunit has one binding site for ACh that is located extracellularly, centered around amino acids 192 and 193, at the interfaces between

the α- and δ-subunits, and the α- and γ- or ε-subunits. Functionally, the ion channel of the AChR is closed in the resting state. When both α-subunit binding sites are occupied, the AChR molecule twists slightly like a Chinese purse, opening the channel transiently, and allowing the rapid passage of cations.

AChRs are normally clustered at high concentrations (15 000 to 20 000/μ^2) at the peaks of folds of the NMJ, opposite the motor nerve's ACh release sites. Clustering of AChRs at the NMJ is dependent on motor innervation, and involves the interaction of several anchoring proteins, including rapsyn, agrin, utrophin, dystroglycan, and MuSK (muscle specific receptor protein kinase). MuSK is of particular interest, since it has recently been shown to be a target for antibodies in some patients with "AChR antibody negative MG" (Hoch et al., 2001; Sanders et al., 2003; McConville et al., 2004; Zhou et al., 2004). AChRs normally undergo continual turnover at the neuromuscular junction (Fambrough, 1979). Motor nerves have an important role in this process, regulating the synthesis, subunit composition, distribution, and degradation of AChRs. In muscles with an intact nerve supply, the turnover of the AChRs is slow with a half life of around 11 days in mice (Ramsay et al., 1992). If the motor nerve is cut, or if neuromuscular transmission is blocked pharmacologically (for example by botulinum toxin or α-BuTx), the turnover is accelerated and there is an increased rate of synthesis of new AChRs (Stanley and Drachman, 1981; Avila et al., 1989; Ramsay et al., 1992). The new receptors in denervated muscles contain γ-subunits instead of ε-subunits, and are distributed over the entire length of the muscle cell membrane (Witzemann et al., 1987). Similarly, in MG or the experimental animal model (EAMG), impairment of AChR transmission results in a compensatory increase in transcription of AChR message (Asher et al., 1988), and increased synthesis of AChRs (Wilson et al., 1983). These dynamic processes of turnover and renewal of junctional AChRs usually permit virtually complete recovery in MG, once the autoimmune attack has been brought under control.

8.1.3. Acetylcholinesterase

Acetylcholinesterase (AChE) is a glycoprotein enzyme that is bound to the basal lamina at the postsynaptic membrane of the NMJ, and is most highly concentrated in the secondary clefts. Its function is to hydrolyze ACh rapidly, and thus terminate each episode of neuromuscular transmission, permitting repeated activation of the muscle fiber. The molecular structure and function of AChE are now known in detail, and this knowledge has facilitated the understanding of genetic mutations causing endplate AChE deficiency (see Chapter 10). Drugs that inhibit AChE permit the released ACh to interact repeatedly with AChRs, and are used to improve neuromuscular transmission in MG. However, failure to remove ACh may cause the AChRs to become *desensitized*, or unresponsive to further application of ACh. Over the longer term, persistent cholinergic stimulation results in excitotoxic damage to the endplate. This may result from the use of excessive amounts of anti-AChE drugs, or from exposure to organophosphate insecticides or "war nerve gases," which produce paralysis by irreversibly blocking AChE.

8.1.4. Immune pathogenesis of MG

It is widely accepted that the neuromuscular abnormalities in MG are due to antibody-mediated processes (Lindstrom et al., 1988; Drachman, 1994; Ragheb and Lisak, 1998). Many lines of evidence support this concept: 1. 80–90% of myasthenic patients have antibodies directed against AChR that are detected by a standard radioimmunoassay (RIA). The RIA measures serum IgG, which binds to human AChR that has been tagged with ^{125}I-labeled α-bungarotoxin (Lindstrom et al., 1976). 2. The pathogenic antibody binds to the target antigen, AChR at neuromuscular junctions, in myasthenic patients (Engel, 1992). 3. Passive transfer of IgG from myasthenic patients to experimental mice reproduces the disease features (Toyka et al., 1975, 1977). 4. Immunization of a wide variety of experimental animals with purified AChR produces an experimental model of MG (experimental autoimmune MG) (Patrick and Lindstrom, 1973; Penn et al., 1976), which has proven useful for testing new therapeutic strategies. 5. Treatments that lower AChR antibody levels result in improvement of the disease (Dau et al., 1979; Hertel et al., 1979).

AChR antibodies reduce the number of available AChRs by three different mechanisms (Drachman et al., 1982). 1. Cross-linking of AChRs by the divalent antibodies, which accelerates endocytosis and degradation of the AChRs by the muscle cells (Kao and Drachman, 1977a; Drachman et al., 1978). 2. Blockade of the receptors' ACh binding sites by antibody. 3. Complement-mediated damage to neuromuscular junctions (Toyka et al., 1977). It is most likely that accelerated degradation and complement-mediated effects are most important pathologically, although the antibody repertoires of different myasthenic patients may have different functional effects. Their particular functional properties are probably related to the specific epitopes of the AChR to which they bind.

However, the ability of the serum to induce loss of available AChR by a combination of these mechanisms corresponds most closely to the clinical severity of the patient's MG (Drachman et al., 1982).

8.1.5. AChR antibody-negative MG

About 10–20% of patients with acquired MG do not have AChR antibodies detectable by RIA. Although this includes patients with mild localized MG, there is also a subgroup with generalized MG, whose disease corresponds to conventional MG with respect to most other clinical, diagnostic, and therapeutic properties (Mossman et al., 1986). Actually, these patients have circulating antibodies that are not detected by the conventional RIA, but do cause accelerated degradation of AChRs in culture systems, and are capable of inducing features of MG by passive transfer to mice (Drachman et al., 1987; Burges et al., 1994). Approximately 40% of these patients have serum antibodies that bind to MuSK, which plays a key role in anchoring AChRs at the neuromuscular junction (Hoch et al., 2001; Evoli et al., 2003; Sanders et al., 2003; McConville et al., 2004; Zhou et al., 2004). Anti-MuSK antibodies have recently been shown to result in a reduction of AChRs at NMJs (Shigemoto et al., 2006). Taken together, these findings indicate that "antibody-negative" MG is an antibody-mediated autoimmune disorder directed against one or more components of the NMJ that are not detected by the standard anti-AChR RIA.

8.1.6. Role of T cells in MG

Although production of the pathogenic antibodies in MG is directly attributable to B cells, T cells play a pivotal role in the disease process by providing help that is essential for the antibody production (Ragheb and Lisak, 1998). The requirement for T cells has been formally demonstrated in EAMG in rats (Lennon et al., 1976), and there is extensive evidence that T cells play a key role in the autoantibody response in human MG (Newsom-Davis et al., 1989). T cells from myasthenic patients respond to stimulation with AChR, and augment the production of AChR antibody production in vitro. AChR-reactive T cell lines or clones have been isolated from the peripheral blood lymphocytes or thymuses of myasthenic patients. In contrast to their role in AChR antibody production, T cells do not act as effector cells in MG. It is well documented that lymphocytes from some normal individuals can also be stimulated by AChR, although AChR-specific T cells are more numerous in myasthenic patients (Sommer et al., 1991). This is consistent with the concept that potentially autoreactive T cells can exist in the normal immune system.

Analysis of AChR-specific T lymphocytes from myasthenic patients has revealed striking heterogeneity in their patterns of responsiveness (Melms et al., 1992; Moiola et al., 1993). The T cells of each individual respond to a great variety of AChR epitopes, and there are significant differences in the epitopes to which T cells of different patients respond. The majority of T cell recognition sites are on the α-subunit, but T cells recognize epitopes on the other subunits as well. Attempts to analyze the repertoire of T cell receptors that recognize AChRs have not shown a consistent or restricted pattern. The striking heterogeneity of AChR-specific T lymphocytes must be taken into account when attempting to design immunotherapeutic approaches aimed specifically at these T cells (Drachman, 1996).

8.1.7. Origin of MG

The origin of the autoimmune response in MG remains an unsolved problem, as is also true in virtually all human autoimmune diseases. In fact, the heterogeneity of the repertoires of the AChR-specific autoantibodies and T cells argues that multiple different factors may trigger the autoimmune response in MG. The thymus has been implicated as a possible site of origin of MG for several reasons. Approximately 75% of MG patients have thymic abnormalities. Of these, 85% have hyperplasia (germinal center formation), and 15% have thymic tumors (Castleman, 1966). Thymectomy apparently results in improvement in a majority of patients. Both T and B lymphocytes from the thymus of myasthenic patients are more responsive to stimulation with AChR than are peripheral blood lymphocytes from the same patients (Sommer et al., 1990). In addition to lymphocytes, thymus glands from normal and myasthenic individuals contain muscle-like ("myoid") cells that express surface AChRs (Kao and Drachman, 1977b; Wekerle et al., 1978). Because of their strategic location within the thymus, surrounded by antigen presenting cells (APCs), and helper T cells, these AChR-bearing myoid cells are thought to be the source of the autoantigen, AChR. Some alteration of the myoid cells or the lymphocytes may break tolerance, and lead to the autoimmune response.

Attempts to implicate viruses as possible agents in precipitating the autoimmune response have been unsuccessful. Viruses could not be cultured from MG thymus tissue in recent-onset cases, and antibody titers against a number of common viruses did not differ from those in matched controls (Aoki et al., 1985).

The hypothesis that MG may be triggered by "molecular mimicry"—that is, an immune response to an infectious agent that resembles the AChR—has some support. Antibodies from 6 of 40 patients with MG recognized a peptide sequence of herpes simplex virus that is similar to a sequence of the AChR α-subunit (Schwimmbeck et al., 1989). Cross-reactivity between bacteria and the AChR has also been reported (Dieperink and Stefansson, 1989). Genetic factors may influence the likelihood of developing MG. There is a weak to moderate association of MG with the HLA antigens B8 and DRW3 in Caucasians (Carlsson et al., 1990), but Japanese and Chinese patients have different HLA associations. A wide variety of other autoimmune diseases have been reported to occur in some myasthenic patients and their relatives, suggesting that a genetic defect in immune regulation may be a predisposing factor in those patients.

8.2. Treatment of MG

The goal of treatment of MG is most simply defined in terms of clinical benefit: i.e., to restore the patient to fully functional status, and maintain the improved condition without recurrence or adverse effects of the treatments. For the great majority of MG patients this goal is attainable if the treatment program is carried out in a rational and systematic fashion. The steps in the treatment program may be divided into: 1. preliminaries; 2. selection of agents to use; 3. avoidance of agents or treatments that pose undue risks; 4. adjusting the treatment parameters as needed for the individual patient throughout the entire disease course, which is commonly lifelong.

8.2.1. Preliminaries

8.2.1.1. Diagnosis

It is essential to establish the diagnosis of MG *unequivocally* because 1. other treatable conditions may closely resemble MG and 2. the treatment of MG usually requires the prolonged use of drugs with the potential for adverse side effects, and in many patients surgical thymectomy. The diagnosis may be suspected on the basis of weakness and fatigability of skeletal muscles in a characteristic distribution, without loss of reflexes or impairment of sensation or other neurologic function. Typically, the extraocular muscles are involved early, giving rise to diplopia and ptosis. Proximal muscles are usually involved more than distal muscles, but virtually any pattern of skeletal muscle weakness may occur. Confirmatory tests include measurement of serum antibodies, electrodiagnostic testing, and response to anticholinesterase agents (Oh et al., 1992).

Approximately 85% of patients with generalized MG, but only 50–60% of patients with myasthenic weakness confined to the extraocular muscles, have antibodies to AChR, as measured by RIA (Lindstrom et al., 1976; Vincent and Newsom-Davis, 1985). As noted above, about 40% of AChR antibody negative patients with generalized myasthenic weakness have antibodies to MuSK, which has extended our diagnostic accuracy (Hoch et al., 2001; Evoli et al., 2003; Sanders et al., 2003; McConville et al., 2004; Zhou et al., 2004).

The presence of significant levels of anti-AChR or anti-MuSK antibodies is diagnostic for MG. Repetitive electrical stimulation of nerves at rates of 3–5 Hz, with recording of muscle potentials, shows decremental responses of 15% or more in *weak* muscles. Single fiber EMG (SFEMG) is a sensitive test, but may give positive responses of "jitter" or blocking in conditions other than MG. Electrodiagnostic tests in non-weak muscles may fail to give positive results. The injection of drugs that inhibit the enzyme AChE allow ACh to interact repeatedly with the limited number of AChRs, producing improvement in the strength of myasthenic muscles. Edrophonium is used most commonly for diagnostic testing because of the rapid onset (30 s) and brief duration (about 5 min) of its effect. Unequivocal improvement in function of one or more *objectively* weak muscles during the brief interval of pharmacologic effect is usually confirmatory of MG, but false-positive tests occur in some patients with other causes of muscle weakness. Because of the risk of bradycardia, syncope, or other cholinergic symptoms, atropine should be drawn up in a syringe and ready for use (for details of these tests see Chapter 7). Finally, there are rare patients in whom these confirmatory diagnostic tests are negative, but who are presumed to have MG on the basis of clinical features.

8.2.1.2. Differential diagnosis

Other conditions that may cause weakness of the cranial and somatic muscles must be considered in the differential diagnosis of MG, including Lambert–Eaton myasthenic syndrome (LEMS), the congenital myasthenias, botulism, drug-induced myasthenia (penicillamine, aminoglycosides, magnesium), intracranial mass lesions or vascular malformations, progressive external ophthalmoplegia, oculopharyngeal dystrophy, and thyrotoxic ophthalmopathy.

Each of these conditions should be considered, and appropriate diagnostic testing carried out. Especially when weakness is limited to the cranial musculature, it is essential to obtain MRI imaging of the brain and orbits to exclude other conditions that can cause similar features (Moorthy et al., 1989).

8.2.1.3. Search for associated conditions

These conditions must be searched for because (a) they may occur with increased incidence in myasthenic patients; (b) they may coexist, and lead to exacerbation of MG; (c) they may influence the choice of treatment methods for MG; (d) drugs that patients may be taking for some other condition may either affect MG directly, or could interact with therapeutic agents used to treat MG.

Myasthenic patients have an increased incidence of several associated disorders. Most common among them are abnormalities of the thymus gland. Approximately 75% of myasthenic patients have thymic abnormalities, as noted above. It is important to evaluate the thymus by CT or MRI scan. A thymic shadow in the anterior mediastinum may be present normally throughout young adulthood, but in a patient over the age of 40 it is highly suspicious for a thymoma unless proven otherwise. At any age, progressive increase in size of a mediastinal soft tissue density on repeated scans suggests the presence of a thymoma. Autoimmune thyroid disease—Hashimoto's thyroiditis and Graves' disease—occurs in 3–8% of myasthenic patients. Since either hyper- or hypothyroidism can exacerbate the weakness of MG (Drachman, 1962), it is important to evaluate both the thyroid status, and the evidence of autoimmune thyroid disease. MG is associated with a variety of other autoimmune diseases, including lupus erythematosus, rheumatoid arthritis, polymyositis, systemic sclerosis, idiopathic thrombocytopenic purpura (ITP), alopecia areata, and poliosis. The appropriate tests for these conditions should be done at the time of diagnosis of MG.

A variety of intercurrent diseases may exacerbate MG, and often present the most challenging problems in treatment. Any infection, overt or occult, can lead to worsening or persistence of MG, sometimes to the point of "myasthenic crisis." It is critical to exclude infections before undertaking treatment. As noted above, deviation from the euthyroid state can exacerbate myasthenic weakness, making it imperative to evaluate the patient's thyroid status by clinical and laboratory testing.

Several unrelated co-morbid conditions may influence the choice of agents used for treatment. Hypertension, diabetes, obesity, GI disorders such as esophageal reflux, ulcer disease, or irritable bowel syndrome, psychological factors, and chronic pulmonary disease (COPD) should all be evaluated before setting up a treatment plan. For example, hypertension must be controlled if adrenal corticosteroids or cyclosporine are used. Diabetes and obesity may be exacerbated by adrenal corticosteroids, which should only be used with caution. GI conditions may be made worse by corticosteroids, anticholinesterase agents, mycophenolate and others. Bone densitometry should be obtained before treatment with steroids, which may cause osteopenia.

A history of the patient's other medications is essential, since various drugs that the patient may take for some other condition can actually precipitate MG (penicillamine, used for systemic sclerosis, rheumatoid arthritis, etc.) or exacerbate pre-existing MG, such as certain antibiotics, anti-arrhythmics, etc. (see below). Drug interactions should be considered. For example, if the patient is taking allopurinol for the treatment of gout, azathioprine should not be used, since allopurinol inhibits metabolic degradation of azathioprine, resulting in very high levels and bone marrow depression.

In short, before undertaking treatment of a patient with MG, the physician should carry out a comprehensive history, clinical examination, and radiological and laboratory evaluation.

8.2.1.4. Assessment of myasthenic status

In order to evaluate the effectiveness of treatment, it is important to assess the patient's myasthenia at baseline and on repeated interval examinations in a systematic manner. Because of the variability of symptoms of MG, the interval history as well as findings on examination and laboratory testing must be taken into account. We use a convenient form to record the history and physical findings. The most useful clinical tests include range of eye movements, forward arm abduction time (up to a full 5 min), forced vital capacity (easily measured in the clinic), and time to development of ptosis on upward gaze. Manual testing of muscles, or preferably quantitative dynamometry (Beck et al., 1999) of limb muscles, especially proximal muscles, is very important. Following the patient's AChR antibody level quantitatively is an excellent surrogate measure of myasthenic status: a reduction in the AChR antibody level provides confirmation of the effectiveness of treatment, while a rise in the antibody level may predict exacerbation, and indicate the need for an increase in immune suppression. For comparison of an individual patient's AChR antibody levels over time, measurement of prior cryopreserved aliquots simultaneously with current serum samples in the same assay is most reliable. A standardized method of quantitative scoring of MG patients' clinical status (QMG) has been described (Jaretzki et al., 2000) and may be useful for large scale evaluation of therapeutic agents in planned clinical trials.

8.2.2. Treatment strategies

Treatment options for MG can be considered in six categories: 1. enhancement of cholinergic transmission; 2. short term immunotherapy—removal of antibodies, or IVIg treatment; 3. immunosuppression; 4. thymectomy; 5. management of associated conditions; and 6. treatment of refractory MG. We will discuss each of these categories below.

Time-linked treatment strategy: in deciding on the treatment strategy for an individual patient, a "time-linked" plan is invaluable. The patient's condition and needs should decide the urgency of treatment— how rapidly improvement must be effected. *Short term treatment*: the development of severe MG (or more often, the referral of a severely ill myasthenic patient) necessitates treatments that may produce improvement rapidly. Alternatively, patients who are leading very active lives and are anxious for a quick result may be treated so as to produce rapid improvement. Agents that may produce rapid short term improvement include anti-ChE drugs such as pyridostigmine, and the short term immunotherapeutic methods of plasmapheresis and intravenous immunoglobulin (IVIg) infusion. *Intermediate term treatment* choices generally produce improvement in weeks to months, and peaking within months to a year. They include various immunosuppressive agents, such as adrenal corticosteroids, and the calcineurin inhibitors Cyclosporine A (CsA) and Tacrolimus (FK506). *Long term treatment* modalities may take many months or even years to provide effective benefit, but have important advantages in terms of the ultimate outcome, and freedom from adverse side effects. Included in this group are the immunosuppressive agents azathioprine and mycophenolate mofetil (MMF), and thymectomy. Most often, combinations of short, intermediate, and long term treatments should be applied. The strategy of combining immunosuppressive agents has three advantages: First, it takes into account the time course of therapy, as described above, with benefits beginning early, and continued for the intermediate and long term. Second, it results in additive immune suppressive effects, while minimizing the adverse side effects of each of the drugs because relatively low doses of each drug can be used. Finally, some combinations of agents may act synergistically because of their different, and possibly complementary, mechanisms of action.

8.2.2.1. Enhancement of cholinergic transmission

Anticholinesterase (anti-ChE) agents inhibit the enzymatic elimination of acetylcholine, thereby prolonging its action at the postsynaptic membrane, and enhancing neuromuscular transmission. They are usually the first line treatment of MG, and historically were discovered first (Walker, 1934; Keesey, 1998). There is no substantial difference in efficacy among the various anti-ChE drugs; oral pyridostigmine bromide (Mestinon®) is the one most widely used in the US. Its beneficial action begins within 15–30 min, and lasts for 3–6 h, but individual responses vary. The dosage schedule should be tailored to the needs of the patient, and should be timed to maximize strength prior to anticipated activities, such as 30–60 min before meals. The initial dosage of pyridostigmine bromide is 30–60 mg every 4–6 h. The dose may be increased to 60 mg or 90 mg every 3 h when awake. The maximum useful dosage rarely exceeds 120 mg every 3 h during the daytime, and higher doses may produce increased weakness. A long-acting pyridostigmine preparation (Timespan® 180 mg) should be used only at bedtime, for patients who are symptomatic at night or in the early morning. It should not be used during the day in place of regular acting pyridostigmine, because of variability of absorption. The side effects of anti-ChE drugs include gastrointestinal hyperactivity with abdominal cramping or diarrhea, increased oral and upper respiratory secretions, and rarely bradycardia. Anticholinergic medications such as atropine/diphenoxylate (Lomotil®), loperamide (Imodium®), or glycopyrrolate (Robinul®) may overcome these muscarinic side effects without diminishing the nicotinic benefit. As a rule, anti-ChE drugs provide at least partial improvement in most patients, but their effects often wane after weeks or months of treatment. Ephedrine is an older medication for MG (Edgeworth, 1930) that may be helpful at a dose of 25 mg twice a day, but is now difficult to obtain because of its propensity to abuse. Its mechanism of action in humans is uncertain, but it is believed to enhance presynaptic release of ACh (Sieb and Engel, 1993).

8.2.2.2. Short term immunotherapy— plasmapheresis and IVIg

In view of the antibody-mediated pathogenesis of MG, plasmapheresis has been used therapeutically. The plasma, which contains the pathogenic antibodies, is mechanically separated from the blood cells, which are returned to the patient. Plasmapheresis produces a short term reduction in autoantibodies, with clinical improvement in many AChR-antibody positive and MuSK-antibody positive patients (Newsom-Davis et al., 1978; Keesey et al., 1981). It is useful as a temporary expedient in seriously affected patients, or to improve the patient's condition prior to surgery

(e.g., thymectomy). A typical course of plasmapheresis consists of 5 or 6 exchanges of 2 to 3 L each, every other day. The need for large-bore venous access, usually requiring the surgical insertion of a double-lumen catheter, and the risk of infection related to the indwelling catheter, limit the use of plasmapheresis.

The indications for IVIg are generally similar to those for plasma exchange: to produce rapid improvement in order to help the patient through a difficult period of myasthenic weakness, or prior to surgery (Gajdos et al., 1984, 1997). IVIg can also be used to produce a rapid effect in patients who are not seriously ill, but are anxious for quick improvement. IVIg treatment has the advantages of not requiring special equipment or the difficulties of obtaining adequate venous access. The usual dose is 2 g/kg, which is typically administered over 5 days (400 mg/kg/day). If well tolerated, subsequent courses of IVIg can be shortened to 3 days. Improvement occurs in approximately 70% of patients (Arsura, 1989; Dalakas, 2004), beginning during treatment or within a few days thereafter, and continuing for weeks to months. The therapeutic mechanism of IVIg in the treatment of MG is uncertain, and several possible mechanisms have been postulated, including binding of anti-idiotypic antibodies to the autoantibodies of MG, accelerated loss of pre-existing antibodies, inhibition of complement binding, etc. (Dalakas, 2004). IVIg treatment has no consistent effect on the measurable amount of circulating AChR antibody. Adverse reactions may include headache, fluid overload, and rarely aseptic meningitis. Pre-existing renal disease may predispose to the rare occurrence of renal shutdown, and the serum creatinine level should be followed during the series of infusions. The high cost of IVIg treatment and limited supplies of IgG may be problematic. No significant difference in benefit was noted in a randomized comparison of IVIg and plasmapheresis in the treatment of exacerbation of myasthenia (Gajdos et al., 1997). However, it is the clinical impression of many in the field that plasmapheresis is more effective and has a more rapid effect in the treatment of myasthenic crisis (Dalakas, 2004).

8.2.2.3. Immunosuppressive agents

Most patients can be restored to full activity with optimum immunosuppressive therapy. An increasing number of immunosuppressive agents including glucocorticoids, azathioprine, cyclosporine, tacrolimus, mycophenolate mofetil, methotrexate, cyclophosphamide, and others are now available. The choice of which drugs or other immunomodulatory treatments to use should be guided by their relative benefits and risks for the individual patient, and by the "time-linked" treatment strategy. As noted above, if immediate improvement is essential either because of the severity of weakness or because of the patient's need to return to activity as soon as possible, plasmapheresis or IVIg treatment should be undertaken. For the intermediate term, adrenal cortico-steroids and cyclosporine generally produce clinical improvement within a period of 1–3 months. The benefi-cial effects of azathioprine and mycophenolate usually begin after many months (up to a year), but these drugs have advantages for the long term treatment of patients with MG. The side effects of each drug may preclude its use in some patients, as indicated below.

8.2.2.3.1. Combinations of treatments

Combinations of treatments can be used to advantage because different agents may have additive immuno-suppressive effects, but different side effects. By com-bining these agents, the beneficial effect is maximized while the adverse side effects are kept to a minimum.

8.2.2.3.2. Adrenal corticosteroids

Adrenal corticosteroids, when used properly, safely produce improvement in myasthenic weakness in the great majority of patients (Johns, 1987; Schneider-Gold et al., 2005), but have a long list of potential side effects that must be guarded against. Corticosteroids exert a wide variety of immunosuppressive and anti-inflammatory actions that may contribute to their therapeutic benefit in MG, including alteration of traf-ficking of lymphocytes, inhibition of production of cytokines and interleukins, and reduction of antibodies by several mechanisms (Barshes et al., 2004; Taylor et al., 2005). Paradoxically, about one-third of MG patients treated initially with a high-dose corticoster-oid regimen develop increased weakness during the early stages of treatment, which may be severe enough to precipitate a myasthenic crisis (Pascuzzi et al., 1984; Johns, 1987). To avoid this problem, we recom-mend a relatively low (15–20 mg/day) initial dose of prednisone, and then a gradual increase by 5–10 mg every 2–3 days as tolerated, until a total dose of about 60 mg/day is reached (Seybold and Drachman, 1974). Prednisone should be administered in a single dose in the morning so as to minimize side effects (which are more pronounced when it is given in divided doses throughout the day), and to mimic the natural diurnal cortisol cycle. After reaching an optimal dose, treatment is continued for 1–3 months or until near-maximal or maximal improvement occurs. The treatment sche-dule is then modified gradually to an alternate-day regi-men, which further reduces side effects, and reduces suppression of endogenous adrenal function. This is

accomplished over weeks to months by raising the dose on one day and lowering it on the alternate day. In some patients, a small dose of prednisone must be given on the "off" day to prevent fluctuations in strength. The ultimate aim of therapy is to maximize the benefits while minimizing the risks. Since the risks are directly related to the dose and duration of steroid use, the smallest effective dose given on alternate days should be determined for each patient by gradually taper-ing the dose (usually by no more than 10 mg every month or so). The combination of other immuno-suppressive agents (see below) with corticosteroids facilitates the reduction of the steroid dose, while maintaining the therapeutic effect on MG.

Potential side effects of steroid therapy include hyperglycemia, hypertension, weight gain, fluid reten-tion, cataract formation, gastrointestinal irritation and ulcers, psychological changes, osteoporosis, aseptic necrosis of bones (the hip), increased risk of infection, suppression of pituitary ACTH secretion, and impaired wound healing (Taylor et al., 2005). Because of these side effects, consistent follow-up is essential. We routinely monitor blood pressure, body weight, cardio-pulmonary function, ophthalmoscopy with a +10 lens to evaluate cataract formation, blood glucose, electro-lytes, bone density, and occult infection. We recommend a low fat low sodium diet, calcium and biphosphonates or vitamin D to prevent osteopenia, and surveillance or treatment for hyperglycemia. When surgery is required for patients who are treated with steroids, the oral admin-istration of retinol (Vitamin A) at a dose of 25 000 IU twice a day may enhance wound healing (Anstead, 1998; Wicke et al., 2000). Inability or unwillingness of a patient to be followed closely is a serious contraindica-tion to the use of steroid therapy.

8.2.2.3.3. Azathioprine

Azathioprine (Imuran®) has been the most widely used non-steroidal immunosuppressive agent for the treatment of MG because of its long track record and relative safety in most patients (Hertel et al., 1979; Palace et al., 1998). It is first metabolized to 6-mercaptopurine (6-MP), and converted to other pro-ducts that interfere with purine synthesis of lympho-cytes, as well as exhibiting other immunosuppressive effects (Taylor et al., 2005). Its therapeutic effect may add to that of glucocorticoids, and usually allows the steroid dose to be reduced (Palace et al., 1998). However, up to 10% of patients are unable to tolerate azathioprine because of idiosyncratic reactions consist-ing of flu-like symptoms of fever and malaise, bone marrow depression, or abnormalities of liver function. Patients with gout must be cautioned to avoid the use of allopurinol, which interferes with the elimination of azathioprine, and may result in severe bone marrow depression. An initial dose of 50 mg/day should be given for one week to test for adverse side effects. If this dose is tolerated, it is increased gradually until the white blood count (WBC) falls to approximately 3000–4000/μL. The typical dosage range is 2–3 mg/kg total body weight (including fat in obese patients). In patients who are receiving steroids concurrently, leukocytosis confounds the use of the WBC count as a measure of treatment. A reduction in the lymphocyte count below 1000/μL and/or an increase of the mean corpuscular volume (MCV) of red blood cells (Witte et al., 1986) may be used as indications of adequacy of azathioprine dosage. The beneficial effect of azathioprine takes 3–6 months to begin and even longer to peak. Long term use of azathioprine has been reported to predispose to malignancies in patients with organ transplants, as is also reported for some other immunosuppressive agents (Buell et al., 2005).

8.2.2.3.4. Cyclosporine

Cyclosporine A, a cyclic polypeptide produced by a fungus, is now used extensively for immunosuppression in transplantation and autoimmune diseases. First shown to be effective for the treatment of MG in an experimental animal model (Drachman et al., 1985), and later in a modest randomized clinical trial (Tindall et al., 1987), it is approximately as effective as azathioprine, and is being used increasingly in the clinical management of MG (Juel and Massey, 2005). CsA inhibits calcineurin, resulting in reduction of IL2 production by T cells, and inhibition of T cell activation (Taylor et al., 2005). Its therapeutic effect in MG appears more rapidly than that of azathioprine. It may be given alone but usually is used as an adjunct to permit reduction of the steroid dose. A microemulsified preparation (cyclosporine modified, Neoral), which is absorbed reliably from the GI tract, should be used rather than the original formulation of CsA. The usual oral dose is 4–5 mg/kg per day, given in two divided doses (to minimize side effects). Side effects of CsA include hypertension, nephrotoxicity, hirsutism, gingival hyperplasia, and GI effects. Blood pressure and serum creatinine levels should be monitored on a regular basis. Cyclosporine has complex interactions with many other drugs (listed on the MGFA web site: http://www.myasthenia.org/information/MGFA_Brochure_Cyclosporine.pdf), and therefore "trough" blood levels of CsA, obtained 12 h after the evening dose, should be measured periodically, and especially after the addition of any new medication. The therapeutic range, as measured by radioimmunoassay, is 150–200 ng/L.

8.2.2.3.5. Tacrolimus

Tacrolimus, also known as FK506 or Prograf, is a calcineurin inhibitor, closely similar to CsA in its therapeutic mechanism. Tacrolimus binds to a receptor (FK binding protein, or FKBP) different from the receptor for CsA (cyclophilin), but interacts with calcineurin in virtually the same way as CsA. It was first used for immunosuppression in organ transplantation, especially liver transplants (Jain et al., 1999). Recent reports indicate its effectiveness in the treatment of MG, and some suggest that it may even be superior (Evoli et al., 2002; Yoshikawa et al., 2002; Konishi et al., 2005; Ponseti et al., 2005). The side effects of nephrotoxicity and hypertension are like those of CsA, but hirsutism and gingival hyperplasia may be less prominent (Cameron and Ghobrial, 2005). The dose of tacrolimus is about 0.075–0.1 mg/kg twice a day, but must be guided by measurement of trough levels. Trough levels should be about 7–10 ng/mL (Ponseti et al., 2005). Both cyclosporine and tacrolimus are very expensive.

8.2.2.3.6. Mycophenolate mofetil

Mycophenolate mofetil (MMF, CellCept), which has been used for immunosuppression in transplant patients, is proving to be extremely useful in the treatment of MG (Chaudhry et al., 2001; Meriggioli et al., 2003). Its mechanism takes advantage of the fact that lymphocytes have only one pathway of purine synthesis, i.e., the de novo pathway, whereas all other cells have an alternative "salvage pathway." Mycophenolate blocks the de novo pathway, and thereby inhibits proliferation of both T and B lymphocytes, but not proliferation of other cells. It may also inhibit antibody formation by B cells. However, it does not kill or eliminate preexisting autoreactive lymphocytes, and therefore clinical improvement in MG and other autoimmune diseases may be delayed until the pre-existing autoreactive lymphocytes spontaneously die, which may take many months to a year. The advantage of mycophenolate lies in its relative lack of adverse side effects, with only occasional production of diarrhea, and uncommon leukopenia, anemia or thrombocytopenia. It reportedly has a lower risk of development of late malignancies than other immunosuppressive agents (Buell et al., 2005). The oral dose is 1 g or 1.5 g twice a day. MMF is likely to become the agent of choice for long-term treatment of myasthenic patients. Unfortunately, the present cost of mycophenolate is very high.

8.2.2.3.7. Thymectomy

As noted above, approximately 75% of MG patients have abnormalities of the thymus: either thymic hyperplasia with germinal center formation (64%), or thymoma (11%). The thymus may play a role in the origin and maintenance of the autoimmune response in MG. There are two different indications for thymectomy in MG: surgical removal of a thymic tumor; and thymectomy as a treatment for MG.

Thymic tumors must be removed because they may spread locally and involve important structures within the chest, although most thymomas are generally histologically benign. If the thymoma is invasive, postoperative radiation therapy is commonly used (Nakahara et al., 1988), and chemotherapy has also been advocated (Park et al., 1994). Favorable responses of thymomas to corticosteroids have been reported (Tandan et al., 1990; Termeer et al., 2001).

In the absence of a tumor, there is now broad consensus that patients with generalized MG who are between the ages of puberty and about 60 years should have thymectomy, because up to 85% of patients eventually experience improvement in their MG after thymectomy (Buckingham et al., 1976; Lanska, 1990; Bulkley et al., 1997; Gronseth and Barohn, 2000). Of these, about 35% achieve drug-free remission, while the remaining 50% show some improvement (Fig. 8.1) (Buckingham et al., 1976). The advantage of thymectomy is that it offers the possibility of long term benefit, although the benefit may only be realized after an interval of many months or years. In some cases thymectomy diminishes or eliminates the need for continued medical treatment. In view of these potential long term benefits, and the negligible risk

in skilled hands, thymectomy has gained widespread acceptance for the treatment of MG, though controlled studies demonstrating the benefit of thymectomy are not available (Gronseth and Barohn, 2000). A randomized multicenter trial of thymectomy has been proposed (Wolfe et al., 2003) and is currently under way, but the prospect of distinguishing the relative benefits of surgical thymectomy and medical immunosuppressive therapy seems daunting.

The Mayo Clinic retrospective report (Buckingham et al., 1976), which preceded the era of immunosuppression for MG, avoided the confounding factors of medical treatment, although it was not a prospective randomized study. It has been suggested that thymectomy should be performed *early* in the disease course to achieve maximum benefit (Monden et al., 1984). Early thymectomy has the theoretical advantage of eliminating the export of long-lived autoreactive lymphocytes from the thymus. There is debate about the age limits for thymectomy in patients without thymoma. Because the thymus often undergoes atrophy after late middle age (~55–65 years) (Perlo et al., 1975), thymectomy is usually not carried out in older patients except for removal of thymoma. Conversely, thymectomy is sometimes delayed in childhood MG until puberty, because of the active role of the thymus in development of the immune system. However, thymectomy carried out in children with MG reportedly did not have adverse effects, monitored on subsequent follow up (Seybold et al., 1971). The value of

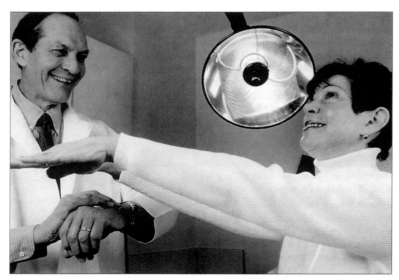

Fig. 8.1. Patient with myasthenia gravis in drug-induced complete remission. She was initially severely disabled. She was treated, with pyridostigmine and thymectomy, followed by prednisone and azathioprine, gradually tapered to a minimal dose of azathioprine (75 mg/day). She has been restored to a full productive life for over 35 years. Complete omission of azathioprine after 28 years of treatment resulted in recurrence of diplopia, which was corrected by reinstatement of the current dose.

thymectomy in AChR antibody negative MG patients has been questioned. Recent reports suggest that anti-MuSK positive patients have limited changes to germinal centers, and do not benefit from thymectomy, while patients whose serologies are negative for both anti-AChR and anti-MuSK antibodies may have thymic abnormalities, and may benefit from thymectomy (Evoli et al., 2003; Leite et al., 2005). Finally, thymectomy is not often carried out in patients with purely ocular involvement, although studies indicate that improvement occurs in this group of patients (Schumm et al., 1985) as well as in those with generalized myasthenic weakness.

Thymectomy should never be performed as an emergency procedure. Unless absolutely necessary, thymectomy should be performed before beginning treatment with immunosuppressive drugs, so as to minimize the risks of infection and delayed wound healing. If MG is severe, or in patients with bulbar or respiratory dysfunction, thymectomy should be carried out only after stabilization of the disease with plasmapheresis, IVIg treatment, or other immunomodulatory therapy. Although various surgical approaches to thymectomy—transcervical, trans-sternal, or "maximal"—continue to be used at different centers, median sternotomy with cervical exploration is presently the standard of care, since it permits maximal removal of all thymic tissue. Newer methods of robotic assisted surgery may eventually replace the trans-sternal approach. Potential complications from thymectomy include the general risks of anesthesia, impaired wound healing, sternal instability, pleural effusion, atelectasis, pneumonia, pulmonary embolism, paresis of phrenic or recurrent laryngeal nerve, and precipitation of myasthenic crisis. Exacerbation of MG may occur following removal of a thymoma (Kuroda et al., 1984; Somnier, 1994), possibly because of the elimination of an immunosuppressive action of the tumor. To minimize the risk of these complications, thymectomy should always be carried out in a hospital where it is performed regularly, and where the staff is experienced in the pre- and post-operative management of myasthenic patients, anesthesia, and surgical techniques of total thymectomy.

Prior to thymectomy, the optimum dose of anti-ChE medication should be established, and the equivalent dose of intravenous medication should be given by continuous infusion until the patient is capable of taking oral medication. We substitute 1 mg of neostigmine IV for each 60 mg tablet of oral pyridostigmine. Post-operative care should include careful attention to pulmonary function. The use of epidural analgesia minimizes post-operative pain and facilitates adequate respiratory function (Kirsch et al., 1991).

8.2.2.3.8. Refractory MG: "rebooting" the immune system with high dose cyclophosphamide

Although most MG patients respond to conventional treatment with the immunosuppressive agents described above, occasional patients either fail to respond to appropriate doses of these agents, or cannot tolerate their adverse side effects. Treatment for these "refractory" patients has previously required resorting to repeated plasmapheresis or IVIg infusion, which provide only temporary benefit, are expensive and inconvenient, and may not provide satisfactory clinical results. Ideally, treatment for these patients should attempt to eliminate the autoimmune response, and provide long term or permanent benefit. Previous experiments in our laboratory using rats with experimental autoimmune MG suggested that complete elimination of the existing immune system, and replacement by means of bone marrow transplantation (BMT), could restore the animals to their pristine immunological state, without residual responsiveness to the antigen AChR (Pestronk et al., 1982, 1983). More recently, we have learned that high-dose cyclophosphamide treatment *without BMT* can be used successfully to eliminate the mature immune system, resulting in durable remissions in a variety of autoimmune diseases (Brodsky et al., 1996, 2000; Moyo et al., 2002). Hematopoietic stem cells are not damaged by this treatment, because they express substantial levels of aldehyde dehydrogenase, which inactivates the active metabolite of cyclophosphamide. In contrast, mature lymphocytes and committed hematopoietic progenitors are rapidly killed by high-dose cyclophosphamide, because they express only low levels of aldehyde dehydrogenase (Gordon et al., 1985; Jones et al., 1995). After the treatment, the undamaged stem cells proliferate, enhanced by GCSF (granulocyte colony stimulating factor), and re-populate the immune system. In principle, the newly developing (or "rebooted") immune system may recognize the autoantigen as "self," thereby inducing tolerance to it. Alternatively, the procedure may simply "reset" the immune system, so that its autoreactive component is significantly diminished.

The current treatment protocol first involves assessment of MG status, and thorough evaluation to exclude general medical problems or occult infection that might pose problems in treatment (see Drachman et al., 2003a for details). The patients are hydrated to prevent bladder irritation by cyclophosphamide, and treated to prevent nausea using prochlorperazine or ondansetron. Cyclophosphamide is administered IV at a dose of 50 mg/kg daily for 4 days. Following the treatment, the patients are housed near the medical center, and are followed every day until the neutrophil count returns to 1000/mm^3. To enhance proliferation of hematopoietic cells and reconstitute the immune system GCSF is administered beginning 6 days after the end of the cyclophosphamide treatment. Packed RBC, platelets, fluids, and antibiotics are given as needed during the 2–3 week period until the patient's hematopoietic and immune systems are sufficiently reconstituted to allow them to return home.

We have recently treated 12 refractory myasthenic patients by "rebooting" the immune system with high dose cyclophosphamide (Hi Cy). All but one of the patients experienced dramatic clinical improvement for variable periods from 5 months to 7 1/2 years, lasting for more than one year in 8 of the patients. Two patients are still in treatment-free remission at 5 1/2 and 7 1/2 years, and five have achieved responsiveness to immunosuppressive agents that were previously ineffective. Eight of the patients were AChR antibody positive, one was MuSK antibody positive, and three were AChR and MuSK antibody negative. Antibodies to the autoantigens AChR or MuSK were typically reduced, but not completely eliminated by Hi Cy treatment. This treatment results in effective, but not necessarily permanent, remission in most refractory myasthenic patients, suggesting that the immune system is in fact "rebooted" but not completely "reformatted" in the computer analogy. We therefore recommend that treatment of refractory MG with Hi Cy be followed with maintenance immunotherapy.

8.2.2.4. Treating MG in special situations

When MG occurs in the setting of other medical issues, it presents special problems in management. In this section we will discuss:

1. Ocular myasthenia
2. Co-morbidities
3. Drug interactions
4. Pregnancy and neonatal MG
5. Myasthenic "crisis"

8.2.2.4.1. Ocular myasthenia

Although the great majority of myasthenic patients experience diplopia and/or ptosis early in the course of the disease, more than 85% go on to develop generalized weakness, usually within the first 3 years. Those patients in whom weakness remains confined to the ocular or palpebral muscles are said to have "ocular myasthenia" (OMG). It is uncertain whether immunological differences predispose to OMG (Wang et al., 2000; Kaminski et al., 2004), but circulating antibody to AChR is detectable in only about 50–70% of OMG patients (Somner et al., 1993). Anti-ChE medications typically are helpful for treating ptosis, but infrequently produce satisfactory improvement of diplopia. Immunosuppressive agents described above usually can restore single vision, though the risks of treatment must be weighed against the benefits. Since diplopia often interferes with reading, driving, computer work, and other activities common to work and recreation, many patients benefit from treatment with immunosuppressive drugs. As noted above, thymectomy is not commonly recommended in pure OMG, although it has been reported to be beneficial (Schumm et al., 1985).

8.2.2.4.2. Co-morbidities

By far the most difficult myasthenic patients to treat are those with complex co-morbidities. Nevertheless, if recognized and dealt with, most such problems can be surmounted.

8.2.2.4.2.1. Infection

Infections of any sort may exacerbate MG, and infection is the most common cause of myasthenic crisis. Infections should be treated empirically as soon as they are recognized; later, when cultures and bacterial sensitivities become available, the most appropriate antibiotics are substituted. Occult infections, such as diverticulitis, hepatitis, dental abscesses, etc., should be sought and treated in patients who respond poorly to immunotherapy. It is particularly important to recognize and treat hepatitis B, since immunosuppression permits proliferation of the viruses. Fortunately, antiviral agents are available to prevent reactivation of hepatitis B, while managing the MG (Yeo and Johnson, 2006).

8.2.2.4.2.2. Obesity

Obesity is a relative contraindication to the use of corticosteroids, and corticosteroid treatment may lead to obesity. It is our practice to pay careful attention to the weight and nutritional management of patients being treated with steroids. Minimizing the corticosteroid dose and using an alternate day regimen are also helpful for controlling weight gain. Obesity may also be a problem in determining the dose of azathioprine, which should usually be calculated on the basis of the total weight, not merely the lean mass.

8.2.2.4.2.3. Diabetes

Hyperglycemia is exacerbated by corticosteroids, and an alternate day steroid schedule may result in fluctuations in serum glucose levels that are difficult to manage. Tacrolimus may also exacerbate hyperglycemia. (Levy and Cole, 2005).

8.2.2.4.2.4. Hypertension

Corticosteroids and the calcineurin inhibitors, cyclosporine and tacrolimus, may increase blood pressure, which should be followed at every visit and managed as needed.

8.2.2.4.2.5. Thyroid disease

Autoimmune thyroid diseases, including Hashimoto's thyroiditis and Graves' disease, occur in 5–8% of patients with MG, and may cause hyper or hypothyroidism. Any departure from the euthyroid state may increase myasthenic weakness (Drachman, 1962), and should be corrected.

8.2.2.4.2.6. Renal disease

Renal disease is a relative contraindication to the use of cyclosporine and tacrolimus, which are nephrotoxic. When treating patients with IVIg, serum creatinine and urea nitrogen should be followed, especially in patients with borderline renal function, since it may rarely cause renal shutdown.

8.2.2.4.2.7. Osteoporosis

Corticosteroids can cause osteopenia, and patients should have periodic bone density measurements, and be treated with calcium, and either biphosphonates or high dose vitamin D (50 000 u twice a week), as needed.

8.2.2.4.3. Drug interactions

Various drugs can exacerbate myasthenic weakness, and should be avoided when possible, or used with care. Individual patients may react differently to some of these drugs, and as always, treatment should be individualized. For an extensive listing of drugs that may be associated with exacerbations of MG see Pascuzzi (2000). Drugs that are most likely to cause exacerbation of MG include antibiotics (aminoglycosides, quinolones, and possibly macrolides), muscle relaxants used during surgery, especially nondepolarizing curariform agents, quinine and quinidine, magnesium, and beta blockers. Many other drugs have been implicated in anecdotal reports, and should be used with caution. In fact, myasthenic patients should be carefully followed when any new drug is introduced. For example, there are recent reports of unexpectedly severe exacerbation of MG following the use of telithromycin (Ketek®), a ketolide antibiotic (Pascuzzi, 2000). Penicillamine used for other autoimmune diseases such as scleroderma or rheumatoid arthritis may trigger typical autoimmune MG, which can persist for many months. Unlike idiopathic MG it eventually subsides after discontinuation of the penicillamine treatment.

Many drugs used for the treatment of MG have important interactions with medications used for other conditions. For example, when allopurinol (used for gout) is given to patients treated with azathioprine, it can lead to severe but generally reversible bone marrow suppression. Cyclosporine has many interactions with a wide variety of other drugs (http://www.myasthenia.org/information/MGFA_Brochure_Cyclosporine.pdf, 2004), and the safest method of avoiding unexpectedly high or low levels is to track the trough (12 h post-dose) cyclosporine serum level periodically, and when adding any new drugs.

8.2.2.4.4. Pregnancy and neonatal MG

The severity of untreated MG varies with pregnancy, and it has been stated that one third of patients improve, one third remain the same, and one third worsen during pregnancy (Plauche, 1991), although other series (quoted in Ciafaloni and Massey, 2004) give varying proportions. The course of MG in any given pregnancy is unpredictable, and myasthenic patients should be under close supervision by the neurologist and obstetrician during and after pregnancy. Birth should be arranged in a center where care of a newborn with neonatal MG is available (see below). During the postpartum period some patients become weaker and are also fatigued as a result of the lack of sleep and stresses associated with care of the newborn. Treatment during pregnancy should aim to maintain the mother's clinical status and to avoid adverse effects of drugs on the fetus. It seems clear that anti-ChE agents, corticosteroids and IVIg are safe for the fetus (Ciafaloni and Massey, 2004). There is a large literature on the effects of immunosuppressive drugs during pregnancy in transplant patients (Armenti et al., 1998). Azathioprine is probably safe, but is listed as a category D agent; cyclosporine and tacrolimus appear to be relatively safe; mycophenolate mofetil is contraindicated during pregnancy. Our practice is to maintain patients on only those drugs that are needed, limited to pyridostigmine and prednisone, with the possibility of adding IVIg if needed.

Transient neonatal MG occurs in 12–20% of infants born to myasthenic mothers, and is manifested by hypotonia, and poor suck and cry, usually occurring within 12–48 h after birth (Papazian, 1992). Neither the mother's clinical status nor the anti-AChR antibody level can predict whether the infant will develop clinical weakness, and it is clear that other factors determine the clinical manifestations in the newborn. Infants of myasthenic mothers should be observed closely for 3–4 days after birth, since signs of weakness may not be present for several days. Neonatal MG is self-limited, and usually resolves within a few weeks, or at most 4 months. Anti-ChE medication is helpful; the oral dose of pyridostigmine syrup is 4–10 mg every 4 h, and the IV dose of neostigmine is 0.05–0.1 mg as needed every 3–4 h, preferably 30 min before feedings. Depending on the severity of weakness, the infant may require ventilatory support and management in a neonatal intensive care unit.

Arthrogryposis multiplex congenita, a condition characterized by congenital fixation of multiple joints (Drachman and Banker, 1961), is due to lack of joint movement during embryonic development, whatever the cause (Murray and Drachman, 1969). Arthrogryposis occurs rarely in infants born to myasthenic mothers who have antibodies directed against the γ- (fetal) subunit of the AChR (Vincent et al., 1995; Polizzi et al., 2000). There is a history of decreased fetal movements. Fetal or neonatal death can occur because of pulmonary hypoplasia and polyhydramnios. Recurrence may be avoided in future pregnancies if the mother is treated with plasmapheresis and immunosuppression (S.-M. Huson, J. Newsom-Davis, A. Vincent, unpublished observations, 2002).

8.2.2.4.5. Myasthenic crisis

Myasthenic crisis is defined as an exacerbation of weakness sufficient to endanger life, due to respiratory failure caused by diaphragmatic and intercostal muscle weakness. In this era of effective treatment of MG, crisis should be a rare occurrence. The most common cause of crisis is intercurrent infection, often in a patient whose previous treatment has been inadequate. Emotional stress, rapid initiation of high dose corticosteroid therapy, or surgery may also precipitate crisis in some myasthenic patients. If there is no obvious cause, a thorough search should be made for an occult source of infection, such as diverticulitis, dental abscess, or opportunistic fungal or viral infections. Infection should be treated immediately, because the patient's mechanical and immunologic defenses can be assumed to be compromised. Empirical antimicrobial therapy based on the most likely infectious agent should be started without delay, and modified as needed when cultures and sensitivities become available. As discussed above, plasmapheresis or IVIg is frequently helpful in hastening recovery. It should be emphasized that thymectomy should never be considered as a treatment for myasthenic crisis, since the surgery is likely to make matters worse, and any potential benefit would only be realized in the distant future. Treatment must be carried out in an intensive care unit staffed with physicians experienced in the management of myasthenic crisis. The physician must take charge of virtually every aspect of the patient's life functions, including neurologic, respiratory, cardiovascular, infectious, immunologic, renal, GI, and psychological, until

the crisis is resolved. Indeed, management of myasthenic crisis is one of the greatest challenges in medicine.

8.3. Future prospects for treatment of MG

Although current treatments for MG are highly effective in most patients, they have the potential for adverse side effects, including overall suppression of the immune system as a whole. Future treatments will fall into two categories: 1. new immunosuppressive agents with improved profiles of safety and/or efficiency; 2. novel treatments designed to inhibit only the autoimmune response to the autoantigen, without otherwise interfering with the immune system.

8.3.1. New immunosuppressive agents

Several newer immunosuppressive agents have recently been developed, and used to prevent rejection of transplants, for treatment of various autoimmune disorders, or for the treatment of malignancies.

8.3.1.1. Rituximab

Rituxan® is a monoclonal antibody that binds to the CD20 membrane marker of B lymphocytes, and has been widely used for the treatment of B cell lymphomas. In principle, since autoantibodies produced by B lymphocytes are responsible for MG, one might anticipate that it would be beneficial, as it is in other autoimmune diseases such as lupus erythematosus (Willems et al., 2006) and pemphigus (G. Anhalt, 2003, personal communication), or in some cases of IgM-related neuropathies (Pestronk et al., 2003). There are only a few reported cases of MG successfully treated with rituximab (Zaja et al., 2000; Wylam et al., 2003). A few personal cases of MG refractory to conventional immunosuppressive agents did not respond to standard oncology dosage treatment with rituximab, although the CD20 B lymphocytes were markedly depleted. In these cases, it is likely that plasma cells, which are not CD20 positive, were responsible for the anti-AChR antibodies.

8.3.1.2. Leflunomide

Arava® acts primarily to block the de novo pathway of pyrimidine synthesis (similar to the action of mycophenolate in purine synthesis), in addition to other anti-inflammatory effects. It has been used successfully in rheumatoid arthritis, Crohn's disease, and systemic lupus erythematosus (Kessel and Toubi, 2002; Silverman et al., 2005), although adverse side effects have been noted. Leflunomide inhibited the development of EAMG in a rat model (Vidic-Dankovic et al., 1995), but there are as yet no reports of its use in human MG. In principle, it should act synergistically with mycophenolate, so as to block both purine and pyrimidine synthesis.

8.3.1.3. Rapamycin (sirolimus)

Rapamune® is an immunosuppressive agent that inhibits T cell proliferation by blocking the IL-2 stimulated cell cycle, and also inhibits antibody production. It has been used in conjunction with the calcineurin inhibitors, particularly tacrolimus, for prevention of transplant rejection. Its action, which blocks the effect of IL-2, is synergistic with that of the calcineurin inhibitors, which block the production of IL-2. There are as yet no reports of its use in MG, and my experience in a few cases has been inconclusive.

8.3.1.4. Tumor necrosis factor blockers

Tumor necrosis factor (TNFα) blockers include etanercept (soluble recombinant TNF receptor with Fc, Enbrel®), and two monoclonal anti-TNFα antibodies—infliximab (Remicade®) and adalimumab (Humira®). These agents are in clinical use for the treatment of rheumatoid arthritis, psoriasis and psoriatic arthritis, and Crohn's disease. Etanercept improves weakness of rats with EAMG (Christadoss and Goluszko, 2002). It has been used in a small pilot trial in 11 MG patients, with improvement of about half, and acute clinical worsening in two, thought to be due to an increase in circulating TNFα (Rowin et al., 2004). It is unclear whether it will be generally useful in MG.

8.3.1.5. Costimulation blockade

Stimulation of helper T cells requires two signals: 1. antigen in the context of Class II (MHC II); and 2. a costimulatory signal provided by the antigen presenting cell (APC). Dendritic cells, macrophages and B cells express the costimulatory molecules CD80 and CD86 on their surfaces, and these costimulatory molecules are up-regulated when the APCs are activated. They interact with a receptor on the T cell surface (CD28), thereby providing the second signal required for T cell activation. If the APCs present antigen to a T cell *without* costimulation, the T cell becomes unable to respond (anergic), and may undergo apoptosis. The costimulatory molecules can be blocked by a soluble form of CTLA4, which is a high affinity receptor derived from T cells. CTLA4Ig has been used clinically in the treatment of rheumatoid arthritis (Genovese et al., 2005) and psoriasis. We tested the effects of CTLA4Ig in EAMG in rats, and found that it inhibited the immune responses to AChR both in vitro and in vivo (McIntosh et al., 1995; McIntosh et al., 1998). New, more potent costimulation blocking agents, Abatacept and Belatacept, derived from CTLA4Ig, have been shown to be effective in treating rheumatoid arthritis and preventing graft rejection (Vincenti and Luggen, 2007). These agents may prove useful in the treatment of MG as well.

8.3.2. Therapeutic strategies

Given the remarkable advances in knowledge of the immunology of MG, it should be possible to design therapeutic strategies that specifically eliminate the autoimmune response to the known antigen(s) AChR (or MuSK), without otherwise affecting the immune system. Indeed, specific therapy is the long-sought "Holy Grail" of immunology. Although practical application of specific immunotherapy for MG is not yet available, several intriguing strategies are in the experimental stages.

1. Oral administration of antigen. This is known to prevent the development of autoimmune diseases. In the case of EAMG, oral administration of *Torpedo* AChR prior to immunization inhibits the subsequent development of EAMG, AChR-reactive T cells, and AChR antibodies (Okumura et al., 1994). Feeding of a syngeneic rat AChR fragment has also been shown to ameliorate ongoing EAMG in rats (Souroujon et al., 2003; Maiti et al., 2004). However, the possible risk of exacerbation of the autoimmune disease by oral antigen suggests caution in application of this strategy in human MG. A human trial of oral treatment of multiple sclerosis with a myelin preparation was disappointingly negative.

2. The strategy of utilizing genetically engineered APCs as "guided missiles" that target AChR-specific T cells by presenting AChR, and kill them by a Fas ligand "warhead," has worked effectively in vitro (Wu et al., 2001; Drachman et al., 2003b), and is being tested in animals with EAMG. It has the potential advantage of utilizing the individual's own APCs to seek and destroy the unique and heterogeneous repertoire of T cells specific for that individual.

3. Altered AChR epitopes have been synthesized that have been shown to inhibit the immune response to native AChR in mice (Ben-David et al., 2005).

4. Immature dendritic cells pulsed with the antigen AChR have been shown to reduce the immune response to subsequent immunization with native AChR in a rat model of EAMG (Li et al., 2005).

8.4. Conclusions

At present, the ability to treat myasthenic patients effectively is so bright that one may suggest that the name "gravis" be dropped altogether. Virtually all myasthenic patients can now be returned to fully productive lives. The physician's quiver is replete with many effective therapeutic arrows, but it requires skill and persistence to optimize their use in the unique circumstances of individual patients with a wide variety of different medical, immunologic and social backgrounds. The ideals of specific immunotherapy, and even a "cure," may emerge from the novel strategies that are currently being pursued.

References

Anstead GM (1998). Steroids, retinoids, and wound healing. Adv Wound Care 11: 277–285.

Aoki T, Drachman DB, Asher DM, et al. (1985). Attempts to implicate viruses in myasthenia gravis. Neurology 35: 185–192.

Armenti VT, Moritz MJ, Davison JM (1998). Drug safety issues in pregnancy following transplantation and immunosuppression: effects and outcomes. Drug Saf 19: 219–232.

Arsura E (1989). Experience with intravenous immunoglobulin in myasthenia gravis. Clin Immunol Immunopathol 53: S170–S179.

Asher O, Neumann D, Fuchs S (1988). Increased levels of acetylcholine receptor alpha-subunit mRNA in experimental autoimmune myasthenia gravis. FEBS Lett 233: 277–281.

Avila OA, Drachman DB, Pestronk AP (1989). Neurotransmission regulates stability of acetylcholine receptors at the neuromuscular junction. J Neurosci 9: 2902–2906.

Barshes NR, Goodpastor SE, Goss JA (2004). Pharmacologic immunosuppression. Front Biosci 9: 411–420.

Beck M, Giess R, Wurffel W, et al. (1999). Comparison of maximal voluntary isometric contraction and Drachman's hand-held dynamometry in evaluating patients with amyotrophic lateral sclerosis. Muscle Nerve 22: 1265–1270.

Ben-David H, Sela M, Mozes E (2005). Down-regulation of myasthenogenic T cell responses by a dual altered peptide ligand via CD4+CD25+-regulated events leading to apoptosis. Proc Natl Acad Sci U S A 102: 2028–2033.

Brodsky RA, Sensenbrenner LL, Jones RJ (1996). Complete remission in severe aplastic anemia after high-dose cyclophosphamide without bone marrow transplantation. Blood 87: 491–494.

Brodsky RA, Petri M, Jones RJ (2000). Hematopoietic stem cell transplantation for systemic lupus erythematosus. Rheum Dis Clin North Am 26: 377–387, viii.

Buckingham J, Howard FJ, Bernatz P, et al. (1976). The value of thymectomy in myasthenia gravis: a computer-assisted matched study. Ann Surg 184: 453–458.

Buell JF, Gross TG, Woodle ES (2005). Malignancy after transplantation. Transplantation 80: S254–S264.

Bulkley GB, Bass KN, Stephenson GR, et al. (1997). Extended cervicomediastinal thymectomy in the integrated management of myasthenia gravis. Ann Surg 226: 324–334.

Burges J, Vincent A, Molenaar PC, et al. (1994). Passive transfer of seronegative myasthenia gravis to mice. Muscle Nerve 17: 1393–1400.

Cameron A, Ghobrial R (2005). Immunosuppressive therapy for liver transplant recipients: the benefits of tacrolimus. Transplantation and Immunology Letter 21: 5–7.

Carlsson B, Wallin J, Pirskanen R, et al. (1990). Different HLA DR-DQ associations in subgroups of idiopathic myasthenia gravis. Immunogenetics 31: 285–290.

Castleman B (1966). The pathology of the thymus gland in myasthenia gravis. Ann N Y Acad Sci 135: 496–503.

Changeux J (1990). Functional Architecture and Dynamics of the Nicotinic Acetylcholine Receptor: An Allosteric Ligand. Raven Press, New York, pp. 21–168.

Chaudhry VV, Cornblath DR, Griffin JW, et al. (2001). Mycophenolate mofetil: a safe and promising immunosuppressant in neuromuscular diseases. Neurology 56: 94–96.

Christadoss P, Goluszko E (2002). Treatment of experimental autoimmune myasthenia gravis with recombinant human tumor necrosis factor receptor Fc protein. J Neuroimmunol 122: 186–190.

Ciafaloni E, Massey JM (2004). Myasthenia gravis and pregnancy. Neurol Clin 22: 771–782.

Dalakas MC (2004). The use of intravenous immunoglobulin in the treatment of autoimmune neuromuscular diseases: evidence-based indications and safety profile. Pharmacol Ther 102: 177–193.

Dau P, Lindstrom J, Cassel C, et al. (1979). Plasmapheresis in myasthenia gravis and polymyositis. In: PC Dau (Ed.), Plasmapheresis and the Immunobiology of Myasthenia Gravis. Houghton Mifflin, Boston, pp. 229–247.

Dieperink ME, Stefansson K (1989). Molecular mimicry and microorganisms: a role in the pathogenesis of myasthenia gravis? Curr Top Microbiol Immunol 145: 57–65.

Drachman D (1962). Myasthenia gravis and the thyroid gland. N Eng J Med 266: 330–333.

Drachman DB (1994). Myasthenia gravis. N Engl J Med 330: 1797–1810.

Drachman DB (1996). Immunotherapy in neuromuscular disorders: current and future strategies. Muscle Nerve 19: 1239–1251.

Drachman D, Banker B (1961). Arthrogryposis multiplex congenita. Arch Neurol 5: 77–93.

Drachman DB, Angus CW, Adams RN, et al. (1978). Myasthenic antibodies cross-link acetylcholine receptors to accelerate degradation. N Engl J Med 298: 1116–1122.

Drachman DB, Adams RN, Josifek LF, et al. (1982). Functional activities of autoantibodies to acetylcholine receptors and the clinical severity of myasthenia gravis. N Engl J Med 307: 769–775.

Drachman DB, Adams RN, McIntosh K, et al. (1985). Treatment of experimental myasthenia gravis with cyclosporin A. Clin Immunol Immunopathol 34: 174–188.

Drachman D, DeSilva S, Ramsay D, et al. (1987). "Sero-negative" myasthenia gravis: a humorally mediated variant of myasthenia. Neurology 37: 214.

Drachman DB, Jones RJ, Brodsky RA (2003a). Treatment of refractory myasthenia: "rebooting" with high-dose cyclophosphamide. Ann Neurol 53: 29–34.

Drachman D, Wu J-M, Miagkov A, et al. (2003b). Specific immunotherapy of experimental myasthenia by genetically engineered APCs: the "guided missile" strategy. Ann N Y Acad Sci 998: 520–532.

Edgeworth H (1930). A report of progress on the use of ephedrine in a case of myasthenia gravis. JAMA 94: 1136.

Engel AG (1992). Myasthenia gravis and myasthenic syndromes. In: LP Rowland, S DiMauro (Eds.), Handbook of Clinical Neurology. Elsevier, Edinburgh, pp. 391–455.

Engel A, Tsujihata M, Lindstrom J, et al. (1976). The motor endplate in myasthenia gravis and in experimental autoimmune myasthenia gravis. A quantitative ultrastructural study. Ann N Y Acad Sci 274: 60–79.

Evoli A, Di Schino C, Marsili F, et al. (2002). Successful treatment of myasthenia gravis with tacrolimus. Muscle Nerve 25: 111–114.

Evoli A, Tonali PA, Padua L, et al. (2003). Clinical correlates with anti-MuSK antibodies in generalized seronegative myasthenia gravis. Brain 126: 2304–2311.

Fambrough D (1979). Control of acetylcholine receptors in skeletal muscle. Physiol Rev 59: 165–227.

Fambrough DM, Drachman DB, Satyamurti S (1973). Neuromuscular junction in myasthenia gravis: decreased acetylcholine receptors. Science 182: 293–295.

Gajdos P, Outin H, Elkharrat D, et al. (1984). High-dose intravenous gammaglobulin for myasthenia gravis. Lancet 1: 406–407.

Gajdos P, Chevret S, Clair B, et al. (1997). Clinical trial of plasma exchange and high-dose intravenous immunoglobulin in myasthenia gravis. Ann Neurol 41: 789–796.

Genovese MC, Becker JC, Schiff M, et al. (2005). Abatacept for rheumatoid arthritis refractory to tumor necrosis factor alpha inhibition. N Engl J Med 353: 1114–1123.

Gordon MY, Goldman JM, Gordon-Smith EC (1985). 4-Hydroperoxycyclophosphamide inhibits proliferation by human granulocyte-macrophage colony-forming cells (GM-CFC) but spares more primitive progenitor cells. Leuk Res 9: 1017–1021.

Grob D, Arsura EL, Brunner NG, et al. (1987). The course of myasthenia gravis and therapies affecting outcome. Ann N Y Acad Sci 505: 472–499.

Gronseth GS, Barohn RJ (2000). Practice parameter: thymectomy for autoimmune myasthenia gravis (an evidence-based review): report of the Quality Standards Subcommittee of the American Academy of Neurology. Neurology 55: 7–15.

Hertel G, Mertens H, Reuther P, et al. (1979). The treatment of myasthenia gravis with azathioprine. In: PC Dau (Ed.), Plasmapheresis and the Immunobiology of Myasthenia Gravis. Houghton Mifflin, Boston, pp. 315–328.

Hoch W, McConville J, Helms S, et al. (2001). Auto-antibodies to the receptor tyrosine kinase MuSK in patients with myasthenia gravis without acetylcholine receptor antibodies. Nat Med 7: 365–368.

Ito Y, Miledi R, Vincent A, et al. (1978). Acetylcholine receptors and endplate electrophysiology in myasthenia gravis. Brain 101: 345–368.

Jain AB, Kashyap R, Rakela J, et al. (1999). Primary adult liver transplantation under tacrolimus: more than 90 months actual follow-up survival and adverse events. Liver Transpl Surg 5: 144–150.

Jaretzki A, 3rd, Barohn RJ, Ernstoff RM, et al. (2000). Myasthenia gravis: recommendations for clinical research standards. Task Force of the Medical Scientific Advisory Board of the Myasthenia Gravis Foundation of America. Neurology 55: 16–23.

Johns TR (1987). Long-term corticosteroid treatment of myasthenia gravis. Ann N Y Acad Sci 505: 568–583.

Jolly F (1895). Ueber Myasthenia gravis pseudoparalytica. Berl Klin Wochenschr 32: 1.

Jones RJ, Barber JP, Vala MS, et al. (1995). Assessment of aldehyde dehydrogenase in viable cells. Blood 85: 2742–2746.

Juel VC, Massey JM (2005). Autoimmune myasthenia gravis: recommendations for treatment and immunologic modulation. Curr Treat Options Neurol 7: 3–14.

Kaminski HJ, Li Z, Richmonds C, et al. (2004). Complement regulators in extraocular muscle and experimental autoimmune myasthenia gravis. Exp Neurol 189: 333–342.

Kao I, Drachman DB (1977a). Myasthenic immunoglobulin accelerates acetylcholine receptor degradation. Science 196: 527–529.

Kao I, Drachman DB (1977b). Thymic muscle cells bear acetylcholine receptors: possible relation to myasthenia gravis. Science 195: 74–75.

Keesey JC (1998). Contemporary opinions about Mary Walker: a shy pioneer of therapeutic neurology. Neurology 51: 1433–1439.

Keesey J, Buffkin D, Kebo D, et al. (1981). Plasma exchange alone as therapy for myasthenia gravis. Ann N Y Acad Sci 377: 729–743.

Kessel A, Toubi E (2002). Leflunomide in systemic lupus erythematosus. Harefuah 141: 355–357, 409.

Kirsch JR, Diringer MN, Borel CO, et al. (1991). Preoperative lumbar epidural morphine improves postoperative analgesia and ventilatory function after transsternal thymectomy in patients with myasthenia gravis. Crit Care Med 19: 1474–1479.

Kistler J, Stroud RM, Klymkowsky MW, et al. (1982). Structure and function of an acetylcholine receptor. Biophys J 37: 371–383.

Konishi T, Yoshiyama Y, Takamori M, et al. (2005). Long-term treatment of generalised myasthenia gravis with FK506 (tacrolimus). J Neurol Neurosurg Psychiatry 76: 448–450.

Kuroda Y, Oda K, Neshige R, et al. (1984). Exacerbation of myasthenia gravis after removal of a thymoma having a membrane phenotype of suppressor T cells. Ann Neurol 15: 400–402.

Lanska DJ (1990). Indications for thymectomy in myasthenia gravis. Neurology 40: 1828–1829.

Leite MI, Strobel P, Jones M, et al. (2005). Fewer thymic changes in MuSK antibody-positive than in MuSK antibody-negative MG. Ann Neurol 57: 444–448.

Lennon VA, Lindstrom JM, Seybold ME (1976). Experimental autoimmune myasthenia gravis: cellular and humoral immune responses. Ann N Y Acad Sci 274: 283–289.

Levy G, Cole E (2005). Immunosuppressive drug therapy for liver transplant recipients: current perspectives on the benefits of cyclosporine. Transplantation and Immunology Letter 21: 3–4.

Li L, Sun S, Cao X, et al. (2005). Experimental study on induction of tolerance to experimental autoimmune myasthenia gravis by immature dendritic cells. J Huazhong Univ Sci Technolog Med Sci 25: 215–218.

Lindstrom JM, Seybold ME, Lennon VA, et al. (1976). Antibody to acetylcholine receptor in myasthenia gravis. Prevalence, clinical correlates, and diagnostic value. Neurology 26: 1054–1059.

Lindstrom J, Shelton D, Fujii Y (1988). Myasthenia gravis. Adv Immunol 42: 233–284.

Maiti PK, Feferman T, Im SH, et al. (2004). Immunosuppression of rat myasthenia gravis by oral administration of a syngeneic acetylcholine receptor fragment. J Neuroimmunol 152: 112–120.

McConville J, Farrugia ME, Beeson D, et al. (2004). Detection and characterization of MuSK antibodies in seronegative myasthenia gravis. Ann Neurol 55: 580–584.

McIntosh KR, Linsley PS, Drachman DB (1995). Immunosuppression and induction of anergy by CTLA4Ig in vitro: effects on cellular and antibody responses of lymphocytes from rats with experimental autoimmune myasthenia gravis. Cell Immunol 166: 103–112.

McIntosh KR, Linsley PS, Bacha PA, et al. (1998). Immunotherapy of experimental autoimmune myasthenia gravis: selective effects of CTLA4Ig and synergistic combination with an IL2-diphtheria toxin fusion protein. J Neuroimmunol 87: 136–146.

Melms A, Malcherek G, Gern U, et al. (1992). T cells from normal and myasthenic individuals recognize the human acetylcholine receptor: heterogeneity of antigenic sites on the alpha-subunit. Ann Neurol 31: 311–318.

Meriggioli MN, Rowin J, Richman JG, et al. (2003). Mycophenolate mofetil for myasthenia gravis: a double-blind, placebo-controlled pilot study. Ann N Y Acad Sci 998: 494–499.

Miledi R, Molenaar PC, Polak RL (1983). Electrophysiological and chemical determination of acetylcholine release at the frog neuromuscular junction. J Physiol 334: 245–254.

Moiola L, Protti MP, Manfredi AA, et al. (1993). T-helper epitopes on human nicotinic acetylcholine receptor in myasthenia gravis. Ann N Y Acad Sci 681: 198–218.

Monden Y, Nakahara K, Kagotani K, et al. (1984). Effects of preoperative duration of symptoms on patients with myasthenia gravis. Ann Thorac Surg 38: 287–291.

Moorthy G, Behrens MM, Drachman DB, et al. (1989). Ocular pseudomyasthenia or ocular myasthenia "plus": a warning to clinicians. Neurology 39: 1150–1154.

Mossman S, Vincent A, Newsom-Davis J (1986). Myasthenia gravis without acetylcholine-receptor antibody: a distinct disease entity. Lancet 1: 116–119.

Moyo V, Smith D, Brodsky I, et al. (2002). High-dose cyclophosphamide for refractory autoimmune hemolytic anemia. Blood 100: 704–706.

Murray PDF, Drachman DB (1969). The role of movement in the development of joints and related structures: the head and neck in the chick embryo. J Embryol Exp Morph 22: 349–371.

Nakahara K, Ohno K, Hashimoto J, et al. (1988). Thymoma: results with complete resection and adjuvant postoperative irradiation in 141 consecutive patients. J Thorac Cardiovasc Surg 95: 1041–1047.

Newsom-Davis J, Vincent A, Wilson SG, et al. (1978). Plasmapheresis for myasthenia gravis. N Engl J Med 298: 456–457.

Newsom-Davis J, Harcourt G, Sommer N, et al. (1989). T-cell reactivity in myasthenia gravis. J Autoimmun 2: 101–108.

Oh SJ, Kim DE, Kuruoglu R, et al. (1992). Diagnostic sensitivity of the laboratory tests in myasthenia gravis. Muscle Nerve 15: 720–724.

Okumura S, McIntosh K, Drachman DB (1994). Oral administration of acetylcholine receptor: effects on experimental myasthenia gravis. Ann Neurol 36: 704–713.

Palace J, Newsom-Davis J, Lecky B (1998). A randomized double-blind trial of prednisolone alone or with azathioprine in myasthenia gravis. Neurology 50: 1778–1783.

Papazian O (1992). Transient neonatal myasthenia gravis. J Child Neurol 7: 135–141.

Park HS, Shin DM, Lee JS, et al. (1994). Thymoma. A retrospective study of 87 cases. Cancer 73: 2491–2498.

Pascuzzi RM (2000). Medications and Myasthenia Gravis. http://www.myasthenia.org/drugs/reference.htm

Pascuzzi RM, Coslett HB, Johns TR (1984). Long-term corticosteroid treatment of myasthenia gravis: report of 116 patients. Ann Neurol 15: 291–298.

Patrick J, Lindstrom J (1973). Autoimmune response to acetylcholine receptor. Science 180: 871–872.

Penn A, Chang H, Lovelace R, et al. (1976). Antibodies to acetylcholine receptors in rabbits: immunological and electrophysiological studies. Ann N Y Acad Sci 274: 354–376.

Perlo VP, Arnason B, Castleman B (1975). The thymus gland in elderly patients with myasthenia gravis. Neurology 25: 294–295.

Pestronk A, Drachman DB, Adams RN (1982). Treatment of ongoing experimental myasthenia gravis with short term high dose cyclophosphamide. Muscle Nerve 5: 79–84.

Pestronk A, Drachman DB, Teoh R, et al. (1983). Combined short-term immunotherapy for experimental autoimmune myasthenia gravis. Ann Neurol 14: 235–241.

Pestronk A, Drachman DB, Self SG (1985). Measurement of junctional acetylcholine receptors in myasthenia gravis: clinical correlates. Muscle Nerve 8: 245–251.

Pestronk A, Florence J, Miller T, et al. (2003). Treatment of IgM antibody associated polyneuropathies using rituximab. J Neurol Neurosurg Psychiatry 74: 485–489.

Plauche WC (1991). Myasthenia gravis in mothers and their newborns. Clin Obstet Gynecol 34: 82–99.

Polizzi A, Huson SM, Vincent A (2000). Teratogen update: maternal myasthenia gravis as a cause of congenital arthrogryposis. Teratology 62: 332–341.

Ponseti JM, Azem J, Fort JM, et al. (2005). Long-term results of tacrolimus in cyclosporine- and prednisone-dependent myasthenia gravis. Neurology 64: 1641–1643.

Ragheb S, Lisak RP (1998). Immune regulation and myasthenia gravis. Ann N Y Acad Sci 841: 210–224.

Ramsay D, Drachman D, Drachman R, et al. (1992). Stabilization of acetylcholine receptors at the neuromuscular synapse: the role of the nerve. Brain Res 581: 198–207.

Rowin J, Meriggioli MN, Tuzun E, et al. (2004). Etanercept treatment in corticosteroid-dependent myasthenia gravis. Neurology 63: 2390–2392.

Ruff RL (1998). Electrophysiology of postsynaptic activation. Ann N Y Acad Sci 841: 57–70.

Sanders D, El-Salem K, Irbid J, et al. (2003). Muscle specific tyrosine kinase (MuSK) positive, seronegative myasthenia gravis (SN-MG). Clinical characteristics and response to therapy. Neurology 60: A418.

Schneider-Gold C, Gajdos P, Toyka KV, et al. (2005). For myasthenia gravis. Cochrane Database Syst Rev (2): CD002828.

Schumm F, Wietholter H, Fateh-Moghadam A, et al. (1985). Thymectomy in myasthenia with pure ocular symptoms. J Neurol Neurosurg Psychiatry 48: 332–337.

Schwimmbeck PL, Dyrberg T, Drachman DB, et al. (1989). Molecular mimicry and myasthenia gravis. An autoantigenic site of the acetylcholine receptor alpha-subunit that has biologic activity and reacts immunochemically with herpes simplex virus. J Clin Invest 84: 1174–1180.

Seybold ME, Drachman DB (1974). Gradually increasing doses of prednisone in myasthenia gravis. Reducing the hazards of treatment. N Engl J Med 290: 81–84.

Seybold ME, Howard FM, Jr., Duane DD, et al. (1971). Thymectomy in juvenile myasthenia gravis. Arch Neurol 25: 385–392.

Shigemoto K, Kubo S, Maruyama N, et al. (2006). Induction of myasthenia by immunization against muscle-specific kinase. J Clin Invest 116: 1016–1024.

Sieb JP, Engel AG (1993). Ephedrine: effects on neuromuscular transmission. Brain Res 623: 167–171.

Silverman E, Spiegel L, Hawkins D, et al. (2005). Long-term open-label preliminary study of the safety and efficacy of leflunomide in patients with polyarticular-course juvenile rheumatoid arthritis. Arthritis Rheum 52: 554–562.

Sommer N, Willcox N, Harcourt GC, et al. (1990). Myasthenic thymus and thymoma are selectively enriched in acetylcholine receptor-reactive T cells. Ann Neurol 28: 312–319.

Sommer N, Harcourt GC, Willcox N, et al. (1991). Acetylcholine receptor-reactive T lymphocytes from healthy subjects and myasthenia gravis patients. Neurology 41: 1270–1276.

Somner N, Melms A, Weller M, et al. (1993). Ocular myasthenia: a critical review of clinical and pathophysiological aspects. Doc Ophthalmol 84: 309–333.

Somnier FE (1994). Exacerbation of myasthenia gravis after removal of thymomas. Acta Neurol Scand 90: 56–66.

Souroujon MC, Maiti PK, Feferman T, et al. (2003). Suppression of myasthenia gravis by antigen-specific mucosal tolerance and modulation of cytokines and costimulatory factors. Ann N Y Acad Sci 998: 533–536.

Stalberg E, Trontely JV, Schwartz MS (1976). Single muscle-fiber recording of the jitter phenomenon in patients with myasthenia gravis and in members of their families. Ann N Y Acad Sci 274: 189–202.

Stanley EF, Drachman DB (1981). Denervation accelerates degradation of junctional acetylcholine receptors. Exp Neuro 73: 390–396.

Tandan R, Taylor R, DiCostanzo DP, et al. (1990). Metastasizing thymoma and myasthenia gravis. Favorable response to glucocorticoids after failed chemotherapy and radiation therapy. Cancer 65: 1286–1290.

Taylor AL, Watson CJ, Bradley JA (2005). Immunosuppressive agents in solid organ transplantation: mechanisms of action and therapeutic efficacy. Crit Rev Oncol Hematol 56: 23–46.

Termeer A, Visser FJ, Mravunac M (2001). Regression of invasive thymoma following corticosteroid therapy. Neth J Med 58: 181–184.

Tindall RS, Rollins JA, Phillips JT, et al. (1987). Preliminary results of a double-blind, randomized, placebo-controlled trial of cyclosporine in myasthenia gravis. N Engl J Med 316: 719–724.

Toyka KV, Drachman DB, Pestronk A, et al. (1975). Myasthenia gravis: passive transfer from man to mouse. Science 190: 397–399.

Toyka KV, Drachman DB, Griffin DE, et al. (1977). Myasthenia gravis. Study of humoral immune mechanisms by passive transfer to mice. N Engl J Med 296: 125–131.

Unwin N (1995). Acetylcholine receptor channel imaged in the open state. Nature 373: 37–43.

Vidic-Dankovic B, Kosec D, Damjanovic M, et al. (1995). Leflunomide prevents the development of experimentally induced myasthenia gravis. Int J Immunopharmacol 17: 273–281.

Vincenti A, Newsom-Davis J (1985). Acetylcholine receptor antibody as a diagnostic test for myasthenia gravis: results in 153 validated cases and 2967 diagnostic assays. J Neurol Neurosurg Psychiatry 48: 1246–1252.

Vincent A, Newland C, Brueton L, et al. (1995). Arthrogryposis multiplex congenita with maternal autoantibodies specific for a fetal antigen. Lancet 346: 24–25.

Vincenti F, Luggen M (2007). T cell costimulation: a rational target in the therapeutic armamentarium for autoimmune diseases and transplantation. Annu Rev Med 58: 347–358.

Walker MB (1934). Treatment of myasthenia gravis with physostigmine. Lancet 1: 1200.

Wang ZY, Diethelm-Okita B, Okita DK, et al. (2000). T cell recognition of muscle acetylcholine receptor in ocular myasthenia gravis. J Neuroimmunol 108: 29–39.

Waud D (1971). A review of pharmacological approaches to the acetylcholine receptors at the neuromuscular junction. Ann N Y Acad Sci 183: 147–157.

Wekerle H, Ketelsen UP, Zurn AD, et al. (1978). Intrathymic pathogenesis of myasthenia gravis: transient expression of acetylcholine receptors on thymus-derived myogenic cells. Eur J Immunol 8: 579–582.

Wicke C, Halliday B, Allen D, et al. (2000). Effects of steroids and retinoids on wound healing. Arch Surg 135: 1265–1270.

Willems M, Haddad E, Niaudet P, et al. (2006). Rituximab therapy for childhood-onset systemic lupus erythematosus. J Pediatr 148: 623–627.

Wilson S, Vincent A, Newsom-Davis J (1983). Acetylcholine receptor turnover in mice with passively transferred myasthenia gravis. II. Receptor synthesis. J Neurol Neurosurg Psychiatry 46: 383–387.

Witte AS, Cornblath DR, Schatz NJ, et al. (1986). Monitoring azathioprine therapy in myasthenia gravis. Neurology 36: 1533–1534.

Witzemann V, Barg B, Nishikawa Y, et al. (1987). Differential regulation of muscle acetylcholine receptor gamma- and epsilon-subunit mRNAs. FEBS Lett 223: 104–112.

Wolfe GI, Kaminski HJ, Jaretzki A, 3rd, et al. (2003). Development of a thymectomy trial in nonthymomatous myasthenia gravis patients receiving immunosuppressive therapy. Ann N Y Acad Sci 998: 473–480.

Wu JM, Wu B, Miagkov A, et al. (2001). Specific immunotherapy of experimental myasthenia gravis in vitro: the "guided missile" strategy. Cell Immunol 208: 137–147.

Wylam ME, Anderson PM, Kuntz NL, et al. (2003). Successful treatment of refractory myasthenia gravis using rituximab: a pediatric case report. J Pediatr 143: 674–677.

Yeo W, Johnson PJ (2006). Diagnosis, prevention and management of hepatitis B virus reactivation during anticancer therapy. Hepatology 43: 209–220.

Yoshikawa H, Mabuchi K, Yasukawa Y, et al. (2002). Low-dose tacrolimus for intractable myasthenia gravis. J Clin Neurosci 9: 627–628.

Zaja F, Russo D, Fuga G, et al. (2000). Rituximab for myasthenia gravis developing after bone marrow transplant. Neurology 55: 1062–1063.

Zhou L, McConville J, Chaudhry V, et al. (2004). Clinical comparison of muscle-specific tyrosine kinase (MuSK) antibody-positive and -negative myasthenic patients. Muscle Nerve 30: 55–60.

http://www.myasthenia.org/information/MGFA_Brochure_Cyclosporine.pdf

Handbook of Clinical Neurology, Vol. 91 (3rd series)
Neuromuscular junction disorders
A.G. Engel, Editor

Chapter 9

The Lambert–Eaton myasthenic syndrome

DONALD B. SANDERS* AND VERN C. JUEL

Duke University Medical School, Durham, NC, USA

9.1. Introduction

The Lambert–Eaton myasthenic syndrome (LEMS) is a rare autoimmune condition in which weakness results from a presynaptic abnormality of acetylcholine (ACh) release at the neuromuscular junction. LEMS was first described in association with lung cancer, and most recent evidence indicates that approximately 40% of patients have small cell lung cancer (SCLC). There is strong evidence that LEMS results from an autoimmune attack against the P/Q-type voltage-gated calcium channels (VGCC) on the presynaptic motor nerve terminals and autonomic ganglia. Because of the protean symptoms and variability in strength, the diagnosis is frequently elusive and many patients have symptoms for months or years before LEMS is suspected.

9.2. Clinical presentation

9.2.1. Symptoms

LEMS usually begins in later life, although children are rarely affected (Table 9.1, Fig. 9.1). The predominant symptoms are weakness in the legs and generalized fatigue. The weak muscles frequently ache and may be tender. Oropharyngeal and ocular muscles are usually spared or only mildly affected (O'Neill et al., 1988; Tim et al., 2000; Wirtz et al., 2002b), but frequent oculobulbar involvement has been reported (Burns et al., 2003). Although symptoms usually begin insidiously, acute onset is not uncommon, especially after an upper respiratory or diarrheal illness (Tim et al., 1998b). Rapid onset has been associated with underlying cancer in some reports (Wirtz et al., 2005) but not in others (Tim et al., 1998a). Many patients go for months or years before the correct diagnosis is made. Although

respiratory symptoms are probably not more common than expected from underlying lung disease, breathing function is usually reduced and occasionally patients present with respiratory failure (Smith and Wald, 1996). Dry mouth is almost always present and frequently precedes other symptoms of LEMS. However, many patients do not mention this symptom unless specifically questioned. Many are also aware of an unpleasant metallic taste. Impotence is common in males and some patients have other symptoms of autonomic dysfunction, such as postural hypotension.

LEMS may be first discovered when prolonged paralysis follows the use of neuromuscular blocking agents during surgery. The weakness of LEMS may be worse when the ambient temperature is elevated or when the patient is febrile.

9.2.2. Physical findings

The weakness demonstrated on examination is usually relatively mild compared to the patient's symptoms. Strength may improve after exercise and then weaken as activity is sustained, but this does not occur in all patients and is demonstrable on examination in only about half (Oh et al., 2005). Tendon reflexes are reduced or absent in most patients, but may be preserved early in the disease. Hypoactive reflexes can frequently be potentiated by having the patient briefly contract the appropriate muscle (Nilsson and Rosén, 1978; O'Neill et al., 1988; Oh et al., 2005). This finding is said to be virtually diagnostic of LEMS.

Pupils may be dilated and respond poorly to light (O'Neill et al., 1988; Wirtz et al., 2001). Edrophonium or pyridostigmine may improve strength in LEMS but the response is rarely as dramatic as in myasthenia gravis (MG).

*Correspondence to: Donald B. Sanders, MD, Professor of Medicine (Neurology), Duke University Medical School, Box 3403, Duke University Medical Center, Durham, NC 27710, USA. E-mail: Donald.Sanders@Duke.edu, Tel: 1-919-684-6078, Fax: 1-919-660-3853.

Table 9.1

Demographics of 96 LEMS patients seen in the Duke MG Clinic since 1980

	CA-LEMS	NCA-LEMS	All LEMS
M:F	22:18	24:32	46:50
VGCC pos:neg	13:4 (76%)	27:9 (75%)	40:13 (75.5%)
Age onset, median	62.5	51.5	58
mean, sd	62.3 ± 10.1	50.4 ± 16.8	55.3 ± 15.6
min–max	40–83	8–77	8–83

CA, associated cancer detected; NCA, no associated cancer detected; VGCC, P/Q type voltage-gated calcium channel antibodies.

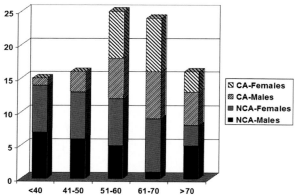

Fig. 9.1. Age onset in 96 LEMS patients seen in the Duke MG Clinic since 1980. CA—associated cancer; NCA—no associated cancer detected. Most patients less than 50 have no associated cancer. With increasing age, more LEMS patients have cancer, but even over 70, cancer is not detected in half the patients.

9.3. Cancer in LEMS

Cancer is present when the disease begins or is found later in 40% of patients (Sanders, 1995) (Table 9.1). Small cell lung cancer is by far the most common associated cancer, and smoking and age at onset are the major risk factors for this neoplasm. The age at onset is higher in cancer-associated LEMS (CA-LEMS) than in those without detected cancer (NCA-LEMS), and more men than women with LEMS have an associated cancer (Wirtz et al., 2002a) (Table 9.1, Fig. 9.1).

Lymphoproliferative malignancies, especially non-Hodgkin's lymphoma, are found in occasional LEMS patients. The association with other cancers has not been

established. Among 96 patients diagnosed with LEMS in the Duke MG Clinic since 1980, 34 had SCLC and 5 had lung tumors of other cell types, felt to be causally associated with LEMS (Table 9.2). Breast cancer developed in three patients, 8 and 12 years after and 4 years before onset of LEMS; one had prostate cancer diagnosed 3 years before LEMS onset, and one patient developed leukemia 11 years after LEMS onset. These cancers were probably coincidental, and not causally related to LEMS.

What is the likelihood that a patient with LEMS has an underlying cancer? If a tumor is not found within the first two years after LEMS symptom onset, then it is unlikely to occur later. In practical terms, this means that a patient less than age 50 at onset of LEMS symptoms with no known tumor after 2 years is unlikely to have an underlying cancer. On the other hand, a chronic smoker with LEMS beginning after age 50 almost certainly has an underlying lung cancer.

9.4. Pathophysiology

The physiology of neuromuscular transmission is studied by measuring the subsynaptic events at the neuromuscular junction with microelectrodes inserted into muscle fibers in vitro (see Chapter 3). Single quanta of ACh released from the motor nerve terminal produce localized depolarizations of the peri-endplate muscle membrane. The amplitude of these miniature endplate potentials (MEPPs) reflects the size of each ACh quantum, as well as the responsiveness of the postsynaptic muscle membrane to ACh. Microphysiological studies demonstrate that MEPP amplitude is normal in LEMS muscle but fewer quanta are released by each nerve depolarization (Lambert and Elmqvist, 1971).

Table 9.2

Cancer type in 96 LEMS patients in the Duke MG Data Registry

Small cell lung cancer (SCLC)	34
Other lung cancer	6
Mixed small/cell/other	2
Non-small cell	2
Carcinoid	1
Neuroendocrine tumor	1
Other tumors, not likely associated*	5
Breast	3
Prostate	1
Leukemia	1

*These tumors occurred many years before or after onset of LEMS and were felt to be coincidental and unrelated to the LEMS.

9.5. Immunopathology

The following observations have suggested that LEMS has an autoimmune etiology:

- LEMS is frequently associated with known autoimmune diseases.
- Treatment with prednisone, plasma exchange (PLEX) or hyper-immune human γ-globulin (IVIg) improves weakness in many LEMS patients.

The conclusive evidence for an autoimmune etiology of LEMS, however, came from passive transfer to mice of the electrophysiologic and morphologic features of LEMS and by localizing LEMS IgG to the active zones. Active zone particles (AZPs), which represent the VGCC, are normally arranged in regular parallel arrays on the presynaptic nerve terminal membrane (Fig. 9.2A). In LEMS, this regular pattern is lost and the AZPs become clustered and reduced in number (Fukunaga et al., 1982) (Fig. 9.2B, C). Studies of mice treated with LEMS IgG revealed that the quantal content of the endplate potential was reduced (Lang et al., 1981, 1983; Kim, 1986) and presynaptic membranes of the treated mice displayed the same clustering and depletion of the AZPs as found in humans (Fukunaga et al., 1983, 1987a), but only divalent LEMS IgG had this effect (Nagel et al., 1988). Confirming the above findings, immunoelectron microscopy studies localized LEMS IgG to the active zones (Fukuoka et al., 1987b). The above findings provided convincing evidence that 1. the P/Q VGCC is the target of pathogenic LEMS autoantibodies, and 2. the antibodies downregulate expression of the VGCC by antigenic modulation. The demonstration of antibodies against the P/Q VGCC

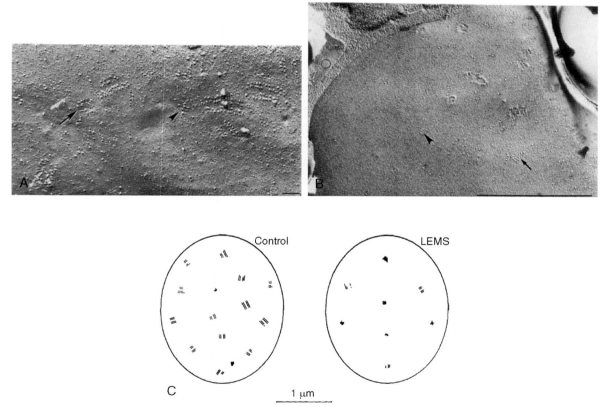

Fig. 9.2. Electron microscopy of freeze-fractured human presynaptic membrane preparations. (From Fukunaga et al., 1982, with permission from *Muscle and Nerve*.) (A) Control presynaptic membrane, P-face ×55 000, bar = 0.1 μm. Intramembrane particles representing VGCC are abundant and organized in active zones with double parallel rows of particles (arrows). (B) LEMS presynaptic membrane, P-face ×61 000, bar = 0.1 μm. Active zones are markedly depleted. A solitary short active zone (arrow) is identified. The cluster of large intramembrane particles (arrowhead) may reflect cross-linkage of VGCC antibody-receptor complexes. (C) Schematic reconstruction of 5 μm² regions of presynaptic membrane P-faces based upon data from membrane preparations in 9 LEMS patients and 14 controls. Control membranes had a mean of 13 active zones and 2 intramembrane clusters, while LEMS membranes had a mean of 3 active zones and 5 intramembrane clusters.

in serum of 90% of non-immunosuppressed LEMS patients closed the chain of evidence that LEMS was mediated by humoral immunity (Lennon et al., 1995).

SCLC cells are of neuroectodermal origin, share a number of antigens with peripheral nervous system tissue, and contain high concentrations of VGCC. LEMS IgG inhibits calcium influx into these cells. In LEMS patients with SCLC, the cancer cells presumably contain antigens that mimic VGCC and induce the production of VGCC antibodies. In NCA-LEMS VGCC antibodies are produced as part of a more general autoimmune state.

9.6. Epidemiology

LEMS is rare, and the frequency in any population is affected by factors that determine the frequency of lung cancer—primarily smoking—and the susceptibility of the population to autoimmune disease in general. The best epidemiological data available, from the Netherlands, demonstrate an annual incidence of 0.4 per million and a prevalence of 2.5 per million in 2003 (Wirtz et al., 2004b). These numbers would indicate that there are fewer than 1000 patients with LEMS in the US at any time. Considering the difficulty in making the correct diagnosis, many patients with LEMS are undiagnosed and these numbers underestimate the true incidence. In our clinic, LEMS was diagnosed in 96 patients since 1980, compared with 949 patients diagnosed with MG, a ratio of 1:10, which is also the experience reported from the Mayo Clinic (Harper and Lennon, 2002).

9.7. Diagnostic procedures

The classical clinical findings of LEMS are weakness, particularly of proximal muscles, reduced or absent muscle stretch reflexes, and dry mouth. The diagnosis can be confirmed in most cases by demonstrating characteristic abnormalities on electrodiagnostic studies (see Section 9.7.1). Not all LEMS patients have all these findings, however, but the diagnosis can be considered secure if the patient has weakness, electromyographic evidence of abnormal neuromuscular transmission and either elevated voltage-gated calcium channel antibodies or small cell lung cancer.

9.7.1. Electrodiagnostic tests

Electrodiagnostic studies (EMG) in LEMS patients usually show characteristic abnormalities. Compound muscle action potentials (CMAPs) recorded with surface electrodes are small, often less than 10% of nor-

mal, and fall further with repetitive nerve stimulation (RNS) at frequencies between 1 Hz and 5 Hz (Fig. 9.3). During stimulation at frequencies from 20 Hz to 50 Hz, the CMAP increases in size and characteristically becomes at least twice the size of the initial response (facilitation). Facilitation can also be demonstrated as an increase in CMAP size immediately after the patient contracts the muscle maximally for 5–10 s (Fig. 9.4). Because these electrodiagnostic abnormalities may be partially masked by low muscle temperature or incomplete relaxation, the muscle should be warmed and rested for several minutes before testing.

In the initial description of LEMS, it was emphasized that doubling of CMAP amplitude after activation should be seen to confirm the diagnosis (Lambert et al., 1961) and this finding is considered to be typical of LEMS (AAEM Quality Assurance Committee American Association of Electrodiagnostic Medicine, 2001). However, in some patients with LEMS the RNS findings are identical to MG, especially when symptoms are mild, or early in the disease process (Lambert, 1987). Also, facilitation may be quite marked in some

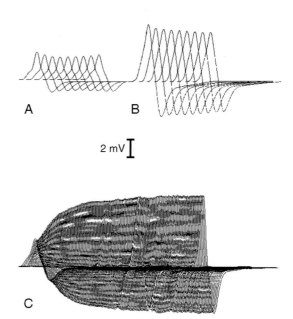

Fig. 9.3. Repetitive nerve stimulation studies in LEMS. A CMAPs recorded from the hypothenar muscles during stimulation of the ulnar nerve at 3/s. The initial CMAP amplitude is less than normal and there is a decrementing response. B Immediately after maximum contraction of the muscle for 10 s, the amplitude of the initial response has increased by more than 100% from A. C During 20/s stimulation the CMAP amplitude falls slightly, then increases by more than 100% of the initial value. (From Sanders, 1993, with permission.)

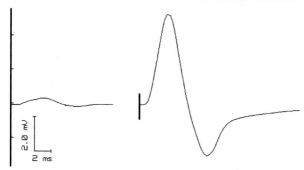

Fig. 9.4. Compound muscle action potentials in LEMS elicited before (left) and immediately after (right) maximum voluntary contraction of the tested muscle for 10 s. (From Sanders, 2005, with permission.)

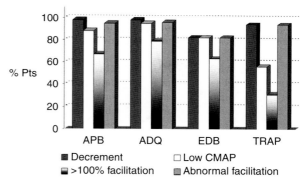

Fig. 9.5. Electrodiagnostic findings in 57 patients with LEMS. The percentage of patients in whom each abnormality was found on repetitive nerve stimulation studies. APB—abductor pollicis brevis; ADQ—abductor digiti quinti; EDB—extensor digitorum brevis; TRAP—trapezius (tested in 34 patients); Decrement—>10% decrement at 3 Hz; Low CMAP—CMAP amplitude less than normal; >100% facilitation—CMAP amplitude increased at least 100% after maximum voluntary contraction for 10 s; Abnormal facilitation—CMAP amplitude increased more than control values after maximum voluntary contraction for 10 s.

MG patients, especially if the tested muscle is atrophic. Thus, no electrodiagnostic criteria will distinguish LEMS from MG in all cases.

The following statements regarding the electrodiagnosis of LEMS are based on our experience (Tim et al., 2000).

- Electrodiagnostic findings vary among muscles, even between two muscles of the same hand. Thus, several muscles should be tested to determine the overall pattern of abnormality.
- Almost all patients have a decrementing response to low frequency nerve stimulation in at least one hand muscle (Fig. 9.5). This finding is not specific for LEMS, because it is typically seen also in MG and is rarely seen in some nerve and muscle diseases.
- The CMAP amplitude is low in most muscles tested. This is also a non-specific finding, commonly occurring also in nerve or muscle disease.
- Facilitation of 100% or more is found in at least one hand or foot muscle in 90% of LEMS patients. The amount of facilitation varies considerably among muscles, but is greater in distal than in proximal muscles.
- If facilitation is greater than 100% in most muscles tested or exceeds 400% in any muscle, the patient almost certainly has LEMS.
- In some LEMS patients there may be no facilitation in any tested muscle, especially if symptoms are mild or have been present for only a short time. In these patients, all available clinical and serological information must be assessed in arriving at the most likely diagnosis. In some cases, follow-up and repeated RNS studies may be necessary to confirm the diagnosis.

- The electrodiagnostic abnormalities are frequently more marked than the clinical findings would suggest (Eaton and Lambert, 1957), whereas the opposite is usually the case in MG (Lambert, 1987).

Needle electromyography in LEMS demonstrates markedly unstable motor unit action potentials, which vary in shape during voluntary activation. This variability is a manifestation of abnormal neuromuscular transmission and can be quantified by single-fiber EMG (SFEMG) measurements of jitter (see Chapter 4). Jitter is markedly increased in LEMS, frequently out of proportion to the severity of weakness, and there is frequent impulse blocking. In many endplates the jitter and blocking decrease as the firing rate increases (Trontelj and Stålberg, 1991; Sanders, 1992). However, this pattern is not seen in all endplates nor in all patients with LEMS (Sanders, 1992; Trontelj and Stålberg, 1992).

9.7.2. Voltage-gated calcium channel antibodies

Human neuronal cell lines and SCLC cell lines both express VGCC that bind the Ω-conotoxin from the snail *Conus geographus*. This toxin binds with high affinity to the P/Q form of VGCC, which is associated with neurotransmitter release. Assays for antibodies to VGCC have been developed using human neuroblastoma or SCLC cell lines as the source of VGCC, which is labeled by binding to ^{125}I-Ω-conotoxin. Immunoprecipitation of conotoxin-bound VGCC complexes demonstrates antibodies in almost 100% of patients with LEMS who have primary lung cancer, and in over 90% of those without evident cancer (Harper and Lennon, 2002). No differences have been found between LEMS patients with or without detectible P/Q VGCC antibodies except that fewer patients with CA-LEMS are seronegative (Nakao et al., 2002). Low titers of VGCC antibodies (VGCC-Abs) are also found in non-LEMS patients with systemic lupus erythematosus or rheumatoid arthritis, conditions in which there are high levels of circulating immunoglobulins (Lang et al., 1993) and in fewer than 5% of patients with MG (Harper and Lennon, 2002).

Because VGCC-Abs may disappear in patients receiving immunosuppressive therapy, the assay is most informative when performed before such treatment. On the other hand, assay for these antibodies may be normal early in the disease and become abnormal later, so repeat testing may be of value if the initial test was normal. VGCC-Ab levels do not correlate with disease severity among patients with LEMS but the antibody levels do fall in individual patients as the disease improves (Leys et al., 1991).

9.8. Other tests

Autonomic function tests are abnormal in most LEMS patients, even when there are no clinical signs of autonomic dysfunction (Khurana, 1993). These tests usually show evidence of sympathetic as well as parasympathetic dysfunction (Khurana et al., 1988; Baker et al., 1994; O'Suilleabhain et al., 1998).

Muscle biopsy in LEMS frequently shows type II muscle fiber atrophy, as in disuse, which is non-specific.

9.9. Associated diseases

LEMS patients with SCLC may have other paraneoplastic syndromes, such as inappropriate ADH secretion (SIADH), sensorimotor neuropathy, or cerebellar degeneration (Kobayashi et al., 1988).

Before VGCC antibodies had been demonstrated in LEMS, the early report of a NCA-LEMS patient with several autoimmune disorders raised the possibility that NCA-LEMS represented an organ-specific autoimmune disorder (Gutmann et al., 1972). A review of 227 LEMS cases in the literature found immunological disorders in 6% of CA-LEMS and 27% of NCA-LEMS (Wirtz et al., 2002a). Thyroid disease was the most commonly reported associated disorder. Sixteen percent of our CA-LEMS patients developed inappropriate antidiuretic hormone secretion, and among the NCA-LEMS patients 16% had another autoimmune disorder or serological evidence for autoimmunity. Hypothyroidism was most common, but vitamin B_{12} deficiency,

rheumatoid arthritis, inflammatory myopathy, and systemic vasculitis were also observed (Tim et al., 2000).

Organ-specific autoantibodies (e.g., thyroid microsomal, thyroglobulin, gastric parietal cell, acetylcholine receptor, striated muscle) have been found in 52–60% of NCA-LEMS sera and in 24–28% of CA-LEMS sera (Lennon et al., 1982; O'Neill et al., 1988). Non-organ specific autoantibodies (e.g., antinuclear, smooth muscle, mitochondrial, rheumatoid factor) were found in 60% of CA-LEMS and 24% of NCA-LEMS (O'Neill et al., 1988). Increased frequency of autoimmune disease has also been reported in maternal relatives of NCA-LEMS patients, but not in relatives of CA-LEMS patients, suggesting that NCA-LEMS shares immunogenetic factors with other autoimmune disorders (Wirtz et al., 2004a).

9.10. Differential diagnosis of LEMS

LEMS patients commonly receive an incorrect diagnosis before LEMS is established (Wirtz et al., 2004b). In patients with cancer, the symptoms of LEMS may be attributed to cachexia, peripheral neuropathy or the effects of treatment. In patients without evident cancer, LEMS symptoms may be dismissed without explanation if little weakness is found on examination, or may be erroneously attributed to myopathy, neuropathy or MG.

Although the clinical presentations of MG and LEMS are usually quite distinct (Wirtz et al., 2002b), the clinical and electrodiagnostic findings may be similar in some patients, in which case distinguishing between these diseases may be challenging (see Chapter 7). Clinical features that strongly suggest MG are prominent ocular muscle weakness, limb weakness that predominates in the arms, and normal muscle stretch reflexes (Table 9.3). Features that favor LEMS include weakness that predominates in the legs, hypoactive or absent reflexes, and autonomic symptoms, especially dry mouth.

If the patient has AChR or MuSK antibodies, the diagnosis of MG is secure. Similarly, if there are antibodies to VGCC in a patient with abnormal neuromuscular transmission, LEMS can be diagnosed with confidence. It has been reported that AChR antibodies are also elevated in up to 13% of patients with LEMS, usually in low concentrations (Lennon, 1997); however, among 96 patients with LEMS in the Duke MG Registry, AChR antibodies were elevated in only one, and that patient had clinical and electrophysiologic findings of a true overlap between MG and LEMS (see Section 9.13).

9.11. Treatment of LEMS

Therapy must be tailored for each patient, based on the severity of weakness, underlying disease(s), life

Table 9.3

Features that distinguish MG from LEMS

	MG	LEMS
Ocular muscle weakness	Usual/severe	Uncommon/mild
Limb muscle weakness	Frequent	Usual
Benefit from cholinesterase inhibitors	Usual	Limited
Autonomic symptoms	None	Dry mouth, impotence
Tendon reflexes	Normal	Reduced or absent
Clinical facilitation	Occasional	Frequent
CMAP amplitude	Normal	Reduced
CMAP facilitation >100%	Uncommon	Usual
Thymoma	10–20%	Rare/none
Lung cancer	Rare/none	50%
MEPP amplitude	Low	Normal
Quantal content	Normal	Reduced

expectancy and response to previous treatment. The treatment plan that follows may serve as a general guide, but will require modification for many patients.

When the diagnosis of LEMS has been confirmed, an extensive search for malignancy should be carried out, including radiographs and CT scan of the chest. Bronchoscopy is recommended during the initial evaluation of patients with LEMS who have a significant risk of lung cancer, especially in smokers and when symptoms have been present for less than 2 years. Bronchoscopy may reveal cancer when results of chest CT and MRI are normal.

The initial treatment should be aimed at any tumor present, since the weakness in CA-LEMS may improve with effective cancer therapy (Jenkyn et al., 1980; Chalk et al., 1990), and in some patients no further treatment for LEMS may be necessary. If no tumor is found, the search for an occult malignancy should be repeated periodically, based on the patient's risk of cancer. Patients less than 50 without a history of chronic smoking have a low risk of cancer, especially if there is evidence for a co-existing autoimmune disease. In these patients extensive surveillance for cancer may not be necessary. Patients over 50 with a history of chronic smoking almost certainly have an underlying lung cancer, which must be assiduously sought.

In patients with cancer, LEMS is usually not the major therapeutic concern nor does it represent the major threat to life. In our experience, immunotherapy of LEMS without effective treatment of an underlying cancer usually produces little or no improvement in strength. There is also a theoretical concern that immunosuppression may reduce the immunologic suppression of tumor growth.

Aggressive immunotherapy is more readily justified in NCA-LEMS.

Cholinesterase inhibitors do not usually produce significant improvement in LEMS although they may improve dry mouth. Pyridostigmine (Mestinon©) (30 mg or 60 mg every 4–6 h) is the preferred agent and should be given for several days before assessing the response.

Guanidine hydrochloride inhibits mitochondrial calcium uptake, which increases the intracellular calcium concentration. This increases the release of ACh from the motor nerve terminal, which produces improvement in strength in many patients with LEMS. Guanidine is taken orally, beginning with a dose of 5–10 mg/kg/day, divided throughout the waking hours. The dose may be increased to a maximum of 30 mg/kg/day, depending upon the clinical response, but side effects may be severe at doses greater than 1 g/day. Pyridostigmine enhances the therapeutic response to guanidine and permits use of a lower dose. Side effects of guanidine seriously limit its clinical use. These include bone marrow suppression, renal tubular acidosis, chronic interstitial nephritis, cardiac arrhythmia, hepatic toxicity, pancreatic dysfunction, peripheral paresthesias, ataxia, confusion, alterations of mood and behavioral changes. Blood tests of hematologic, hepatic and renal function must be performed frequently as long as patients are taking guanidine.

Aminopyridines increase neurotransmitter release at central and peripheral synapses by blocking the delayed potassium conductance (Yeh et al., 1976). Clinical trials have demonstrated that 3,4-diaminopyridine (DAP) improves strength and autonomic function in most patients with LEMS (McEvoy et al., 1989; Sanders et al., 2000; Maddison and Newsom-Davis, 2003).

In our experience, more than 85% of LEMS patients have significant clinical benefit from DAP; in over half of these, the improvement is marked (Tim et al., 2000). The effect of DAP begins about 20 min after an oral dose, the effect of each dose lasts about 4 h, and the maximum response to a given dosage may not be seen for 2–3 days. DAP is given orally in dosages of 5–25 mg, 3 or 4 times a day. The optimal dose and dosing schedule vary considerably and must be determined for each patient. In most patients, pyridostigmine enhances and prolongs the duration of action of DAP and permits use of lower doses. The optimal dose of DAP, taken with pyridostigmine, is usually between 15 mg and 60 mg per day.

Patients with or without underlying cancer benefit from DAP. Side-effects are minimal and usually are limited to brief perioral and digital paresthesias if the dose is 10–15 mg or more. Gastrointestinal cramps and diarrhea may occur when DAP is taken with pyridostigmine, and can be minimized by reducing the dose of pyridostigmine. Seizures may occur with doses greater than 100 mg/day, and asthma attacks have been induced in patients with pre-existing asthma. A patient who inadvertently took six times the therapeutic dose of DAP (60 mg ×6) had seizures and cardiac arrhythmia, which resolved within 24 h without apparent sequelae (Boerma et al., 1995).

DAP should not be given to patients with known seizures. There is also a theoretical possibility that DAP could cause cardiac arrhythmia, although no such effects have been reported, and no effect on the electrocardiogram was found during a controlled trial (Sanders et al., 2000). Organ toxicity has not been reported, even in patients who have taken DAP for more than 10 years. However, because the clinical experience is still limited, periodic blood tests of liver, kidney and hematologic function are recommended to assure that no such side-effects develop.

Experience indicates that DAP is a safe, effective and valuable treatment for LEMS. It has not been approved for clinical use in the US, but is available to physicians on a treatment use basis for individual patients. Information about the application process can be obtained from Jacobus Pharmaceutical Co., Inc., Princeton, NJ, USA, Fax 1-609-799-1176.

If the previously discussed treatments are not effective and the weakness is relatively mild, the physician must determine if aggressive immunotherapy is justified, bearing in mind that even with optimum immunosuppression, most LEMS patients continue to have significant dysfunction. When weakness is severe, plasma exchange or high dose intravenous immunoglobulin (IVIg) may be used to induce relatively rapid, albeit transitory, improvement (see below). Immunosuppressants can be added in an attempt to produce more sustained improvement. Prednisone and azathioprine (AZA) are the most frequently used immunosuppressants, given alone or together (Maddison et al., 2001).

Plasma exchange produces temporary improvement in many patients with LEMS (NIH Consensus Conference Statement, 1986) but repeated courses are usually necessary to sustain the improvement. IVIg also induces clinically significant temporary improvement in many patients (Rich et al., 1997). The frequency with which improvement occurs and the response to repeated courses of plasma exchange or IVIg have yet to be determined.

9.11.1. Medications that exacerbate LEMS

Drugs that exacerbate MG have similar effects in LEMS (see Chapter 12, Drugs and Other Toxins with Adverse Effects on the Neuromuscular Junction). Competitive neuromuscular blocking agents, such as d-tubocurarine and pancuronium, have an exaggerated and prolonged effect on LEMS, as on MG. In the first reported case thought to represent LEMS, neuromuscular dysfunction was initially recognized when prolonged apnea followed administration of succinylcholine during anesthesia (Anderson et al., 1953). There are reports of LEMS becoming worse after administration of magnesium and intravenous iodinated radiographic contrast agents (Gutmann and Takamori, 1973; Streib, 1977; van den Bergh et al., 1986). In general, patients with LEMS should be observed for worsening after any new medication is begun.

9.12. Prognosis

The prognosis in patients with LEMS is largely determined by the presence and type of any underlying cancer, the presence and severity of any associated autoimmune disease, and the severity and distribution of weakness. Patients with rapidly progressive symptoms usually have more severe disease. Effective treatment of underlying cancer leads to sustained improvement, or even complete remission of weakness, in many patients. The long-term prognosis in these patients is determined by the recurrence rate for the cancer. It has been reported that SCLC has a better prognosis when associated with LEMS (Maddison et al., 1999). This could be because LEMS leads to earlier tumor detection and treatment, or it could reflect more effective immunologic surveillance. In NCA-LEMS, long-term outcome was correlated with initial clinical muscle strength measurements but not with anti-VGCC antibody levels or electrophysiological findings (Maddison et al., 2001). Judiciously-selected treatment with combinations of symptomatic agents and immunosuppression can improve function significantly in many LEMS patients, but most will continue to have some disability despite all therapeutic measures.

9.13. MG/LEMS overlap syndrome

There are many reports of patients with various overlapping features of MG and LEMS. These include: clinical features of one condition but facilitation, or lack thereof, typical of the other; clinical and electrodiagnostic patterns typical of one condition initially, but changing to the other later; or electrodiagnostic patterns typical of MG in one muscle, and of LEMS in another. However, low amplitude CMAPs with marked facilitation should not be taken as unequivocal evidence of a presynaptic block since this combination can also be seen with postsynaptic block, such as that produced by curare (Hutter, 1952), some severe congenital myasthenic syndromes (Harper, 2002), and MG with severe muscle atrophy. Taking into consideration also that findings on repetitive nerve stimulation in some LEMS patients resemble those in MG, especially when symptoms are mild, or early in the disease process (Lambert, 1987), it is apparent that the findings on RNS depend on the severity, as well as the mechanism, of the neuromuscular transmission defect, and that "anomalous" RNS findings do not constitute a true overlap.

Six patients have been reported who appear to have a true MG/LEMS overlap syndrome, with antibodies to both the AChR and VGCC (Newsom-Davis et al., 1991; Katz et al., 1998; Kanzato et al., 1999; Oh and Sher, 2005). Of the 96 LEMS patients seen in the Duke MG Clinic since 1980, only one had both antibodies, and that patient also had clinical and electrodiagnostic features that overlapped between the two conditions.

These overlap syndromes could represent outliers of either MG or LEMS, with nonpathogenic antibodies against the epitope typically targeted by the other, as has been suggested (Katz et al., 1998). However, the simplest explanation is that two autoimmune diseases coexist, a not uncommon event, each targeting a different anatomic site at the neuromuscular junction. The contribution of each disorder could be resolved by microphysiologic and ultrastructural studies of the neuromuscular junction or passive transfer experiments, but such studies are not usually available to guide therapeutic decisions.

The ultimate diagnosis in patients with mixed features of MG and LEMS may be moot because many treatments are the same for both conditions. Exceptions are that we do not search for cancer other than thymoma in MG, and thymectomy would not be considered as potential treatment in LEMS.

References

AAEM Quality Assurance Committee American Association of Electrodiagnostic Medicine (2001). Practice parameter for repetitive nerve stimulation and single fiber EMG evaluation of adults with suspected myasthenia gravis or Lambert–Eaton myasthenic syndrome: summary statement. Muscle Nerve 24: 1236–1238.

Anderson HJ, Churchill-Davidson HC, Richardson AT (1953). Bronchial neoplasm with myasthenia. Prolonged apnea after administration of succinylcholine. Lancet ii: 1291–1293.

Baker MK, Low PA, McEvoy KM (1994). Quantification of autonomic dysfunction in Lambert–Eaton syndrome by composite autonomic scoring scale. Neurology 44: A220.

Boerma CE, Rommes JH, van Leeuwen RB, et al. (1995). Cardiac arrest following an iatrogenic 3,4-diaminopyridine intoxication in a patient with Lambert–Eaton myasthenic syndrome. J Toxicol Clin Toxicol 33: 249–251.

Burns TM, Russell JA, LaChance DH, et al. (2003). Oculobulbar involvement is typical with Lambert–Eaton myasthenic syndrome. Ann Neurol 53: 270–273.

Chalk CH, Murray NM, Newsom-Davis J, et al. (1990). Response of the Lambert–Eaton myasthenic syndrome to treatment of associated small-cell lung carcinoma. Neurology 40: 1552–1556.

Eaton LM, Lambert EH (1957). Electromyography and electric stimulation of nerves in diseases of the motor unit. JAMA 163: 1117–1124.

Fukunaga H, Engel AG, Osame M, et al. (1982). Paucity and disorganization of presynaptic membrane active zones in the Lambert–Eaton myasthenic syndrome. Muscle Nerve 5: 686–697.

Fukunaga H, Engel AG, Lang B, et al. (1983). Passive transfer of Lambert–Eaton myasthenic syndrome with IgG from man to mouse depletes the presynaptic membrane active zones. Proc Natl Acad Sci U S A 80: 7636–7640.

Fukuoka T, Engel AG, Lang B, et al. (1987a). Lambert–Eaton myasthenic syndrome: I. Early morphological effects of IgG on the presynaptic membrane active zones. Ann Neurol 22: 193–199.

Fukuoka T, Engel AG, Lang B, et al. (1987b). Lambert–Eaton myasthenic syndrome: II. Immunoelectron microscopy localization of IgG at the mouse motor end-plate. Ann Neurol 22: 200–211.

Gutmann L, Takamori M (1973). Effect of Mg^{++} on neuromuscular transmission in the Eaton–Lambert syndrome. Neurology 23: 977–980.

Gutmann L, Crosby TW, Takamori M, et al. (1972). The Eaton–Lambert syndrome and autoimmune disorders. Am J Med 53: 354.

Harper CM (2002). Congenital myasthenic syndromes. In: WF Brown, CF Bolton, MJ Aminoff (Eds.), Neuromuscular Function and Disease. W.B. Saunders Company, Philadelphia, pp. 1687–1695.

Harper CM, Lennon VA (2002). The Lambert–Eaton myasthenic syndrome. In: HJ Kaminski (Ed.), Current Clinical Neurology: Myasthenia Gravis and Related Disorders. Humana Press, Totowa, NJ, pp. 269–291.

Hutter OF (1952). Post-tetanic restoration of neuromuscular transmission blocked by d-tubocurarine. J Physiol 118: 216–227.

Jenkyn LR, Brooks PL, Forcier RJ, et al. (1980). Remission of the Lambert–Eaton syndrome and small cell anaplastic carcinoma of the lung induced by chemotherapy and radiotherapy. Cancer 46: 1123–1127.

Kanzato N, Motomura M, Suehara M, et al. (1999). Lambert–Eaton myasthenic syndrome with ophthalmoparesis and pseudoblepharospasm. Muscle Nerve 22: 1727–1730.

Katz JS, Wolfe GI, Bryan WW, et al. (1998). Acetylcholine receptor antibodies in the Lambert–Eaton myasthenic syndrome. Neurology 50: 470–475.

Khurana RK (1993). Paraneoplastic autonomic dysfunction. In: PA Low (Ed.), Clinical Autonomic Disorders. Little, Brown Co., Boston, pp. 506–511.

Khurana RK, Koski CL, Mayer RF (1988). Autonomic dysfunction in Lambert–Eaton myasthenic syndrome. J Neurol Sci 85: 77–86.

Kim YI (1986). Passively transferred Lambert–Eaton syndrome in mice receiving purified IgG. Muscle Nerve 9: 523–530.

Kobayashi H, Matsuoka R, Kitamura S, et al. (1988). Bronchogenic carcinoma with subacute cerebellar degeneration and Eaton–Lambert syndrome: an autopsy case. Jpn J Med 27: 203–206.

Lambert EH (1987). General discussion. Ann N Y Acad Sci 505: 380–381.

Lambert EH, Elmqvist D (1971). Quantal components of end-plate potentials in the myasthenic syndrome. Ann N Y Acad Sci 183: 183–199.

Lambert EH, Rooke ED, Eaton LM, et al. (1961). Myasthenic syndrome occasionally associated with bronchial neoplasm: neurophysiologic studies. In: HR Viets (Ed.), Myasthenia Gravis. Charles C. Thomas, Springfield, pp. 362–410.

Lang B, Newsom-Davis J, Wray DW, et al. (1981). Autoimmune aetiology for myasthenic (Lambert–Eaton) syndrome. Lancet 2: 224–226.

Lang B, Newsom-Davis J, Prior C, et al. (1983). Antibodies to motor nerve terminals: an electrophysiological study of a human myasthenic syndrome transferred to mouse. J Physiol 344: 335–345.

Lang B, Johnston I, Leys K, et al. (1993). Autoantibody specificities in Lambert–Eaton myasthenic syndrome. Ann N Y Acad Sci 681: 382–393.

Lennon VA (1997). Serological profile of myasthenia gravis and distinction from the Lambert–Eaton myasthenic syndrome. Neurology 48: S23–S27.

Lennon VA, Lambert EH, Whittingham S, et al. (1982). Autoimmunity in the Lambert–Eaton syndrome. Muscle Nerve 5: S21–S25.

Lennon VA, Kryzer TJ, Griesmann GE, et al. (1995). Calcium-channel antibodies in the Lambert–Eaton syndrome and other paraneoplastic syndromes. N Engl J Med 332: 1467–1474.

Leys K, Lang B, Johnston I, et al. (1991). Calcium channel autoantibodies in the Lambert–Eaton myasthenic syndrome. Ann Neurol 29: 307–314.

Maddison P, Newsom-Davis J (2003). Treatment for Lambert–Eaton myasthenic syndrome. Cochrane Database of Syst Rev CD003279.

Maddison P, Newsom-Davis J, Mills KR, et al. (1999). Favourable prognosis in Lambert–Eaton myasthenic syndrome and small-cell lung carcinoma. Lancet 353: 117–118.

Maddison P, Lang B, Mills K, et al. (2001). Long term outcome in Lambert–Eaton myasthenic syndrome without lung cancer. J Neurol Neurosurg Psychiatry 70: 212–217.

McEvoy KM, Windebank AJ, Daube JR, et al. (1989). 3,4-Diaminopyridine in the treatment of Lambert–Eaton myasthenic syndrome. N Engl J Med 321: 1567–1571.

Nagel A, Engel AG, Lang B, et al. (1988). Lambert–Eaton myasthenic syndrome IgG depletes presynaptic membrane active zone particles by antigenic modulation. Ann Neurol 24: 552–558.

Nakao YK, Motomura M, Fukudome T, et al. (2002). Seronegative Lambert–Eaton myasthenic syndrome: study of 110 Japanese patients. Neurology 59: 1773–1775.

Newsom-Davis J, Leys K, Vincent A, et al. (1991). Immunological evidence for the co-existence of the Lambert–Eaton myasthenic syndrome and myasthenia gravis in two patients. J Neurol Neurosurg Psychiatry 54: 452–453.

NIH Consensus Conference Statement (1986). The utility of therapeutic plasmapheresis for neurological disorders. JAMA 256: 1333–1337.

Nilsson O, Rosén I (1978). The stretch reflex in the Eaton–Lambert syndrome, myasthenia gravis and myotonic dystrophy. Acta Neurol Scand 57: 350–357.

Oh SJ, Sher E (2005). MG and LEMS overlap syndrome: case report with electrophysiological and immunological evidence. Clinic Neurophysiol 116: 1167–1171.

Oh SJ, Kurokawa K, Claussen GC, et al. (2005). Electrophysiological diagnostic criteria of Lambert–Eaton syndrome. Muscle Nerve 32: 515–520.

O'Neill JH, Murray NM, Newsom-Davis J (1988). The Lambert–Eaton myasthenic syndrome. A review of 50 cases. Brain 111: 577–596.

O'Suilleabhain P, Low PA, Lennon VA (1998). Autonomic Dysfunction in the Lambert–Eaton myasthenic syndrome: serologic and clinical correlates. Neurology 50: 88–93.

Rich MM, Teener JW, Bird SJ (1997). Treatment of Lambert–Eaton syndrome with intravenous immunoglobulin. Muscle Nerve 20: 614–615.

Sanders DB (1992). The effect of firing rate on neuromuscular jitter in Lambert–Eaton myasthenic syndrome. Muscle Nerve 15: 256–258.

Sanders DB (1993). Clinical neurophysiology of disorders of the neuromuscular junction. J Clin Neurophysiol 10: 167–180.

Sanders DB (1995). Lambert–Eaton myasthenic syndrome: clinical diagnosis, immune-mediated mechanisms, and update on therapy. Ann Neurol 37(S1): S63–S73.

Sanders DB, Massey JM, Sanders LL, et al. (2000). A randomized trial of 3,4-diaminopyridine in Lambert–Eaton myasthenic syndrome. Neurology 54: 603–607.

Sanders DB (2005). Electrophysiological study of disorders of the neuromuscular transmission. In: Aminoff MJ (ed.), Electrodiagnosis in Clinical Neurology. Elsevier/Churchill Livingstone, Philadelphia, pp. 335–355.

Smith AG, Wald J (1996). Acute ventilatory failure in Lambert–Eaton myasthenic syndrome and its response to 3,4-diaminopyridine. Neurology 46: 1143–1145.

Streib EW (1977). Adverse effects of magnesium salt cathartics in a patient with the myasthenic syndrome (Lambert–Eaton syndrome). Ann Neurol 2: 175–176.

Tim RW, Massey JM, Sanders DB (1998a). Lambert–Eaton myasthenic syndrome (LEMS). Clinical and electrodiagnostic features and response to therapy in 59 patients. Ann N Y Acad Sci 841: 823–826.

Tim RW, Massey JM, Sanders DB (1998b). Lambert–Eaton myasthenic syndrome: diagnostic findings and response to treatment in 70 patients. In: EV Stålberg, AW de Weerd, J Zidar (Eds.), 9th European Congress of Clinical Neurophysiology. Moduzzi Editore, Bologna, pp. 329–334.

Tim RW, Massey JM, Sanders DB (2000). Lambert–Eaton myasthenic syndrome. Electrodiagnostic findings and response to treatment. Neurology 54: 2176–2178.

Trontelj JV, Stålberg E (1991). Single motor end-plates in myasthenia gravis and LEMS at different firing rates. Muscle Nerve 14: 226–232.

Trontelj JV, Stålberg E (1992). The effect of firing rate on neuromuscular jitter in Lambert–Eaton myasthenic syndrome: a reply. Muscle Nerve 15: 258.

van den Bergh P, Kelly JJ, Carter B, et al. (1986). Intravascular contrast media and neuromuscular junction disorders. Ann Neurol 19: 206–207.

Wirtz PW, de Keizer RJ, de Visser M, et al. (2001). Tonic pupils in Lambert–Eaton myasthenic syndrome. Muscle Nerve 24: 444–445.

Wirtz PW, Smallegange TM, Wintzen AR, et al. (2002a). Differences in clinical features between the Lambert–Eaton myasthenic syndrome with and without cancer: an analysis of 227 published cases. Clinic Neurol Neurosurg 104: 359–363.

Wirtz PW, Sotodeh M, Nijnuis M, et al. (2002b). Difference in distribution of muscle weakness between myasthenia gravis and the Lambert–Eaton myasthenic syndrome. J Neurol Neurosurg Psychiatry 73: 766–768.

Wirtz PW, Bradshaw J, Wintzen AR, et al. (2004a). Associated autoimmune diseases in patients with the Lambert–Eaton myasthenic syndrome and their families. J Neurol 251: 1255–1259.

Wirtz PW, van Dijk JG, van Doorn PA, et al. (2004b). The epidemiology of the Lambert–Eaton myasthenic syndrome in the Netherlands. Neurology 63: 397–398.

Wirtz PW, Wintzen AR, Verschuuren JJ (2005). The Lambert–Eaton myasthenic syndrome has a more progressive course in patients with lung cancer. Muscle Nerve 32: 226–229.

Yeh JZ, Oxford CH, Wu CH, et al. (1976). Interactions of aminopyridines with potassium channels of squid axon membranes. Biophys J 16: 77–81.

Handbook of Clinical Neurology, Vol. 91 (3rd series)
Neuromuscular junction disorders
A.G. Engel, Editor

Chapter 10

Congenital myasthenic syndromes

ANDREW G. ENGEL*

*3M McKnight Professor of Neuroscience, Mayo Clinic College of Medicine, Consultant,
Department of Neurology, Mayo Clinic, Rochester, MN, USA*

Congenital myasthenic syndromes (CMSs) are inherited disorders of neuromuscular transmission associated with abnormal weakness and fatigability on exertion. In each CMS, the safety margin of neuromuscular transmission is compromised by one or more specific mechanisms. To facilitate understanding these mechanisms, this chapter begins with a brief overview of the classical anatomic and physiologic aspects of neuromuscular transmission.

10.1. Basic concepts and definitions

10.1.1. Components of the neuromuscular junction

The neuromuscular junction consists of presynaptic and postsynaptic regions separated by the synaptic space. Each presynaptic region is made up of a nerve terminal covered by a Schwann cell process. Each postsynaptic region is composed of junctional folds that overlie a specialized region of the muscle fiber, the junctional sarcoplasm. The synaptic space includes a single primary and multiple secondary synaptic clefts lined by basal lamina.

Acetylcholine (ACh) is stored in the nerve terminal in synaptic vesicles (Jones and Kwanbunbumpen, 1970; Heuser and Reese, 1973). An average synaptic vesicle contains 6000–8000 ACh molecules (Kuffler and Yoshikami, 1975; Hartzell et al., 1976). The contents of the synaptic vesicles are discharged into the synaptic space by exocytosis (Heuser and Reese, 1973; Heuser et al., 1979). A transmitter quantum is the amount of ACh released from a single synaptic vesicle.

The endplate-specific form of acetylcholinesterase (AChE) is positioned in the synaptic basal lamina at a density of about 2500 sites/μm^2 (McMahan et al.,

1978; Salpeter et al., 1978). The acetylcholine receptor (AChR) is concentrated on the terminal expansions of the junctional folds, where its packing density is close to 104/μm^2 (Matthews-Bellinger and Salpeter, 1978; Hirokawa and Heuser, 1982). Voltage-gated sodium channels of the $Na_v1.4$ type are concentrated in the depth of the junctional folds (Flucher and Daniels, 1989; Ruff, 1996).

10.1.2. Events after release of a single ACh quantum

In the resting state, there is a steady but random release of transmitter quanta from the nerve terminal associated with exocytosis of individual synaptic vesicles (Fatt and Katz, 1952; Martin, 1977). Focally released ACh molecules diffuse into the synaptic space, but most are not hydrolyzed initially by AChE due to saturation of AChE by the high concentration of ACh (Fertuck and Salpeter, 1976; Salpeter, 1983). The peak concentration of ACh that reaches the postsynaptic membrane is close to 1 mM (Stiles et al., 1996, 1999). Under normal conditions and with AChE fully active, ACh molecules in a single quantum exert their effect within a distance of 0.8 μm from their site of release (Hartzell et al., 1975). AChE limits the number of collisions of ACh with AChR and also the radius of spread of ACh. When AChE is inactive, the lateral spread of ACh is increased, so that each ACh molecule can sequentially bind to multiple AChRs and open multiple ion channels before leaving the synaptic space by diffusion (Katz and Miledi, 1973).

The depolarization and the concomitant current flow induced by a single quantum give rise to the miniature endplate (EP) potential (MEPP) and miniature

*Correspondence to: Dr Andrew G. Engel, MD, Department of Neurology, Mayo Clinic, Rochester, MN 55905, USA. E-mail: age@mayo.edu, Tel: 1-507-284-5102, Fax: 1-507-284-5831.

EP current (MEPC), respectively. The amplitude of the MEPP is a function of the number of AChR channels opened by the quantum, the depolarization per channel opening, and the input resistance of the muscle fiber (Katz and Thesleff, 1957b; Martin, 1976, 1977). The amplitude of the MEPC is a function of the number of AChR channels opened and the mean current flow per opening. The number of channel openings is a function of the number of ACh in the quantum, the number of available AChR, and the geometry of the synaptic space, which allows rapid diffusion of most ACh molecules from their site of release to AChR. The duration of the MEPP depends on the duration of channel opening events (Katz and Miledi, 1972; Anderson and Stevens, 1973), the functional state of AChE (Katz and Miledi, 1973) and the cable properties of the muscle fiber surface membrane (Fatt and Katz, 1952). The duration of the MEPC is independent of the cable properties of the muscle fiber surface membrane; otherwise, its duration is affected by the same factors that determine the duration of the MEPP (Martin, 1977).

Once dissociated from AChR, ACh is rapidly hydrolyzed by AChE to choline and acetate. Choline is taken up by the nerve terminal by a high-affinity, sodium-dependent and hemicholinium-sensitive choline transporter (Beech et al., 1980; Apparsundaram et al., 2000; Okuda et al., 2000). ACh is resynthesized by choline acetyltransferase (ChAT) and is then transported into the synaptic vesicles by the vesicular ACh transporter (VAChT) (Parsons et al., 1982; Reimer et al., 1998) in exchange for protons delivered to the synaptic vesicle by a proton pump (McMahon and Nicholls, 1991; Reimer et al., 1998).

10.1.3. Transmitter release by a single nerve impulse

Depolarization of the nerve terminal by nerve impulse is followed by an influx of calcium ions into the terminal through voltage-sensitive calcium channels, and it is this influx that mediates transmitter release (Katz and Miledi, 1969; Miledi, 1973; Llinás and Nicholson, 1975; Charlton et al., 1982). The calcium ingress into the nerve terminal also results in facilitation, so that the probability of release by a subsequent impulse is increased. The effects of calcium are antagonized by magnesium (Katz and Miledi, 1967; Hubbard et al., 1968).

The details of the mechanism by which calcium triggers synaptic vesicle exocytosis are still not fully understood. However, it is now clear that the increased calcium concentration in the nerve terminal releases the synaptic vesicles from cytoskeletal constraints

and affects the interaction of several proteins which, together, form a synaptic vesicle fusion complex (also see Chapter 3).

Nerve stimulation results in synaptic vesicle exocytosis adjacent to the active zones of the presynaptic membrane (Heuser et al., 1979). In the freeze-fractured presynaptic membrane, the active zones are represented by double parallel rows of large (10–12 nm) intramembrane particles that correspond to the voltage-sensitive Ca^{2+} channels in the active zones. This assumption is supported by the pattern of localization of fluorescent γ-conotoxin, a ligand for voltage-sensitive calcium channels at the frog motor nerve terminal (Robitaille et al., 1990; Tarelli et al., 1991).

The number of quanta released by nerve impulse (m) depends on the probability of release (p) and on at least one additional factor designated as n, according to the formula $m = np$ (del Castillo and Katz, 1954). The factor n was originally defined as the number of quantal units capable of responding to the nerve impulse, but it more likely indicates the number of readily releasable quanta (Elmqvist and Quastel, 1965), the number of active release sites in the nerve terminal (Zucker, 1973; Wernig, 1975), or a combination of these variables.

The amplitude of the EPP is affected by the same factors that affect the amplitude of the MEPP and by the number of quanta released by nerve impulse. When the EPP exceeds the threshold for activating the $Na_v1.4$ sodium channels in the depth of the synaptic folds, it triggers a muscle fiber action potential (Martin, 1977). A high concentration of AChRs on crests of the folds (Salpeter, 1987) and of $Na_v1.4$ in the depth of the folds (Flucher and Daniels, 1989; Ruff, 1996) ensures that excitation is propagated beyond the endplate (Martin, 1994; Wood and Slater, 2001). The safety margin of neuromuscular transmission is a function of the difference between the depolarization caused by the EPP and the depolarization required to activate $Na_v1.4$. All congenital or acquired defects of neuromuscular transmission identified to date have been traced to one or more factors that render the EPP subthreshold for activating $Na_v1.4$, or to a defect in $Na_v1.4$ that renders it unresponsive to EPPs of normal amplitude.

10.1.4. Transmitter release by repetitive nerve stimulation

Repetitive stimulation of the endplate under physiological conditions results in a frequency-dependent depression of the EPP amplitude, and of the safety margin of transmission, to a certain plateau. The decline has been attributed to a decrease of m, the quantum content of the EPP, due to a decrease in the number of readily releasable synaptic vesicles, and the plateau to equilibrium between quantal release and mobilization (Elmqvist and Quastel, 1965). This might be an oversimplification, for a decrease in p (Christensen and Martin, 1970) or in the number of ACh molecules per quantum might also occur during repetitive stimulation.

Under conditions of low quantal release (as in a high-magnesium or low-calcium medium), repetitive nerve stimulation increases transmitter release (Martin, 1977). Four temporally distinct stimulation-dependent processes facilitate transmitter release. Although facilitation is best studied under conditions of low quantal release, it also occurs under physiological conditions and tends to antagonize the process of depression. The temporal profiles of the opposing processes explain why a neuromuscular transmission defect is most readily demonstrated at a low frequency (2–3 Hz) stimulation, and why a transient improvement and then a worsening of the defect occur after tetanic stimulation.

In clinical electromyography (EMG), the transmission defect is demonstrated by repetitive supramaximal stimulation of a motor nerve and recording of the evoked compound muscle action potential (CMAP) by an electrode placed on the surface of the muscle. The amplitude of the evoked potential is proportionate to the number of muscle fibers activated by the nerve impulse. As neuromuscular transmission fails, the EPP becomes subthreshold for triggering the muscle fiber action potential at an increasing number of junctions, and consequently the amplitude of the CMAP decreases. This is referred to as the decremental EMG response.

10.1.5. The saturating disk model of neuromuscular transmission

The preceding sections reviewed the factors that can alter the safety margin of neuromuscular transmission. To understand how the safety margin is compromised, it is useful to consider the endplate as a composite of units that respond to ACh quanta. Each unit, or disk, represents that region of the postsynaptic membrane on which a single quantum exerts its effect. Within the disk, effective interaction between the ACh quantum and the postsynaptic membrane is assured by 1. positioning of the presynaptic release sites in relation to the junctional folds, 2. the high density of ACh binding sites on the crests of the junctional folds, and 3. the lower density but uniform distribution of AChE throughout the synaptic basal lamina (Salpeter, 1987).

After a quantum is released from the nerve terminal, ACh concentration is highest at the exocytotic site and gradually decreases as ACh diffuses into the synaptic space. By the time ACh has spread over about 0.2 μm of the junctional folds, its average concentration (about 1–3 mM) is still sufficiently high to swamp AChE. Further, by the time a quantal packet spreads over a distance of 0.3 μm along the top and down the side of the folds, all its ACh molecules will bind to AChR at a saturating concentration. The small size of the saturating disks assures that they do not overlap. Therefore only a small proportion of all available AChR is saturated with ACh when up to several hundred quanta are released by a nerve impulse. Also, since the presynaptic release sites are discrete and vary from impulse to impulse (Heuser et al., 1979; Heuser and Reese, 1981), different sets of disks become saturated at finite intervals during normal activity. This prevents desensitization of AChR from continued exposure to ACh.

From the above discussion it follows that factors that govern the safety margin can be grouped into the following main categories: 1. factors that affect the number of ACh molecules per synaptic vesicle, 2. factors that affect quantal release mechanisms, and 3. factors that affect the efficacy of individual quanta. Factors affecting quantal release and size were discussed above. Quantal efficacy depends on the endplate geometry, the density and functional state of AChE in the synaptic space, the density of AChR on the junctional folds, the kinetic properties of AChR, and the kinetic properties of $Na_v1.4$.

10.2. Classification of congenital myasthenic syndromes

The presently recognized CMSs stem from defects in presynaptic, synaptic basal lamina, and postsynaptic molecules, and several distinct types of presynaptic and postsynaptic CMSs exist. Table 10.1 shows a site-of-defect classification of 253 CMS kinships. This classification is useful but is still tentative because additional types of CMS probably exist, and because the basis of some presynaptic CMSs, or CMSs with AChR deficiency but no mutations in AChR, rapsyn or Dok-7, is still unresolved.

With few exceptions (Croxen et al., 2002a), the slow-channel syndromes are caused by dominant gain-of-function mutations; in the single identified patient with sodium channel myasthenia, the mode of inheritance has not been established. All other CMSs are caused by recessive, loss-of-function mutations.

10.3. Clinical features of congenital myasthenic syndromes

Generic diagnosis of a CMS is often possible on the basis of myasthenic symptoms since birth or early

Table 10.1

Classification of congenital myasthenic syndrome (CMS) based on site of defect*

	Index cases
Presynaptic defects (7%)	
Choline acetyltransferase deficiency**	13
Paucity of synaptic vesicles and reduced quantal release	1
Lambert–Eaton syndrome like	2
Other presynaptic defects	2
Synaptic basal lamina-associated defects (14%)	
Endplate AChE deficiency**	36
Postsynaptic defects (73%)	
Kinetic abnormality of AChR with/without AChR deficiency**	52
AChR deficiency with/without minor kinetic abnormality**	93
Rapsyn deficiency**	38
Kinetic defect in $Na_v1.4$**	1
Plectin deficiency	1
Synaptopathy (6%)	
Dok-7 myasthenia**	14
Total (100%)	253

*Classification based on cohort of CMS patients investigated at the Mayo Clinic between 1988 and 2007. A single patient with CMS cause by mutations in MuSK has also been described by Chevessier et al. (2004).
**Gene defects identified.
AChE, acetylcholinesterase; AChR, acetylcholine receptor.

Table 10.2

Investigation of congenital myasthenic syndromes

Clinical
History, examination, response to AChE inhibitor
EMG: conventional, stimulation studies, SFEMG
Serologic tests (tests for antibodies against AChR, MuSK, and calcium channels and tests for botulism)
Morphologic studies
Routine histochemical studies
Cytochemical and immunocytochemical localizations of AChE, AChR, agrin, β_2-laminin, utrophin, and rapsyn at the endplate
Estimate of the size, shape and two-dimensional profile of AChE-reactive endplates or endplate regions on teased muscle fibers
Quantitative electron microscopy and electron cytochemistry
Endplate-specific ^{125}I-α-bungarotoxin-binding sites
In vitro electrophysiology studies
Conventional microelectrode studies: MEPP, MEPC, evoked quantal release (*m, n, p*)
Single-channel patch-clamp recordings: channel types and kinetics
Molecular genetic studies
Mutation analysis (if candidate gene or protein identified)
Linkage analysis (if no candidate gene or protein recognized)
Expression studies (if mutation identified)

AChE, acetylcholinesterase; AChR, acetylcholine receptor; EMG, electromyography; MEPC, miniature endplate current; MEPP, miniature endplate potential; MuSK, muscle specific tyrosine kinase; *m*, number of ACh quanta released by nerve impulse; *n*, number of readily releasable ACh quanta; *p*, probability of quantal release; SFEMG, single fiber EMG.

childhood, a typical pattern of the distribution of weakness with involvement of the cranial muscles and a high-arched palate, a history of similarly affected relatives, a decremental EMG response of the CMAP on repetitive low-frequency (2–3 Hz) stimulation of its motor nerve, and negative tests for antibodies against the acetylcholine receptor, the P/Q type calcium channel, and the muscle specific receptor tyrosine kinase (MuSK). Some CMSs, however, are sporadic or present in later life, a decremental EMG response may not be present in all muscles or at all times, and the weakness may be restricted in distribution and not involve cranial muscles. In some CMSs, a specific diagnosis can be made by simple histologic or EMG studies. In other CMSs, in vitro electrophysiologic, ultrastructural, and immunocytochemical investigations are needed for accurate diagnosis (see Table 10.2).

On examination, the most important clue to a defect in neuromuscular transmission is increasing weakness on sustained exertion, also referred to as fatigable

weakness. This can be documented by observing increasing ptosis during sustained upward gaze, measuring the arm abduction time, and counting the number of deep-knee bends the patient can perform as well as noting the progressive difficulty the patient has in performing this task. Patients with severe involvement of the truncal muscles rapidly develop postural scoliosis on standing and shift their weight from one foot to another (Hutchinson et al., 1993). Selectively severe weakness of cervical and of wrist and finger extensor muscles is found in older patients with endplate AChE deficiency (Hutchinson et al., 1993) and in the slow-channel syndrome (Engel et al., 1982). The pupillary light reflexes are delayed in some patients with endplate AChE deficiency (Hutchinson et al., 1993). Ocular muscle involvement can be absent or mild in some cases of endplate AChE deficiency (Hutchinson et al., 1993), the slow-channel syndrome (Engel et al., 1982), rapsyn deficiency (Ohno et al., 2002; Burke et al., 2003) and in Dok-7 myasthenia (Beeson et al., 2006; Slater et al., 2006). The tendon reflexes are usually preserved, but can be hypoactive in endplate AChE deficiency, in the slow-channel CMS when there is a severe endplate myopathy (Engel et al., 1993) and in Dok-7 myasthenia. Arthrogryposis can be associated with mutations of the AChR δ-subunit (Brownlow et al., 2001), the fetal AChR γ-subunit (Hoffmann et al., 2006; Morgan et al., 2006), and rapsyn (Ohno et al., 2002).

Worsening of symptoms by an intercurrent febrile illness can occur in any CMS, but is especially apparent in the CMS caused by choline acetyltransferase (ChAT) or rapsyn deficiency. A history of sudden episodes of apnea is a distinguishing feature of ChAT deficiency (Mora et al., 1987; Ohno et al., 2001; Byring et al., 2002) and sodium channel myasthenia (Tsujino et al., 2003).

10.3.1. The intravenous edrophonium test

The test can be negative in patients with ChAT deficiency between episodes of worsening, is always negative in endplate AChE deficiency, and is inconsistently positive in the slow-channel syndrome. A negative edrophonium test does not exclude the diagnosis of CMS; a positive test can be consistent with the diagnosis of CMS but does not differentiate it from acquired autoimmune myasthenia gravis.

10.3.2. Electromyography studies

The diagnosis must be supported by a decremental EMG response at low-frequency (2–3 Hz) stimulation in at least one muscle or by abnormal jitter and blocking on single-fiber EMG (SFEMG). The decremental response can be absent in rested muscles of patients in ChAT deficiency, sodium channel myasthenia, some cases of rapsyn deficiency, and in infants with endplate AChR deficiency. In these cases, a decremental response at 2 Hz can be elicited by prolonged 10 Hz or briefer tetanic stimulation, or by exercise for several minutes (Mora et al., 1987; Ohno et al., 2001; Byring et al., 2002). Alternatively, the defect of neuromuscular transmission can be demonstrated by single-fiber EMG.

A single nerve stimulus evokes a repetitive CMAP in patients taking AChE inhibitors, in organophosphate poisoning, in endplate AChE deficiency (Engel et al., 1977; Hutchinson et al., 1993) and in the slow-channel CMS (Engel et al., 1982). However, in endplate AChE deficiency the repetitive response can be absent during infancy, and in the slow-channel CMS it can be absent in patients with a severe endplate myopathy. The interval between the first and subsequent potentials is 5–10 ms, and the second and subsequent potentials decrease more rapidly than the first. Therefore, the

repetitive CMAP is best elicited in patients not exposed to AChE inhibitors, after a period of rest, and with single nerve stimuli. The amplitude of the first evoked CMAP is usually normal, but a low-amplitude CMAP that facilitates severalfold on exercise is a feature of the Lambert–Eaton-like syndrome CMS (Bady et al., 1987). In patients with complete endplate AChR deficiency, edrophonium has no effect on the repetitive CMAP or on the extent of the EMG decrement, whereas in slow-channel syndrome edrophonium may elicit additional repetitive CMAPs after a single nerve stimulus and can improve the EMG decrement at 2–3 Hz stimulation.

Observations in the EMG laboratory can also provide an objective estimate of responsiveness to AChE inhibitors or other cholinergic agents. For example, one can compare the decrement recorded from the same site of a given muscle before and within 5 min after an intravenous dose of edrophonium, or between 30 min and 60 min after an oral dose of 3,4-diaminopyridine.

10.3.3. Serologic tests

In nearly all cases, a positive test for an anti-AChR, an anti-MuSK, or an anti-calcium channel antibody excludes the diagnosis of a CMS, but a CMS patient with predisposing HLA haplotypes has developed seropositive myasthenia gravis in later life (Croxen et al., 2002b). A negative AChR antibody test in a sporadic case of CMS does not exclude autoimmune myasthenia gravis (MG) because a high proportion of juvenile patients with autoimmune MG are seronegative (Youssef, 1983; Andrews et al., 1993). Seronegative autoimmune MG can sometimes be excluded by the clinical data or by the EMG findings. The absence of immune deposits (IgG and complement) from the endplate argues against seronegative autoimmune MG and so does the demonstration of an in vitro electrophysiologic abnormality that is different from that found in autoimmune MG. A favorable response to plasmapheresis has been interpreted as evidence for autoimmune MG.

10.3.4. Response to therapy

The response to therapy in a given CMS depends on the etiology. Patients with a defect in ACh synthesis, or with low-expressor mutations or a fast-channel kinetic abnormality in AChR, or with low-expressor mutations in rapsyn generally benefit from anticholinesterase medications, and may derive additional benefit from 3,4-diaminopyridine (3,4-DAP). Patients with slow-channel syndromes respond transiently to these measures, or do not respond, or show worsening of their symptoms. Patients with endplate AChE deficiency are refractory to, and are worsened by, AChE inhibitors. A favorable response to plasmapheresis has been interpreted as evidence for autoimmune MG.

10.4. Presynaptic CMS

Four types of presynaptic CMS have been described to date: 1. CMS caused by defects in ChAT associated with episodic apnea (Ohno et al., 2001); 2. a CMS with paucity of synaptic vesicles and reduced quantal release (Walls et al., 1993); 3. a CMS resembling the Lambert–Eaton syndrome (Bady et al., 1987); and 4. a CMS with reduced quantal release due to an undefined mechanism (Maselli et al., 2001; Milone et al., 2006).

10.4.1. CMS caused by defects in ChAT

10.4.1.1. Clinical features

The clinical features of this disorder were recognized more nearly five decades ago under the rubric of familial infantile myasthenia (Greer and Schotland, 1960; Robertson et al., 1980), but it was not differentiated from MG until the autoimmune origin of MG was established and electrophysiologic and morphologic differences were demonstrated between MG and the congenital syndrome (Hart et al., 1979; Engel and Lambert, 1987; Mora et al., 1987).

Greer and Schotland (1960) described the clinical features of the disease and in Conomy et al. (1975) referred to it as "familial infantile myasthenia." Because all CMSs can be familial and because most CMSs present in infancy, the term "familial infantile myasthenia" has become a nonspecific term and a source of confusion (Deymeer et al., 1999). Because the distinguishing clinical feature is sudden and unexpected episodes of severe dyspnea and bulbar weakness culminating in apnea, the disease has also been referred to as CMS with episodic apnea (CMS-EA). Initial studies of the clinical syndrome revealed no endplate AChR or AChE deficiency but suggested impaired resynthesis or vesicular packaging of ACh (Engel and Lambert, 1987; Mora et al., 1987).

Some patients present at birth with hypotonia and severe bulbar and respiratory weakness requiring ventilatory support (Fig. 10.1). This gradually improves, but is followed by apneic attacks and bulbar paralysis in later life precipitated by infections, fever, or excitement, or occurring with no apparent cause. Between these episodes, patients may have no, mild, or moderately severe myasthenic symptoms. Other patients are

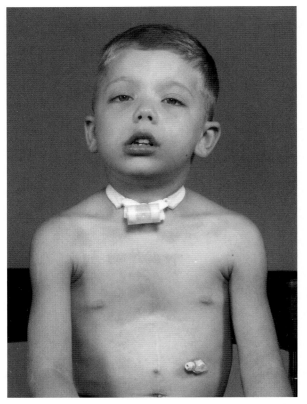

Fig. 10.1. CMS caused by mutation in choline acetyl transferase. This 5-year-old boy has had numerous apneic episodes since birth and has mild to moderately severe myasthenic symptoms between these episodes. Note ptosis, esotropia, compensatory head tilt, facial diplegia, tracheostomy, and percutaneous gastrostomy. (From Engel et al., 1999, with permission of Oxford University Press.)

normal at birth and develop apneic attacks during infancy or childhood. Some children, following an acute episode, experience prolonged respiratory insufficiency that may last for weeks (Kraner et al., 2003). A worsening of symptoms on exposure to cold was also reported (Maselli et al., 2003b). This finding could be related to a negative effect of the decreased temperature on the catalytic efficiency of the mutant enzyme. Phenotypic heterogeneity can occur within a given kinship (Byring et al., 2002) or in unrelated patients carrying identical mutations (Barisic et al., 2005). Intrafamily phenotypic variability is illustrated by a kinship in which two siblings died suddenly at 2 months and 11 months of age during febrile episodes; one was asymptomatic and the other had only mild ptosis prior to death. A third sibling began having abrupt episodes of dyspnea and cyanosis at age 14 months precipitated by fever or vaccination; at age 32 months, she developed ptosis and abnormal fatigue on exertion which led to the diagnosis of a myasthenic disorder (Byring et al., 2002).

With increasing age, the exacerbations become less frequent. After age 10, some patients only complain of easy fatigability on sustained exertion; others have mild to moderate weakness of cranial, limb, and respiratory muscles even at rest, resembling patients with mild to moderately severe autoimmune MG. The tendon reflexes remain normally active. There is no loss of muscle bulk, and a permanent myopathy does not occur (Greer and Schotland, 1960; Conomy et al., 1975; Robertson et al., 1980; Gieron and Korthals, 1985; Mora et al., 1987).

10.4.1.2. Electrophysiologic features

A decremental response at 2 Hz stimulation and single-fiber EMG abnormalities similar to those observed in MG are present in muscles weak when tested. The EMG decrement, when present, can be corrected by edrophonium. Weakness and EMG abnormalities can be induced in some but not all muscles by exercise. Subtetanic stimulation at 10 Hz for 5–10 min of weak or non-weak muscles results in progressive decline of the evoked CMAP to less than 50% of its initial amplitude followed by slow recovery over the next 10 min (Engel and Lambert, 1987; Mora et al., 1987; Byring et al., 2002). The slow recovery of the CMAP after 10 Hz stimulation is characteristic of CMS-EA; a marked decline of the CMAP during subtetanic stimulation also occurs in patients with EP AChE or AChR deficiency but in these patients the CMAP returns to the baseline within 1–2 min.

10.4.1.3. Endplate studies

The number of AChRs per endplate and postsynaptic ultrastructure are normal, but morphometric analysis indicates that the synaptic vesicles are smaller than normal in rested muscle (Mora et al., 1987). Microelectrode studies of intercostal muscle EPs in vitro show the MEPP amplitude to be normal in the rested state, but it decreases abnormally after 10 Hz stimulation for 5 min. The amplitude of the EPP also decreases abnormally during 10 Hz stimulation and then recovers slowly over the next 10–15 min (Fig. 10.2) whereas the quantal content of the EPP is essentially unaltered (Mora et al., 1987; Byring et al., 2002). An abnormal decline of the EPP during 10-Hz stimulation can also occur in other CMSs, but in these CMSs the EPP amplitude returns to baseline within 1–2 min.

10.4.1.4. Molecular studies

The slow recovery of the synaptic response to ACh after subtetanic stimulation pointed to a defect in the resynthesis or vesicular packaging of ACh and implicated four candidate genes: the presynaptic high-affinity choline transporter (Apparsundaram et al., 2000; Okuda et al., 2000), ChAT (Oda et al., 1992), the vesicular ACh transporter (VAChT) (Erickson et al., 1994), and the vesicular proton pump (Reimer et al., 1998). In 2001, mutation analysis in five CMS-EA patients uncovered no mutations in VAChT but revealed 10 recessive mutations in ChAT (Ohno et al., 2001). One mutation (523insCC) was a null mutation; three others (I305T, R420C, E441K) markedly reduced ChAT expression in COS cells. Kinetic studies of nine

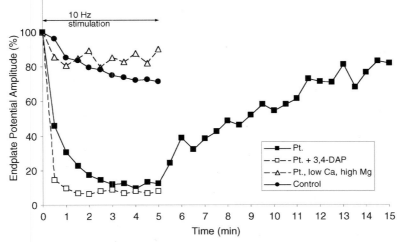

Fig. 10.2. CMS caused by mutation in choline acetyl transferase. Ten Hz stimulation for 5 min results in rapid abnormal decline of the endplate potential which then recovers slowly over the next 10 min. 3,4-diaminopyridine (3,4-DAP), which accelerates ACh release, enhances the defect, whereas a low Ca^{2+}/high Mg^{2+} solution, which reduces ACh release, prevents the abnormal decline of the EPP. Pt, patient. (From Engel, 2003, with permission.)

bacterially expressed and purified missense mutants revealed that one (E441K) lacked catalytic activity, and eight (L210P, P211A, I305T, R420C, R482G, S498L, V506L, R560H) had significantly impaired catalytic efficiencies. Subsequently, four additional recessive mutations have been reported (I336T, V194L, R548X, and S694C) (Kraner et al., 2003; Maselli et al., 2003b; Schmidt et al., 2003; Barisic et al., 2005). Further studies of other CMS-EA patients in the author's laboratory revealed seven additional mutations in ChAT.

Figure 10.3 shows a stereo image of the atomic structural model of ChAT with all presently identified mutations mapped on the model. Eight mutations (V194L, L210P, P211A, E441K, R560H, T608N, and S694C) localize to the substrate binding site, or at or near to the catalytic site of ChAT; the remaining mutations likely alter enzyme activity allosterically or alter the folding or stability of the enzyme.

Interestingly, no patients harboring ChAT mutations had central or autonomic nervous system symptoms. The simplest explanation of this paradox would be that the identified mutations reside in an EP-specific isoform of ChAT but this is unlikely: there are five alternative ChAT transcripts with at least three different promoters in humans (Eiden, 1998), but the observed mutations occur in the common coding region of all recognized ChAT isoforms. A possible explanation is that presynaptic levels of ChAT or sub-strate availability render ChAT rate limiting for ACh synthesis when increased impulse transmission is increased at the EP but not at other cholinergic synapses.

It is also important to note that defects in the pre-synaptic high-affinity choline transporter (Apparsun-daram et al., 2000; Okuda et al., 2000), the vesicular ACh transporter (Erickson et al., 1994), or the vesicu-lar proton pump (Reimer et al., 1998) may have similar phenotypic consequences, but mutations of these proteins have not been detected to date.

10.4.1.5. Therapy

Anticholinesterase medications benefit patients with myasthenic symptoms between respiratory crises and also prevent or mitigate the crises. Therefore prophy-lactic anticholinesterase therapy is advocated even for patients asymptomatic between crises. Parents of affected children must be indoctrinated to anticipate sudden worsening of the weakness and possible apnea with febrile illnesses, excitement, or overexertion. They also should be able to administer appropriate doses of prostigmine or pyridostigmine intramuscu-larly, and use an inflatable rescue bag with a fitted mask in a crisis and during transport to hospital. Long-term nocturnal apnea monitoring is indicated in any patient in whom CMS-EA is suspected (Byring et al., 2002).

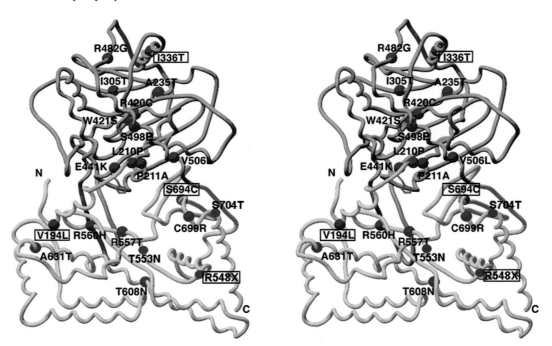

Fig. 10.3. ChAT mutations in CMS patients mapped on stereo image of structural model of rat ChAT (PDB code1Q6X). The active site is in a solvent accessible tunnel at the interface of the N (upper) and C (lower) domains. Histidine at active site is shown in stick representation. Residue numbers correspond to human sequence. The indicated mutations, except those in boxes, were identified in the author's laboratory.

10.4.2. Paucity of synaptic vesicles and reduced quantal release

Only one patient suffering from this disorder has been described (Walls et al., 1993). This patient's clinical and EMG features were indistinguishable from those of patients with autoimmune myasthenia gravis but the onset was at birth anti-AChR antibodies were absent, there was no endplate AChR deficiency, and electron microscopy revealed no postsynaptic abnormality. A presynaptic defect was indicated by a decrease to about 20% of the quantal content of the EPP (m). The decrease in m was due to a decrease in the number of readily releasable quanta (n), which was associated with a decrease in the numerical density of synaptic vesicles to about 20% of normal in unstimulated nerve terminals (Walls et al., 1993, Fig. 66-5). The patient's symptoms were improved by pyridostigmine.

In this disorder the clinical consequences stem from the paucity of synaptic vesicles in the nerve terminal. Synaptic vesicle precursors associated with different sets of synaptic vesicle proteins are produced in the perikaryon of the anterior horn cell and are carried distally along motor axons to the nerve terminal by kinesin-like motors (Bööj et al., 1986; Kiene and Stadler, 1987; Llinás et al., 1989; Okada et al., 1995). Mature vesicles containing a full complement of vesicular proteins are assembled in the nerve terminal (Okada et al., 1995) and are then packed with ACh. After ACh has been released by exocytosis, the vesicle membranes are recycled and then repacked with ACh (Südhof and Jahn, 1991). In the present syndrome, the reduction in synaptic vesicle density could arise from 1. a defect in the formation of synaptic vesicle precursors in the anterior horn cell, 2. a defect in the axonal transport of one or more species of precursor vesicles, 3. impaired assembly of the mature synaptic vesicles from their precursors, or 4. impaired recycling of the synaptic vesicles in the nerve terminal. That synaptic vesicle density was reduced, even in unstimulated nerve terminals, argues against a defect in vesicle recycling.

10.4.3. Lambert–Eaton-like syndrome

One young child was reported with this syndrome in 1987 (Bady et al., 1987). The CMAP amplitude was abnormally small but facilitated severalfold on tetanic stimulation, and the symptoms were improved by guanidine. A second patient observed at the Mayo Clinic was a 6-month-old girl with severe bulbar and limb weakness, hypotonia, areflexia, and respirator dependency since birth. The EMG showed a low-amplitude CMAP that facilitated 500% on high-frequency stimulation and decremented 40% on low-frequency stimulation. Studies of an anconeus muscle specimen revealed no endplate AChR deficiency. Electron microscopy of the endplates showed structurally intact presynaptic and postsynaptic regions, no deficiency of AChR, and abundant synaptic vesicles in the nerve terminals. The MEPP amplitude was normal for muscle fiber size. The quantal content of the EPP, m, was less than 10% of normal at 1 Hz stimulation, and 40 Hz stimulation increased m by 300%. Thus, the in vitro electrophysiologic findings were like those in the Lambert–Eaton syndrome (Lambert and Elmqvist, 1971). Consistent with this, the EMG abnormalities were improved by 3,4-DAP, an agent that increases the number of ACh quanta released by nerve impulse (Lundh et al., 1984), but the patient remained weak and respirator dependent. The molecular basis of this CMS could reside in an abnormality of the presynaptic voltage-gated calcium channel or in a component of the synaptic vesicle release complex. Mutation analysis of *CACNA1A*, the gene encoding the pore-forming α_1 subunit of the $Ca_v2.1$, or P/Q type, calcium channel expressed by the nerve terminal membrane, revealed no mutations.

10.4.4. Other presynaptic defects

10.4.4.1. Severe CMS with reduced quantal release

Milone et al. (2006) reported two highly debilitating cases of CMS: one was that of a 7-year-old boy and the other of a 48-year-old man. Quantal release was compromised in both. The older patient, however, also had postsynaptic abnormalities associated with EP AChR deficiency and was eventually found to carry two pathogenic mutations in Dok-7 (see Section 10.6.8). The younger patient was respirator dependent since birth, had severe weakness of all skeletal muscles, and was areflexic except at the ankles (Fig. 10.4). EMG studies showed a decremental response, which was improved by edrophonium but not by high frequency stimulation. Microelectrode studies of intercostal EPs showed that the MEPP amplitude was normal but the quantal component of the EPP (m) was reduced to 25% of normal due to a decrease in both n and p. Single channel recordings revealed no abnormality of the AChR channel and there was no EP AChR deficiency. Endplate ultrastructure was preserved. A search for mutations in components of the synaptic vesicle release complex and in other candidate proteins concerned with quantal release failed to identify the molecular basis of the disease. Initially, the patient responded partially to pyridostigmine and 3,4-DAP but became refractory to both medications after 2 months (Milone et al., 2006).

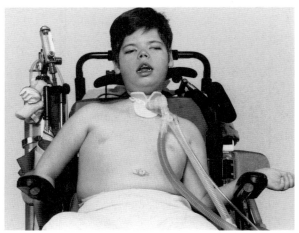

Fig. 10.4. Severe presynaptic CMS due to decreased quantal release in a 7-year-old boy. Note severe ptosis, facial weakness, open mouth, ventilatory support, scoliotic posture, and gastrostomy. An extensive search for mutations in components of the synaptic vesicle release complex failed to uncover the molecular basis of this patient's illness. (From Milone et al., 2006, with permission.)

10.4.4.2. Presynaptic CMS with central nervous system symptoms

Maselli and coworkers (Maselli et al., 2001) reported three sporadic patients, two presenting in early infancy and one after the age of 5 years, with myasthenic symptoms that spared the external ocular muscles. All three had other neurological symptoms that included trunkal or limb ataxia and, in one case, horizontal nystagmus. Unlike in Lambert–Eaton syndrome patients, none had abnormally small first-evoked CMAPs, and the decremental response on 2 Hz stimulation was not improved by stimulation at higher frequencies. None had endplate AChR deficiency. The nerve terminals were of normal size and the synaptic vesicles were normally abundant. Microelectrode studies revealed a decreased quantal content of the EPP (m). In one patient, this was associated with a significantly decreased probability of quantal release (p); in another patient, there was <50%, but still significant, decrease in the number of readily releasable quanta (n). No mutations were detected in the α1 and β2 subunits of the P/Q-type Ca^{2+} channel, syntaxin 1A, synaptobrevin 1, SNAP 25, or Rab3A (Maselli et al., 2003a). One of the three patients responded well to combined treatment with pyridostigmine and 3,4-DAP, one showed only mild improvement to combined therapy with pyridostigmine and ephedrine, and one failed to respond adequately to pyridostigmine.

10.5. Synaptic basal-lamina-associated CMS

The synaptic basal lamina harbors several molecules that regulate the development and function of the neuromuscular junction, as, for example, α2- and β2-laminin, agrin, and AChE. Defects in any of these proteins could instigate a CMS but defects only in ColQ, the collagenic structural component of AChE, are known to cause a CMS.

10.5.1. Endplate acetylcholinesterase deficiency

10.5.1.1. Clinical features

Human endplate AChE deficiency was first recognized in 1977 in a 16-year-old male with life-long myasthenic symptoms refractory to AChE inhibitors (Engel et al., 1982). AChE was absent from the endplates by enzyme cytochemical and immunocytochemical criteria, and electron cytochemical studies revealed no reaction product for the enzyme in the synaptic space. The distinguishing clinical feature of this CMS is failure to respond to, or being worsened by, AChE inhibitors. In most patients, weakness and abnormal fatigability are present since birth or early childhood and are highly disabling (Engel et al., 1982; Hutchinson et al., 1993; Ohno et al., 1998c; Ohno et al., 2000a). Poor suck, cry, and episodes of respiratory distress can occur in infancy. Motor milestones are delayed. The weakness affects the facial, cervical, axial, and limb muscles (Fig. 10.5). Ophthalmoparesis is present but not in all patients. The axial muscles are severely involved, so that on standing the patient may show increasing lordosis and scoliosis after a few seconds. Fixed scoliosis and severe weakness and atrophy of the dorsal forearm and intrinsic hand muscles occur in older patients. The tendon reflexes are hypoactive or normally reactive. Some patients have an abnormally slow pupillary light response without other autonomic deficits (Hutchinson et al., 1993). In some patients the disease presents in childhood and becomes disabling only in the second decade (Donger et al., 1998; Ohno et al., 1999b; Bestue-Cardiel et al., 2005) or later in life (Shapira et al., 2002). Infrequently, severe symptoms from birth are followed by improvement during adolescence (Ishigaki et al., 2003). Phenotypic heterogeneity with regard to age of onset, progression, and severity of symptoms can occur within and between kinships carrying the homozygous G240X (Shapira et al., 2002) or heterozygous (Ishigaki et al., 2003) *COLQ* mutations. These observations imply that modifying genes, polymorphisms, or environmental factors can mitigate or worsen the consequences of EP AChE deficiency.

10.5.1.2. Electrophysiologic features

The EMG shows a decremental response at 2 Hz as well as at higher frequencies of stimulation. Nerve stimulation evokes a repetitive CMAP; a second response occurs 5–10 ms after the first and is of lower amplitude and decrements faster than the first response (Fig. 10.6A).

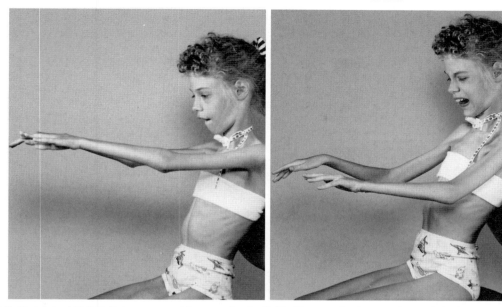

Fig. 10.5. Endplate AChE deficiency caused by mutation in ColQ. Note ptosis, decreased muscle bulk and inability to elevate arms for more than a few seconds.

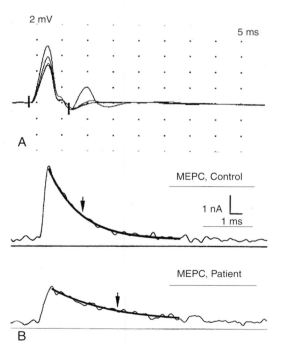

Fig. 10.6. EP AChE deficiency. (A) Decremental EMG response and repetitive compound muscle action potential recorded from thenar muscle during 2 Hz stimulation of the median nerve. The second response decrements more rapidly than the first and appears only once. (B) Representative miniature endplate currents (MEPCs) from a patient with EP AChE deficiency and a control subject. The best-fit exponential curve is superimposed on the decay phase of each current. Arrows indicate decay time constants. The patient MEPC is smaller and decays more slowly than the control MEPC. (From Hutchinson et al., 1993, with permission.)

The repetitive response disappears at stimulation frequencies greater than 0.2 Hz, or with mild activity. Therefore, it can be overlooked unless a well rested muscle is tested by single stimuli. The repetitive CMAP is attributed to the prolonged lifetime of ACh in the synaptic space; this allows each ACh to bind to more than one AChR and thereby prolong the synaptic response beyond the absolute refractory period of the muscle fiber.

In vitro microelectrode studies reveal MEPPs of normal or reduced amplitude, but MEPPs of higher than normal amplitude would be expected when AChE is absent from the endplate. Consistent with the absence of AChE, the decay time constant of the MEPP and MEPC is prolonged (Fig. 10.6B). AChE inhibitors have no effect on the amplitude or decay time of the synaptic response (Engel et al., 1977; Hutchinson et al., 1993). The quantal content of the EPP is markedly decreased due to a decreased number of releasable quanta (n); the probability of quantal release (p) is normal or higher than normal (Engel et al., 1977; Hutchinson et al., 1993; Ohno et al., 1998c; Ohno et al., 2000a; Shapira et al., 2002). Patch-clamp analysis of single-channel currents indicates that the conductance and kinetic properties of the AChR channel are normal (Ohno et al., 1998c; Shapira et al., 2002).

10.5.1.3. Morphologic features

Conventional histologic studies of muscle show type 2 fiber atrophy, or type 1 fiber preponderance, or both, or are normal. In most cases, AChE is absent from the endplate by light microscopic criteria (Engel et al., 1977; Hutchinson et al., 1993; Shapira et al., 2002) but traces of AChE were found in some patients harboring a C-terminal mutation in ColQ (Donger et al., 1998). Electron cytochemical studies show absence (Engel et al., 1977; Hutchinson et al., 1993; Shapira et al., 2002) (Fig. 10.7) or only a trace of AChE (Jennekens et al., 1992) in the synaptic space. Immunoreactivity for AChE with polyclonal and several monoclonal AChE antibodies is absent or barely detectable (Hutchinson et al., 1993).

The nerve terminals are abnormally small (Figs. 10.7B and 10.8A and B). At many endplates, Schwann cell processes intrude into the primary synaptic cleft and partially or even completely cover the presynaptic membrane, further reducing the surface available for ACh release from the nerve terminal. The smallness of the nerve terminals and their partial occlusion by Schwann cell processes readily explains the decreased quantal content of the EPP. At some EPs, the junctional folds are studded with myriad pinocytotic vesicles and labyrinthine membranous networks (Fig. 10.8A). At other EPs, the junctional folds are degenerating and shed AChR-rich fragments into the synaptic space (Fig. 10.8B). The total number of AChRs per EP is normal or reduced. Some of the junctional nuclei are degenerating and some are apoptotic.

10.5.1.4. Pathogenesis

Although ACh release is restricted by the smallness of n, the increased synaptic lifetime of the released AChE still results in cationic overloading of the postsynaptic region and degeneration of junctional folds with concomitant loss of AChR. The safety margin of neuromuscular transmission is compromised by 1. the smallness of n, 2. a degree of AChR deficiency, 3. desensitization of AChR from prolonged exposure to ACh during physiological activity (Katz and Thesleff, 1957a; Magleby and Pallotta, 1981), and 4. progressive depolarization of the endplate region during physiological activity. The depolarization of the endplate region may be similar to that observed in organophosphate poisoning (Maselli and Soliven, 1991), arising from the temporal summation of the prolonged EPPs at physiological rates of motor nerve firing. The depolarization of the endplate region inactivates the voltage-gated sodium channels at the junction (Ruff et al., 1988) and can block generation of the muscle fiber action potential.

10.5.1.5. Molecular pathogenesis

The endplate species of AChE is an asymmetric enzyme composed of homotetramers of globular (G) catalytic subunits attached to a collagenic tail subunit (Massoulié et al., 1993). The catalytic subunit has two carboxyl-terminal splice variants, AChET and AChEH, expressed in muscle and erythrocytes, respectively (Massoulié et al., 1999). The collagenic tail subunit is formed by the triple helical association of three collagen-like strands, ColQ, encoded by *COLQ*, each of which can bind a homotetramer of AChET to form the asymmetric A4, A8, and A12 moieties of the asymmetric enzyme (Bon et al., 1997) (Fig. 10.9A and B). Expression of globular and

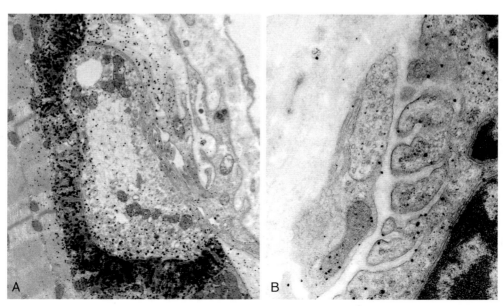

Fig. 10.7. Electron cytochemical localization of AChE at a control (A) and patient (B) EP. At the control EP, heavy reaction product fills the synaptic space and extends into the adjacent regions. At patient EP there is no reaction product for AChE in the synaptic space. (A), ×14 000; (B), ×25 900.

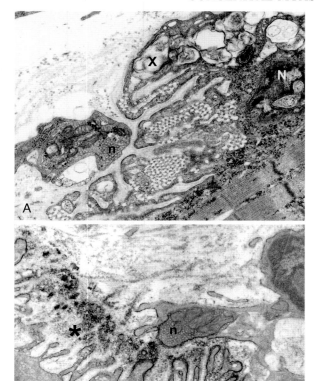

Fig. 10.8. EP regions in patient with EP AChE deficiency. In (A), note myriad pinocytotic vesicles and labyrinthine membranous networks in the junctional folds, degenerating fold (X), and an apoptotic nucleus in the junctional sarcoplasm. In (B), AChR is visualized with peroxidase-labeled α-bgt. AChR reactive debris is shed from degenerating junctional folds (asterisk). In both A and B, the nerve terminals (n) are small relative to the size of the postsynaptic region. (A), ×15 400; (B), ×28 900. (From Engel et al., 1999, with permission of Oxford University Press.)

asymmetric forms of AChE in muscle, or in COS cells transfected with *ACHET* and *COLQ* cDNA, is readily monitored by density gradient centrifugation of tissue or cell extracts (Fig. 10.9C and D).

Conserved domains of ColQ include an N-terminal proline-rich attachment domain (PRAD) that associates with an AChET tetramer, a central collagen domain composed of GXY triplets (where X and Y are any amino acid), and a carboxyl-terminal region enriched in charged residues and cysteines required for the assembly of the ColQ strands in a triple helix (Prockop and Kivirikko, 1995) (Fig. 10.9A). Anchorage of the asymmetric enzyme in the synaptic space is assured by two cationic heparan sulfate proteoglycan binding domains within the collagen domain (Deprez and Inestrosa, 1995) and by residues in the carboxyl-terminal

domain (Ohno et al., 2000a; Kimbell et al., 2004). The tail subunit is anchored to the synaptic basal lamina by at least two binding partners: the heparan sulfate proteoglycan perlecan (Arikawa-Hirasawa et al., 2002), which binds in turn dystroglycan, and the extracellular domain of MuSK (Cartaud et al., 2004). Association with these binding partners predicts close proximity of the extracellular asymmetric enzyme to the postsynaptic membrane. All naturally occurring mutations in the EP species of AChE observed to date reside in ColQ.

No fewer than 24 *COLQ* mutations have been identified to date (Donger et al., 1998; Ohno et al., 1998c, 1999b, 2000a; Shapira et al., 2002; Ishigaki et al., 2003) (Fig. 10.9B). Density gradient centrifugation of extracts of COS cells cotransfected with wild-type $AChE_T$ and wild-type or mutant *COLQ* cDNA reveals whether $AChE_T$ associates with ColQ and whether the mutant ColQ can assemble as a triple helix. This type of analysis combined with endplate studies demonstrates four major types of mutations in ColQ. 1. Mutations involving PRAD prevent attachment of $AChE_T$ to ColQ and yield a sedimentation profile identical to that obtained after transfection with AChET alone (Fig. 10.9E and I). So, mutant ColQ, if expressed, fails to bind catalytic subunits (Ohno et al., 1998c, 2000a) and no asymmetric AChE is formed. 2. Mutations that truncate the collagen domain prevent triple helical association of ColQ strands; instead, an insertion incompetent truncated single strand of ColQ linked to an AChET tetramer is formed that sediments at 10.5S (Ohno et al., 1998c, 2000a) (Fig. 10.9F and J). 3. A carboxyl-terminal mutant, 1082delC, produces a single-stranded insertion incompetent enzyme (Ohno et al., 1998c) on account of the 64 hydrophobic residues that follow the frame-shifting point mutation (Ohno et al., 2000a) (Fig. 10.9G and K, left). 4. Other C-terminal mutations produce either reduced (R315X) (Ohno et al., 1999b) or normal amounts of the triple-helical asymmetric enzyme (Fig. 10.9H and K, right) which is generally insertion incompetent (Kimbell et al., 2004).

10.5.1.6. Diagnosis

A lifelong history of weakness and fatigability of all muscles, a delayed pupillary light response, a decremental EMG response, and refractoriness or an adverse reaction to anticholinesterase drugs should suggest the correct diagnosis. A repetitive CMAP response to single nerve stimulus in a patient not exposed to anticholinesterase drugs indicates endplate AChE deficiency or a slow-channel syndrome, but is not seen in all cases of endplate AChE deficiency. The diagnosis of endplate AChE deficiency is established by showing that AChE is absent from all endplates by cytochemical or immunocytochemical criteria. In vitro electrophysiological

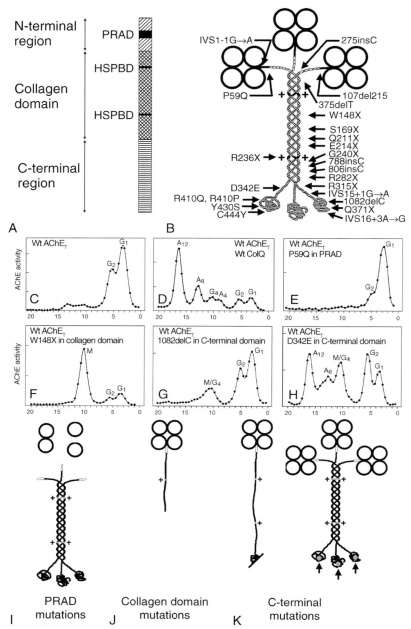

Fig. 10.9. (A) Schematic diagram showing domains of a ColQ strand. (B) Schematic diagram showing the A12 species of asymmetric AChE with 24 identified ColQ mutations. (C–H) Density gradient profiles of AChE extracted from COS cells transfected with wild-type AChET and different types of CoLQ mutants. (I–K) Schematic diagrams of the abnormal species of AChE formed in transfected HEK cells. In (E) and (I) note that disruption of the PRAD domain produces a sedimentation profile identical with that obtained after transfection with AChET alone. Thus, AChET fails to attach to ColQ and no asymmetric AChE is formed. In (F) and (J), note that the asymmetric A4, A8, or A12 moieties are absent and there is a prominent −10.5 S mutant (M) peak, representing a G4 tetramer of the catalytic subunit linked to the truncated ColQ peptide. In (G) and the left diagram in (K), note the presence of a small M peak but absence of peaks corresponding to triple-stranded asymmetric enzymes. In (H) and the right diagram in (K), note that both an M peak and asymmetric AChE are present. PRAD, proline-rich attachment domain; HSPBD, heparan sulfate proteoglycan binding domain. (From Engel et al., 1999, with permission of Oxford University Press.)

studies can further confirm the diagnosis by demonstrating the typical abnormalities of the endplate potentials and reduced quantal release by nerve impulse.

10.5.1.7. Therapy

Presently, there is no satisfactory drug therapy for endplate AChE deficiency. Anticholinesterase medications should be avoided because they are ineffective, and because AChE deficient patients appear to have enhanced sensitivity to their muscarinic side-effects. If the diagnosis of AChE deficiency is not suspected, refractoriness to an anti-AChE medication may prompt the physician to increase the dose; this, in turn, may result in excessive bronchial secretions and worsen the patient's clinical state. Ephedrine sulfate was reported to help some patients (Bestue-Cardiel et al., 2005). Alternate-day prednisone therapy had a slight beneficial effect in two patients but was ineffective in one and appeared to worsen the symptoms in another. Prednisone does not change the AChE deficiency or the electrophysiologic abnormalities; its mode of action remains unknown. A respirator dependent infant was improved by intermittent blockade of AChR by atracurium, an agent that protects AChR from overexposure to ACh, allowing for temporary withdrawal of respiratory support (Breningstall et al., 1996).

10.6. Postsynaptic syndromes

The presently identified postsynaptic CMSs arise from defects in AChR, rapsyn, MuSK, Dok-7, plectin, and the voltage-gated sodium channel of adult muscle, $Na_v1.4$. Rapsyn, under the influence of agrin and MuSK, maintains a high concentration of AChR in the postsynaptic membrane by linking the AChR to the subsynaptic cytoskeleton. MuSK as well as Dok-7 are important for maturation and maintenance of the neuromuscular junction. Plectin is an intermediate filament linker protein, concentrated at sites of mechanical stress. Because most postsynaptic CMSs are caused by defects in AChR, we will begin with a brief overview of its structure activation.

10.6.1. AChR structure

Muscle AChR is an integral membrane protein composed of five homologous subunits: two of α, one of β and δ, and one of ϵ in adult AChR, or one of γ instead of ϵ in fetal AChR. The genes encoding α, δ, and γ are at different loci on chromosome 2q, and those encoding β and ϵ are at different loci on chromosome 17p. The subunits are highly homologous, have similar secondary structures, fold similarly, and are organized like barrel staves around a central cation-selective channel. Each subunit has an N-terminal extracellular domain that comprises about 50% of the primary sequence, four transmembrane domains (M1–M4), a large cytoplasmic domain between M3 and M4, and a small C-terminal extracellular domain.

The two ACh binding sites are formed at interfaces between subunits: α and α–δ in embryonic and denervated muscle, and α–ϵ and α–δ in adult muscle, and residues from both α and non-α subunits contribute to binding of ACh and its antagonists (Corringer et al., 2000). Seven linearly distinct loops within each α and non-α subunits (loops A–G) contribute to each site (Galzi et al., 1990; Czajkowski and Karlin, 1995; Chiara et al., 1998; Wang et al., 2000a).

Since 2001, crystallography studies of the ACh binding protein (AChBP) of invertebrate species have provided a model for the ligand binding domain of AChR at 2.1–2.7 Å resolution (Brejc et al., 2001; Celie et al., 2004, 2005; Hansen et al., 2004; Ulens et al., 2006), and cryoelectron microscopy of *Torpedo* AChR revealed its binding and pore domains at 4 Å resolution (Unwin, 2005). These reports rationalized previous structure-function studies and enabled mutagenesis-based homology modeling of the human AChR ligand binding domain (Sine et al., 2002b). Three points relevant to the CMS emerged from these reports: 1. CMS mutations could now be mapped on an atomic structural model of the receptor (Fig. 10.10); 2. knowledge of the atomic structural model of nearly the entire receptor, however, does not reveal the conformational changes that occur in microdomains of the receptor during ligand binding, in the transitional state between binding and gating, and during gating or desensitization; 3. in some instances the atomic structural model can predict the functional consequences of a mutation, but more frequently the converse is true: the functional consequences of a mutation illuminate the kinetic significance of a given domain of the receptor (Ohno et al., 1996; Wang et al., 1997, 1999; Milone et al., 1998; Sine et al., 2002a; Shen et al., 2003, 2005).

The cryoelectron microscopy studies envision the closed pore of the receptor as a radially tapering path shaped by an inner ring of five α-helices that correspond to M2 domains of the five AChR subunits. The inner ring is surrounded by an outer ring of 15 α-helices that coil around each other and separate the inner ring from membrane lipids. The gate of the channel is predicted to consist of hydrophobic residues in the inner ring, positioned at the level of the center of the lipid bilayer. Entry of ACh into the ligand binding domain is postulated to trigger rotation of protein chains on opposite sides of the pore entrance that

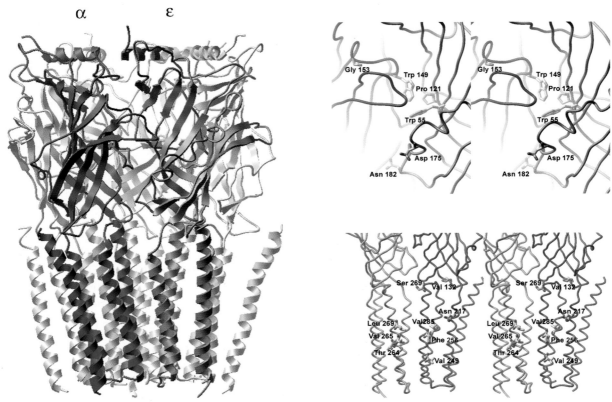

Fig. 10.10. Structural model of the adult human muscle AChR. Left panel shows joined ligand binding and pore domains with the cytoplasmic M3–M4 linker omitted. Note the predominantly β-sheet structure of the binding domain (upper portion) and α-helical structure of the pore domain (lower portion), with the α-subunit magenta and ε-subunit yellow. Top right panel shows a close-up stereo view of the ACh binding site with key binding sites Trp α149 and ε55 highlighted in stick representation to indicate the approximate position of ACh binding. The remaining highlighted residues are mutated in several cases of CMS (see text). Bottom right panel shows a close-up stereo view of the pore domains of the α- and ε-subunits rotated 180° compared to the left panel and with the remaining subunits removed for clarity. The highlighted residues are mutated in several cases of CMS. (From Engel and Sine, 2005, with permission.)

would effect rotational movement of the M2 helices to open the channel pore (Miyazawa et al., 2003). Cryoelectron microscopy also suggests that the M3 and M4 domains of the subunits have a fenestrated basket-like structure that extends into the cytoplasm to provide attachment sites for cytoskeletal components (Miyazawa et al., 1999).

The conformational changes that occur during transition from the closed to the open conformation of the receptor are not well understood. Extensive studies based on rate equilibrium-free energy relationships reveal a conformational wave that involves sequential synchronous movement of dozens of rigid residues, with segments closer to the binding site moving first and those nearest to the channel pore moving last (Grosman et al., 2000; Mitra et al., 2004, 2005; Zhou et al., 2005). The sites of interactions between different receptor segments that move in the transitional state have been investigated by mutant cycle analysis, which reveals energetic coupling between residues

(Horovitz and Fersht, 1990). This revealed a pathway that links agonist binding to channel opening in the *Torpedo* AChR α-subunit: energetic coupling was detected between invariant arginine and glutamate residues in nearby β-sheets at the base of the extracellular binding domain and conserved proline and serine residues at the top of the channel-forming M2 α-helix (Lee and Sine, 2005). Similar studies of residues located at interfaces of the α/δ and α/ε subunits have revealed strong energetic coupling between the tyrosine residue (Y127) in each α-subunit and asparagine residues in the nearby ε (N39) and δ (N41) subunits. These couplings assure near synchronous movements of the α, δ and ε subunits, promoting rapid and efficient gating of the receptor (Mukhtasimova and Sine, 2007).

10.6.2. Mechanisms of receptor activation by ACh

The linear scheme of receptor activation shown below includes rates of agonist association (k_{+1} and k_{+2}) and dissociation (k_{-1} and k_{-2}) for two bindings steps, and rates of channel opening (β) and closing (α):

$$A + R \xrightleftharpoons[k_{-1}]{k_{+1}} AR + A \xrightleftharpoons[k_{-2}]{k_{+2}} A_2R \xrightleftharpoons[\alpha]{\beta} A_2R^*$$

In the above equation, A is the agonist, R is the resting channel state, and R* is the open-channel state; k_{-1}/k_{+1} defines K_1 and k_{-2}/k_{+2} defines K_2, the dissociation constants for agonist binding to the monoliganded and diliganded closed receptor. The ratio β/α defines the gating equilibrium constant γ, which is a measure of gating efficiency. The above scheme is a subset of the Monod–Wyman–Changeux (MWC) description (1965) of allosteric protein function shown below.

$$
\begin{array}{ccccc}
R^* + A & \underset{}{\overset{K_1^*}{\rightleftharpoons}} & AR^* + A & \underset{}{\overset{K_2^*}{\rightleftharpoons}} & A_2R^* \\
\theta_0 \Updownarrow & & \theta_1 \Updownarrow & & \theta_2 \Updownarrow \\
R + A & \underset{K_1}{\rightleftharpoons} & AR + A & \underset{K_2}{\rightleftharpoons} & A_2R
\end{array}
$$

This scheme assigns a higher agonist affinity to open compared to closed states and accommodates additional transitions, such as opening of the unliganded and monoliganded receptors as well as agonist dissociation from open channel states. Except for opening of the monoliganded receptor, the additional transitions are difficult to detect when recording channel events from wild-type receptors, but these events become apparent when recording from kinetic mutants of AChR.

10.6.3. Slow-channel syndromes

The slow-channel syndromes are caused by gain-of-function missense mutations. The syndrome was recognized by Engel and coworkers (1982) by its distinct phenotypic features: dominant inheritance, selective weakness of cervical, scapular, and finger extensor muscles, mild ophthalmoparesis, and variable weakness of other muscles. As in endplate AChE deficiency, single nerve stimuli evoked a repetitive CMAP that decremented abnormally on repetitive nerve stimulation and the synaptic response to ACh was prolonged, but there was no loss of AChE from the endplate.

10.6.3.1. Clinical features

Some slow-channel CMSs present in early life and cause severe disability by the end of the first decade (Milone et al., 1997); others present later in life and progress gradually or in an intermittent manner, remaining quiescent for years or decades between periods of worsening (Engel et al., 1982, 1996b; Sine et al., 1995).

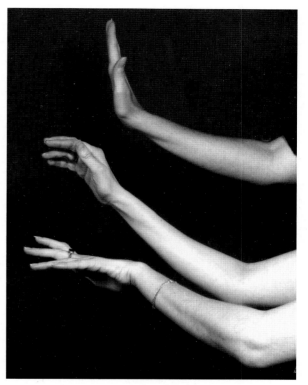

Fig. 10.11. Slow-channel syndrome patient attempting to extend wrists and fingers as shown by examiner (on top). Note atrophy of patient's forearm muscles.

Most patients show selectively severe involvement of cervical and wrist and finger extensor muscles (Figs. 10.11 and 10.12). Except for the more severely affected patients, the cranial muscles are only mildly affected. The weakness and fatigability can fluctuate, but not as rapidly as in autoimmune MG. The tendon reflexes are usually normal but can be reduced in severely affected limbs. The more severely affected muscles become atrophic. Progressive spinal deformities and respiratory embarrassment are common complications during the evolution of the illness.

10.6.3.2. Electrophysiologic features

Single nerve stimuli evoke repetitive CMAPs, a phenomenon also noted in congenital endplate AChE deficiency. The consecutive spikes of the repetitive CMAP occur at 5–10-ms intervals, each smaller than the preceding one, and disappear after a brief voluntary contraction. A decremental EMG response at 2–3 Hz stimulation is present in clinically affected muscles. The motor unit potentials fluctuate in shape and amplitude during voluntary activity.

The synaptic potentials and currents are markedly prolonged and decay biexponentially (Fig. 10.13C) owing to expression of both wild-type and mutant AChRs at

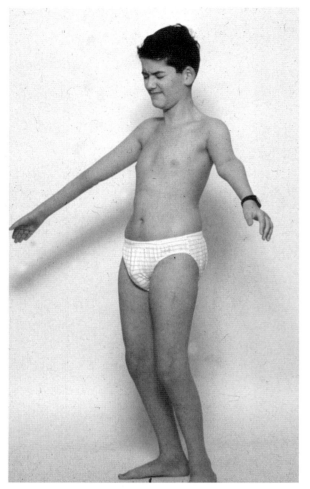

Fig. 10.12. Slow-channel syndrome caused by the εL269F mutation. The patient's arms dropped from the horizontal and his knees buckled after 15 s.

the endplate (Ohno et al., 1995; Sine et al., 1995; Engel et al., 1996b). Proof of this came from single-channel patch-clamp recordings from patient EPs that showed a dual population of AChR channels, one with normal and one with prolonged opening episodes (Fig. 10.13B), reflecting presence of both wild-type and mutant receptors (Ohno et al., 1995; Engel et al., 1996b; Milone et al., 1997). It was also noted that the mutant channels opened even in the absence of ACh (Ohno et al., 1995; Milone et al., 1997), as predicted by the allosteric scheme of receptor activation, causing a continuous cation leak into the postsynaptic region.

10.6.3.3. Morphologic features

Light microscopic histochemical studies show type 1 fiber predominance, isolated or small groups of atrophic fibers of either histochemical type, tubular aggregates, and vacuoles in fiber regions near endplates. Other biopsy specimens show abnormal variation in fiber size,

variable fiber splitting, and, in some instances, mild to moderate increase of endomysial or perimysial connective tissue. AChE activity is present at all endplates. In the more severely affected muscles, the configuration of the endplate is often abnormal, with multiple small, discrete regions distributed over an extended length of the muscle fiber (Fig. 10.14A). Calcium overloading of the postsynaptic region can be demonstrated at some endplates with the glyoxal-bis-(2-hydroxyanil) or the alizarin red stains.

On electron microscopy, at many endplates the junctional folds contain myriad pinocytotic vesicles and labyrinthine membranous networks (Fig. 10.15A). In the more severely affected muscles, the junctional folds are degenerating, the synaptic space is widened and contains electron-dense debris (Fig. 10.14B and C, and 10.15B). Some of the highly abnormal postsynaptic regions are denuded of their nerve terminals (Fig. 10.15E). Unmyelinated nerve sprouts appear near some endplates. The intramuscular nerves are normal. Degenerative changes also occur in the junctional sarcoplasm in nearby fiber regions. These consist of the accumulation of membrane-bound vesicles (Fig. 10.14C), degenerating and apoptotic nuclei (Fig. 10.15E), focal myofibrillar degeneration, and the appearance of large membrane-bound vacuoles. AChR is lost from endplates that show degeneration of the junctional folds (Fig. 10.15D).

10.6.3.4. Pathogenetic mechanisms

The prolonged as well as spontaneous openings of the AChR channel result in an abnormal ingress of cations into the junctional folds and nearby muscle fiber regions. Because a fraction of the current is carried by calcium (Takeuchi, 1963; Evans, 1974), transient or permanent calcium excess occurs in the junctional folds and nearby fiber regions.

For the normal adult human AChR, 7% of the synaptic current is carried by Ca^{2+}; this is higher than for human fetal AChR or for muscle AChR of other species, and predisposes to postsynaptic Ca^{2+} overloading when the synaptic current is prolonged. Slow-channel mutations in the α-subunit do not augment the already high Ca^{2+} permeability of the receptor (Fucile et al., 2006), but slow-channel mutations in the ε-subunit do (Castro et al., 2007) and thereby potentiate the deleterious effects of the prolonged synaptic currents and the intrinsically high Ca^{2+} permeability of the human receptor. The focal Ca^{2+} excess exerts a deleterious effect on cellular proteins and membranes through activation of proteases such as the calpains, by promoting free radical production by activation of lipases or nitric oxide synthase (Mattson et al., 1995), and promotes apoptosis through activation of caspases and endonucleases (Eastman, 1995; McGahon et al., 1995).

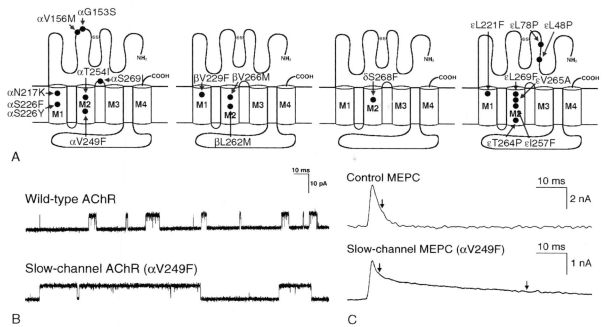

A

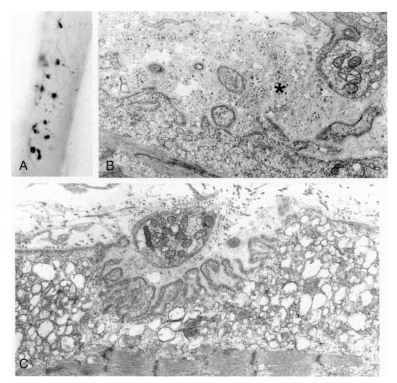

B

C

Fig. 10.13. (A) Schematic diagram of AChR subunits with slow-channel mutation. The mutations occur in the extracellular and transmembrane domains of the different subunits. (B) Examples of single-channel currents from wild-type and slow-channel (αV249F) AChRs expressed in HEK cells. (C) Miniature endplate currents (MEPC) recorded from endplates of a control subject and a patient harboring the αV249F slow-channel mutation. The slow-channel MEPC decays biexponentially due to expression of both wild-type and mutant AChRs at the endplate, so one decay time constant is normal and the other markedly prolonged. (From Engel et al., 2004, with permission.)

Fig. 10.14. Structural changes at slow-channel endplates. (A) Muscle fiber of patient harboring the ϵT264P mutation reacted for cholinesterase. The normal pretzel-shaped synaptic contact area is replaced by myriad small contact areas spread over an extended length of the fiber. (B and C) Endplate regions of patient harboring the ϵL269F mutation. In (B), note replacement of most junctional folds by degenerate globular residues with resultant widening of the synaptic space (asterisk). In (C), note widening of the synaptic space and accumulation of membrane bound vesicles in the junctional sarcoplasm. (A), ×600; (B), ×14 000; (C), ×9500. (Panel (B) is reproduced from Engel et al., 1999, with permission.)

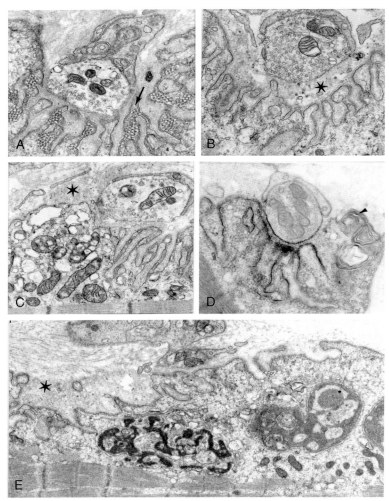

Fig. 10.15. Endplate pathology in a patient harboring the αV249F slow-channel mutation. (A) Many junctional folds are honeycombed by membranous networks. This is a common ultrastructural reaction of the EP in states of cholinergic overactivity. (B) Degeneration of the junctional folds leaves globular debris in the widened synaptic space (asterisk). (C) The junctional sarcoplasm at the left is filled with degenerating organelles; star indicates remnants of degenerated junctional folds. (D) Localization of EP AChR with peroxidase labeled α-bgt. Note loss of AChR from degenerating junctional folds (arrowhead). (E) The junctional sarcoplasm harbors nuclei in early and advanced stages of apoptosis. Star indicates remnants of degenerated junctional folds. (A) ×16 000, (B) ×19 000, (C) ×15 500, (D) ×21 000, (E) ×13 100. (From Milone et al., 1997, with permission.)

This readily explains degeneration of the junctional folds, nuclear apoptosis, and other features of the end-plate myopathy. Some of the morphologic findings at slow-channel endplates are similar to those noted at mouse muscle endplates after exposure to carbachol, a cholinergic agonist, and the carbachol induced changes can be prevented by exclusion of calcium from the extracellular fluid (Leonard and Salpeter, 1982).

The MEPP amplitude is reduced because degeneration of the junctional folds causes loss of AChR and widening of the synaptic space; enlargement of the synaptic space results in dilution and loss by diffusion of ACh before it can reach the junctional folds. The safety margin of neuromuscular transmission is compromised by the decreased MEPP amplitude, a depolarization block of AChR during physiologic activity owing to staircase summation of the markedly prolonged EPPs, and in some cases by desensitization of the receptor (Milone et al., 1997).

10.6.3.5. Molecular pathogenesis

The abnormal kinetic properties of AChR predicted that the slow-channel syndrome stemmed from mutations in AChR subunits. Since 1995, no fewer than 18 slow-channel mutations have been uncovered (Sine et al., 1995; Engel et al., 1996b; Gomez et al., 1996,

1998; Croxen et al., 1997; Milone et al., 1997; Wang et al., 1997; Ohno et al., 1998d, 2000b, Gomez et al., 2002; Shen et al., 2002a; Hatton et al., 2003). The different mutations occur in different AChR subunits and in different functional domains of the subunits (Fig. 10.13A).

In the kinships observed to date, mutations in the channel domain had more severe phenotypic consequences than those at the ACh binding site, but there were also variations in phenotypic expressivity between and within kinships harboring the same mutation. Thus, although suggestive, phenotypic severity is not a fully reliable predictor of mutation site.

Patch-clamp studies at the EP, mutation analysis, and expression studies in human embryonic kidney (HEK) cells indicate that the αG153S mutation near the extracellular ACh binding site (Fig. 10.10) (Sine et al., 1995) and the αN217K (Wang et al., 1997) and the εL221F (Hatton et al., 2003) mutations in the N-terminal part of the M1 domain act mainly by enhancing affinity for ACh. This slows dissociation of ACh from the binding site and results in repeated channel reopenings during the prolonged receptor occupancy. Another slow-channel mutation near the ACh binding site, αV156M, probably has similar effects, although its mechanistic consequences were not investigated (Croxen et al., 1997). Mutations in the M2 domain that lines the channel pore, such as βV266M, εL269F, εT264P and αV249F, promote the open state by affecting channel opening and closing steps (Ohno et al., 1995; Engel et al., 1996b; Milone et al., 1997), especially by slowing the channel closing rate α and variably speeding the channel opening rate β.

Some M2 domain mutations also increase affinity for ACh; this is most marked in the case of αV249F (Milone et al., 1997), pronounced with εL269F (Engel et al., 1996b), εT264P (Ohno et al., 1995), and not apparent with βV266M (Engel et al., 1996b). For a further discussion of the mechanistic consequences of the slow-channel mutations at the single channel level, the reader is referred to recent reviews by Engel et al. (2003a) and Sine and Engel (2006).

10.6.3.6. Diagnosis

The clinical diagnosis is supported by dominant inheritance, selective distribution of the weakness and fatigability, and the decremental and repetitive CMAP. However, some slow-channel mutations that increase the duration of channel opening burst less than 4-fold, like εP245L (Ohno et al., 1997), have milder consequences and are transmitted by recessive inheritance. A repetitive CMAP also occurs in endplate AChE deficiency or after exposure to anticholinesterase agents. Normal reactivity for AChE at the endplate excludes the diagnosis of endplate AChE deficiency. In vitro electrophysiological studies confirm the diagnosis by demonstrating abnormally slowly and biexponentially decaying MEPCs and abnormally prolonged opening events of single AChR channels.

Misdiagnoses in patients with the slow-channel syndrome have included Möbius syndrome, peripheral neuropathy, radial nerve palsy, motor neuron disease, syringomyelia, mitochondrial myopathy, limb-girdle dystrophy, facioscapulohumeral dystrophy, and myotonic dystrophy. After careful assessment of the clinical and EMG features, each of the above entities can be excluded. For example, fluctuating ocular palsies and selectively severe weakness and fatigability of forearm muscles are not features of facioscapulohumeral or limb-girdle dystrophy; none of the patients have systemic manifestations of myotonic dystrophy or action or percussion myotonia, and the repetitive CMAP is entirely different from electrical myotonia. The EMG findings are different from those observed in motor neuron disease or peripheral neuropathy. The histochemical findings may suggest a primary myopathy or neuropathy. However, the presence of vacuoles and tubular aggregates near the endplates should suggest the possibility of cationic overload of the endplate due to a prolonged opening time of the AChR channel.

10.6.3.7. Therapy

Anticholinesterase drugs can provide temporary improvement but are ineffective or harmful in the long run. By further increasing the number of normal and abnormal receptors activated by ACh, AChE inhibitors enhance cationic overloading of the endplate and likely accelerate the progression of the endplate myopathy.

Long-lived open-channel blockers of AChR shorten the openings of the AChR channel and are thus ideally suited to treat the slow-channel syndrome. Sieb and coworkers (1996) demonstrated that quinidine is a long-lived open-channel blocker of AChR, and Fukudome and coworkers (1998) showed that clinically attainable levels of the drug normalize the prolonged opening episodes of slow-channel mutants expressed in HEK cells (Fig. 10.16). Based on this clue, Harper and Engel (1998) treated slow-channel patients with 200 mg quinidine sulfate 3–4 times daily, producing serum levels of 0.7–2.5 μg/mL (2.1–7.7 μM/L), and found that the patients improved gradually by clinical and EMG criteria. Subsequently, Garcia-Colunga and coworkers (1997) showed that fluoxetine can block neuronal AChR channels, and Fukudome and coworkers found that fluoxetine is also a long-lived open-channel blocker of the muscle AChR channel. Next, Harper and

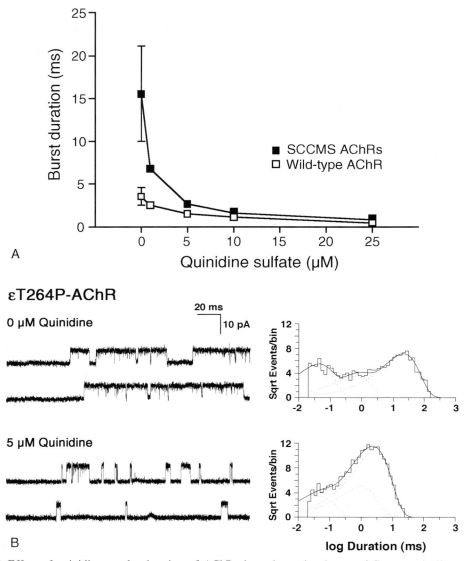

Fig. 10.16. (A) Effect of quinidine on the duration of AChR channel opening bursts of five genetically engineered slow-channel mutants (solid squares) and wild-type AChR (open squares) expressed in HEK cells. Vertical lines indicate SD. Note that 5 μM of quinidine normalizes the duration of the slow-channel bursts. (B) The effect of 5 μM quinidine on channel events generated by the εT264P slow-channel mutant of AChR. The abnormally long bursts characteristic of the slow-channel mutant become much shorter in the presence of 5 μM quinidine. The burst duration histograms indicate that quinidine left-shifts the dominant component of the burst duration. (From Fukudome et al., 1998, with permission.)

coworkers (2003) showed that fluoxetine was effective in adult slow-channel patients at doses of 60–80 mg/day. The safe use of either medication requires monitoring their level in serum and close observation of the patient for possible side effects. Fluoxetine has been reported to increase the risk of suicide-related behaviors in depressed children and adolescents (Whittington et al., 2005; Bailly, 2006). Therefore caution is required when the medication is used in this age group, and should not be used in patients with signs of depression.

10.6.4. Fast-channel syndromes

Except for one patient whose disease was caused by a dominant negative mutation (Webster et al., 2004), the fast-channel syndromes are caused by recessive, loss-of-function mutations that reside in the AChR α-, δ-, and ε-subunits. The mutations decrease affinity for ACh, or reduce gating efficiency, or destabilize channel kinetics, or act by a combination of these mechanisms. Each of these derangements results in abnormally brief channel opening events that are reflected by an abnormally fast decay of the synaptic response.

10.6.4.1. Clinical features

The symptoms resemble those of autoimmune myasthenia gravis, but are mild when the main effect is on gating efficiency (Wang et al., 1999), moderately severe when channel kinetics are unstable (Milone et al., 1998; Wang et al., 2000b), and severe when affinity for ACh, or both affinity and gating efficiency, are impaired (Ohno et al., 1996; Brownlow et al., 2001; Shen et al., 2001, 2003). A patient in the last category who carries an αV132L Cys-loop mutation plus a second null mutation in the α-subunit has had life-threatening myasthenic symptoms since birth requiring frequent ventilator support. At 4 years of age, she could not hold her head erect, stand, or walk, had marked eyelid-ptosis and facial diplegia, was unable to close her mouth, and could not speak, or swallow (Fig. 10.17).

10.6.4.2. Electrophysiologic features

The common electrophysiologic features of the fast-channel CMSs are rapidly decaying low-amplitude endplate currents (Fig. 10.18A) and abnormally brief

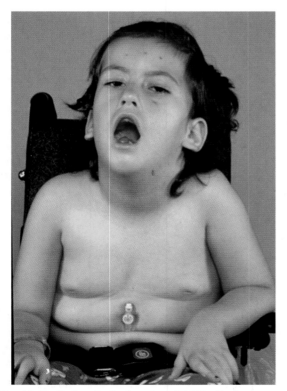

Fig. 10.17. Patient harboring the αV132L Cys-loop mutation at age 4. Note lack of head control, eyelid ptosis, facial diplegia, open mouth, and gastrostomy. (From Shen et al., 2003, with permission.)

channel activation episodes (Fig. 10.18B). The amplitude of the synaptic response is reduced by a decreased probability of channel opening, abnormal activation kinetics, and in the case of the αV132L mutation, also by failure of ACh quanta to saturate AChR (Shen et al., 2003). In the CMS caused by the ε1254ins18 and αV285I mutations, decreased expression of the mutant receptor also contributes to the reduced synaptic response.

10.6.4.3. Morphologic features

The low-affinity fast-channel syndromes caused by εP121L near the ACh binding site (Ohno et al., 1996) and αV132L in the Cys-loop of the receptor (Shen et al., 2003) leave no anatomic footprint; the structural integrity of the EP is maintained, and there is no EP AChR deficiency. Those syndromes caused by the εN182Y or the εD175N mutation in the extracellular domain (Sine et al., 2002a), αV285I in the M3 domain (Wang et al., 1999), and ε1254ins18 in the long cytoplasmic loop of the ε-subunit (Milone et al., 1998) are associated with variable decrease of AChR expression. These patients display multiple small EP regions dispersed over an extended length of the fiber surface, and some of the postsynaptic regions are simplified.

10.6.4.4. Molecular pathogenesis

After discovery of the εP121L fast-channel mutation, no fewer than seven other fast-channel mutations have been documented (Milone et al., 1998; Wang et al., 1999, 2000b; Brownlow et al., 2001; Sine et al., 2002a; Shen et al., 2003) in the ligand binding domain (εN182Y, εD175N and δE59K), in the signature Cys-loop (αV132L), in the M3 domain (αV285I), and the long cytoplasmic loop (ε1254ins18 and εA411P) (Figs. 10.18C and 10.10). In each case, the mutant allele causing the kinetic abnormality was accompanied by a null mutation in the second allele, so that the kinetic mutation determined the phenotype.

10.6.4.4.1. Low-affinity fast-channel syndromes

Four identified kinetic mutations fall into this group. Two different substitutions of residue 121 in the extracellular domain of the ε subunit, εP121L (Ohno et al., 1996) and εP121T (Shen et al., 2001), result in abnormally brief channel events, reduce the amplitude of the quantal response by decreasing the probability of channel openings, decrease the number of channel reopenings in bursts of openings, and decrease the affinity for ACh in the open channel state (Fig. 10.10). The εP121L mutation also reduces gating efficiency by reducing β, the channel opening rate. In contrast,

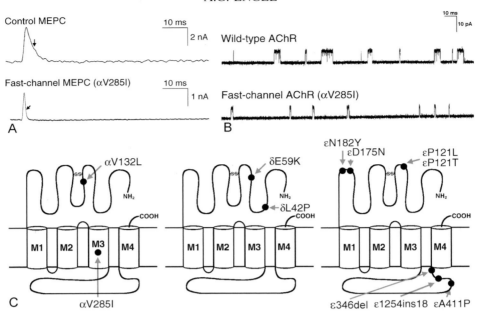

Fig. 10.18. (A) Fast-channel mutations result in endplate currents that decay abnormally fast due to abnormally brief channel opening events. Arrows point to the MEPC decay time constants. (B) The mutations occur in different sites of the α-, δ-, and ε-subunits. (From Engel et al., 2004, with permission.)

εP121T mutation does not alter gating efficiency, but reduces closed-state affinity for ACh and thereby stabilizes the closed state.

The third mutation in this group, αV132L, occurs in the α-subunit, in the most highly conserved domain of the AChR superfamily, the disulfide-bridged β-hairpin formed between cysteine 128 and cysteine 142, or Cys-loop, and results in severe disability. This mutation markedly impairs ACh binding to the resting closed state of the receptor, decreasing binding affinity for the second binding step 30-fold, but attenuates gating efficiency only ~2-fold. Mutation of the equivalent valine residue in the δ-subunit impairs channel gating ~4-fold but has little effect on ACh binding, and corresponding mutations in the β- and ε-subunits are without effect. The unique functional contribution of the α-subunit Cys-loop is attributed to its direct connection via a β-strand to αW149 at the center of the ligand binding domain (Shen et al., 2003) (Figs. 10.10 and 10.19).

The fourth mutation in this group, δE59K, is in the extracellular domain of the δ-subunit. It is of special interest as it causes multiple congenital joint contractures owing to fetal hypomotility in utero (Brownlow et al., 2001).

10.6.4.4.2. Fast-channel syndrome due to a selective abnormality of gating

Replacement of a valine by an isoleucine at residue 285 in the M3 domain of the α-subunit (αV285I)

selectively reduced gating efficiency by depressing the channel opening rate β and enhancing the channel closing rate α. The αV285I mutation also decreases AChR expression, which further impaired the safety margin of neuromuscular transmission (Wang et al., 1999).

10.6.4.4.3. Fast-channel syndromes due to unstable (mode-switching) kinetics

Two mutations causing unstable channel kinetics have been identified. The ε1254ins18 mutation, which is an in-frame duplication of codons 413 to 418 (STRDQE) in the long cytoplasmic loop of ε, also reduces AChR expression at the EP (Milone et al., 1998). Patch-clamp recording from the patient EPs revealed abnormally brief activation episodes during steady-state ACh application. When the mutation was expressed in HEK cells and exposed to desensitizing concentrations of ACh, the kinetic behavior of clusters of opening appearing between periods of desensitization changed abruptly, so that normal modes alternated with three abnormal and inefficient modes in which the receptor opened more slowly and closed more rapidly than normal (Milone et al., 1998). The second mutation in this group was a nearby missense mutation in the ε-subunit, εA411P, also accompanied by a null mutation so that εA411P determined the phenotype. When expressed in HEK cells, different clusters of channel openings differed widely in their activation kinetics, so that the

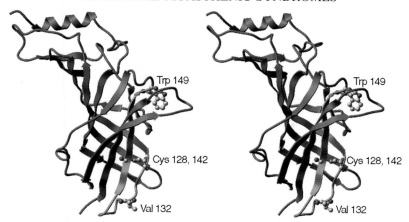

Fig. 10.19. Location of V132 in the AChR α-subunit. View of a structural model of the human α-subunit is shown in magenta with the Cys-loop and contiguous β-strand 7 highlighted in green. Ball and stick representations indicate Val 132 within the Cys-loop, cysteines 128 and 142 that form the loop, and Trp 149 at the center of the α-subunit portion of the binding pocket. (From Shen et al., 2003, with permission.)

spread in the distribution of the channel opening and closing rates was greatly expanded (Wang et al., 2000b). That both ε1254ins18 and εA411P occur in the amphipathic helix region of the long cytoplasmic loops of the ε-subunit highlights the importance of this region for assuring the fidelity of channel kinetics.

10.6.4.5. Diagnosis

The specific diagnosis of a fast-channel syndrome requires in vitro microelectrode studies to show abnormally rapidly decaying MEPCs at voltage-clamped EPs, or the recording of abnormally brief channel openings from EP AChRs or from genetically engineered mutants expressed in HEK cells.

10.6.4.6. Therapy

A markedly attenuated postsynaptic response to ACh is common to all fast-channel mutations. Increasing the postsynaptic response is therefore the logical therapy. Indeed, patients with fast-channel CMSs generally respond well to combined therapy with 3,4-DAP, which increases the number of quanta released by nerve impulse, and cholinesterase inhibitors, which increase the number of receptors activated by each quantum. Patients with a normal density of AChR on the junctional folds respond best, for a decreased density of receptors on the folds entails a proportionate reduction in the number of receptors that can be saturated by any given quantum.

The above review of the features of the slow- and fast-channel syndromes indicates that they are physiologic opposites. Table 10.3 summarizes the divergent features of the two syndromes.

10.6.5. Mutations causing AChR deficiency with or without minor kinetic abnormality

10.6.5.1. Clinical features

The clinical phenotypes vary from mild to severe. Patients with recessive mutations in the ε-subunit are generally less affected than those with mutations in other subunits, but some harboring ε-subunit mutations can also be severely affected. The sickest patients have severe ocular, bulbar, and respiratory muscle weakness from birth and survive only with respiratory support and gavage feeding. They may be weaned from a respirator and begin to tolerate oral feedings during the first year of life, but have bouts of aspiration pneumonia and may need intermittent respiratory support during childhood and adult life. Motor milestones are severely delayed; they seldom learn to negotiate steps and can walk for only a short distance. Older patients close their mouth by supporting the jaw with the hand and elevate their eyelids with their fingers (Fig. 10.20A). Facial deformities, prognathism, malocclusion, and scoliosis or kyphoscoliosis become noticeable during the second decade. Muscle bulk is reduced. The tendon reflexes are normal or hypoactive.

The least affected patients pass their motor milestones with slight or no delay and show only mild ptosis and limited ocular ductions. They are often clumsy in sports, fatigue easily, and cannot run well, climb rope, or do pushups. In some instances, a myasthenic disorder is suspected only when the patient develops prolonged respiratory arrest on exposure to a curariform drug during a surgical procedure.

Patients with intermediate clinical phenotypes experience moderate physical handicaps from early childhood.

Table 10.3

Kinetic abnormalities of AChR

	Slow-channel syndromes	Fast-channel syndromes
Endplate currents	Slow decay	Fast decay
Channel opening events	Prolonged	Brief
Open states	Stabilized	Destabilized
Closed states	Destabilized	Stabilized
Mechanisms[*]	Increased affinity	Decreased affinity
	Increased β	Decreased β
	Decreased α	Increased α
		Mode-switching kinetics
Pathology	Endplate myopathy from cationic overloading	No anatomic footprint
Genetic background	Dominant gain-of-function mutations	Recessive loss-of-function mutations
Response to therapy	Long-lived open channel blockade of AChR with quinidine or fluoxetine	3,4-DAP and AChE inhibitors

β, channel opening rate; α, channel closing rate.
*Different combinations of mechanisms operate in the individual slow- and fast-channel syndromes.

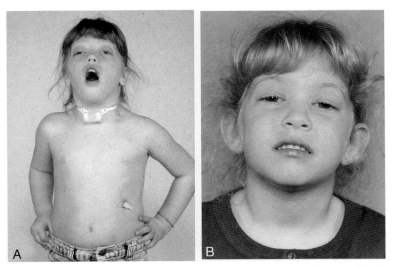

Fig. 10.20. Patient in (A) had a severe and eventually fatal CMS caused by two recessive mutations in the AChR β-subunit: a null mutation, and a 3-codon deletion (β426del EQE) that hindered subunit assembly. Note severe ptosis, facial diplegia, open mouth, and tracheostomy and gastrostomy tubes. Patient in (B) is less severely affected. She carries two null mutations in the ε-subunit but expresses AChR containing the γ- instead of the ε-subunit at her EPs.

Ocular palsies and ptosis of the lids become apparent during the first year of life. They fatigue easily, walk and negotiate stairs with difficulty, cannot keep up with their peers in sports, but can perform most activities of daily living (Fig. 10.20B).

10.6.5.2. Endplate studies

Morphologic studies show an increased number of EP regions distributed over an increased span of the muscle fiber. AChR expression at the EP is markedly attenuated and patchy (Fig. 10.21). The integrity of the junctional folds is preserved, but some EP regions are simplified and smaller than normal. The quantal response at the EP, indicated by the amplitude of MEPP and MEPC, is reduced, but quantal release by nerve impulse is frequently higher than normal. In patients with low-expressor or null mutations of the ε-subunit, single-channel patch-clamp recordings (Milone et al., 1996; Ohno et al., 1997, 2003a) and immunocytochemical studies (Engel et al., 1996a) reveal presence of the fetal γ-AChR at the EP.

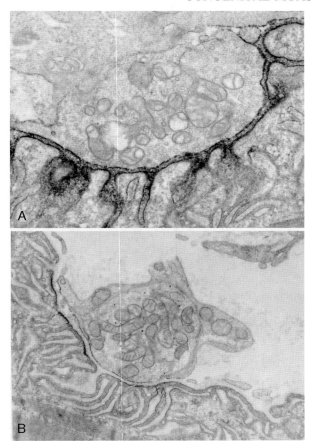

Fig. 10.21. AChR expression (dark reaction product) at a normal EP (A) and at EP from patient harboring two low-expressor mutations in the AChR α-subunit (B).

10.6.5.3. Molecular pathogenesis

CMSs with severe EP AChR deficiency result from different types of homozygous or, more frequently, heterozygous recessive mutations of the AChR subunit genes. The mutations are concentrated in the ε-subunit (Fig. 10.22). There are two possible reasons for this. 1. Expression of the fetal type γ-subunit, although at a low level, can partially compensate for the absence of the ε-subunit (Engel et al., 1996a; Ohno et al., 1997; Milone et al., 1998) (see Fig. 10.21), whereas patients harboring null mutations in subunits other than ε might not survive for lack of a substituting subunit. 2. The gene encoding the ε-subunit, and especially exons coding for the long cytoplasmic loop, have a high GC content that can predispose to DNA rearrangements.

Different types of recessive mutations causing severe endplate AChR deficiency have been identified. Some mutations cause premature termination of the translational chain. These mutations are frameshifting (Engel et al., 1996a; Ohno et al., 1997, 1998b; Abicht et al., 1999; Croxen et al., 1999; Middleton et al.,

1999; Shen et al., 2002b, 2003), occur at a splice site (Ohno et al., 1998b; Middleton et al., 1999), or produce a stop codon directly (Ohno et al., 1997). An important mutation in this group is the 1369delG in the ε-subunit that results in loss of a C-terminal cysteine, C470, crucial to both maturation and surface expression of the adult receptor (Ealing et al., 2002). Thus any mutation that truncates the ε-subunit upstream of C470 is predicted to inhibit ε expression.

A second type of recessive mutation is point mutations in the Ets binding site, or N-box, of the promoter region of the ε-subunit gene: ε-154G>A (Abicht et al., 2002), ε-155G>A (Ohno et al., 1999a), and ε-156C>T (Nichols et al., 1999). The N-box represents the end point of a signaling cascade driven by neuregulin through ERBB receptors. ERBB receptors phosphorylate mitogen-activated protein (MAP) kinases. Phosphorylated MAP kinases phosphorylate GABPα and GABPβ (members of the Ets family of transcription factors), which then bind to the N-box (Duclert et al., 1996; Fromm and Burden, 1998; Schaeffer et al., 1998). That these mutations impair AChR expression is direct evidence that the neuregulin signaling pathway participates in the regulation of synapse-specific transcription at the human EP.

There are also missense mutations in a signal peptide region (εG-8R (Ohno et al., 1996) and εV-13D (Middleton et al., 1999)), and missense mutations involving residues essential for assembly of the pentameric receptor. Mutations of the latter type were observed in the ε-subunit at an N-glycosylation site (εS143L) (Ohno et al., 1996), in Cys 128 (εC128S), a residue that is an essential part of the C128–C142 disulfide loop in the extracellular domain (Milone et al., 1998), in arginine 147 (εR147L), which is part of a short extracellular span of residues that contributes to subunit assembly (Ohno et al., 1997), in Thr 51 (εT51P) (Middleton et al., 1999), and in the long cytoplasmic loop of the β-subunit causing the deletion of three codons (Quiram et al., 1999). Another important missense mutation is δE381K in the long cytoplasmic loop of the δ-subunit, which causes clinical symptoms typical of rapsyn deficiency. Cotransfection of the δE381K-AChR with wild-type rapsyn showed reduced coclustering of the mutant receptor with rapsyn compared to wild type indicating the importance of δGlu381 as an AChR binding partner for rapsyn (Müller et al., 2006b).

Finally, another group of low-expressor missense mutations lead to production of channels with minor kinetic defects. The kinetic consequences of these mutations are modest and overshadowed by low expression of the mutant gene. For example, εR311W in the long cytoplasmic loop between M3 and M4 decreases endplate AChR below 10% of normal and also shortens the length

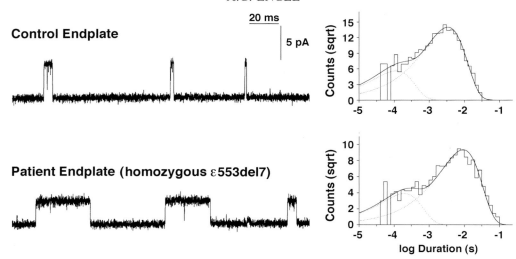

Fig. 10.22. Single channel currents recorded from a control EP and from EP of patient harboring two null mutations in the AChR ε-subunit. Currents at the patient EP have a lower amplitude and longer duration than currents at the control EP, signaling the presence of fetal AChR harboring the γ- instead of the ε-subunit. The dominant component of the burst duration histogram is shifted to the right for the patient. (From Engel et al., 2004, with permission of McGraw-Hill.)

of channel opening events three-fold; P245L in ε M1 and δP250Q in δ M1 both decrease AChR expression, but εP245L shortens whereas δP250Q prolongs channel opening events (Ohno et al., 1997; Shen et al., 2002b).

It also noteworthy that homozygous low-expressor ε-subunit mutations are endemic in Mediterranean or other Near Eastern countries (Ohno et al., 1998a; Middleton et al., 1999), and that the frameshifting ε1267delG mutation occurring at homozygosity is endemic in gypsy families (Ohno et al., 1998b; Abicht et al., 1999; Croxen et al., 1999) where it derives from a common founder (Abicht et al., 1999).

For other mutations observed in AChR subunit genes and the appropriate references, the reader is referred to a recently published gene table (Ohno and Engel, 2004a).

10.6.5.4. Escobar syndrome

This is a prenatal myasthenic syndrome caused by recessive, nonsense, frameshift, splice site, or missense mutations in the fetal γ-subunit of AChR. In humans, γ-AChR appears on myotubes around the 9th developmental week and becomes concentrated at nascent nerve–muscle junctions around the 16th developmental week. Subsequently the γ-subunit is replaced by the adult ε-subunit and is no longer present at fetal EPs after the 31st developmental week (Hesselmans et al., 1993). Thus pathogenic mutations of the γ-subunit result in hypomotility in utero mostly during the 16th and 31st developmental weeks. The clinical consequences at birth are multiple joint contractures, small muscle bulk, multiple pterygia (webbing of the neck,

axilla, elbows, fingers, or popliteal fossa), campodactily, rocker-bottom feet with prominent heels, and characteristic facies with mild ptosis and a small mouth with downturned corners. Myasthenic symptoms are absent after birth because by then the normal ε-subunit is expressed at the EPs (Hoffmann et al., 2006; Morgan et al., 2006).

10.6.6. CMS caused by defects in rapsyn

The major function of rapsyn is to concentrate AChR in the postsynaptic membrane. The discovery of the rapsyn deficiency syndromes was prompted by the observation that some CMS patients had EP AChR deficiency but carried no mutations in any AChR subunit.

10.6.6.1. Rapsyn function and structure

Rapsyn (receptor associated protein of the synapse), under the influence of agrin, Dok-7 and MuSK, concentrates AChR in the postsynaptic membrane and links it to the subsynaptic cytoskeleton through dystroglycan (Froehner et al., 1990; Cartaud et al., 1998; Okada et al., 2006). Rapsyn knock-out mice cluster AChR poorly and fail to accumulate AChR at the endplate (Gautam et al., 1995). In myotubes, agrin, MuSK, and Dok-7, and possibly other myotube specific mechanisms, regulate rapsyn aggregation (Willman and Fuhrer, 2002), but rapsyn expressed in heterologous systems self-aggregates and can then recruit AChRs, dystroglycan and MuSK. In *Torpedo* electric organ (Marchand et al., 2000) and in transfected COS cells (Marchand et al., 2002), rapsyn is cotransported with AChR to the cell surface, and in

COS cells the cotransport utilizes lipid rafts (Marchand et al., 2002). Rapsyn can bind to the long cytoplasmic loop of each AChR subunit (Maimone and Merlie, 1993; Maimone and Enigk, 1999), but it remains unclear whether the binding occurs before or after surface expression.

The primary structure of rapsyn predicts distinct structural domains: a myristoylation signal at the N-terminus required for membrane association (Ramarao and Cohen, 1998); seven tetratrico peptide repeats (TPRs; codons 6–279) that subserve rapsyn self-association (Ramarao and Cohen, 1998; Ramarao et al., 2001); a coiled-coil domain (codons 298–331),

the hydrophobic surface of which can bind to determinants within the long cytoplasmic loop of each AChR subunit (Bartoli and Cohen, 2001; Ramarao et al., 2001); a Cys-rich RING-H2 domain (codons 363–402) that binds to the cytoplasmic domains of β-dystroglycan (Bartoli et al., 2001) and mediates the MuSK induced phosphorylation of AChR (Lee et al., 2002); and a serine phosphorylation site at codon 406 (Fig. 10.23). Transcription of rapsyn in muscle is under the control of helix–loop–helix myogenic determination factors that bind to the *cis*-acting E-box sequence in the *RAPSN* promoter (Ohno et al., 2003b) (Fig. 10.24).

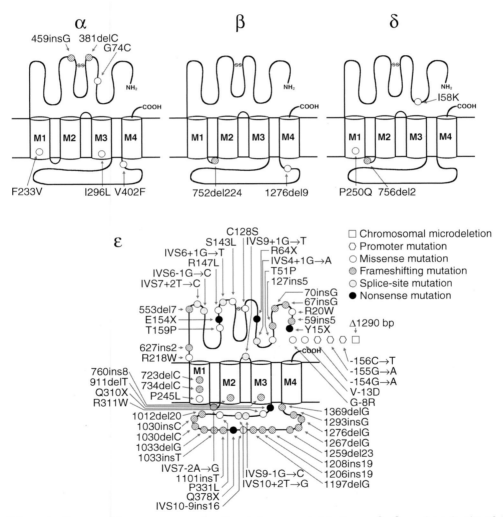

Fig. 10.23. Schematic diagram of low-expressor and null mutations reported in the α-, β-, δ-, and ε-subunits of AChR. Note that most mutations appear in the ε-subunit and especially in the long cytoplasmic loop between M3 and M4. Square indicates a chromosomal microdeletion; hexagons are promoter mutations; open circles are missense mutations; closed circles are nonsense mutations; shaded circles are frameshifting mutations; dotted circles are splice-site mutations. The most likely consequence of a splice-site mutation is skipping of a flanking exon; therefore the splice-site mutations point to N-terminal codons of the predicted skipped exons. (From Engel et al., 2003, with permission.)

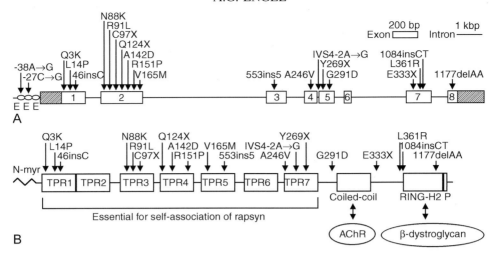

A

B

Essential for self-association of rapsyn

Fig. 10.24. Schematic diagram showing structure of the *RAPSN* gene (A), domains of rapsyn (B), and identified mutations. Seven tetratricopetide repeats (TPRs) are required for rapsyn self-association; the coiled-coil domain binds to the long cytoplasmic loop of AChR subunits; the RING-H2 domain links rapsyn to β-dystroglycan. Shaded areas in (A) indicate untranslated regions in *RAPSN*. E, E-box. (From Engel and Sine, 2005, with permission.)

10.6.6.2. Clinical features

In most patients, myasthenic symptoms usually present at birth or infancy. Some patients are born with arthrogryposis owing to hypomotility in utero (Ohno et al., 2002; Burke et al., 2003) (Fig. 10.25). Motor milestones are typically delayed and fatigable weakness persists during life. Respiratory infections or other intercurrent febrile illnesses precipitate increased weakness and respiratory crises that can result in anoxic encephalopathy (Ohno et al., 2002; Burke et al., 2003; Banwell et al., 2004). In an otherwise asymptomatic

patient who was homozygous for the N88K mutation, weakness and respiratory insufficiency became apparent only with febrile illnesses (Skeie et al., 2006). When the mutations are in the open reading frame of *RAPSN*, the distribution of weakness is similar to that in autoimmune myasthenia gravis, except the ocular ductions tend to be spared and there is selectively severe weakness of the anterior tibial muscles (Skeie et al., 2006). Few patients present in the second or third decade, have a milder course, and are homozygous for the N88K mutation (Burke et al., 2003; Cossins et al., 2006)

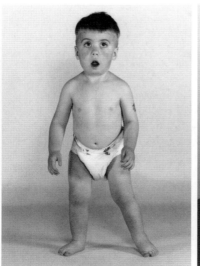
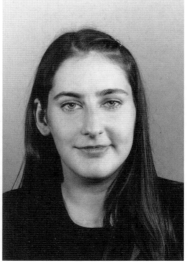

Fig. 10.25. A two-year-old boy and a 27-year-old woman are both homozygous for the N88K rapsyn mutation. In the two-year-old boy, note bilateral eyelid ptosis, facial diplegia, open mouth, and contractures at the knees and elbows. The 27-year-old woman shows only mild eyelid ptosis and mild fatigable weakness on exertion.

(Fig. 10.25). The clinical course is stable and essentially benign, but one patient observed by the authors experienced worsening of her weakness and increased respiratory embarrassment during pregnancy and the postpartum period.

Facial deformities associated with prognathism and malocclusion are pronounced in Near-Eastern Jewish patients who carry an E-box mutation (−38A>G) in the *RAPSN* gene (Ohno et al., 2003b). These patients have mild to severe weakness of the masticatory muscles, moderate to severe eyelid ptosis without ophthalmoparesis, facial weakness, and slurred or hypernasal speech. Cervical, trunkal and limb muscles are usually spared.

10.6.6.3. Electrophysiologic features

A decremental EMG response is present in some but not all patients. The decremental response on 2-Hz stimulation can appear only after subtetanic stimulation for 5 min or SFEMG is required to uncover the defect of neuromuscular transmission (Ohno et al., 2002). Similar EMG findings were reported in the Near-Eastern Jewish patients with facial malformations (Goldhammer et al., 1990; Sadeh et al., 1993).

In vitro electrophysiologic studies show a higher than normal quantal release in some patients. Consistent with the endplate AChR deficiency, the MEPP and MEPC amplitudes are reduced. Single-channel patch-clamp recordings show no kinetic abnormality of the AChR channel.

10.6.6.4. Morphologic features

The EPs, like those of patients with low-expressor mutation of the AChR, show a reduced expression of rapsyn and a proportionately reduced expression of AChR (Fig. 10.26B). In some patients, however, the number of AChRs per endplate is only mildly reduced (Ohno et al., 2002). The cholinesterase reaction reveals multiple small endplate regions dispersed over an increased span of individual muscle fibers. Ultrastuctural studies show shallow postsynaptic folds, few secondary clefts, and smaller than normal nerve terminals and postsynaptic regions but the structural integrity of the pre- and postsynaptic regions is preserved (Fig. 10.26A and B) (Ohno et al., 2002, 2003b).

10.6.6.5. Molecular pathogenesis

Mutations have now been detected in each translated domain of *RAPSN* as well as in the untranslated *RAPSN* E-box (Ohno et al., 2002, 2003b; Burke et al., 2003; Dunne and Maselli, 2003; Müller et al., 2003, 2004b, 2006b; Yasaki et al., 2004; Cossins et al., 2006) (Fig. 10.24A and B). Among the first four identified

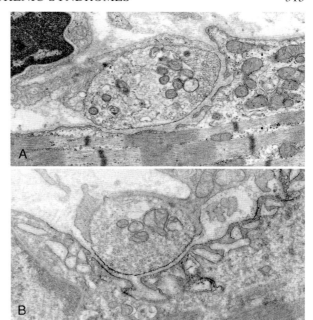

Fig. 10.26. (A) and (B) Endplate regions from patients harboring mutations in rapsyn. The postsynaptic regions are simpler than normal, displaying shallow or no junctional folds. AChR expression, indicated by black reaction product in (B), is patchy and attenuated.

patients with rapsyn deficiency, one carried L14P in TPR1 and N88K in TPR3; two were homozygous for N88K; and one carried N88K and 553ins5, which frameshifts in TPR5. Expression studies in HEK cells showed that none of the mutations hindered rapsyn self-association but all three diminished coclustering of AChR with rapsyn (Ohno et al., 2002). That missense mutations in TPR domains decrease coclustering of AChR with rapsyn implies that they exert an allosteric effect on the coiled-coil or RING-H2 domains, or that they affect rapsyn folding and stability, or reduce rapsyn transport to the cell surface. A recent study noted different effects of different *RAPSN* mutants in expression systems, namely decreased stability due to K372del, decreased ability to associate with AChR due to A25V, impaired capacity to self-associate due to R91L, or unstable clustering under the influence of agrin due to N88K and L361R (Cossins et al., 2006).

Nearly all Indo-European patients with mutations in the translated region of *RAPSN* carry the N88K mutation on at least one allele; other mutations in the translated region are dispersed over different rapsyn domains. There is evidence for an ancient Indo-European founder for N88K (Richard et al., 2003; Müller et al., 2004a), but not all patients with the N88K mutation carry the same haplotype (Richard et al., 2003; Ohno and Engel, 2004b).

Mutations also occur in the E-box of the *RAPSN* promoter (Fig. 10.24A). The E-box elements have a consensus sequence of CANNTG; they are targets of myogenic determination factors and therefore participate in modulating *RAPSN* expression. The two identified mutations in *RAPSN* E-box elements ($-38A>G$ and $-27C>G$) are first examples of E-box mutations in humans. The $-38A>G$ mutation was homozygous in seven Oriental Jewish kinships with characteristic facial malformations and was traced to a common founder (Ohno et al., 2003b).

10.6.6.6. Genotype–phenotype correlations

The mild phenotype associated with the $-38A>G$ mutation appears to be homogeneous but there is no clear genotype–phenotype correlation for other rapsyn mutations. Among two patients homozygous for the same N88K mutation, one had severe myasthenic symptoms and joint contractures at the age of 2 years but the other had only mild weakness at the age of 27 years (see Fig. 10.25). One patient heterozygous for N88K and L14P was as severely affected as another patient homozygous for N88K; and one patient who harbors N88K and 553ins5 and was born with arthrogryposis, but has only mild weakness at age 11. A recent study, however, suggested that patients carrying N88K at homozygosity were less severely affected than those who carry N88K at heterozygosity (Cossins et al., 2006). However, the fact remains that identical mutations can have different phenotypic effects in different patients; this may be due to polymorphisms in functionally related genes that can mitigate or worsen the effects of the mutations.

10.6.6.7. Diagnosis

The diagnosis can be suspected on clinical grounds in the presence of congenital joint contractures, worsening of symptoms and respiratory crises precipitated by febrile illness, only mild or no limitation of the ocular ductions, and selectively severe weakness of the anterior tibial muscles. The definitive diagnosis depends on mutation analysis of *RAPSN*. In Indo-European patients this can begin by screening for the N88K mutation; some patients, however, do not carry this mutation and then the entire gene needs to be sequenced (Müller et al., 2006a). If this also fails to reveal a mutation, one needs to search for mutations in the long cytoplasmic loop of the δ-subunit, the consequences of which can mimic those of mutations in rapsyn (Müller et al., 2006b).

10.6.6.8. Therapy

Most patients respond well to anticholinesterase medications; some derive additional benefit from the use of 3,4-DAP (Banwell et al., 2004), and two patients observed by the author benefited from the added use of ephedrine.

10.6.7. CMS caused by MuSK deficiency

MuSK (a muscle specific receptor tyrosine kinase), under the influence of agrin and Dok-7, acts on rapsyn to cluster AChR in the postsynaptic membrane. In addition, MuSK plays a role in organizing the postsynaptic protein scaffold and promotes maturation of the developing neuromuscular junction.

A heteroallelic frameshift (220insC) and a missense (V789M) mutation were documented in a CMS patient whose EPs were deficient in AChR and MuSK. The frameshift mutation prevents MuSK expression; the missense mutation diminishes the expression and stability of MuSK (Chevessier et al., 2004) and impairs the interaction of MuSK with Dok-7 (Okada et al., 2006). Forced expression of the V789M mutant in mouse muscle decreases AChR expression at the EP and appears to cause aberrant axonal outgrowth (Chevessier et al., 2004). The patient responded to combined treatment with pyridostigmine and 3,4-diaminopyride (Chevessier et al., 2004).

10.6.8. Dok-7 myasthenia

10.6.8.1. Clinical features

Recently, Slater and coworkers (2006) described their findings in eight patients from seven kinships suffering from limb-girdle myasthenia. All had progressive weakness in a proximal limb-girdle distribution that began in the first or second decade of life, a decremental EMG response on 3 Hz stimulation, and a favorable response to anticholinesterase medications. The oculobulbar muscles were spared except for slight facial weakness and ptosis in some patients. None were noted to have fatigable weakness and none had detectable anti-AChR antibodies. Thus they differed from most myasthenic patients with anti-AChR antibodies in whom oculobulbar involvement heralds the onset of the disease and who typically experience increased weakness after exertion.

Shortly after this report, two other studies cast further light on limb-girdle myasthenia. The first report by Okada and coworkers (2006) described a novel postsynaptic protein, Dok-7 ("downstream of kinase-7"), which activates MuSK alone or in combination with agrin, and thereby promotes clustering of AChRs by rapsyn at EPs. A second report by Beeson and coworkers (2006) described *DOK-7* mutations in 19 CMS patients, 7 of whom were initially described by Slater. In this larger group, all had limb-girdle weakness with lesser face, jaw or neck muscle involvement; some patients presented at birth, 3 had limited ocular ductions, and 8 had dysphagia.

A subsequent study of 16 CMS patients harboring Do-7 mutations observed at the Mayo Clinic showed a still wider clinical spectrum (Selcen et al., 2008). The age at onset of symptoms ranged from the first day of life to 5 years (mean, 1.6 years, median, 1 year). The clinical course varied from mild static weakness limited to limbgirdle muscles to severe generalized progressive disease. All experienced short-term fatigability on exertion. The tendon reflexes were decreased in the arms, legs, or both. Ten patients experienced intermittent worsenings lasting from days to weeks. Three patients had been hypomotile in utero, and one was unusual in having severe ptosis, facial weakness and bulbar symptoms but only slight shoulder muscle weakness. Seven patients had significant respiratory embarrassment. The overall course was progressive in 12 (Fig 10.27).

10.6.8.2. Electrophysiologic features

A decremental EMG response can be detected in all patients but not in all muscles, with the trapezius, facial, and deltoid muscles yielding the most consistent results. SFEMG studies have been positive in all tested patients.

In vitro microelectrode studies of the EP consistently show a decreased quantal content (m) of the EPP and a decreased amplitude of the MEPP. The amplitude of the MEPC is normal (Slater et al., 2006) or variably reduced (Selcen et al., 2008).

10.6.8.3. Morphologic features

In the 8 patients investigated by Slater and coworkers (2006) there were no light microscopic abnormalities in the muscle fibers but in the 14 patients observed at the Mayo Clinic, type 1 fiber preponderance, type 2 fiber atrophy, isolated necrotic and regenerating fibers, and pleomorphic oxidative enzyme decreases or target formations were variable associated features (Selcen et al., 2008). In both studies, the EP area was small relative to muscle fiber size, with each EP consisting of one to multiple small synaptic contacts. Because of the small size of the EPs, Dok-7 myasthenia has been dubbed as a "synaptopathy."

Ultrastructural studies of EPs of 6 patients studied by Slater (2006) demonstrated simplified junctional folds and a concomitant shortening of the postsynaptic membrane (Slater et al., 2006). A further study of 464 EP regions of 289 EPs in the Mayo cohort of 14 patients revealed disintegrating junctional folds in 32% (Figs. 10.28 and 10.29A and B), denuded postsynaptic regions with nearby nerve sprouts in 18% (Figs. 10.29B and 10.30B), partial occupancy of the postsynaptic region in 22%, and degenerating postsynaptic organelles in 18% (Fig. 10.29B) of the EP regions

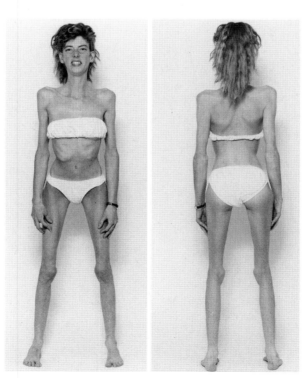

Fig. 10.27. Patient harboring two frame-shift mutations in Dok-7. Note ptosis, markedly reduced muscle bulk, severe lordosis and adduction deformity of the knees.

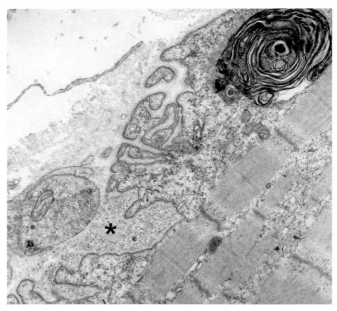

Fig. 10.28. EP region in Dok-7 myasthenia. Note severe focal degeneration of junctional folds (asterisk) and large myeloid structure in the junctional sarcoplasm. ×25 900.

(Selcen et al., 2007). Interestingly, few EPs in each patient appeared structurally normal (Fig. 10.30A). These findings indicate an EP myopathy and are evidence of ongoing destruction and remodeling of the EP.

The AChR content of the EPs was reduced in proportion to the reduced size of the EPs and, at some EPs, by concomitant loss of AChR from degenerating junctional folds (Fig. 10.30B).

10.6.8.4. Pathogenetic mechanisms

The basic abnormality is smallness, immaturity and ongoing degeneration and regeneration of the EPs. The low quantal content of the EPP (m) is appropriate for the small size of the EP but inappropriate for the size of the muscle fiber. The decreased amplitude of the MEPP can be attributed to a decreased input resistance of the simplified postsynaptic region; the MEPC is independent of the input resistance of the postsynaptic region but is likely lowered at some EPs due to degeneration of the junctional folds and by the altered EP geometry. The AChR content of the EP is reduced approximately in proportion to EP size, or more if there is degeneration of the junctional folds. The combined decrease of m and of the MEPP results in an approximately 50% reduction of the EPP and lowers the safety margin of neuromuscular transmission.

10.6.8.5. Molecular pathogenesis

Dok-7 is a 504 amino-acid protein. Like other members of the Dok family, it is a modular protein with a pleckstrin-homology (PH) domain in exons 1–3, a phosphotyrosine binding (PTB) domain in exons 4 and 5, and an SRC homology 2 (SH2) target motif in its last exon, exon 7 (Okada et al., 2006). The PH and PTB domains enable Dok proteins to couple to tyrosine kinases whereas the unique C-termini of Dok proteins contain docking sites for effectors (Crowder et al., 2004).

The PTB domain of Dok-7 interacts with a PTB target motif in MuSK to instigate intense autophosphorylation of MuSK. Dok-7 is essential for MuSK activation in myotubes; it is expressed in the central EP region of mouse diaphragm at day 14.5 of embryonic development when AChRs cluster in a nerve- and agrin-independent manner. Forced expression of Dok-7 in C2 myotubes induces phosphorylation of MuSK and thereby phosphorylation of the AChR β-subunit, and enhances expression of AChR in clusters (Okada et al., 2006).

Most mutations of *DOK-7* occur in exon 7; a frequent mutation here is 1124_1127dupTGCC, that converts an alanine at codon 378 to a serine and results in a stop codon 29 nucleotides downstream. All except one of the other mutations identified by Beeson and coworkers (2006) were frameshifting, but in some patients the second mutation remained elusive. In the Mayo cohort of 14 patients, mutation analysis based on sequencing of genomic DNA and, when needed of mRNA, revealed two heteroallelic mutations in each patient. Four of these were previously reported (Beeson et al., 2006); 12 were novel comprising 2 missense mutations, 4 frameshifting

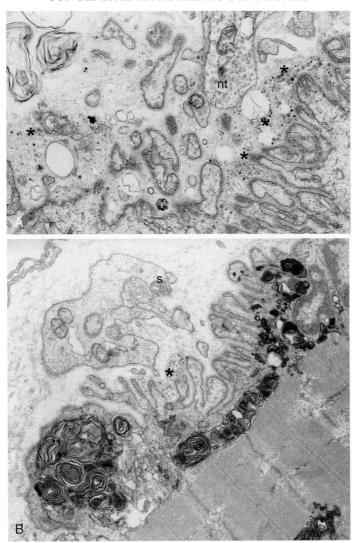

Fig. 10.29. Dok-7 myasthenia. (A) Note extensive degeneration of the junctional folds resulting in accumulation of globular debris (asterisks) and widening of the synaptic space; highly degenerate EP region on the left has been abandoned by its nerve terminal. (B) Note extensive accumulation of myeloid structures in the junctional sarcoplasm, focal degeneration of the junctional folds (asterisk), and absence of nerve terminal above the folds. A nerve sprout (s) partly surrounded by Schwann cell is present above the EP. nt, nerve terminal. (A) ×18 800, (B) ×17 300.

duplications/deletions, 1 intron inclusion, 3 resulting in exon-skipping, and 2 at canonical splice-sites (Selcen et al., 2007). Neither study has revealed consistent phenotype–genotype correlations.

10.6.8.6. Diagnosis

A clinical phenotype of limb-girdle weakness, abnormal fatigability on exertion and sparing of the external ocular and of other cranial muscles can suggest the correct diagnosis, but in some patients the distribution of the weakness is more widespread and involves oculobulbar and distal as well as proximal muscles. EP studies can point to the correct diagnosis by revealing small EPs

relative to the size of the muscle fibers, mild to moderate reduction of the quantal content of the EPP, the MEPP amplitude, and the AChR content per EP. A further and laboriously obtained clue is absence of mutations in any of the AChR subunits or rapsyn, but it was this clue that led to the identification of most cases of Dok-7 myasthenia documented to date.

The definitive diagnosis rests on identifying two recessive mutations in *DOK-7*. In patients in whom analysis of genomic DNA reveals only one mutation, the DNA rearrangements must be searched for in untranslated regions and in mRNA isolated from EP enriched muscle segments.

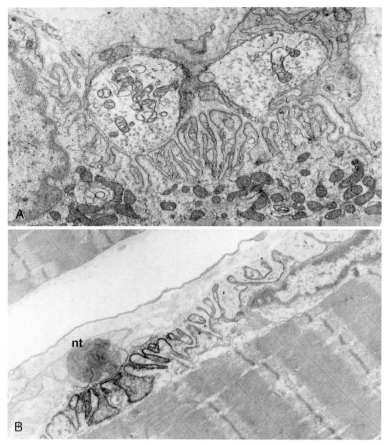

Fig. 10.30. Dok-7 myasthenia. (A) The imaged EP region shows no structural abnormality. (B) EP region reacted for AChR. Right side of the postsynaptic region is degenerating and is denuded of its nerve terminal. Left side of the postsynaptic region reacts for AChR but the overlying nerve terminal (nt) is degenerating.

The differential diagnosis includes autoimmune myasthenia gravis with a limb-girdle distribution (Oh and Kuruoglu, 1992; Azulay et al., 1994; Rodolico et al., 2002), as well as other and as yet uncharacterized forms of congenital limb-girdle myasthenia. The latter group includes patients whose muscle fibers harbor prominent tubular aggregates of the sarcoplasmic reticulum (Johns et al., 1973; Dobkin and Verity, 1978; Azulay et al., 1994; Furui et al., 1997; Zephir et al., 2001; Rodolico et al., 2002; Colomer et al., 2006). Interestingly, the authors found that living members of the first limb-girdle myasthenia kinship described by McQuillen (1966) carry no mutation in *DOK-7*.

10.6.8.7. Therapy

Anticholinesterase dugs are effective in some patients, but only few experience long-term improvement and some deteriorate even after a few days of therapy. 3,4-DAP benefited three out of eight patients and worsened one patient. Ephedrine improved five out of five patients but the improvement was temporary

in one (Beeson et al., 2006; Slater et al., 2006). Similar responses to therapy were observed in a second group of patients (Selcen et al., 2007).

10.6.8. Sodium channel myasthenia

Only one patient with this syndrome has been observed to date. The clinical and EMG features in this case closely mimicked those observed in the CMS caused by mutations in CHAT, but CHAT harbored no mutations. In vitro electrophysiologic studies pointed to $Na_v1.4$, the adult muscle sodium channel, as the site of the defect, and this was confirmed by mutation analysis and expression studies (Tsujino et al., 2003).

10.6.8.1. Clinical features

A 20-year-old normokalemic woman had abrupt attacks of respiratory and bulbar paralysis since birth lasting 3–30 min recurring 1–3 times per month. She survived only because she has been on an apnea monitor since infancy and received ventilatory support during apneic attacks. Her motor development was delayed, she always fatigued easily, and had droopy eyelids. At age 20, she had eyelid ptosis, limited ocular ductions, as well as facial, trunkal and limb muscle weakness worsened by activity; she could walk less than half a block, and could elevate her arms to the horizontal for only 20 s. She had a high-arched palate, adduction deformity of the knees and ankles, and increased lumbar lordosis (Fig. 10.31). She was mentally retarded and had mild cerebral atrophy attributed to previous hypoxic episodes. Tests for anti-AChR antibodies were negative. The patient's mother and sister were asymptomatic. No clinical data or DNA were available from the patient's father.

10.6.8.2. Nerve stimulation studies

Two Hz stimulation did not decrement the CMAP in rested muscle (Fig. 10.32A), but elicited a 50% decrement after a conditioning train of 10 Hz stimuli for 1 min (Fig. 10.32B). In a healthy subject, 2 Hz stimulation elicited no decrement before (Fig. 10.32E) or after (Fig. 10.32F) 10 Hz stimulation for 1 min.

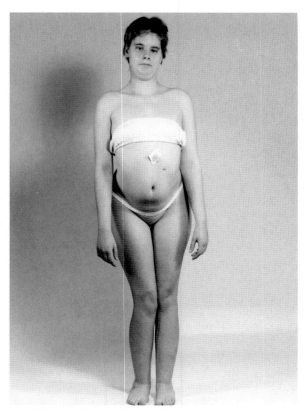

Fig. 10.31. Patient with myasthenic syndrome caused by mutation of the $Na_v1.4$ sodium channel. Note asymmetric ptosis, strabismus, lumbar lordosis, and adduction deformities of knees and ankles. (From Engel et al., 2004, with permission.)

In the patient, 10 Hz stimulation for 5 min (Fig. 10.32C), or 50 Hz stimulation for 2 s (Fig. 10.32D), decremented the CMAP, by about 85%. In a healthy subject, 10 Hz stimulation for 5 min reduced the CMAP by only ~35% (Fig. 10.32G), and 50 Hz stimulation for 2 s caused pseudofacilitation (increased amplitude with proportionate decrease in area) (Fig. 10.32H). These findings were similar to those observed in the CMS caused by mutations in CHAT.

10.6.8.3. Morphologic features

An intercostal muscle specimen showed mild type 1 fiber atrophy. The random distribution of the histochemical fiber types was maintained. None of the intercostal muscle fibers harbored vacuoles of the type observed in periodic paralysis. The configuration of cholinesterase reacted EPs and the number of AChRs per EP were normal. EP ultrastructure was also normal and the density and distribution of AChR on the junctional folds was normal. Immunolocalization of sodium channels with an anti-pan sodium channel antibody showed similar surface membrane and similarly enhanced synaptic expression at patient and control muscle fibers.

10.6.8.4. Electrophysiologic studies in vitro

The muscle fiber membrane potential was similar to that recorded from control muscle fibers. EPPs of the order of 40 mV depolarized the membrane potential to −40 mV or more but failed to trigger action potentials. The MEPP amplitude and quantal content of the EPP were normal. Ten Hz stimulation for 5 min decreased the EPP by only 13% (normal <30%). Patch-clamp recordings from three EPs revealed normal conductance and kinetics of the AChR channel. These findings indicated that the stimulation-dependent decrement of the CMAP was not due to impaired resynthesis of ACh and pointed to a defect in the muscle sodium channel.

10.6.8.5. Molecular pathogenesis

Mutation analysis of *SCN4A*, the gene encoding the muscle sodium channel $Na_v1.4$, revealed two heteroallelic missense mutations: S246L in the cytoplasmic link between the S4 and S5 segments of domain I, and V1442E in the extracellular link between the S3 and S4 segments of domain IV (Fig. 10.33A). Both S246 and V1442 are conserved across $Na_v1.4$ channels of different species.

Expression studies in HEK cells revealed normal expression of the mutant channels. The salient finding consisted of a hyperpolarizing shift in the voltage dependence of fast inactivation; this was marked (−33 mV) for the V1442E mutant and milder (−7 mV) for the S246L mutant (Fig. 10.33B). The hyperpolarizing shift

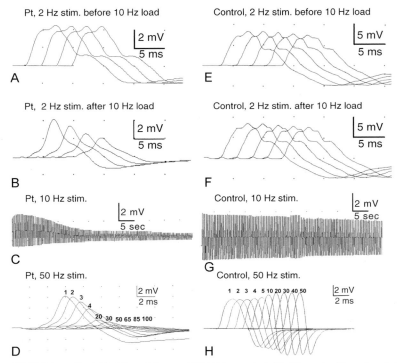

Fig. 10.32. Hypothenar CMAP in patient (A–D) and thenar CMAP in control (E–H) evoked by stimulation at 2 Hz, 10 Hz, and 50 Hz. The patient shows no decrement at 2 Hz stimulation unless it is preceded by a 10 Hz stimulation for 5 min. In the patient, 10 Hz stimulation for 1 min or 50 Hz stimulation for 2 s reduces the CMAP by 85%. Control CMAP decrements slightly after 10 Hz stimulation, pseudofacilitates after 50 Hz stimulation, and is unaffected by 2 Hz stimulation before or after a 10 Hz conditioning train. Numbers in (D) and (H) indicate nth CMAPs elicited during 50 Hz stimulation. (From Tsujino et al., 2003, with permission.)

caused by the V1442E mutation predicts that nearly all V1442E channels at the endplate are fast-inactivated, and hence inexcitable, at a normal resting membrane potential of −80 mV. To determine whether use-dependent sodium channel inactivation might contribute to the abnormal decrement of the CMAP at high frequency stimulation, the response to a 50 Hz train of 3 ms pulses was measured in vitro. This revealed a precipitous drop of 30% of the normalized peak current amplitude during the first few pulses for the V1442E mutant, whereas wild-type and S246L channels showed only a 5% decrease (Fig. 10.33C). The rapid decrement can be attributed to trapping of V1442E channels in the fast-inactivated state because recovery at −100 mV was slowed three-fold for this mutant. These studies indicate that sodium channel myasthenia is caused by loss-of-function mutations in *SCN4A*.

10.6.8.6. Relation to other sodium channel disorders

The phenotype in this CMS differs from that of periodic paralyses caused by previously identified muta-

tions of *SCN4A*. In sodium channel myasthenia the onset is neonatal, the disorder is normokalemic, the attacks selectively involve bulbar and respiratory muscles, physiologic rates of stimulation decrement the CMAP abnormally, and the muscle fiber membrane potential is normal when action potential generation fails. Periodic paralyses stemming from mutations in *SCN4A* present later in life, the attacks typically spare cranial, bulbar, and respiratory muscles, the serum potassium level increases or declines during attacks in most cases, mild exercise for brief periods does not decrement the CMAP, and the resting membrane potential of the muscle fiber is decreased when action potential generation fails (Engel et al., 1965; Lehmann-Horn and Jurkat-Rott, 1999).

Sodium channel myasthenia also differs from most other sodium channel disorders involving skeletal muscle, which are typically associated with a gain-of-function consisting of an excessive inward sodium current whereas the present syndrome is associated with loss of function consisting of a markedly diminished inward sodium current. However, a subset of

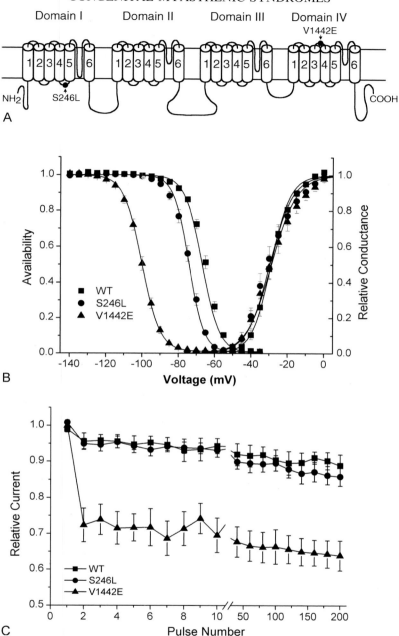

Fig. 10.33. (A) Scheme of skeletal muscle sodium channel $Na_v1.4$ encoded by *SCN4A* and the identified mutations. (B) Gating behavior of mutant and wild-type sodium channels expressed in HEK cells. Channel availability (left) after a 300 ms prepulse is left-shifted -33 mV for the V1442E channel, and -7 mV for the S246L channel, whereas activation (right) is unchanged. (C) Normalized peak current amplitude in response to a 50 Hz train of 3 ms depolarizations to -10 mV from a holding potential of -100 mV. The peak current amplitude falls rapidly during the first few pulses for the V1442E mutant but decreases only 5% for wild-type and S246L channels. (From Tsujino et al., 2003, with permission.)

hypokalemic periodic paralyses caused by mutations of Arg 672 is also associated with loss of function and a hyperpolarizing shift of fast inactivation, but the shift is only -10 mV and does not prevent action potential generation (Struyk et al., 2000).

10.6.8.7. Therapy

After the defect in $Na_v1.4$ was established, the patient was treated with pyridostigmine, which improved her endurance, and with acetazolamide, which prevented further attacks of respiratory and bulbar weakness.

10.6.9. CMS-caused plectin deficiency

Plectin is a highly conserved and ubiquitously expressed intermediate filament-linking protein concentrated at sites of mechanical stress, such as the postsynaptic membrane of the endplate, the sarcolemma, Z-disks in skeletal muscle, hemidesmosomes in skin, and intercalated disks in cardiac muscle. Pathogenic mutations in plectin are associated with a simplex variety of epidermolysis bullosa, a progressive myopathy, and a myasthenic syndrome (Banwell et al., 1999).

A patient with epidermolysis bullosa simplex had a progressive myopathy, abnormal fatigability involving ocular, facial and limb muscles, a decremental EMG response, and no anti-AChR antibodies. Plectin expression was absent in muscle and severely decreased in skin. Morphologic studies revealed necrotic and regenerating fibers and a wide spectrum of ultrastructural abnormalities: large accumulations of heterochromatic and lobulated nuclei, rare apoptotic nuclei, numerous cytoplasmic and few intranuclear nemaline rods, disarrayed myofibrils, thick-filament loss, vacuolar change, and pathologic alterations in membranous organelles. Many EPs had an abnormal configuration with chains of small regions over the fiber surface, and a few EPs displayed focal degeneration of the junctional folds. The EP AChR content was normal. In vitro electrophysiologic studies showed normal quantal release by nerve impulse, small MEPPs, and expression of fetal as well as adult AChR at the endplates. Pyridostigmine failed to improve the patient's symptoms, but 3,4-DAP improved her strength and endurance (Banwell et al., 1999).

Acknowledgment

Work in the author's laboratory was supported by NIH Grant NS6277 and by a research grant from the Muscular Dystrophy Association.

References

Abicht A, Stucka R, Karcagi V, et al. (1999). A common mutation (ε1267delG) in congenital myasthenic patients of Gypsy ethnic origin. Neurology 53: 1564–1569.

Abicht A, Stucka R, Schmidt C, et al. (2002). A newly identified chromosomal microdeletion and an N-box mutation of the AChRεγgene cause a congenital myasthenic syndrome. Brain 125: 1005–1013.

Anderson CR, Stevens CF (1973). Voltage clamp analysis of acetylcholine produced end-plate current fluctuations at frog neuromuscular junction. J Physiol 235: 655–691.

Andrews PI, Massey JM, Sanders DB (1993). Acetylcholine receptor antibodies in juvenile myasthenia gravis. Neurology 43: 977–982.

Apparsundaram S, Ferguson SM, George AL Jr, et al. (2000). Molecular cloning of a human, hemicholinium-3-sensitive choline transporter. Biochem Biophys Res Commun 276: 862–867.

Arikawa-Hirasawa E, Rossi SG, Rotundo RL, et al. (2002). Absence of acetylcholinesterase at the neuromuscular junction of perlecan-null mice. Nat Neurosci 5: 119–123.

Azulay J-P, Pouget J, Figarella-Branger D, et al. (1994). Chronic limb-girdle weakness and myasthenia. Rev Neurol 150: 377–381.

Bady B, Chauplannaz G, Carrier H (1987). Congenital Lambert–Eaton myasthenic syndrome. J Neurol Neurosurg Psychiatry 50: 476–478.

Bailly D (2006). Efficacy of selective serotonin reuptake inhibitor treatment in children and adolescents. Presse Med 35: 1293–1302.

Banwell BL, Russel J, Fukudome T, et al. (1999). Myopathy, myasthenic syndrome, and epidermolysis bullosa simplex due to plectin deficiency. J Neuropathol Exp Neurol 58: 832–846.

Banwell BL, Ohno K, Sieb JP, et al. (2004). Novel truncating RAPSN mutation causing congenital myasthenic syndrome responsive to 3,4-diaminopyridine. Neuromuscul Disord 14: 202–207.

Barisic N, Muller JS, Paucic-Kirincic E, et al. (2005). Clinical variability of CMS-EA (congenital myasthenic syndrome with episodic apnea) due to identical CHAT mutations in two infants. Eur J Paediatr Neurol 9: 7–12.

Bartoli M, Cohen JB (2001). Identification of the modular domains of rapsyn binding to nicotinic acetylcholine receptor (AChR) and to dystroglycan. Soc Neurosci Abstr 27: Program No. 904. 16.

Bartoli M, Ramarao MK, Cohen JB (2001). Interactions of the rapsyn RING-H2 domain with dystroglycan. J Biol Chem 276: 24911–24917.

Beech RL, Vaca K, Pilar G (1980). Ionic and metabolic requirements for high-affinity choline uptake and acetylcholine synthesis in nerve terminals of a neuromuscular junction. J Neurochem 34: 1387–1398.

Beeson D, Higuchi O, Palace J, et al. (2006). Dok-7 mutations underlie a neuromuscular junction synaptopathy. Science 313: 1975–1978.

Bestue-Cardiel M, de-Cabazon-Alvarez AS, Capablo-Liesa JL, et al. (2005). Congenital endplate acetylcholinesterase deficiency responsive to ephedrine. Neurology 65: 144–146.

Bon S, Coussen F, Massoulié J (1997). Quaternary associations of acetylcholinesterase. II. The polyproline attachment domain of the collagen tail. J Biol Chem 272: 3016–3021.

Bööj S, Larsson P-A, Dahllöf A-G, et al. (1986). Axonal transport of synapsin I and cholinergic synaptic vesicle-like material. Further immunohistochemical evidence for transport of axonal cholinergic transmitter vesicles in motor neurons. Acta Physiol Scand 128: 155–165.

Brejc K, van Dijk WV, Schuurmans M, et al. (2001). Crystal structure of Ach-binding protein reveals the ligand-binding domain of nicotinic receptors. NAT 411: 269–276.

Breningstall GN, Kuracheck SC, Fugate JH, et al. (1996). Treatment of congenital endplate acetylcholinesterase deficiency by neuromuscular blockade. J Child Neurol 11: 345–346.

Brownlow S, Webster R, Croxen R, et al. (2001). Acetylcholine receptor δ subunit mutations underlie a fast-channel myasthenic syndrome and arthrogryposis multiplex congenita. J Clin Invest 108: 125–130.

Burke G, Cossins J, Maxwell S, et al. (2003). Rapsyn mutations in hereditary myasthenia. Distinct early- and late-onset phenotypes. Neurology 61: 826–828.

Byring RF, Pihko H, Shen X-M, et al. (2002). Congenital myasthenic syndrome associated with episodic apnea and sudden infant death. Neuromuscul Disord 12: 548–553.

Cartaud A, Coutant S, Petrucci TC, et al. (1998). Evidence for in situ and in vitro association between β-dystroglycan and the subsynaptic 43K rapsyn protein. Consequence for acetylcholine receptor clustering at the synapse. J Biol Chem 273: 11321–11326.

Cartaud A, Strochlic L, Guerra M, et al. (2004). MuSK is required for anchoring acetylcholinesterase at the neuromuscular junction. J Cell Biol 165: 505–515.

Castro AD, Martinello K, Grassi F, et al. (2007). Pathogenic point mutations in a transmembrane domain of the ε subunit increase the Ca^{2+} permeability of the human endplate ACh receptor. J Physiol 579: 671–677.

Celie PHN, van Rossum-Fikkert SE, van Dijk WJ, et al. (2004). Nicotine and carbamylcholine binding to nicotinic acetylcholine receptors as studied in AChBP crystal structures. Neuron 41: 907–914.

Celie PHN, Klaassen RV, van Rossum-Fikkert SE, et al. (2005). Crystal structure of acetylcholine-binding protein from Bulinus truncatus reveals the conserved structural scaffold and sites of variation in nicotinic acetylcholine receptors. J Biol Chem 280: 26457–26466.

Charlton MP, Smith SJ, Zuker R (1982). Role of presynaptic calcium ions and channels in synaptic facilitation and depression at the squid giant synapse. J Physiol 323: 173–193.

Chevessier F, Faraut B, Ravel-Chapuis A, et al. (2004). MuSK, a new target for mutations causing congenital myasthenic syndrome. Hum Mol Genet 13: 3229–3240.

Chiara DC, Middleton RE, Cohen JB (1998). Identification of tryptophan 55 as the primary site of [3H]nicotine photoincorporation in the gamma subunit of Torpedo nicotinic acetylcholine receptor. FEBS Lett 423: 223–226.

Christensen BN, Martin AR (1970). Estimates of probability of transmitter release at the mammalian neuromuscular junction. J Physiol 210: 933–945.

Colomer J, Muller JS, Vernet A, et al. (2006). Long-term improvement of slow-channel myasthenic syndrome with fluoxetine. Neuromuscul Disord 16: 329–333.

Conomy JP, Levisohn M, Fanaroff A (1975). Familial infantile myasthenia gravis: a cause of sudden death in young children. J Pediatr 87: 428–429.

Corringer JP, Le Novère N, Changeux J-P (2000). Nicotine receptors at the amino acid level. Annu Rev Pharmacol Toxicol 40: 431–458.

Cossins J, Burke G, Maxwell S, et al. (2006). Diverse molecular mechanisms involved in AChR deficiency due to rapsyn mutations. Brain 129: 2773–2783.

Crowder RJ, Enomoto H, Yang M, et al. (2004). Dok-6, a novel p62 Dok family member, promotes Ret-mediated neurite outgrowth. J Biol Chem 279: 42072–42081.

Croxen R, Newland C, Beeson D, et al. (1997). Mutations in different functional domains of the human muscle acetylcholine receptor α subunit in patients with the slow-channel congenital myasthenic syndrome. Hum Mol Genet 6: 767–774.

Croxen R, Newland C, Betty M, et al. (1999). Novel functional ε-subunit polypeptide generated by a single nucleotide deletion in acetylcholine receptor deficiency congenital myasthenic syndrome. Ann Neurol 46: 639–647.

Croxen R, Hatton CJ, Shelley C, et al. (2002a). Recessive inheritance and variable penetrance of slow-channel congenital myasthenic syndromes. Neurology 59: 162–168.

Croxen R, Vincent A, Newsom-Davis J, et al. (2002b). Myasthenia gravis in a woman with congenital AChR deficiency due to ε-subunit mutations. Neurology 58: 1563–1565.

Czajkowski C, Karlin A (1995). Structure of the nicotinic receptor acetylcholine binding site. J Biol Chem 270: 3160–3164.

del Castillo J, Katz B (1954). Quantal components of the end-plate potential. J Physiol 124: 560–573.

Deprez PN, Inestrosa NC (1995). Two heparin-binding domains are present on the collagenic tail of asymmetric acetylcholinesterase. J Biol Chem 270: 11043–11046.

Deymeer F, Serdaroglu P, Özdemir C (1999). Familial infantile myasthenia: confusion in terminology. Neuromuscul Disord 9: 129–130.

Dobkin BH, Verity MA (1978). Familial neuromuscular disease with type 1 fiber hypoplasia, tubular aggregates, cardiomyopathy, and myasthenic features. Neurology 28: 1135–1140.

Donger C, Krejci E, Serradell P, et al. (1998). Mutation in the human acetylcholinesterase-associated gene, COLQ, is responsible for congenital myasthenic syndrome with end-plate acetylcholinesterase deficiency. Am J Hum Genet 63: 967–975.

Duclert A, Savatier N, Schaeffer L, et al. (1996). Identification of an element crucial for the sub-synaptic expression of the acetylcholine receptor epsilon-subunit gene. J Biol Chem 271: 17433–17438.

Dunne V, Maselli RA (2003). Identification of pathogenic mutations in the human rapsyn gene. Hum Genet 48: 204–207.

Ealing J, Webster R, Brownlow S, et al. (2002). Mutations in congenital myasthenic syndromes reveal an ε subunit C-terminal cysteine, C470, crucial for maturation and surface expressions of adult AChR. Hum Mol Genet 11: 3087–3096.

Eastman A (1995). Assays for DNA fragmentatin, endonucleases, and intra cellular pH and Ca^{2+} associated with apoptosis. In: LM Schwartz, BA (Eds.), Methods in Cell Biology, Vol 46, Cell Death, pp. 41–55.

Eiden LE (1998). The cholinergic gene locus. J Neurochem 70: 2227–2240.

Elmqvist D, Quastel DMJ (1965). A quantitative study of end-plate potentials in isolated human muscle. J Physiol 178: 505–529.

Engel AG, Lambert EH (1987). Congenital myasthenic syndromes. Electroencephalogr Clin Neurophysiol Suppl 39: 91–102.

Engel, AG, Ohno K, and Sine SM (1999). Congenital myasthenic syndromes. In: AG Engel (Ed.), Myasthenia Gravis and Myasthenic Disorders, Oxford, New York, pp. 251–297.

Engel AG, Potter CS, Rosevear JW (1965). Clinical and electromyographic studies in a patient with primary hypokalemic periodic paralysis. Am J Med 38: 626–640.

Engel AG, Lambert EH, Gomez MR (1977). A new myasthenic syndrome with end-plate acetylcholinesterase deficiency, small nerve terminals, and reduced acetylcholine release. Ann Neurol 1: 315–330.

Engel AG, Lambert EH, Mulder DM, et al. (1982). A newly recognized congenital myasthenic syndrome attributed to a prolonged open time of the acetylcholine-induced ion channel. Ann Neurol 11: 553–569.

Engel AG, Hutchinson DO, Nakano S, et al. (1993). Myasthenic syndromes attributed to mutations affecting the epsilon subunit of the acetylcholine receptor. Ann N Y Acad Sci 681: 496–508.

Engel AG, Ohno K, Bouzat C, et al. (1996a). End-plate acetylcholine receptor deficiency due to nonsense mutations in the ε subunit. Ann Neurol 40: 810–817.

Engel AG, Ohno K, Milone M, et al. (1996b). New mutations in acetylcholine receptor subunit genes reveal heterogeneity in the slow-channel congenital myasthenic syndrome. Hum Mol Genet 5: 1217–1227.

Engel AG, Ohno K, Sine SM (2003). Congenital myasthenic syndromes: Progress over the past decade. Muscle Nerve 27: 4–25.

Engel AG, Ohno K, Sine SM (2003a). Sleuthing molecular targets for neurological diseases at the neuromuscular junction. Nat Rev Neurosci 4: 339–352.

Engel AG, Sine SM (2005). Current understanding of congenital myasthenic syndromes. Curr Opin Pharmacol 5: 308–321.

Engel AG (2004). Congenital myasthenic syndromes. In: AG Engel, C Franzini-Armstrong (Eds.), Myology, 3rd ed. McGraw-Hill, New York, pp. 1755–1790.

Erickson JD, Varoqui H, Eiden LE, et al. (1994). Functional identification of a vesicular acetylcholine transporter and its expression from a "cholinergic" gene locus. J Biol Chem 269: 21929–21932.

Evans RH (1974). The entry of labelled calcium into the innervated region of the mouse diaphragm muscle. J Physiol 240: 517–533.

Fatt P, Katz B (1952). Spontaneous subthreshold activity at motor nerve endings. J Physiol 117: 109–128.

Fertuck HC, Salpeter MM (1976). Quantitation of junctional and extrajunctional acetylcholine receptors by electron microscope autoradiography after 125I-α-bungarotoxin binding at mouse neuromuscular junctions. J Cell Biol 69: 144–158.

Flucher BE, Daniels MP (1989). Distribution of Na+ channels and ankyrin in neuromuscular junctions is complementary to that of acetylcholine receptors and the 43 Kd protein. Neuron 3: 163–175.

Froehner SC, Luetje CW, Scotland PB, et al. (1990). The postsynaptic 43K protein clusters muscle nicotinic acetylcholine receptors in Xenopus oocytes. Neuron 5: 403–410.

Fromm L, Burden SJ (1998). Synapse-specific and neuregulin-induced transcription require an Ets site that binds GABPα/GABPβ. Genes Dev 12: 3074–3083.

Fucile S, Sucapane A, Grassi A, et al. (2006). The human adult subtype AChR channel has high Ca^{2+} permeability. J Physiol (London) 573: 35–43.

Fukudome T, Ohno K, Brengman JM, et al. (1998). Quinidine normalizes the open duration of slow-channel mutants of the acetylcholine receptor. Neuroreport 9: 1907–1911.

Furui E, Fukushima K, Sakashita T, et al. (1997). Familial limb-girdle myasthenia with tubular aggregates. Muscle Nerve 20: 599–603.

Galzi J-L, Revah F, Black D, et al. (1990). Identification of a novel amino acid α-tyrosine 93 within the cholinergic ligand-binding sites of the acetylcholine receptor by photoaffinity labeling. J Biol Chem 265: 10430–10437.

Garcia-Colunga J, Awad JN, Miledi R (1997). Blockage of muscle and neuronal nicotinic acetylcholine receptors by fluoxetine (Prozac). Proc Natl Acad Sci U S A 94: 2041–2044.

Gautam M, Noakes PG, Mudd J, et al. (1995). Failure of postsynaptic specialization to develop at neuromuscular junctions of rapsyn-deficient mice. Nat 377: 232–236.

Gieron MA, Korthals JK (1985). Familial infantile myasthenia gravis. Report of three cases with follow-up into adult life. Arch Neurol 42: 143–144.

Goldhammer Y, Blatt I, Sadeh M, et al. (1990). Congenital myasthenia associated with facial malformations in Iraqi and Iranian Jews. Brain 113: 1291–1306.

Gomez CM, Maselli R, Gammack J, et al. (1996). A beta-subunit mutation in the acetylcholine receptor gate causes severe slow-channel syndrome. Ann Neurol 39: 712–723.

Gomez CM, Maselli R, Staub J, et al. (1998). Novel δ and β subunit acetylcholine receptor mutations in the slow-channel syndrome demonstrate phenotypic variability. Soc Neurosci Abstr 24: 484.

Gomez CM, Maselli R, Vohra BPS, et al. (2002). Novel delta subunit mutation in slow-channel syndrome causes severe weakness by novel mechanism. Ann Neurol 51: 102–112.

Greer M, Schotland M (1960). Myasthenia gravis in the newborn. Pediatrics 26: 101–108.

Grosman C, Zhou M, Auerbach A (2000). Mapping the conformational wave of acetylcholine receptor channel gating. NAT 403: 773–776.

Hansen SB, Talley TT, Radic Z, et al. (2004). Structural and ligand binding characteristics of an acetylcholine-binding protein from Aplysia californica. J Biochem (Tokyo) 279: 24197–24202.

Harper CM, Engel AG (1998). Quinidine sulfate therapy for the slow-channel congenital myasthenic syndrome. Ann Neurol 43: 480–484.

Harper CM, Fukudome T, Engel AG (2003). Treatment of slow channel congenital myasthenic syndrome with fluoxetine. Neurology 60: 170–173.

Hart Z, Sahashi K, Lambert EH, et al. (1979). A congenital, familial, myasthenic syndrome caused by a presynaptic defect of transmitter resynthesis of mobilization. Neurology 29: 559.

Hartzell HC, Kuffler SW, Yoshikami D (1975). Postsynaptic potentiation: interaction between quanta of acetylcholine at the skeletal neuromuscular synapse. J Physiol 251: 427–463.

Hartzell HC, Kuffler SW, Yoshikami D (1976). The number of acetylcholine molecules in a quantum and the interaction between quanta at the subsynaptic membrane of the skeletal neuromuscular synapse. Symp Quant Biol 40: 175–186.

Hatton CJ, Shelley C, Brydson M, et al. (2003). Properties of the human muscle nicotinic receptor, and of the slow-channel myasthenic syndrome mutant εL221F, inferred from maximum likelihood fits. J Physiol 547: 729–760.

Hesselmans LFGM, Jennekens FGI, Vand Den Oord CJM, et al. (1993). Development of innervation of skeletal muscle fibers in man: relation to acetylcholine receptors. Anat Rec 236: 553–562.

Heuser JE, Reese TS (1973). Evidence for recycling of synaptic vesicle membrane during transmitter release at the frog neuromuscular junction. J Cell Biol 57: 315–344.

Heuser JE, Reese TS (1981). Structural changes after transmitter release at the frog neuromuscular junction. J Cell Biol 88: 564–580.

Heuser JE, Reese TS, Dennis MJ, et al. (1979). Synaptic vesicle exocytosis captured by quick freezing and correlated with quantal transmitter release. J Cell Biol 81: 275–300.

Hirokawa N, Heuser JE (1982). Internal and external differentiations of the postsynaptic membrane at the neuromuscular junction. J Neurocytol 11: 487–510.

Hoffmann K, Muller JS, Stricker S, et al. (2006). Escobar syndrome is a prenatal myasthenia caused by disuption of the acetylcholine receptor fetal gamma subunit. Am J Hum Genet 79: 303–312.

Horovitz A, Fersht A (1990). Strategy for analyzing the cooperativity of intramolecular interactions in peptides and proteins. J Mol Biol 214: 613–617.

Hubbard JI, Jones SF, Landau EM (1968). On the mechanism by which calcium and magnesium affect the release of transmitter by nerve impulses. J Physiol 196: 75–87.

Hutchinson DO, Walls TJ, Nakano S, et al. (1993). Congenital endplate acetylcholinesterase deficiency. Brain 116: 633–653.

Ishigaki K, Nicolle D, Krejci E, et al. (2003). Two novel mutations in the *COLQ* gene causing endplate acetylcholinesterase deficiency. Neuromuscul Disord 13: 236–244.

Jennekens FGI, Hesselmans LFGM, Veldman H, et al. (1992). Deficiency of acetylcholine receptors in a case of endplate acetylcholinesterase deficiency: a histochemical investigation. Muscle Nerve 15: 63–72.

Johns TR, Campa JF, Adelman LS (1973). Familial myasthenia with 'tubular aggregates' treated with prednisone. Neurology 23: 426.

Jones SF, Kwanbunbumpen S (1970). The effects of nerve stimulation and hemicholinium on synaptic vesicles at the mammalian neuromuscular junction. J Physiol 207: 31–50.

Katz B, Miledi R (1967). The release of acetylcholine from nerve endings by graded electrical pulses. Proc R Soc London Ser B 167: 23–38.

Katz B, Miledi R (1969). Tetrodotoxin-resistant electrical activity in presynaptic terminals. J Physiol 203: 459–487.

Katz B, Miledi R (1972). The statistical nature of the acetylcholine potential and its molecular components. J Physiol 224: 665–699.

Katz B, Miledi R (1973). The binding of acetylcholine to receptors and its removal from the synaptic cleft. J Physiol 231: 549–574.

Katz B, Thesleff S (1957a). A study of the 'desensitization' produced by acetylcholine at the motor end-plate. J Physiol 138: 63–80.

Katz B, Thesleff S (1957b). On the factors which determine the amplitude of the miniature end-plate potential'. J Physiol 137: 267–278.

Kiene L-M, Stadler H (1987). Synaptic vesicles in electromotoneurones. I. Axonal transport, site of transmitter uptake and processing of a core proteoglycan during maturation. EMBO J 6: 2209–2215.

Kimbell LM, Ohno K, Engel AG, et al. (2004). C-terminal and heparin-binding domains of collagenic tail subunit are both essential for anchoring acetylcholinesterase at the synapse. J Biol Chem 279: 10997–11005.

Kraner S, Lufenberg I, Strassburg HM, et al. (2003). Congenital myasthenic syndrome with episodic apnea in patients homozygous for a *CHAT* missense mutation. Arch Neurol 60: 761–763.

Kuffler SW, Yoshikami D (1975). The number of transmitter molecules in the quantum: an estimate from iontophoretic application of acetylcholine at the neuromuscular synapse. J Physiol 251: 465–482.

Lambert EH, Elmqvist D (1971). Quantal components of end-plate potentials in the myasthenic syndrome. Ann N Y Acad Sci 183: 183–199.

Lee WY, Sine SM (2005). Principal pathway coupling agonist binding to channel gating in nicotinic receptors. Nat 438: 243–247.

Lee YI, Swope SL, Ferns MJ (2002). Rapsyn's C-terminal domain mediates MuSK-induced phosphorylation of the AChR. Mol Biol Cell 13: 395a.

Lehmann-Horn F, Jurkat-Rott K (1999). Voltage-gated ion channels and hereditary disease. Physiol Rev 79: 1317–1372.

Leonard JP, Salpeter MM (1982). Calcium-mediated myopathy at neuromuscular junctions of normal and dystrophic muscle. Exp Neurol 46: 121–138.

Llinás R, Nicholson C (1975). Calcium in depolarization secretion coupling: an aequorin study in squid giant synapse. Proc Natl Acad Sci U S A 72: 187–190.

Llinás R, Sugimori M, Lin J-W, et al. (1989). ATP-dependent directional movement of rat synaptic vesicles injected into the presynaptic terminal of squid giant synapse. Proc Natl Acad Sci U S A 86: 5656–5660.

Lundh H, Nilsson O, Rosen I (1984). Treatment of Lambert–Eaton syndrome: 3,4-diaminopyridine and pyridostigmine. Neurology 34: 1324–1330.

Magleby KL, Pallotta BS (1981). A study of desensitization of acetylcholine receptors using nerve-released transmitter in the frog. J Physiol 316: 225–250.

Maimone MM, Enigk RE (1999). The intracellular domain of the nicotinic acetylcholine receptor α subunit mediates its coclustering with rapsyn. Molec Cell Neurosci 14: 340–354.

Maimone MM, Merlie JP (1993). Interaction of the 43 Kd postsynaptic protein with all subunits of the muscle nicotinic acetylcholine receptor. Neuron 11: 53–66.

Marchand S, Bignami F, Stetzkowski-Marden F, et al. (2000). The myristoylated protein rapsyn is cotargeted with the nicotinic acetylcholine receptor to the postsynaptic membrane via the exocytic pathway. J Neurosci 20: 521–528.

Marchand S, Devillers-Thiéry A, Pons S, et al. (2002). Rapsyn escorts the nicotinic acetylcholine receptor along the exocytic pathway via association with lipid rafts. J Neurosci 22: 8891–8901.

Martin AR (1976). Current concepts of pre- and postjunctional mechanisms in neuromuscular transmission. Ann N Y Acad Sci 274: 3–5.

Martin AR (1977). Junctional transmission. II. Presynaptic mechanisms. In: Handbook of the Nervous System. Vol. 1. Amer Physiol Soc, Bethesda, pp. 329–355.

Martin AR (1994). Amplification of neuromuscular transmission by postjunctional folds. Proc R Soc Lond B Biol Sci 258: 321–326.

Maselli RA, Soliven BC (1991). Analysis of the organo phosphate-induced electromyographic response to repetitive nerve stimulation: paradoxical response to edrophonium and d-tubocurarine. Muscle Nerve 14: 1182–1188.

Maselli RA, Kong DZ, Bowe CM, et al. (2001). Presynaptic congenital myasthenic syndrome due to quantal release deficiency. Neurology 57: 279–289.

Maselli RA, Books W, Dunne V (2003a). Effect of inherited abnormalities of calcium regulation on human neuromuscular transmission. Ann N Y Acad Sci 998: 18–28.

Maselli RA, Chen D, Mo D, et al. (2003b). Choline acetyltransferase mutations in myasthenic syndrome due to deficient acetylcholine resynthesis. Muscle Nerve 27: 180–187.

Massoulié J, Pezzementi L, Bon S, et al. (1993). Molecular and cellular biology of cholinesterases. Prog Neurobiol 41: 31–91.

Massoulié J, Anselmet A, Bon S, et al. (1999). The polymorphism of acetylcholinesterase: post-translational processing, quaternary associations and localization. Chem Biol Interact 119–120: 29–42.

Matthews-Bellinger J, Salpeter MM (1978). Distribution of acetylcholine receptors at frog neuromuscular junctions with a discussion of some physiological implications. J Physiol 279: 197–213.

Mattson MP, Barger SW, Begley JG, et al. (1995). Calcium, free radicals, and excitotoxic neuronal death in primary cell culture. In: LM Schwartz and BA Osborne (Eds.), Methods in Cell Biology, Vol 26, Cell death, pp. 187–216.

McGahon AJ, Martin SM, Bissonette RP, et al. (1995). The end of the (cell) line: Methods for the study of apoptosis in vitro. In: LM Schwartz and BA Osborne (Eds.), Methods in Cell Biology, Vol 46, Cell death, pp. 153–185.

McMahan UJ, Sanes JS, Marshall LM (1978). Cholinesterase is associated with the basal lamina at the neuromuscular junction. NAT 271: 172–174.

McMahon HT, Nicholls DG (1991). The bioenergetics of neurotransmitter release. Biochim Biophys Acta 1059: 243–264.

McQuillen MP (1966). Familial limb-girdle myasthenia. Brain 89: 121–132.

Middleton L, Ohno K, Christodoulou K, et al. (1999). Congenital myasthenic syndromes linked to chromosome 17p are caused by defects in acetylcholine receptor ε subunit gene. Neurology 53: 1076–1082.

Miledi R (1973). Transmitter release by injection of calcium ions into nerve terminals. Proc R Soc London Ser B 183: 421–425.

Milone M, Ohno K, Pruitt JN, et al. (1996). Congenital myasthenic syndrome due to frameshifting acetylcholine receptor epsilon subunit mutation. Soc Neurosci Abstr 22: pp. 1942.

Milone M, Wang H-L, Ohno K, et al. (1997). Slow-channel syndrome caused by enhanced activation, desensitization, and agonist binding affinity due to mutation in the M2 domain of the acetylcholine receptor alpha subunit. J Neurosci 17: 5651–5665.

Milone M, Wang H-L, Ohno K, et al. (1998). Mode switching kinetics produced by a naturally occurring mutation in the cytoplasmic loop of the human acetylcholine receptor ε subunit. Neuron 20: 575–588.

Milone M, Fukuda T, Shen X-M, et al. (2006). Novel congenital myasthenic syndromes associated with defects in quantal release. Neurology 66: 1223–1229.

Mitra A, Bailey TD, Auerbach A (2004). Structural dynamics of the M4 transmembrane segment during acetylcholine receptor gating. Structure 12: 1909–1918.

Mitra A, Tascione R, Auerbach A, et al. (2005). Plasticity of Acetylcholine Receptor Gating Motions via Rate–Energy Relationships. Biophys J 89: 3071–3078.

Miyazawa A, Fujiyoshi Y, Unwin N (1999). Nicotinic acetylcholine receptor at 46 Å resolution: transverse tunnels in the channel wall. J Mol Biol 288: 765–786.

Miyazawa A, Fujiyoshi Y, Unwin N (2003). Structure and gating mechanism of the acetylcholine receptor pore. NAT 424: 949–955.

Monod J, Wyman J, Changeux J-P (1965). On the nature of allosteric transitions: a plausible model. J Mol Biol 12: 88–118.

Mora M, Lambert EH, Engel AG (1987). Synaptic vesicle abnormality in familial infantile myasthenia. Neurology 37: 206–214.

Morgan NV, Brueton LA, Cox P, et al. (2006). Mutations in the embryonal subunit of the acetylcholine receptor (CHNRG) cause lethal and Escobar variants of the multiple pterygium syndrome. Am J Hum Genet 79: 390–395.

Mukhtasimova N, Sine SM (2007). An inter-subunit trigger of channel gating in the muscle nicotinic receptor. J Neurol Sci 27: 4110–4119.

Müller JS, Mildner G, Müller-Felber W, et al. (2003). Rapsyn N88K is a frequent cause of CMS in European patients. Neurology 60: 1805–1811.

Müller JS, Abicht A, Burke G, et al. (2004a). The congenital myasthenic syndrome mutation RAPSN N88K derives from an ancient Indo-European founder. J Med Genet 41: www.jemedgenet.com/cgi/content/full/41/8/e104.

Müller JS, Abicht A, Christen H-J, et al. (2004b). A newly identified chromosomal microdeletion of the rapsyn gene causes a congenital myasthenic syndrome. Neuromuscul Disord 14: 744–749.

Müller JS, Baumeister SK, Rasic VM, et al. (2006a). Impaired receptor clustering in congenital myasthenic syndrome with novel RAPSN mutations. Neurology 67: 1159–1164.

Müller JS, Baumeister SK, Schara U, et al. (2006b). CHRND mutation causes a congenital myasthenic syndrome by impairing co-clustering of the acetylcholine receptor with rapsyn. Brain 129: 2784–2793.

Nichols PR, Croxen R, Vincent A, et al. (1999). Mutation of the acetylcholine receptor ε-subunit promoter in congenital myasthenic syndrome. Ann Neurol 45: 439–443.

Oda Y, Nakanishi I, Deguchi T (1992). A complementary DNA for human choline acetyltransferase induces two forms of enzyme with different molecular weights in cultured cells. Brain Res Mol Brain Res 16: 287–294.

Oh SJ, Kuruoglu R (1992). Chronic limb-girdle myasthenia gravis. Neurology 42: 1153–1156.

Ohno K, Engel AG (2004a). Congenital myasthenic syndromes: gene mutations. Neuromuscul Disord 14: 117–122.

Ohno K, Engel AG (2004b). Lack of founder haplotype for the rapsyn mutation: N88K is an ancient founder mutation or arises from multiple founders. J Med Genet online 41: e8.

Ohno K, Hutchinson DO, Milone M, et al. (1995). Congenital myasthenic syndrome caused by prolonged acetylcholine receptor channel openings due to a mutation in the M2 domain of the ε subunit. Proc Natl Acad Sci U S A 92: 758–762.

Ohno K, Wang H-L, Milone M, et al. (1996). Congenital myasthenic syndrome caused by decreased agonist binding affinity due to a mutation in the acetylcholine receptor ε subunit. Neuron 17: 157–170.

Ohno K, Quiram P, Milone M, et al. (1997). Congenital myasthenic syndromes due to heteroallelic nonsense/missense mutations in the acetylcholine receptor ε subunit gene: identification and functional characterization of six new mutations. Hum Mol Genet 6: 753–766.

Ohno K, Anlar B, Ozdemir C, et al. (1998a). Frameshifting and splice-site mutations in acetylcholine receptor ε subunit gene in 3 Turkish kinships with congenital myasthenic syndromes. Ann N Y Acad Sci 841: 189–194.

Ohno K, Anlar B, Özdirim E, et al. (1998b). Myasthenic syndromes in Turkish kinships due to mutations in the acetylcholine receptor. Ann Neurol 44: 234–241.

Ohno K, Brengman JM, Tsujino A, et al. (1998c). Human endplate acetylcholinesterase deficiency caused by mutations in the collagen-like tail subunit (ColQ) of the asymmetric enzyme. Proc Natl Acad Sci U S A 95: 9654–9659.

Ohno K, Milone M, Brengman JM, et al. (1998d). Slow-channel congenital myasthenic syndrome caused by a novel mutation in the acetylcholine receptor ε subunit. Neurology 50: A432.

Ohno K, Anlar B, Engel AG (1999a). Congenital myasthenic syndrome caused by a mutation in the Ets-binding site of the promoter region of the acetylcholine receptor ε subunit gene. Neuromuscul Disord 9: 131–135.

Ohno K, Brengman JM, Felice KJ, et al. (1999b). Congenital endplate acetylcholinesterase deficiency caused by a nonsense mutation and an A-to-G splice site mutation at position +3 of the collagen-like tail subunit gene (COLQ): how does G at position +3 result in aberrant splicing? Am J Hum Genet 65: 635–644.

Ohno K, Engel AG, Brengman JM, et al. (2000a). The spectrum of mutations causing endplate acetylcholinesterase deficiency. Ann Neurol 47: 162–170.

Ohno K, Wang H-L, Shen X-M, et al. (2000b). Slow-channel mutations in the center of the M1 transmembrane domain of the acetylcholine receptor α subunit. Neurology 54 (Suppl 3): A183.

Ohno K, Tsujino A, Brengman JM, et al. (2001). Choline acetyltransferase mutations cause myasthenic syndrome associated with episodic apnea in humans. Proc Natl Acad Sci U S A 98: 2017–2022.

Ohno K, Engel AG, Shen X-M, et al. (2002). Rapsyn mutations in humans cause endplate acetylcholine receptor deficiency and myasthenic syndrome. Am J Hum Genet 70: 875–885.

Ohno K, Milone M, Shen X-M, et al. (2003a). A frameshifting mutation in CHRNE unmasks skipping of the preceding exon. Hum Mol Genet 12: 3055–3066.

Ohno K, Sadeh M, Blatt I, et al. (2003b). E-box mutations in RAPSN promoter region in eight cases with congenital myasthenic syndrome. Hum Mol Genet 12: 739–748.

Okada K, Inoue A, Okada M, et al. (2006). The muscle protein Dok-7 is essential for neuromuscular synaptogenesis. Science 312: 1802–1805.

Okada Y, Yamazaki H, Sekine-Aizawa Y, et al. (1995). The neuron-specific kinesin superfamily protein KIF1A is a unique monomeric motor for anterograde axonal transport of synaptic vesicle precursors. Cell 81: 769–780.

Okada K, Inoue A, Okada M, et al. (2006). The muscle protein Dok-7 is essential for neuromuscular synaptogenesis. Science 312: 1802–1805.

Okuda T, Haga T, Kanai Y, et al. (2000). Identification and characterization of the high-affinity choline transporter. Nat Neurosci 3: 120–125.

Parsons SM, Carpenter RS, Koenigsberger R, et al. (1982). Transport in the cholinergic synaptic vesicle. Fed Proc 41: 2765–2768.

Prockop DJ, Kivirikko KI (1995). Collagens: molecular biology, diseases, and potentials for therapy. Annu Rev Biochem 64: 403–434.

Quiram P, Ohno K, Milone M, et al. (1999). Mutation causing congenital myasthenia reveals acetylcholine receptor β/δ subunit interaction essential for assembly. J Clin Invest 104: 1403–1410.

Ramarao MK, Cohen JB (1998). Mechanism of nicotinic acetylcholine receptor cluster formation by rapsyn. Proc Natl Acad Sci U S A 95: 4007–4012.

Ramarao MK, Bianchetta MJ, Lanken J, et al. (2001). Role of rapsyn tetratricopeptide repeat and coiled-coil domains in self-association and nicotinic acetylcholine receptor clustering. J Biol Chem 276: 7475–7483.

Reimer RJ, Fon AE, Edwards RH (1998). Vesicular neurotransmitter transport and the presynaptic regulation of quantal size. Curr Opin Neurobiol 8: 405–412.

Richard P, Gaudon K, Andreux F, et al. (2003). Possible founder effect of rapsyn N88K mutation and identification of novel rapsyn mutations in congenital myasthenic syndromes. J Med Genet 40: 81e.

Robertson WC, Chun RWM, Kornguth SE (1980). Familial infantile myasthenia. Arch Neurol 37: 117–119.

Robitaille R, Adler EM, Charlton MP (1990). Strategic location of calcium channels at transmitter release sites of frog neuromuscular synapses. Neuron 5: 773–779.

Rodolico C, Toscano A, Autunno M, et al. (2002). Limb-girdle myasthenia: clinical, electrophysiological and morphological features in familial and autoimmune cases. Neuromuscul Disord 12: 964–969.

Ruff RL (1996). Sodium channel slow inactivation and the distribution of sodium channels on skeletal muscle fibres enable the performance properties of different skeletal muscle fiber types. Acta Physiol Scand 156: 159–168.

Ruff RL, Simoncini L, Stühmer W (1988). Slow sodium channel inactivation in mammalian muscle: a possible role in regulating excitability. Muscle Nerve 11: 502–510.

Sadeh M, Blatt I, Goldhammer Y (1993). Single fiber EMG in a congenital myasthenic syndrome associated with facial malformations. Muscle Nerve 16: 177–180.

Salpeter MM (1983). Molecular organization of the neuromuscular synapse. In: EX Albuquerque, and AT Eldefrawi (Eds.), Myasthenia Gravis. Chapman and Hall, New York, pp. 105–129.

Salpeter MM (1987). Vertebrate neuromuscular junctions: General morphology, molecular organization, and functional consequences. In: MM Salpeter (Ed.), The Vertebrate Neuromuscular Junction. Alan Liss, New York, pp. 1–54.

Salpeter MM, Rogers AW, Kasprzak H, et al. (1978). Acetylcholinesterase in the fast extraocular muscle of the mouse by light and electron microscopy autoradiography. J Cell Biol 78: 274–285.

Schaeffer L, Duclert N, Huchet-Dymanus M, et al. (1998). Implication of a multisubunit Ets-related transcription factor in synaptic expression of the nicotinic acetylcholine receptor. EMBO J 17: 3078–3090.

Schmidt C, Abicht A, Krampfl K, et al. (2003). Congenital myasthenic syndrome due to a novel missense mutation in the gene encoding choline acetyltransferase. Neuromuscul Disord 13: 245–251.

Selcen D. Milone M, Shen X-M, et al. (2008). Dok-7 myasthenia: phenotypic and molecular genetic studies in 16 patients. Annals of Neurology, in press.

Shapira YA, Sadeh ME, Bergtraum MP, et al. (2002). Three novel *COLQ* mutations and variation of phenotypic expressivity due to G240X. Neurology 58: 603–609.

Shen X-M, Ohno K, Milone M, et al. (2001). Fast-channel syndrome. Neurology 56(Suppl. 3): A60.

Shen X-M, Ohno K, Adams C, et al. (2002a). Slow-channel congenital myasthenic syndrome caused by a novel epsilon subunit mutation in the second AChR transmembrane domain. J Neurol Sci 199(Suppl. 1): S96.

Shen X-M, Ohno K, Fukudome T, et al. (2002b). Congenital myasthenic syndrome caused by low-expressor fast-channel AChR δ subunit mutation. Neurology 59: 1881–1888.

Shen X-M, Ohno K, Tsujino A, et al. (2003). Mutation causing severe myasthenia reveals functional asymmetry of AChR signature Cys-loops in agonist binding and gating. J Clin Invest 111: 497–505.

Shen X-M, Ohno K, Sine SM, et al. (2005). Subunit-specific contribution to agonist binding and channel gating revealed by inherited mutation in muscle AChR M3–M4 linker. Brain 128: 345–355.

Sieb JP, Milone M, Engel AG (1996). Effects of the quinoline derivatives quinine, quinidine, and chloroquine on neuromuscular transmission. Brain Res 712: 179–189.

Sine SM, Engel AG (2006). Recent advances in Cys-loop receptor structure and function. NAT 440: 448–455.

Sine SM, Ohno K, Bouzat C, et al. (1995). Mutation of the acetylcholine receptor α subunit causes a slow-channel myasthenic syndrome by enhancing agonist binding affinity. Neuron 15: 229–239.

Sine SM, Shen X-M, Wang H-L, et al. (2002a). Naturally occurring mutations at the acetylcholine receptor binding site independently alter ACh binding and channel gating. J Gen Physiol 120: 483–496.

Sine SM, Wang H-L, Bren N (2002b). Lysine scanning mutagenesis delineates structure of nicotinic receptor binding domain. J Biol Chem 277: 29210–29223.

Skeie GO, Aurlien H, Müller JS, et al. (2006). Unusual features in a boy with rapsyn N88K mutation. Neurology 67: 2262–2263.

Slater CR, Fawcett PRW, Walls TJ, et al. (2006). Pre- and postsynaptic abnormalities associated with impaired neuromuscular transmission in a group of patients with "limb-girdle myasthenia." Brain 127: 2061–2076.

Stiles JR, Van Helden D, Bartol TM, et al. (1996). Miniature endplate current rise times <100 μs from improved dual recordings can be modeled with passive acetylcholine diffusion from a synaptic vesicle. Proc Natl Acad Sci U S A 93: 5747–5752.

Stiles JR, Kovyazina IV, Salpeter EE, et al. (1999). The temperature sensitivity of miniature endplate currents is mostly goverened by channel gating: evidence from optimized recordings and Monte Carlo simulations. Biophys J 77: 1177–1187.

Struyk AF, Scoggan KA, Bulman DE, et al. (2000). The human muscle Na channel mutation R699H associated with hypokalemic periodic paralysis enhances slow inactivation. J Neurosci 20: 8610–8617.

Südhof TC, Jahn R (1991). Proteins of synaptic vesicles involved in exocytosis and membrane recycling. Neuron 6: 665–677.

Takeuchi N (1963). Effects of calcium on the conductance change of the end-plate membrane during the action of the transmitter. J Physiol 167: 141–155.

Tarelli FT, Passafaro M, Clementi F, et al. (1991). Presynaptic localization of omega-conotoxin-sensitive calcium channels at the frog neuromuscular junction. Brain Res 547: 331–334.

Tsujino A, Maertens C, Ohno K, et al. (2003). Myasthenic syndrome caused by mutation of the SCN4A sodium channel. Proc Natl Acad Sci U S A 100: 7377–7382.

Ulens C, Hogg RC, Celie PH, et al. (2006). Structural determinants of selective α-conotoxin binding to a nicotinic acetylcholine receptor homolog AChBP. Proc Natl Acad Sci U S A 103: 3615–3620.

Unwin N (2005). Refined structure of the nicotinic acetylcholine receptor at 4 Å resolution. J Mol Biol 346: 967–989.

Walls TJ, Engel AG, Nagel AS, et al. (1993). Congenital myasthenic syndrome associated with paucity of synaptic vesicles and reduced quantal release. Ann N Y Acad Sci 681: 461–468.

Wang H-L, Auerbach A, Bren N, et al. (1997). Mutation in the M1 domain of the acetylcholine receptor alpha subunit decreases the rate of agonist dissociation. J Gen Physiol 109: 757–766.

Wang H-L, Milone M, Ohno K, et al. (1999). Acetylcholine receptor M3 domain: stereochemical and volume contributions to channel gating. Nat Neurosci 2: 226–233.

Wang D, Chirar DC, Xie Y, et al. (2000a). Probing the structure of the nicotinic acetylcholine receptor with 4-benzoylbenzoyl choline, a novel photoaffinity competitive antagonist. J Biol Chem 275: 28666–28674.

Wang H-L, Ohno K, Milone M, et al. (2000b). Fundamental gating mechanism of nicotinic receptor channel revealed by mutation causing a congenital myasthenic syndrome. J Gen Physiol 116: 449–460.

Webster R, Brydson M, Croxen R, et al. (2004). Mutation in the AChR channel gate underlies a fast channel congenital myasthenic syndrome. Neurology 62: 1090–1096.

Wernig A (1975). Estimates of statistical release parameters from crayfish and frog neuromuscular junctions. J Physiol 244: 207–221.

Whittington CJ, Kendall T, Pilling S (2005). Are the SSRIs and atypical antidepressants safe and effective for children and adolescents? Curr Opin Psychiat 18: 21–25.

Willman R, Fuhrer C (2002). Neuromuscular synaptogenesis. Cell Mol Life Sci 59: 1296–1316.

Wood SJ, Slater CP (2001). Safety factor at the neuromuscular junction. Prog Neurobiol 64: 393–429.

Yasaki E, Prioleau C, Barbier J, et al. (2004). Electrophysiological and morphological characterization of a case of autosomal recessive congenital myasthenic syndrome with acetylcholine receptor deficiency due to a N88K rapsyn mutation homozygous mutation. Neuromuscul Disord 14: 24–32.

Youssef S (1983). Thymectomy for myasthenia gravis in children. J Pediatr Surg 18: 537–541.

Zephir H, Stojkovic T, Maurage C-A, et al. (2001). Tubular aggregate congenital myopathy associated with a neuromuscular block. Rev Neurol 157: 1293–1296.

Zhou Y, Pearson JE, Auerbach A (2005). Phi-value analysis of a linear, sequential reaction mechanism: theory and application to channel gating. Biophys J 89: 3680–3685.

Zucker RS (1973). Changes in the statistics of transmitter release during facilitation. J Physiol 229: 787–810.

Handbook of Clinical Neurology, Vol. 91 (3rd series)
Neuromuscular junction disorders
A.G. Engel, Editor
© 2008 Elsevier B.V. All rights reserved

Chapter 11

Botulism

ERIC A. JOHNSON [1]* AND CESARE MONTECUCCO [2]

[1]*Department of Bacteriology, Food Research Institute, University of Wisconsin, Madison, WI, USA*
[2]*Dipartimento di Scienze Biomediche Sperimentali, Università di Padova, Padova, Italy*

11.1. Introduction

Botulism is an acute neuroparalytic disease of humans and animals caused through the action of botulinum neurotoxins (BoNTs) primarily acting at the neuromuscular junction (NMJ) of somatic nerves that innervate cranial and skeletal muscle. This results in the blockade of release of acetylcholine (ACh) with ensuing denervation and accompanying muscle paralysis and atrophy. BoNT also blocks neurotransmission at cholinergic parasympathetic and postganglionic sympathetic nerves, affecting smooth muscle activity and glandular and secretory functions and impairing certain autonomic activities. Botulism generally presents with symptoms of fatigability affecting bulbar and ocular musculature and, in severe cases, weakness of the neck, limbs, torso and ensuing generalized paralysis. Botulism can be life-threatening, generally due to respiratory paralysis and failure and occasionally due to secondary infections or cardiac arrest. Although botulism is considered an acute intoxication, the duration of paralysis can last for weeks to months and complete recovery requires restoration of neurotransmission and muscle function. During the past century, death caused by botulism has decreased from ca. 70% to ca. 10% worldwide due primarily to clinical recognition of the disease, prompt administration of antitoxin, intensive nursing care, mechanical ventilation, parenteral feeding and control of secondary infections. Botulism outbreaks have had dramatic and devastating impacts on human and animal populations in which they occur (Meyer, 1956; Dolman, 1964).

Botulism is a true toxemia, caused solely through the action of BoNT at cholinergic nerve terminals. BoNTs are protein toxins of 150 kDa produced by neurotoxigenic bacteria of the genus Clostridium. Seven serotypes (A, B, C, D, E, F and G) are currently distinguished (Sugiyama, 1980; Sakaguchi, 1983; DasGupta, 1989; Schiavo et al., 2000). BoNTs are the most poisonous substances known and, currently, there is no antidote to botulism other than passive administration of antitoxin within hours after toxin exposure or immunization of at-risk individuals prior to exposure (Arnon et al., 2005). Since botulism is an extremely rare disease, general immunization of human populations is not practical and would prevent the pharmaceutical use of BoNT for treatment of human disease (Johnson, 1999).

Six clinical forms of botulism are recognized (Hatheway, 1995; Centers for Disease Control, 1998; Cherington, 2004): 1. classic foodborne botulism; 2. wound botulism; 3. intestinal botulism including infant botulism; 4. inhalational botulism; 5. botulism of unknown source; and 6. inappropriate administration of botulinum toxin during its use as a pharmaceutical agent (iatrogenic botulism). Intentional botulism poisoning by oral or inhalation exposure such as in a bioterrorist event could be considered as a seventh class with potentially severe consequences (Hatheway and Dang, 1994; Caya et al., 2004). Foodborne botulism through ingestion of BoNT by the oral route is the most prevalent natural form of botulism that occurs worldwide. However, currently the most common route of exposure of humans to BoNTs is by injection for medicinal treatment of a variety of neurological disorders and therapeutic uses, a remarkable development of this toxin (Scott, 1989; Schantz and Johnson, 1992; Jankovic and Hallett, 1994; Johnson, 1999; Moore and Naumann, 2003). A very large number of injections are performed each year in humans

---

*Correspondence to: Dr Eric A. Johnson, Department of Bacteriology, Food Research Institute, University of Wisconsin, 1550, Linden Drive, Madison, WI 53711, USA. E-mail: eajohnson@wise.edu, Tel: 1-608-263-7944, Fax: 1-608-262-9865.

and the disease syndromes being treated continue to expand at a rapid rate.

The primary objective of this chapter is to address the pathophysiology of botulism with emphasis on the basic science governing the clinical effects, diagnosis, treatment and recovery. Recent aspects regarding epidemiology, pathophysiology and molecular mechanisms of BoNTs are briefly described. Several excellent and in-depth reviews on the biochemistry, structure and pharmacology of BoNT are available (Schiavo et al., 2000; Brin et al., 2002; Moore and Naumann, 2003; Jahn and Scheller, 2006) and the reader is referred to these treatises for in-depth descriptions of these subjects.

11.2. Brief history of botulism as a neuromuscular disorder

Botulism is a presynaptic myasthenic neuromuscular syndrome exhibiting muscle weakness as its primary clinical sign. As such, it shares similarities with other myasthenic syndromes such as myasthenia gravis and Lambert–Eaton syndrome as well as a number of other congenital and acquired diseases and chemical and biological intoxications (Kaminski, 2003; Meriggioli et al., 2005; Holmes et al., 2006). Botulism likely occurred as a dreaded food poisoning in ancient cultures, including the 10th century edict of Emperor Leo VI of Byzantium (886–911), who forbid the preparation of raw sausages (Wright, 1955; Koenig, 1971; Smith and Sugiyama, 1988). The symptoms of botulism were described as a muscle-weakening syndrome by Justinus Kerner (1786–1862) in persons who had consumed uncooked blood sausages (Kerner, 1820; Devriese and Devriese, 2001; Ergguth, 2004). Despite the recognition of the clinical aspects of the disease, the responsible toxic agent remained elusive until 1895, when the toxigenic bacterium (Bacillus botulinus) and the causative toxin (botulinum neurotoxin, BoNT) were described by Emile Pierrre van Ermengem in a remarkable series of experiments from a food poisoning outbreak in Belgium (van Ermengem, 1897a, b, 1979; Devriese and Devriese, 2001). In the mid-to-late 1900s it was established that botulism also could result from wound and intestinal infections in humans and that botulism affected a variety of animals (Johnson and Goodnough, 1988; Smith and Sugiyama, 1988; Hatheway, 1995). Transmission of BoNT in stable aerosols in bioterrorism events has been evaluated and even attempted in modern times and botulism occurrence from bioterrorist events is considered to be a serious concern (Hatheway and Dang, 1994; Caya et al., 2004; Bigalke and Rummel, 2005).

Botulism is a rare disease, and it has been studied less extensively than many other neuromuscular disorders.

It is often considered of low priority in the differential diagnoses of myasthenic disorders except under special circumstances such as in foodborne botulism outbreaks that affect several individuals from a single food source. Being rare, many physicians and neurologists have not encountered botulism in their practices. As such, less information is available regarding certain clinical aspects and pathophysiology of botulism compared to more common myasthenic syndromes.

11.3. Sources of botulinum neurotoxins

Botulinum neurotoxins are produced by a heterogeneous group of clostridial bacteria that differ widely in genetic and metabolic characteristics (Popoff, 1995; Hatheway and Johnson, 1998; Franciosa et al., 2003; Johnson, 2007). The exceptional feature of neurotoxigenic clostridia is their formation of a characteristic neurotoxin of extraordinary potency for humans and certain animals (botulinum and tetanus neurotoxins) (Sugiyama, 1980; Sakaguchi, 1983; Schiavo et al., 2000). Other key features of the neurotoxigenic clostridia are their anaerobic metabolism and the production of spores, which have high resistance to chemicals and physical agents (Hatheway and Johnson, 1998; Setlow and Johnson, 2007). The resistant spores are widely distributed in the biosphere and are disseminated in dust, waters, vapors, sewage and various fomites such as insects from which they readily contaminate most environments including soils, waters, humans and animals, households and buildings, as well as commodities such as foods (Hatheway and Johnson, 1998; Johnson, 2007). Under permissive nutritional and physical conditions (anaerobiosis, low acid, pH > 4.5, relatively low concentrations of salt and sugar and nutrient sufficiency) the spores germinate to form vegetative cell populations and elicit BoNT (Smith and Sugiyama, 1988; Franciosa et al., 2003; Johnson, 2007). The natural habitats of neurotoxigenic clostridia are soils and sediments and the intestinal contents of certain insects and animals (but not healthy humans) (Popoff, 1995; Hatheway and Johnson, 1998; Johnson, 2005c). Unlike many other pathogenic bacteria, neurotoxigenic clostridia are saprophytic and do not have an obligatory relationship with an animal host (Hatheway and Johnson, 1998; Johnson, 2005c).

Recognized species of neurotoxigenic clostrida are *Clostridium botulinum* (a large collection of heterogeneous strains that have the common property of producing BoNT) and rare strains of *Clostridium butyricum* and *Clostridium baratii* (Hatheway, 1995; Popoff, 1995; Johnson and Goodnough, 1998; Franciosa et al., 2003; Johnson, 2005a, c). The heterogeneous nature of the neurotoxigenic clostridia suggests that genes for BoNT have been laterally transferred by plasmid exchange or bacteriophage infection to distinct clostridial species throughout evolution and possibly in contemporary time since most of the new toxigenic species have been isolated from the human intestine (Popoff, 1995; Johnson, 2005b).

Since the primary target of BoNTs is the neuromuscular junction of eukaryotes and particularly vertebrates that evolved billions of years after the initial appearance of the clostridia, the evolution of the BoNT toxin is an intriguing question. Our present view certainly represents only a snapshot in millions of years of evolution. Nucleotide and amino acid sequence studies of the gene as well as structural analyses of the neurotoxins has shown that the BoNT family of toxins comprises a group of highly chimeric molecules of various origins (Niemann, 1991; Lacy and Stevens, 1999; Lacy et al., 1998). Structural and amino acid sequence analyses have shown that BoNT contains segments of genes/proteins from a myriad of organisms (Lacy and Stevens, 1999). Certain properties of BoNTs, especially their synthesis as a polyprotein in a protein complex (Johnson and Bradshaw, 2001; DasGupta, 2006), and similarities in mechanisms of cellular uptake related to certain viruses, suggest that neurotoxigenic clostridia may have acquired portions of the BoNT gene from a neurotropic viral source. Several of the BoNT gene complexes were shown to be associated with mobile genetic elements including bacteriophages, plasmids, transposons and IS (insertion) elements that can be transferred to other bacterial cells and populations (Johnson and Bradshaw, 2001; Johnson, 2005b). Thus, it is likely that the evolutionary diversity of the BoNTs will continue to expand and it is anticipated that additional clostridial species and perhaps other groups of bacteria will be discovered that produce functional BoNTs poisonous to humans and animals.

BoNTs are currently categorized into seven immunologically distinguishable serotypes (serotypes A–G), whereby polyclonal antibodies raised against purified BoNTs neutralize the toxicity of the homologous but not the heterologous serotypes in the mouse bioassay (Hatheway, 1988; Giménez and Giménez, 1993). The mouse bioassay, first introduced in 1939 for detection of botulism in humans (Schneider and Fisk, 1939), is the principal method for assaying and serotyping BoNTs. In the currently used intraperitoneal mouse bioassay (Schantz and Kautter, 1978; Hatheway, 1988; Centers for Disease Control, 1998; Solomon et al., 2001), the LD50 for a 20 g mouse is ca. 7–12 pg for purified BoNT/A and is ca. 20–36 pg for BoNT/A-complex (Schantz and Johnson, 1992; Malizio et al., 2000). All seven serotypes of BoNTs have an intraperitoneal specific toxicity of $\sim 10^8$ LD50 per mg in mice (Sugiyama, 1980), but the toxicity for different animal species including humans varies markedly according to serotype and route of exposure (Morton, 1961; Schantz and Johnson, 1992).

The mouse bioassay has certain drawbacks including the need for large numbers of mice, 2–4 days to obtain definitive results and specimens such as stools and foods may contain lethal substances unrelated to BoNT (Hatheway, 1988). For example, pyridostigmine that had been administered to a patient originally thought to have myasthenia gravis was lethal to mice and presented difficulties in the diagnosis of botulism (Horowitz et al., 1976). Therefore, the assay must be carefully performed with proper controls and the use of serotype-specific antibodies to definitively identify the lethal substance as BoNT (Hatheway, 1988). Several other methods provide biological assays of BoNTs including neuronal cells, tissue preparations such as mouse or rat hemidiaphragm, and others (Habermann and Dreyer, 1986; Habermann, 1989; Johnson, 2005a; Pellett et al., 2007).

Most neurotoxigenic clostridia strains produce a single serotype of BoNT, while some strains produce more than one serotype or have silent unexpressed genes for a different serotype of BoNT (Hatheway, 1995; Franciosa et al., 2003; Johnson, 2005a). Recently, strains of C. botulinum have been recognized that produce subtypes of BoNT within a given serotype that differ substantially in amino acid composition, structure and biological activity compared to the primordial toxin (Smith et al., 2005; Arndt et al., 2006b). The serotypes of BoNT that cause human botulism are A, B, E and (rarely) F (Wright, 1955; Koenig, 1971; Woodruff et al., 1992; CDC, 1998; Sobel, 2005). All serotypes of BoNTs tested can cause botulism when administered intravenously or by inhalation and they differ markedly in potency by these routes (LeClaire and Pitt, 2005; Pitt and LeClaire, 2005). The different serotypes also vary in clinical properties including time to onset of symptoms, autonomic effects, severity and duration of the disease and time to recovery (Koenig, 1971; Woodruff et al., 1992; Hatheway and Dang, 1994; CDC, 1998). In general, BoNT/A causes the most severe and long-lasting and BoNT/E the shorter-lasting human botulism.

When BoNT/A-complex is injected in striated muscle, paresis commences within 2–8 days and lasts for 2–3 months when its effects begin to diminish (Dressler and Saberi, 2005; Johnson et al., 2006). The onset and duration of paralysis not only varies with toxin serotype and animal model, but also among patients. The extent of paresis is correlated with the dose of BoNT injected and these parameters can be optimized for the pathological condition to be treated

(Dressler and Rothwell, 2000). The duration of action shows a correlation primarily at low doses injected (Dressler and Saberi, 2005). When high doses are used, the duration appears to maximize at ~3 months for BoNT/A. Different preparations of BoNT/A and BoNT/B may have different potencies and therapeutic effects. Certain BoNT/A-complexes prepared and formulated by different methods are approved for clinical use and these appear to differ in their therapeutic efficacy (e.g., see recent review by Wenzel et al., 2007).

Some autonomic symptoms appear to be more prominent with BoNT/B than with BoNT/A (Dressler and Benecke, 2003). Autonomic effects between BoNT/A-complex and BTX/B-complex were compared in a double-blind, randomized trial in patients being treated for cervical dystonia (Tintner et al., 2005). BoNT/B-complex exhibited greater autonomic effects than BoNT/A-complex as indicated by decreased saliva production and increased severity of constipation, but not other autonomic functions such as orthostatic hypotension, heart rate or heart rate variation with respiration. Factors contributing to the difference in autonomic symptoms between the two serotypes may include the different quantities of BoNT/B to BoNT/A (50:1) used, which in turn determines toxin spreading from the site of injection, increased susceptibility of the cholinergic autonomic terminals to BoNT/B than BoNT/A and a greater systemic response to BoNT/B. One study in dogs indicated that BoNT/A-complex inhibited cholinergic ganglionic neurotransmission in dog heart (Tsuboi et al., 2002), but other studies showed no effects on heart rate (Claus et al., 1995; Meichsner and Reichel, 2005).

11.4. Toxicity and antitoxins

BoNTs are the most potent protein toxins known and their toxicity depends on the route of entry into the human body. They can enter the blood through the intestine, wounds and mucosal membranes. The estimated intravenous and intramuscular human lethal doses of BoNTs are 0.1–1 ng per kg body weight (Gill, 1982; Schantz and Johnson, 1992; Hatheway and Dang, 1994), whilst more than a one thousand times lower toxicity is detected using the oral route (Morton, 1961; Hatheway and Dang, 1994; Larson and Johnson, unpublished review 2005); for aerosol exposure, the lethal dose has been estimated to be 1–75 ng per kg depending on the serotype and efficiency of exposure (Pitt and LeClaire, 2005). These estimates are based mainly on primate exposure studies and investigations of quantities of toxin in foods implicated in foodborne botulism (Lamanna, 1959; Morton, 1961; Schantz and Johnson, 1992; Hatheway and Dang, 1994; Larson and

Johnson, unpublished review 2005). It is expected that infants and children have substantially increased sensitivity to intoxication due to the reduced size of certain NMJs, including those innervating the respiratory diaphragm, paralysis of which can be linked to death.

The number of BoNT molecules required to cause intoxication, morbidity and death of animals and humans is an intriguing subject. For example, when considered in terms of total body cells, it has been estimated that 20–70 ng or $\sim 8 \times 10^{10}$ to 3×10^{11} molecules of botulinum neurotoxin (molecular mass = 150 kDa) is sufficient to produce lethality in a ca. 70 kg adult human (Lamanna, 1959). It has been estimated that ca. 10 molecules of BoNT/A are sufficient to cause blockade of neurotransmitter releases at a NMJ (Boroff et al., 1974). It is well known that stimulation of nerve activity enhances the toxicity of BoNT in tissue preparations which can influence toxicity (Hughes and Whaler, 1962). It should be noted that much lower amounts of BoNTs are sufficient to lead to death of animals in the wilderness as even minor impairment of functions can be lethal, as in the case of the diplopia of birds with respect to flight and landing abilities. With the recent elucidation of receptor molecules for certain serotypes, it has become evident that presynaptic activity is necessary for uptake and poisoning of cells and nerves in vivo (reviewed in Verderio et al., 2006). Once synaptic activity subsides, additional BoNT cannot enter the poisoned neuron and will be directed to nonpoisoned nerve cells. Thus, *C. botulinum* has evolved a cunning means of pathogenesis through synthesis of BoNT, since when synaptic activity is shut down by intracellular toxin activity, uptake by poisoned nerves is also prevented and this in turn promotes spread of BoNT to active neurons.

Antitoxins to botulinum neurotoxins have been used extensively for characterization of BoNTs and for treatment of individuals with botulism (Tacket et al., 1984; Arnon et al., 2006). In 1897, Kempner first demonstrated that antitoxins against BoNT/A could be raised in goats by injection of inactivated crude botulinum toxin. His findings that BoNTs are antigenic proteins and that antitoxins against the toxins could reduce the severity of botulism has been confirmed and forms the mainstay of prophylaxis on intoxication (Kempner, 1897). Antitoxin antisera prepared against different BoNTs neutralize the homologous but not the heterologous serotype and a polyvalent antitoxin antiserum appears necessary for therapy. Antitoxins are presently used to confirm the identity of BoNTs and intravenous administration provides a first-line defense that is protective against botulism, lessens the symptoms and shortens the hospital stay (Tacket et al., 1984; Mayers et al., 2001; Chang and Ganguly, 2003; Arnon et al., 2006).

Recently, BabyBig® has been approved in the USA for administration to infants with botulism (Arnon et al., 2006).

Since botulism occurs rarely in humans, it is not practical to routinely immunize human populations. Natural immunity has not been observed in humans, even in individuals who have experienced repeated botulism. However, antibody formation is an important consideration in the treatment of humans with BoNT for therapeutic uses (Borodic, 2007). The possibility of developing an immune response is related to the quantity of antigen presented and the frequency of exposure (Hatheway and Dang, 1994; Borodic et al., 1996; Borodic, 2007). The dose of toxin required to elicit an antibody response is not known, yet clinical experience indicates that it is higher than the lethal dose. Humans who routinely handle BoNTs can be effectively immunized by pentavalent toxoid available from the CDC and other international governmental agencies (CDC, 1998).

11.5. General properties of botulinum neurotoxin

Biochemical and structural investigations of BoNT and TeNT and their domains have provided considerable insight into their evolution and mode of action (DasGupta, 1989; Schiavo et al., 2000; Hanson and Stevens, 2002; Swaminathan and Eswaramoorthy, 2002). BoNTs are synthesized as inactive single chain molecules of 150 kDa, that assume their characteristic high toxicity by proteolytic activation into a ca. 100 kDa heavy chain (HC) and a ca. 50 kDa light chain (LC) that remain linked by a single disulfide bond (DasGupta, 1989; Schiavo et al., 2000). Reduction of the disulfide bond is necessary for maximal catalytic activity in vitro and in vivo and may be a rate-limiting step in catalytic action (Schiavo et al., 1990; de Paiva et al., 1993; Antharavally et al., 1998). The carboxy-terminus HC comprises the structural domain for receptor binding to gangliosides and to proteins (Schiavo et al., 2000; Nishikawa et al., 2004; Chai et al., 2006; Jin et al., 2006; Uotso et al., 2006; Baldwin and Barbieri, 2007) and the N-terminus of the HC contains the function for channel formation and translocation of the LC from endosomes to the neuronal cytosol (Hoch et al., 1985; Schiavo et al., 2000; Koriazova and Montal, 2003). The LC is a Zn^{2+}-dependent endopeptidase that selectively cleaves neuronal substrates involved in synaptic vesicle trafficking and membrane fusion (Montecucco and Schiavo, 1995; Schiavo et al., 2000).

BoNTs occur naturally in toxin complexes, commonly referred to as progenitor toxins (Sakaguchi, 1983; Schantz and Johnson, 1992; Johnson and Bradshaw, 2001). In these complexes, BoNT is associated with non-toxic proteins, primarily non-toxic non-hemagglutinin (NTNH), hemagglutinin in certain serotypes, uncharacterized proteins and RNA (Sakaguchi, 1983; Schantz and Johnson, 1992; Inoue et al., 1996; Johnson and Bradshaw, 2001; Dineen et al., 2003, 2004). The structure of the complexes seems dependent upon the genetic composition and expression of the complex components (Sakaguchi, 1983; Johnson and Bradshaw, 2001; Dineen et al., 2003, 2004) as well as purification methods (Sakaguchi, 1983; Schantz and Johnson, 1992). The biochemical, biophysical and structural aspects of the toxin complexes are only beginning to become known (Hanson and Stevens, 2002). The non-toxic proteins in the complexes provide protection during experimental manipulations and from acid and proteases during passage through the gastrointestinal tract (Sugii et al., 1977; Sakaguchi, 1983; Schantz and Johnson, 1992). The different complexes also differ in their safety margins and therapeutic indexes from the perspective as a protein drug for human treatment (Aoki, 2002; Yoneda et al., 2005).

Purified BoNTs can be purified from the toxin complexes by established techniques (DasGupta and Rasmussen, 1983; DasGupta and Sathyamoorthy, 1984; Malizio et al., 2000). An important factor contributing to the structure and function of BoNTs has been the availability of highly purified neurotoxins free of accessory proteins, contaminating proteases or other enzymes. The isolated neurotoxin can be unstable, prone to aggregation, zinc removal, protease modification and auto-fragmentation under certain conditions (DasGupta and Dekleva, 1990; DasGupta et al., 2005; DasGupta, 2006; Keller, 2006; Paik et al., 2006). The loss of activity of BoNTs has negatively affected in vitro and animal studies as well as use of BoNTs for therapy (Schantz and Johnson, 1992; Gartlan and Hoffman, 1993; McLellan et al., 1996).

Three-dimensional structures have been obtained by crystallography for the holotoxins of types BoNT/A and BoNT/B in solution (Lacy and Stevens, 1999; Swaminathan and Eswaramoorthy, 2000, 2002; Hanson and Stevens, 2002) and for all seven serotypes of L chains (not including subtypes) (e.g., Arndt et al., 2006a). The structure of BoNT/A was initially achieved by Stevens and colleagues in 1998 at 3.3-Å resolution (Lacy et al., 1998) (Fig. 11.1) and BoNT/B by Swaminathan and colleagues in 2000 at 1.8-Å (Swaminathan and Eswaramoorthy, 2000). BoNT/A and BoNT/B have similar structures consisting of three distinct domains (Lacy and Stevens, 1999; Swaminathan and Eswaramoorthy, 2000, 2002; Hanson and Stevens, 2002). These domains represent the carboxy terminus of the heavy chain (HCC) (binding domain),

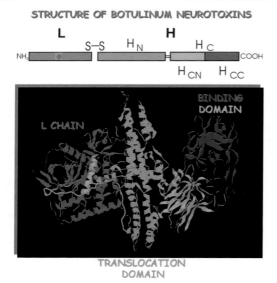

Fig. 11.1. Linear depiction (top) and three-dimensional structure (bottom) of the 150 kDa botulinum neurotoxin type A. The toxin is produced as a single chain protein, which is activated to the di-chain form by proteolysis. Three primary domains, receptor binding domain, translocation domain and the catalytic domain, are present in the neurotoxin.

amino terminus of the heavy chain (HCN) (translocation or channel domain) and the light chain (LC) (catalytic domain). The structural depiction of functional domains is consistent with the toxic activity of the BoNTs determined by various biochemical and physiological approaches and with its mechanism of cell intoxication. The major differences in 3-D structure between the two serotypes are mainly in the receptor binding and catalytic domains, which are anticipated by the differences in the amino acid sequences in these regions and their known binding to different protein receptors and catalytic activity on different SNARE proteins. Subtle differences in the translocation domain and the belt surrounding the catalytic site have also been recognized. The structure complexity has increased with the findings of subtypes of BoNTs (Smith et al., 2005; Arndt et al., 2006b) and it will be interesting to determine whether these newly found subtypes have biological properties that are distinct from the prototype BoNTs, thus increasing the pathogenic spectrum of BoNTs.

11.6. Clinical aspects

11.6.1. Types of botulism

The primary target of BoNTs is the NMJ of the peripheral nervous system and BoNT also binds to preganglionic sympathetic and parasympathetic nerve endings, postganglionic parasympathetic nerve endings and efferent motor nerve endings (Simpson, 2000). Botulism is a blood-borne toxicosis and the susceptibility of animals to different serotypes varies considerably across species. In humans, the primary serotypes of BoNT responsible for botulism are A, B, E and, rarely, F. The different forms of botulism have been categorized mainly by the route by which BoNT enters the bloodstream and the age of the subject. The times of onset, duration of action, symptoms and clinical course varies depending on the serotype of BoNT and the type of botulism, with serotype A causing a more dangerous and long-lasting disease.

11.6.2. Foodborne botulism

Foodborne botulism is caused by the consumption of pre-formed BoNT-complexes in foods. In some foodborne outbreaks, several persons are intoxicated by sharing contaminated food which can be of value in recognizing an outbreak, while the majority of outbreaks affect a single person (CDC, 1998; Shapiro et al., 1998; Sobel et al., 2004). In the United States, botulism is one of the most precisely recognized foodborne illnesses, since all hospitalized cases must be reported to the Centers for Disease Control and Prevention in Atlanta (CDC, 1998). Fortunately, foodborne botulism is quite rare worldwide, but similar to other acute diseases it is undoubtedly under-reported in that mild cases probably are not diagnosed (Woodruff et al., 1992). Certain countries currently do not have adequate public health facilities for botulism diagnosis and treatment, but efforts are being made to develop surveillance and treatment programs in these areas (Shapiro et al., 1998; Villar et al., 1999). The establishment of networks to provide access to botulinum antitoxins could also reduce morbidity and mortality (Abgueguen et al., 2003).

The incidence of foodborne botulism varies markedly by geographic region worldwide (Hauschild and Dodds, 1993; Hatheway, 1995; Johnson and Goodnough, 1998; Shapiro et al., 1998; Sobel, 2005). This regional incidence is related to the serotype and prevalence of spores in the soil and associated foods, as well as food preservation and consumption practices within a region. The principal regions of the world with reported foodborne botulism have been reviewed (Hauschild and Dodds, 1993; Johnson and Goodnough, 1998). Worldwide, case fatality rates from foodborne botulism have been estimated to range from 5–15%, with a mean of 10% (Varma et al., 2004). In the United States, type A has caused the most severe botulism and incidence of fatalities (5–7% deaths), compared to types B and E (1–3% deaths). The incidence and characteristics of foodborne botulism in the United Kingdom (McLauchlin et al., 2006), Thailand (Ungchusak et al.,

2007), South Africa (Arntzen et al., 2004), Republic of Georgia (Varma et al., 2004) and Argentina (Villar et al., 1999) have recently been described. With an increasingly globalized food supply and changes in food consumption, countries are observing types of botulism previously uncommon for that region (e.g., Boyer et al., 2001).

11.6.3. Wound botulism

Wound botulism results from the infection of a wound with *C. botulinum* and subsequent localized production of BoNT in the wound and its entry into the blood-stream (Dezfulian, 1989; Maselli et al., 1997; Werner et al., 2000; Gordon and Lowy, 2005). Wound botu-lism is suspected following trauma or a superficial wound without obvious infection and no history of consumption of botulinogenic food. Although adult tetanus and wound botulism occur under similar pre-disposing conditions, wound botulism is much more rare than tetanus, even though the general population is not immunized against BoNT. *C. botulinum* strains appear to have a weak ability to grow in wounds compared to C. tetani. Like other forms of botulism, wound botulism is quite rare and only about 1000 cases have been reported since its recognition in 1943 (Davis, 1951; Werner et al., 2000). Wound botu-lism has recently increased in incidence and geogra-phical distribution due to its association with intranasal use of cocaine and subcutaneous injection of heroin (MacDonald et al., 1986; Elston et al., 1991; Werner et al., 2000). An unfortunate case of wound botulism was reported in a 5-year-old boy who died from toxin produced in a tooth abscess (Weber et al., 1993). Most wound botulism cases are caused by *C. botulinum* type A producing BoNT/A in the wound, which is absorbed into the bloodstream. A distinguishing feature of wound botulism compared to foodborne botulism is the longer incubation time of 4–14 days (Merson and Dowell, 1973), presumably reflecting the need for *C. botulinum* to colonize the wound and grow to sufficient levels to produce quanti-ties of toxin required for illness.

Rare cases of wound botulism cases have occurred following intestinal surgery and disruption of the integrity of the intestine and composition of intestinal microflora (Chia et al., 1986; McCroskey and Hathe-way, 1991). This form of botulism was initially sus-pected in a patient who had undergone ileojejunal bypass for obesity (English et al., 1981). Botulinum toxin is produced in these intestinal lesions and absorbed into the blood. Since wound botulism is rare, misdiagnosis and delay or failure in treatment have been encountered (Werner et al., 2000; Reller et al.,

2006). Like other forms of botulism, predictors of sur-vival in wound botulism are rapid diagnosis, prompt administration of antitoxin and mechanical venti-lation for persons with respiratory failure (Werner et al., 2000; Sandrock and Murin, 2001; Reller et al., 2006).

11.6.4. Infant botulism

In 1976, infant botulism was suspected in two babies in California that had clinical signs of weakness char-acteristic of floppy babies (Pickett et al., 1976). The clinical diagnosis of botulism was confirmed by the detection of *C. botulinum* and BoNT in the feces of the suspected infants (Midura and Arnon, 1976). Initi-ally, it was considered that the babies had consumed food containing preformed BoNT, but such a food source could not be identified (Midura and Arnon, 1976; Marx, 1978). In vivo formation of BoNT in the intestine and absorption of BoNT into the blood was hypothesized (Midura and Arnon, 1976; Pickett et al., 1976). Subsequently it was recognized that infant botulism occurs from the ingestion of spores of neurotoxigenic clostridia that germinate, multiply and produce BoNT in the intestinal tract of the baby. BoNT is then absorbed through the intestine and enters the general circulation and is carried to peripheral cholinergic synapses. Thus, infant botulism is a type of infection rather than a true intoxication as in food-borne botulism. Infant botulism is not a new disease and retrospective analyses of idiopathic floppy baby syndromes indicated that it has occurred for many years (Arnon et al., 1979).

Infant botulism is now recognized as the most com-mon cause of botulism in the USA, with about 70 hos-pitalized cases annually (Arnon, 2004; Sobel, 2005). Nearly half of the cases have been reported from Cali-fornia, probably due to the relatively high incidence of type A *C. botulinum* spores and the vigorous surveil-lance program for infant botulism in this state (Arnon, 2004). Infant botulism has been documented world-wide in all populated continents except Africa (Arnon, 2004). Certain risk factors have been identified includ-ing feeding of honey, which can be contaminated with spores (Tanzi and Gabay, 2002). Dust and other envir-onmental sources are also known to harbor *C. botuli-num* spores (Nevas et al., 2005). Infant botulism has occurred in distinct geographic regions, probably due to the incidence of spores and other factors such as genetic disposition (Long et al., 1985; Arnon, 2004). Nearly all cases of infant botulism are caused by *C. botulinum* strains producing BoNT/A and BoNT/B. In the United States, infant botulism caused by type A is most common in the Western United States, whilst type B has been prevalent in regions of the Eastern United States (Long et al., 1985; Arnon, 2004). The severity of infant botulism varies according to the serotype of BoNT, with BoNT/A generally causing a more severe and long-lasting disease-syndrome than BoNT/B (Arnon, 2004).

Neurotoxigenic strains of *Clostridium butyricum* and *Clostridium baratii* producing variants of BoNT/E and BoNT/F, respectively, have also been implicated in infant botulism in the United States, Italy and other regions of the world (Hatheway, 1993, 1995; Franciosa et al., 2003). Neurotoxigenic *C. butyricum* and *C. baratii* have recently been detected in expanding geographical regions and may be associated with foodborne as well as infant botulism. Atypical neurotoxigenic variant strains have mostly been isolated from intestinal botulism (Tabita et al., 1991; Hatheway, 1995). These findings suggest that the intestinal tract under certain conditions may be a permissive environment for gene exchange and for evolution of new variants of neurotoxigenic clostridia and it is likely that more neurotoxigenic species may be discovered from this source in the future.

The ability of *C. botulinum* to colonize infants is probably related to perturbations of intestinal flora during infancy and during weaning, as well as the presence of inhibitory factors such as bile acids and innate immunity (Arnon, 2004). The study of *C. botulinum* colonization in animal models has supported the notion that the ability to colonize is dependent on the number and species of competitor microbes present in the intestinal tract, particularly the large bowel (Sugiyama and Mills, 1978; Sugiyama, 1979; Arnon, 2004). Infant botulism usually affects babies 1–6 months of age, but can also manifest only a few hours after birth and (rarely) as long as 10–12 months of age (Arnon, 2004; Fox et al., 2005; Keet et al., 2005). The median age at onset is 10–12 weeks and 95% of the cases have occurred prior to 6 months of age, although cases have been observed up to 10 months (Arnon, 2004; Fox et al., 2005). The illness affects both sexes and all major ethnic and racial groups (Arnon, 2004).

The severity of the clinical syndrome may vary from relatively mild observed in outpatients who show minor weakness and failure to thrive to a rapid and fatal illness resembling sudden infant death syndrome (SIDS) (Arnon et al., 1981; Byard et al., 1992; Böhnel et al., 2001; Bartram and Singer, 2004; Böhnel and Gessler, 2005; Fox et al., 2005; Mitchell and Tseng-Ong, 2005; Nevas et al., 2005). It has been postulated that fulminant cases of botulism may be responsible for a small percentage (5%) of sudden infant death syndrome cases (Marx, 1978; Arnon et al., 1981; Bartram and Singer, 2004; Fischer et al., 2004; Böhnel

and Gessler, 2005). The involvement of infant botulism in SIDS has been a matter of considerable debate. Recent clinical data indicate that rapid onset infant botulism can be a catastrophic presentation of the disease, but with rapid recovery (Keet et al., 2005; Nevas et al., 2005; Tseng-Ong and Mitchell, 2005). Rapid onset of infant botulism has also occurred by BoNT/F produced by *C. baratii* in extremely young patients (9 and 14 days old) (Hoffman et al., 1982; Paisley et al., 1995). The typical presentation of infant botulism is familiar to most pediatric neurologists, but atypical symptoms and sudden and severe features may be obscure or delay the diagnosis (Keet et al., 2005; Mitchell and Tseng-Ong, 2005). Complications of infant botulism during hospitalization and treatment have included sepsis, otitis media, aspiration pneumonia, inappropriate secretion of antidiuretic hormone and adult respiratory distress syndrome (Long et al., 1985). Muscle and nerve biopsies were performed on an infant with botulism, which helped to exclude myopathy or metabolic causes of paralysis (Keet et al., 2005). Studies in animals have demonstrated atrophy of muscle fibers in severe botulism cases, which regenerated during the recovery phase. It has been suggested that chronic neuropathic changes may persist following botulism (Keet et al., 2005), but further investigation is needed in this area to confirm this observation.

11.6.5. Intestinal botulism in adolescents and adults

Intestinal botulism has also occurred in susceptible adolescents and adults, especially following intestinal surgery and antibiotic administration, which can alter the gut's microbial ecology and predispose the patient to colonization and possibly provide wounds for colonization. Infections by *C. botulinum* in adults has been supported by the finding of botulinum toxin and organisms in the feces over a several month period (Hatheway, 1995). Intense immunosuppression and bowel sterilizing regimens in a 3-year-old girl with neuroblastoma were postulated to enable colonization by *C. botulinum* types A and B with ensuing infant botulism (Shen et al., 1994). An intestinal botulism case in a 12-year-old girl associated with an unusual strain of *C. botulinum* type Ab was reported in Japan (Kobayashi et al., 2003).

In foodborne cases, a slow onset of botulism symptoms and a long delay of toxin detection in serum and stool may predispose adults to colonization of the large bowel with *C. botulinum* spores. Thus, there may be a transition between different forms of botulism. In a foodborne case involving chopped garlic in oil that contained type BoNT/B and *C. botulinum* type B, relatively mild and progressive development of botulism occurred over several weeks in patients containing type B toxin and organisms (St. Louis et al., 1988). In a foodborne botulism case occurring in France, type B toxin was found in serum from individuals for up to 122 days after ingestion of toxic food (Sebald and Saimot, 1973). These observations suggest that *C. botulinum* type B could colonize the intestine of adults and continue to produce toxin over several weeks to months. *C. botulinum* type B may have a greater ability than type A to colonize the intestinal tract, which likely explains why more than 50% of the infant botulism cases in the USA involve type B, while type A foodborne botulism is three times more prevalent than type B. The ecology of intestinal botulism is complex and the disease may involve more than one species of toxigenic clostridia including C. difficile, C. perfringens, *C. botulinum*, *C. baratii* and *C. butyricum* that produce various toxins and change the gut flora. C. difficile colonization was found in cases of infant botulism (Schechter et al., 1999), suggesting that certain permissive conditions may promote intestinal colonization by pathogenic clostridia.

11.6.6. Botulism of undetermined etiology

Botulism of undetermined etiology refers to diagnosed cases in patients 1 year of age or older in whom no plausible food vehicle or intestinal or wound colonization can be demonstrated (Bartlett, 1986; Hatheway, 1993; Sobel et al., 2004). *C. botulinum* and its toxin have been observed in the stools of these patients for long time periods (3 weeks and in some cases up to 6 months) (Hatheway, 1993). This form of the disease has occurred in adults following colonization of the digestive tract by *C. botulinum* with production of BoNT and these infections may follow surgery or other procedures that disrupt the GI microflora or inflict intestinal wounds (Chia et al., 1986; Hatheway, 1993). Intestinal botulism and endogenous antibody production occurred in an adult with underlying Crohn's disease (Griffin et al., 1997). Intestinal botulism was also observed in a 3-year-old female with neuroblastoma following autologous bone marrow transplantation, possibly indicating immune suppression leading to susceptibility to botulism (Shen et al., 1994). Following an incident of foodborne botulism in a 12-year-old girl, obstinate constipation was endured for more than 6 months and *C. botulinum* and BoNT/A was detected in stool specimens for several months (Kobayashi et al., 2003). These cases indicate that intestinal colonization by *C. botulinum* can occur following foodborne botulism.

11.6.7. Inhalational botulism

Owing to their high toxicity, BoNTs have been considered as biological weapons including as aerosol preparations (Franz et al., 1993; Bigalke and Rummel, 2005; LeClaire and Pitt, 2005; Pitt and LeClaire, 2005). Since respiratory exposure is not a known natural route of intoxication, virtually no human data on susceptibility are available (Pitt and LeClaire, 2005). Exposure of non-human primates has demonstrated that intoxication can occur by the respiratory route through mucosal membranes (Pitt and LeClaire, 2005). As with foodborne botulism, crude toxin complexes are more potent than purified BoNTs. The toxicity varies with serotype and BoNT/F and BoNT/C appear to be slightly more toxic than BoNT/A (LeClaire and Pitt, 2005; Pitt and LeClaire, 2005). Extrapolations from animal data suggest that BoNT is exceedingly potent by the aerosol route with an estimate LD50 of 1–75 ng per kg with the potency decreasing in the following order: BoNT/F > BoNT/C = BoNT/A > BoNT/D >> BoNT/B in rhesus macaques; no data are available for BoNT/E and BoNT/G (LeClaire and Pitt, 2005; Pitt and LeClaire, 2005). Respiratory failure occurred in 5 hours to 2 days with 90% lethality. A case of human botulism was attributed to inhalation of BoNT in a laboratory accident (Holzer, 1962).

11.6.8. Iatrogenic botulism

Iatrogenic botulism, sometimes referred to as inadvertent botulism, refers to botulism resulting from therapeutic use of botulinum toxin (Chertow et al., 2006). Rare cases of systemic weakness and botulism have been observed in patients treated with BoNT for medicinal purposes (Bakheit et al., 1997; Bhatia et al., 1999; Duffey and Brown, 2006). Quantitation of systemic weakness was assessed in a 34-year-old amateur weight-lifter treated for a gait disorder (Duffey and Brown, 2006). Although the gait disorder was successfully treated with 1000 units (11 U/kg) of BoNT/A-complex, the individual experienced 35–50% reduction in upper body strength, which resolved over a period of ~12 weeks. This case illustrates the possibility that locally injected BoNT may spread systemically and cause generalized weakness. Recently, four cases of iatrogenic botulism were acquired in patients treated for cosmetic purposes with BoNT that had not been approved by the FDA (Chertow et al., 2006). The patients may have been injected with as much as 8 million U of

BoNT/A-complex, which is 2857 times the estimated lethal dose for humans. Available evidence indicates that the toxin was obtained from a wholesale source and was repackaged and marketed at a bargain price. This occurrence emphasizes the potency of toxin and extreme care and scrutiny must be taken in the use of BoNT in medical practice.

This recent incident of iatrogenic botulism provided vivid evidence of the course of severe botulism in humans (Chertow et al., 2006). Initially, four suspected cases of botulism were reported to the Centers for Disease Control and Prevention on November 4, 2004. The patients had been injected with a highly concentrated, unlicensed preparation of botulinum neurotoxin type A for treatment of wrinkles. The vial used to treat the patients contained ~100 µg of BoNT/A, which is an amount estimated to be sufficient to kill more than 1000 adult humans if disseminated evenly. A fatal case of botulism was suspected due to a lidocaine-BoNT-complex mixture (Li et al., 1999), although the presence of human serum albumin could have also caused an immunologic reaction.

11.6.9. Animal botulism

Botulism commonly strikes domestic and wild animal populations, particularly birds and fish, where it can cause devastating epidemics with deaths of thousands to millions of animals (Smith and Sugiyama, 1988; Eklund, 1995; Lindström et al., 2004; Yule et al., 2006), and is the most prevalent form of botulism worldwide. BoNTs types C, D and F are involved as well as A, B and E, as seen in human botulism. Botulism of domestic animals not only causes economic losses but it is also a risk factor for BoNT transmission to humans. Food contaminated with BoNT has also been shown to cause botulism in various domestic or captive animals such as cattle, horses, lions and monkeys (Smith and Sugiyama, 1988). Depending on the animal species, botulism can be caused by contaminated food or water, ingestion of forage poisoned with BoNT from dead animals or by colonization of the intestinal tract by *C. botulinum*. Among fish and birds, botulism outbreaks can involve millions of cases and the diseases may take the appearance of an epidemic because insect larvae grow in the decomposing cadavers and accumulate BoNT, which is non-toxic to the invertebrates. Birds and fish are eager to eat the larvae and consequently become intoxicated and die, providing a rich anaerobic medium for the growth of *C. botulinum* and with consequent toxin accumulation in insect eggs and larvae. A self-perpetuating and escalating cycle is thus established and many animals can die rapidly, particularly among dense populations. In regions where animal botulism is common, animals often carry *C. botulinum* in their digestive tract which rapidly grows in the cadavers and becomes highly toxic and rich in spores (Smith and Sugiyama, 1988).

11.7. Clinical presentation

Irrespective of the type of botulism, the primary clinical signs are similar:

- Symmetrical cranial neuropathies;
- Difficulty swallowing, dry mouth, difficulty speaking, facial ptosis;
- Blurred near vision, blurred distant vision, dilated or non-reactive pupils, diplopia, drooping eyelids;
- Descending bilateral flaccid paralysis, generalized muscle weakness progressing to neck, limbs and torso.

The characteristic symptoms of botulism can principally be ascribed to the blockade of neurotransmission at neuromuscular junctions of skeletal muscle, with ensuing flaccid paralysis (Dickson, 1918; Koenig, 1971; Tacket and Rogawski, 1989; Cherington, 1998, 2004). The incubation period from exposure to BoNTs to onset of symptoms ranges from a few hours to as long as 10 days, but typically present within 12–72 hours in foodborne botulism (Hatheway and Dang, 1994; Cherington, 1998, 2004). The incubation period in foodborne botulism is inversely correlated with the quantity of toxin ingested (Gangarosa et al., 1971). The incubation time for wound and infant botulism is usually several days due to the time needed for *C. botulinum* to colonize the wound or intestine and produce toxin that is then absorbed into the circulation. There have been notable exceptions of rapid onset and rapid recovery (Fox et al., 2005; Keet et al., 2005). The time to onset for inhalational botulism has been reported to be 12–80 hours based on limited non-human primate experiments (LeClaire and Pitt, 2005).

After absorption into the blood, the neurotoxin binds to motor nerve endings as well as to parasympathetic nerve endings that release ACh and cause flaccid paralysis and preganglionic and parasympathetic postganglionic autonomic blockade. The first indications are usually bulbar and ocular weakness and generalized fatigue. The ocular symptoms include diplopia, mydriasis and loss of the light reflex and of accommodation. Occasionally there is also anisocoria. As the intoxication proceeds, weakness of the levator palpebrae and facial muscles becomes noticeable; speech becomes slurred and eventually anarthria ensues. Paralysis of pharyngeal, laryngeal and masticatory muscles results in dysphagia, dysphonia, stridor, nasal regurgitation of liquids and a sensation of suffocation or actual suffocation. Paralysis of the facial muscles give the patient a dull appearance and they become unable to respond to stimuli. Weakness of the respiratory muscles and particularly of the diaphragm can result in respiratory failure and death. Descending weakness progresses for 4–8 days and then plateaus. Vomiting and abdominal pain may precede or follow the paralysis. The non-ocular autonomic symptoms include decreased salivation and a dry mouth, anhydrosis, particularly of the palms and the soles, obstipation, urinary retention and cardiovascular instability. The body temperature is generally normal or slightly subnormal. Representative portrayals of mild and severe botulism are shown in Fig. 11.2.

Despite the involvement of cranial nerves, most cases do not show cognitive or sensory abnormalities. The face often has an expression-less or sagging appearance because of the relaxed tone of the facial muscles. In severe cases the patient lies helpless, resembling a generalized paralysis or coma. The tendon reflexes are intact or slightly decreased. The patient may be able to initiate effective muscular contraction such as opening the eyes or raising the head or an extremity once or twice but cannot repeat the act. The inability of the patient to express their discomfort can cause hysterical attacks and mental depression. Occasionally patients experience a headache, which can persist. It is unusual for the patient to suffer any pain. Dryness of the mouth and impaired salivary and lacrimal secretions can persist for several months (Jenzer et al., 1975; Goode and Shearn, 1982; Dressler and Benecke, 2003; Chertow et al., 2006). The severe muscular weakness, the anxiety and helplessness, the difficulty in swallowing, the attacks of strangling, the struggle for breath and the unsuccessful attempts to articulate constitute an unforgettable clinical picture.

The progressive muscle weakening is a striking hallmark of botulism. Humans with mild cases of botulism also may exhibit poor coordination of the arms and legs. The patient becomes gradually weaker, fatigued and finally death occurs, generally by respiratory failure (Gangarosa et al., 1971; Koenig, 1971; Tacket and Ragawski, 1989; Shapiro et al., 1998). The requirement for endotracheal intubation and ventilatory support is an indicator of the severity of the disease in patients (Woodruff et al., 1992; Hatheway and Dang, 1994; Sandrock and Murin, 2001; Anderson et al., 2002). Woodruff et al. (1992) found that intubation was necessary for 67% of patients with type A botulism, 52% with type B and 39% with type E. Of patients that were intubated, 72% represented isolated cases, while only 54% were intubated from outbreak-associated illness. This suggests that certain patients with mild cases of botulism are often not hospitalized and may remain undiagnosed.

The severity of symptoms and duration of botulism in cell and animal models depends on the serotype of BoNT. In cultured primary neuronal cells

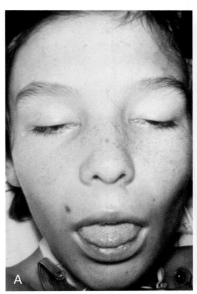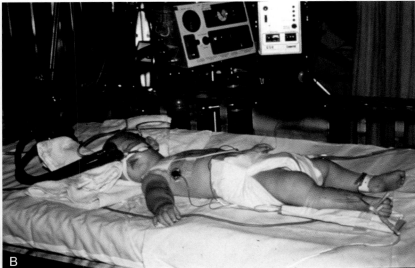

Fig. 11.2. Portrayal of typical symptoms of mild and severe botulism. (A) Photograph of boy is from the CDC collection and provided by Charles Hatheway (deceased). (B) Photograph of infant is courtesy of Stephen Arnon.

(Keller et al., 1999), animal models (Adler et al., 2001; Billante et al., 2002; Foran et al., 2003; Keller, 2006) and in humans with natural botulism or treated for medicinal purposes (Sellin et al., 1983a, b; Sloop et al., 1997; Brin et al., 2002; Eleopra et al., 2004; Gupta et al., 2005) the severity and duration of symptoms relates to the type of toxin in the following order: BoNT/A = BoNT/C1 > BoNT/B > BoNT/F > BoNT/E in cultured primary neuronal cells (Keller et al., 1999), in animal models (Adler et al., 2001; Billante et al., 2002; Foran et al., 2003; Keller, 2006) (Table 11.1) and in humans with natural botulism or after being treated for medicinal purposes (Sellin et al., 1983a, b; Sloop et al., 1997; Brin et al., 2002; Eleopra et al., 2004; Gupta et al., 2005).

Although the different forms of botulism show similar clinical signs and symptoms, there are certain distinctions. Early in foodborne botulism, patients may have gastrointestinal symptoms such as nausea, vomiting, abdominal cramps and diarrhea (Hughes et al., 1981). These symptoms are probably not due to BoNT but from food contaminants. Infant botulism differs from other forms of botulism in the ages of the affected individuals and the infection process by neurotoxigenic clostridia within the large bowel. The incubation period is often several days to weeks, reflecting the ability of *C. botulinum* to colonize, grow and produce toxin within the large intestine. In some infants an acute onset over several hours is followed by rapid recovery (Keet et al., 2005). The disease usually begins with severe constipation lasting 3 days or longer that precedes the appearance of other neurologic signs

by one or more days (Arnon, 2004). Following constipation, the infant develops cranial nerve palsies resulting in oculomotor weakness, eyelid ptosis, a weak suck and hypotonia. In the more severe cases, the infant becomes lethargic and loses head control. The disease progresses to a generalized flaccid paralysis which may involve the respiratory muscles and culminate in apnea. Type A toxin is associated with greater morbidity and a slower recovery than type B or E toxin (Arnon, 2004).

11.8. Diagnosis of botulism

The diagnosis of botulism relies on the clinical findings which include prominent oculobulbar signs and laboratory detection of BoNT from appropriate specimens (Table 11.2) (Hughes et al., 1981; Cherington, 1998, 2004; Shapiro et al., 1998; Arnon, 2004). The initial diagnosis of botulism is based on the characteristic clinical presentation as described in the previous section (CDC, 1998; Cherington, 1998, 2004).

The definitive laboratory diagnosis of botulism requires detection of BoNT in plasma, serum and gastrointestinal contents (stool and vomitus) and food or other sources by the mouse bioassay as described above. Isolation of *C. botulinum* from foods and clinical specimens including vomitus and feces is also supportive in the diagnosis of botulism (Hatheway, 1988; CDC, 1998). Since botulism is a rare disease, toxin and organism diagnostic tests should be performed in a suitable reference laboratory that has the necessary experience and reference toxins, antitoxins and standard cultures for the procedures, such as the Communicable Disease Center National Botulism Laboratory (404-639-2206; 404-639-2888) or qualified local and state public health laboratories (http://www.cdc.gov/other.htm#states or http://www.astho.org/state.html).

Regrettably, for many botulism cases, laboratory studies are of no aid in establishing a diagnosis since the sensitivity of detection of BoNT decreases rapidly

Table 11.1

Potencies and durations of different serotypes of botulinum neurotoxins (BoNTs) acting on cerebellar granule neurons from rats

BoNT[a] blockade of transmitter release	BoNT concentration causing 50% of inhibition [pico Molar (pM)]	Duration (t1/2) (days ± SD)
BoNT/A	10	>>31
BoNT/B	100	9.84 ± 2.12
BoNT/C1	13	>>25
BoNT/E	43	0.73 ± 0.11
BoNT/F	1350	1.76 ± 0.28
TeNT	6.5	Not studied

[a]BoNTs were purified as 150 kDa BoNTs and were completely activated.
After Foran et al. (2003).

Table 11.2

Diagnosis of botulism

Clinical diagnosis	Recognition of clinical symptoms and signs
	Neurological examination, including electromyography
Laboratory confirmation	Demonstration of botulinal neurotoxin in serum, stool, gastric aspirate, or food.
	Culturing *C. botulinum* from stool, wound, or food

with time (Koenig, 1971; Woodruff et al., 1992). Due to delays in specimen collection and analysis or to the presence of mouse lethal substances in samples other than BoNT, laboratory detection of BoNT is often not conclusive (a positive test is present in ~30% of samples obtained more than 2 days after toxin exposure) (Cherington, 1998). A detailed survey of 494 cases of foodborne botulism in the United States from 1975–1988 illustrates the complexities of a definitive diagnosis of botulism (Woodruff et al., 1992). In this study, BoNT/A caused botulism illness in 148 patients (48%), type B in 89 (29%) and type E in 72 (23%). Among the type B outbreaks, 55 cases occurred from a single restaurant outbreak and affected patients mostly under 40 years of age (Terranova et al., 1978), whereas the largest outbreaks for type A and E affected 27 and seven persons, respectively. The median onset period for all patients was 1 day (ranges: type A, 0–7 days; type B, 0–5 days; type E, 0–2 days). Overall, type E patients had the shortest incubation period and type B patients the longest. Type A patients were more likely to require intubation. Of the 105 patients with an onset time of less than 1 day, 59% required intubation and artificial respiration compared to 44% of the 54 patients with longer incubaton periods. Overall, the greater severity of botulism of the reported sporadic cases suggests that sporadic cases are frequently misdiagnosed or not reported to health authorities (Woodruff et al., 1992).

Of patients for which adequate clinical specimens were submitted to the CDC, 67% were confirmed as having botulism by toxin assay or culture. Specimens from patients with type A botulism were more frequently positive for toxin in serum and stool than were those patients with types B and E botulism (Woodruff et al., 1992). BoNT testing results were positive in 126 (37%) of 349 sera and 65 (23%) of 288 stool samples; 27 stool samples gave non-specific deaths in the mouse bioassay (these samples were not neutralized by antitoxin). Serum toxin assays were more likely to be positive if sera were collected soon after toxin ingestion; BoNT was detected in >60% of serum samples obtained during the first 2 days but in only 13–28% of specimens obtained thereafter. Similarly, BoNT was detected in 50% of stool samples obtained within 1 day, but in <20% after 5 days. These results support the notion that different types of botulinal toxins produce distinct clinical manifestations and are diagnosed in the laboratory with different degrees of success. Type A botulism is more severe, as indicated by the increased need for intubation. However, type E botulism patients had the shortest incubation period. These observations are consistent with other studies using indicators of severity other than respiratory support (USPHS, 1979; Hughes et al., 1981; CDC, 1998).

The clinical and pharmacokinetic mechanisms governing these differences are not clear. It is not known if there are race differences in toxin absorption, activation and stability or action. However, short incubation times are common in type E cases and were mostly observed in Alaskan Natives. An investigation of a type B outbreak recorded more severe illness among patients of Chinese descent (St. Louis et al., 1988). After intraperitoneal injection of mice, the onset of symptoms was most rapid with type E toxin and slowest with type B toxin (Sugiyama, 1980; Woodruff et al., 1992). In rats, larger doses of types B and E than type A toxin are required to induce paralysis (Sellin et al., 1983a, b). The administration of antitoxin as well as the pharmacokinetics of absorption, distribution through the lymphatic system and rate and affinity of binding to and internalization within target nerves (Habermann and Dreyer, 1986) likely affect the chance of detecting BoNT in serum samples. The toxin titers in clinical specimens are often too little to definitively confirm the presence of BoNT with serotype specific antisera. Detection of neurotoxigenic organisms also supports the diagnosis, but a positive culture alone does not confirm it since spores are ubiquitously distributed and can be occasionally isolated from the stools of healthy humans and from foods and other environmental sources (Hatheway, 1988; CDC, 1998; Shapiro et al., 1998).

Electrodiagnostic testing can provide presumptive evidence of botulism and is particularly useful in those patients with clinical signs of botulism but with negative mouse bioassay results (Hatheway and Dang, 1994; Cherington, 1998, 2004; Dumitru et al., 2002; Crawford, 2003). EMG abnormalities are observed as the disease progresses but may not be present at onset of symptoms. The amplitude of the compound muscle action potential (CMAP) gradually decreases in the clinically affected muscles, but motor and sensory nerve conduction are usually normal. The most common electrophysiological abnormality in an affected muscle is a low amplitude CMAP in response to a single supra-maximal nerve stimulus (Maselli et al., 1997; Dumitru et al., 2002; Crawford, 2003; Cherington, 2004). Electrodiagnostic findings typical of botulism include normal motor nerve velocity, normal sensory nerve amplitudes, velocities and latencies and a pattern of brief, small amplitude and polyphasic motor unit potentials, and generally an incremental response (facilitation) to repetitive stimulation at high frequencies, with a decremental response at lower frequencies. Single-fiber EMG studies often show increased jitter in posterior cervical and extremity muscles, which diminish on blocking (Cherington, 1988, 2004; Dumitru et al., 2002). Guidelines for electrodiagnostic testing for botulism have been outlined (Cherington, 1990, 1998, 2004; Maselli et al., 1997; Crawford, 2003). Acute care pediatric electromyography can be useful in diagnosing infant botulism among floppy baby syndromes (Gutierrez et al., 1994; Jones and Darras, 2000; Crawford, 2003; Cherington, 2004; Swoboda and Jones, 2006), although pitfalls may occur, particularly in early evaluation (Sheth et al., 1999). Unlike certain other NMJ diseases such as myasthenia gravis and Lambert–Eaton syndrome, botulism is an acute intoxication caused solely by exposure to BoNT; therefore genetic tests or a search for anti-acetylcholine receptor or anti-MuSK antibodies are futile.

11.8.1. Differential diagnosis

The definitive diagnosis of botulism requires differentiation from other neuromuscular disorders including sepsis, meningitis, myasthenia gravis, Guillain–Barré syndrome, Miller–Fisher syndrome, Lambert-Eaton syndrome, stroke, tick paralysis, snake venom poisoning, diphtheritic neuropathy, nerve agent poisoning, Streptococcus pharyngitis, diabetic complications, inflammatory myopathy and CNS infections or tumors, particularly of the brainstem (Table 11.3) (Cherington, 1998, 2004; Dimitru et al., 2002; Arnon, 2004; Caya et al., 2004). Acute flaccid paralysis from polioviruses and other enteroviruses have been misdiagnosed as infant botulism (Kelly et al., 2006). A summary of illnesses requiring differential diagnosis from botulism is presented in Table 11.3. In a recent study, clinical mimics of infant botulism were classified into five broad categories: muscular atrophy, metabolic disorders, other infectious diseases, miscellaneous and probable infant botulism lacking laboratory confirmation (Francisco and Arnon, 2007).

11.9. Treatment of botulism

The mainstay of treatment is intensive nursing care, with careful attention to respiratory failure, need for enteric feeding and cardiac arrest (Woodruff et al., 1992; Arnon, 2004; Cherington, 2004; CDC, 2006). Passive immunization has long been known to lessen the symptoms of botulism and length of clinical course and reduce the incidence of fatalities (Dack and Wood, 1928; Hatheway et al., 1984; Tacket et al., 1984; Mayers et al., 2001; Chang et al., 2003; Arnon et al.,

Table 11.3

Differential diagnosis of botulism from other disorders (Caya et al., 2004; Meriggioli et al., 2004; CDC, 2006)

Adults and children	Infants
Meningitis	Sepsis, meningitis
Guillain–Barré syndrome (GB)	Guillain–Barré syndrome (GB)
Myasthenia gravis	Myasthenia gravis
Lambert–Eaton syndrome	Acute infantile neuropathy
Cerebrovascular accidents	Meningitis/encephalitis
Acute intermediate porphyria	Metabolic disorders, e.g., electrolyte imbalance
Carcinomatosis of cranial nerves	Reye's syndrome
Neoplasm of CNS	Neoplasm
Tick paralysis	Congenital myopathy
Diphtheritic neuropathy	Enteric virus
Polymyelitis	Poliomyelitis
Miller–Fisher variant of GB	Werdnig–Hoffman disease
Food poisoning (e.g., saxitoxin)	Leigh disease
Chemical neurotoxin exposure	Chemical neurotoxin exposure
Mushroom poisoning	Food poisoning
Neuronal viral infection	Neuronal viral infection

2006). When administered within hours following intoxication, antitoxin can markedly reduce morbidity and mortality. Until recently antitoxin treatment has relied on equine-derived products with associated side-effects in about 9% of patients (Black and Gunn, 1980). Equine antitoxin has a half-life in serum of about 5–7 days (Hatheway et al., 1984), whilst human-derived antitoxins may have a longer half-life (Arnon et al., 2006). Recently, human-derived botulism immune globulin (BabyBig®) was shown to reduce the severity and duration of the symptoms, length of hospital stay and associated hospital costs (Arnon et al., 2006). BabyBig® was derived from human donors who had been immunized with botulinum toxoid and the antibody fraction was isolated and formulated for parenteral administration (Arnon et al., 2006). Its supply is currently limited and use is restricted to infants, but efforts are under way to produce additional quantities of antibodies from immunized human donors or to develop antibody producing cell lines with human-compatible antibodies to avoid side-effects caused by the equine antitoxin. New technologies are in progress to develop humanized antibodies of low immunogenicity and side-effects compared to rodent-derived antibodies (Dessain et al., 2004; Lonberg, 2005).

The severity of botulism has been increased with concomitant treatment with certain antimicrobial agents, particularly aminoglycosides and macrolides. These should be avoided in myasthenic illnesses including botulism since they can potentiate muscle paralysis (Pittinger and Adamson, 1972; L'Hommedieu et al., 1979; Santos et al., 1981; Wang et al., 1984; Howard, 1990; Barclay and Begg, 1994). Consequently, botulinum toxin treatment for pharmaceutical purposes is contraindicated in patients with myasthenia gravis, Lambert–Eaton syndrome and possibly other myasthenic disorders. Injection of BoNT-complex in patients has unmasked underlying myasthenic and other neurological disorders (Erbguth et al., 1993; Mezaki et al., 1996; Tuite and Lang, 1996; Tarsy et al., 2000; Thobois et al., 2001; Gioltzoglou et al., 2005; Iwase and Iwase, 2006). Adverse heart rate variability was also detected in a set of patients treated with BoNT/A-complex or BoNT/B-complex (Meichsner and Reichel, 2005). Other cardiovascular and rheumatologic drugs known to adversely affect patients with MG and LES should also be avoided in patients with botulism or in healthy individuals treated with BoNT for cosmetic or therapeutic purposes (Howard, 1990).

11.10. Recovery from botulism and clinical predictors of mortality

Recovery from botulism is slow and tedious. A retrospective review of cases in the USA found a mean of 58 days of mechanical ventilation for type A and 26 days for type B (Colice, 1987). Recovery of speech and the ability to swallow recurs relatively early. Muscular weakness, vertigo and constipation diminish more slowly and may persist for several months. The oculobulbar disturbances are usually the last symptoms to clear. Some patients continue to experience weakness, fatigue and symptoms of impaired autonomic nervous system dysfunction such as dry mouth, constipation and impotence even after 1–2 years following onset of botulism (Goode and Shearn, 1982; Colebatch et al., 1989; Cherington, 1990; Dressler and Benecke, 2003). Communication during recovery is impaired, including inability to speak or write due to ventilatory support and extreme weakness. Agitation, depression and anxiety are common among patients with severe botulism (Cohen and Anderson, 1986).

Clinical predictors of morbidity and mortality from botulism have been evaluated (Mann et al., 1981; Woodruff et al., 1992; Hatheway and Dang, 1994; Nishiura, 2007). The incubation period is related to case fatality and index and early onset cases show the greatest incidence of death (Nishiura, 2007). Early administration of antitoxin reduces morbidity and deaths and is a predictor of the need for mechanical respiration (Tacket et al., 1984; Sandrock and Murin, 2001). Patients with shortness of breath and impaired gag reflex were 23 times more likely to succumb than patients without these signs (Varma et al., 2004). Death from botulism has generally been attributed to ventilatory weakness and respiratory arrest (Hughes et al., 1981; Wilcox et al., 1990; Woodruff et al., 1992). In severe cases of botulism, ventilator muscles may require up to a year to regain full strength (Wilcox et al., 1990). However, deaths also occur by causes not directly involved in airway sufficiency. In a study of causes of death among 19 patients with type A botulism, seven were attributed to respiratory arrest or associated ventilator malfunction and aspiration pneumonia, while surprisingly six were attributed to cardiac arrest (Tacket et al., 1984). It appears that reduction of fatalities related to botulism would benefit from more detailed scrutiny of the causes involved. In common with foodborne botulism, infant botulism caused by BoNT/A is often the most severe in symptoms and time required for patient recovery. In California, a study showed that the mean hospital stay for patients with type A infant botulism was 5.6 weeks, whereas the mean hospital stay for babies with type B infant botulism was 3.7 weeks (Arnon, 2004). Fortunately death in hospitalized cases has been rare and babies recover completely with no permanent weakness or neurologic abnormalities. When death or chronic morbidity has occurred, it has usually resulted from infections or other secondary complications.

Cases of severe botulism with neuropathic features have been reported (Chang and Robinson, 2000; Mackle et al., 2001). Disease sequelae including infectious diseases such as pneumonia have been reported. Stimulation of murine B cells to secrete immunoglobulins by "lipoteichoic acid-like" molecules from *C. botulinum* has been suspected (Campos-Neto et al., 1995), but this needs confirmation. Muscle and nerve biopsies have rarely been performed on patients with botulism, though such analyses can help to exclude myopathy or metabolic causes of paralysis (Keet et al., 2005). Studies in animals have demonstrated atrophy of muscle fibers in severe botulism cases, which regenerated during the recovery phase. It has been suggested that chronic neuropathic changes may persist following botulism (Keet et al., 2005).

11.11. Pathophysiology of botulism and cellular mechanisms of botulinum neurotoxins

Animal models and tissue preparations have traditionally been employed to study the pathophysiology of botulism (Drachman, 1971; Habermann and Dreyer, 1986; Simpson, 2000). The specificity and action of

BoNTs for different tissues and cell types depends on the receptor systems, the trafficking mechanisms and the isoforms of SNARE proteins present in the cells (Schiavo et al., 2000). In this section of the chapter, molecular and tissue effects are described with an emphasis on new developments. It follows the series of actions in the sequence that is believed to occur in botulism poisoning.

11.11.1. Adsorption of botulinum toxin into the lymphatic system

Poisoning caused by botulism involves entry of BoNT into the general circulation either through absorption from the gastrointestinal system, in wound infections or by inhalation. An intriguing aspect of BoNTs is their high oral toxicity as occurs in traditional food-borne botulism (Bonventre, 1979; Sakaguchi, 1983). The estimated lethal dose for humans of BoNT/A by oral ingestion is 0.1–1 μg per kg body weight (Schantz and Johnson, 1992; Hatheway and Dang, 1994), while the systemic toxicity by intramuscular injections in monkeys has been estimated at 39 U/kg (~400 pg) (Scott and Suzuki, 1988). These data suggest about one-thousandth of the toxin ingested is effectively absorbed into systemic circulation, while other estimates have suggested that the ratio of oral to parenteral toxicity in various species of animals is 10^4:10^6 (Smith, 1977). Oral toxicity varies considerably depending on the serotype and the animal species. It has been estimated that $\sim 10^{11}$–10^{12} ($\sim$1–2 μg) molecules of BoNT/A that enter the systemic circulation is sufficient to produce neurologic symptoms and death (Lamanna, 1959; Bonventre, 1974). Boroff et al. (1984) estimated that $\sim$10 molecules of BoNT are necessary to cause intoxication of a NMJ in the frog, but this is certainly an estimate as the quantitative dose would depend on the size and safety margin of the particular NMJs and motor endplate.

Although oral poisoning is the major cause of human botulism (Shapiro et al., 1998), surprisingly little is known regarding the mechanisms of BoNT passage through and absorption from the GI tract and its entry into the lymph and blood of general circulation (Bonventre, 1979; Simpson, 2000). It has been demonstrated that the toxin complexes (progenitor toxins) are more stable during oral passage than is the purified neurotoxin (Ohishi et al., 1977; Sugiyama, 1980; Sakaguchi, 1983; Fujinaga, 2006). The non-toxic proteins of the toxin complexes including hemagglutinins (HA) and non-toxic, non-hemagglutinin protect the toxin from digestive enzymes and low pH. During passage, activation of single chain BoNT precursor proteins from non-proteolytic types such as BoNT/E probably occurs by limited proteolysis in the stomach or in the brush border of the enterocytes (Bonventre, 1979). Such activation of types B, D, E, F and G increases toxicity by 10–100-fold (Sugiyama, 1980; DasGupta, 1989). BoNTs are also inactivated with loss of toxicity by exposure to high concentrations and/or extended times to trypsin and certain other proteases and thus controlled conditions and the use of soybean trypsin inhibitor are needed for careful cleavage to the dichain form in vitro (Sugiyama, 1980; DasGupta, 1989).

How such a large protein (150 kDa) penetrates the intestinal barrier is an interesting question that has not been resolved (Simpson, 2000; Fujinaga, 2006). The quantity of BoNT needed to induce neurologic symptoms is extremely low (fM levels) and it is possible that a sufficient quantity crosses the polarized epithelial monolayer from the apical side to the baso-lateral side (transcytosis) via non-specific mechanisms similar to absorption of certain other proteins. BoNTs are mainly absorbed in the upper small intestine and lesser amounts from the ileum and stomach in various animal models (Dack, 1926; Heckly et al., 1960; Maksymowych et al., 1999; Simpson, 2000). It has been shown that intestinal crypt cells may be a preferential site of transcytosis (Coueson et al., 2008). Small quantities of BoNT may also enter the circulation from other locations within the gastrointestinal tract such as mucosal surfaces of the mouth, esophagus and through intestinal lesions (Lamanna et al., 1967). In inhalational botulism, BoNT is absorbed from the upper respiratory tract by poorly understood mechanisms. C. botulinum colonizes the large bowel in infant and adult intestinal botulism, but it is unclear if the ileum is the major site of absorption. In a mouse model, as few as 10 botulinum spores were able to colonize the ileum and toxin was detected in the feces, but the mice remained asymptomatic, suggesting that BoNT is poorly absorbed from the ileum (Sugiyama, 1979).

Bonventre (1979) presented evidence that BoNT is absorbed by an endocytic process in which the toxin reaches the microvillus membrane and is engulfed in pinocytic vesicles. Some vesicles fuse with lysosomes and the protein is subsequently degraded, while other vesicles will reach the surface of lateral cells and reach the interstitial regions. This pinocytic process is analogous to the mechanism by which neonates absorb immunoglobulins from colostrum and is less prevalent in children and adults than in infants. Bonventre (1979) further proposed that there may be specific receptors for BoNTs in the lumen of the gut and this hypothesis has been supported in more recent studies from various investigators (Maksymowych and Simpson, 2004; Ahsan et al., 2005). Indeed, it has been documented that polysialogangliosides and the protein SV2 are involved in the apical uptake of BoNT/A (Coueson et al., 2008) and that the transcytosis of BoNTs via specific receptors is energy-dependent (Ahsan et al., 2005). The traversal process was visualized in the human gut epithelial cell line (T-84) by labeling BoNT/A with Alexa dye 488 (Ahsan et al., 2005).

Very little is known of the mechanisms involved in the absorption of BoNT into the vasculature from mucosal membranes, from wounds and following intramuscular injection. BoNT likely enters directly into the bloodstream by diffusion from wounds and on intramuscular injection, but the actual mechanism is unclear. Circulating BoNT has been detected in less than 50% of human wound botulism cases (Merson and Dowell, 1973; Hikes and Manoli, 1981), suggesting that the infection is relatively short or that sufficient quantities of BoNT to elicit an immune response are not produced.

11.11.2. Systemic distribution of BoNT

BoNT enters the lymphatic system from the intestine, wounds, mucous membranes or from intramuscular locations and travels via blood to neuronal targets. The different specificity of the serotypes for different cell types mainly depends on the receptor systems (Schiavo et al., 2000; Simpson, 2000). Since BoNT dissociates from the complex proteins at $pH \geq 7.2$ (Sakaguchi et al., 1984), it would occur free in the bloodstream following absorption. The pharmacokinetics of BoNTs in the bloodstream have been poorly studied, particularly in humans. Information is lacking on the mechanisms for transport, metabolism and elimination. In our laboratory, on injections of high concentrations of BoNT 10^6 and 10^5 LD50s into the tail vein of mice, symptoms of botulism are noticeable in $\sim$30 and $\sim$60 minutes, respectively (Malizio et al., 2000). Thus, compared to certain other toxins, especially small molecular weight organic chemical toxins such as saxitoxin and tetrodotoxin (where mice die in minutes following injection) (Schantz and Johnson, 1992), the onset requires several hours, probably due to the large size of BoNT and the multiple steps involved in intoxication.

Few studies have addressed pharmacokinetic properties of BoNTs including mechanisms of metabolism, elimination and detoxification. Such studies have been hindered by the extraordinary potency of BoNTs, which are physiologically active and potentially lethal at femtomolar concentrations, which imposes limitations in detection in in vivo and PK evaluations. Borodic et al. (1994) investigated regional toxin spread in a rabbit-back model showing that diffusion gradients are formed at 5–10 U (1 U = 1 mouse LD50), but

the gradient collapsed at 1 U (Borodic et al., 1994). The diffusion and tissue distribution of BoNT/A and the 900 kDa BoNT/A-complex labeled with ^{125}I were investigated following injection into the gastrocnemius muscle of rats and the eyelids of rabbits (Tang-Liu et al., 2003). No generalized symptoms or systemic effects were observed. In rats, most of the toxin, whether complex or neurotoxin, remained in the regions of the injection site. Radioactivity detected in distant tissues including thyroid, skin and contralateral muscle appeared to be attributed to low molecular weight peptides or free ^{125}I-iodide, suggesting that breakdown of the toxin occurred. Very low concentrations of ^{125}I-iodide were detected even in the brain. Following injection into rabbit eyelids, very low levels of ^{125}I-BoNT/A-complex or free ^{125}I-BoNT/A were detected in distant tissues, including the eye (Tang-Liu et al., 2003). These results suggested that BoNT/A and BoNT/A-complex, when administered at physiological levels, do not diffuse significantly from the injection site, reducing the potential for systemic effects. Illicit injection of high amounts of BoNT/A-complex into the forehead in cosmetic procedures led to systemic botulism in humans, but these levels are much higher than occurs in natural botulism or in proper medical treatments (Chertow et al., 2006).

An assessment of the systemic pharmacokinetics of BoNT was recently studied in mice, rats and rabbits (Ravichandran et al., 2006). Native BoNT and toxin modified by diethyl pyrocarbonate to inactivate histidine residues in the active site (Rossetto et al., 1992) and by iodination were used. Ex vivo experiments involving incubation of BoNT in blood indicated that the toxin was not proteolytically modified or did not undergo major structural changes. BoNT recovered from rat blood was not diminished in its metalloprotease activity and retained its ability to block exocytosis in the phrenic nerve-hemidiaphragm preparations (Ravichandran et al., 2006). These experiments supported the conclusion that BoNT retained full functional activity and biologic structure during incubation in rat blood. In order to reach nerve terminals, BoNT must exit from the bloodstream, which probably depends on the toxin being free and not bound to albumin or other blood proteins. It was estimated that $\sim$70% was free and available for traversal from the blood. The half-life of ^{125}I-BoNT administered intravenously in the tail vein of mice was extrapolated to be $\sim$239 minutes in blood and 231 minutes in serum, and that elimination half-life was ca. 4 hours. In rats, the half-lives in blood and serum of rats was 260 and 255 minutes, respectively. As expected, incubation of BoNT with neutralizing antibodies prior to injection prevented botulinum intoxication for more than 4 days. In antibody chase experiments of 10 or 20 minutes post-challenge decreased the survival time to ca. 22 and 4 hours, respectively, compared to the time to death of 100 minutes in mice challenged without an antibody chase. The tissue disposition of the antiserum-toxin accumulated in the liver was 30–40% and 5–7% in the spleen. These results supported the notion that toxin-specific antibodies strongly promote clearance of toxin from the circulation. This ability would be expected to depend on the affinity and number of antibodies and may be slower with monoclonals against BoNT. BoNT alone was also found in the liver (ca. 7%), spleen (ca. 1%) and kidney (ca. 2%), whereas negligible toxin was detected in the heart or brain. Blood is an important conduit for delivery of the toxin to its sites of action including cholinergic nerve endings. This study also confirmed that the time window of neutralization by antisera administration is small.

11.12. Cellular mechanisms of action of BoNTs at nerve terminals

11.12.1. Background

The cellular mechanisms of BoNTs of activity remained enigmatic for several decades, began to be revealed in the 1950s and 1960s and were gradually elucidated by new techniques and concepts, particularly advanced techniques for imaging tissue, electrophysiological methods, the theory of quantal release of acetylcholine at the synaptic membrane and eventually genetic analyses and structural analyses of the BoNTs (Heuser, 1976; Katz, 1966; Thesleff, 1976; Niemann, 1991; Schiavo et al., 2000). The morphology and structural basis of synaptic vesicle discharge and reformation was illuminated by electron microscopy and freeze fracture, particularly at the frog neuromuscular junction (Heuser, 1976). These studies provided a "panoramic view" of the morphology of the nerve terminal and were important in defining the active zone. The classic study of Burgen et al. (1949) demonstrated that partially purified BoNT/A-complex produced an irreversible paralysis of the isolated rat phrenic-nerve diaphragm after a latent period. They also showed that much higher concentrations (500 times) of BoNT/B-complex were necessary compared to BoNT/A-complex to paralyze the phrenic nerve-diaphragm of the rat, but that guinea pigs and isolated guinea pig phrenic nerve preparations were both highly sensitive to both type A and B toxins. Importantly, they showed that conduction in the nerve was unaffected by BoNT, that the motor endplates remained sensitive to applied acetylcholine, that the output of acetylcholine on motor nerve stimulation was greatly reduced and that the toxin does not affect the enzymes acetylating choline or cholinesterase. This seminal study showed that BoNT bound irreversibly to nerve fibers and prevented release of acetylcholine, resulting in the neuromuscular block (Burgen et al., 1949). Brooks (1953, 1954) subsequently confirmed that conduction in nerve trunks or in muscle fibers was not affected by the toxin even on direct stimulation and that the toxin produced neuromuscular paralysis by interfering with "conduction" proximal to the site of ACh release. The results of these studies implied that botulinum toxin interferes directly with the release of ACh from nerve endings.

The cellular mechanisms of BoNT toxicity and blockade of neurotransmitter release follows a complex multistep process (Montecucco et al., 1994): (a) receptor binding; (b) receptor mediated endocytosis inside synaptic vesicles; (c) translocation of the L chain from the acidic vesicle lumen into the cytoplasm; and (d) catalytic activity of the BoNT LCs on SNARE substrates (Fig. 11.3). Several excellent reviews have described these steps, particularly the intracellular activity of the toxins on SNARE substrates (Schiavo et al., 2000; Jahn and Scheller, 2006); therefore the sections described below will focus mainly on new developments.

11.12.2. Receptors for BoNTs in neuronal cells

Several protein toxins are known to have specific protein cellular receptors, with cholera and diphtheria being classic examples (van Heyningen, 1974; Chang et al., 1975). In addition, polysialogangliosides often participate as membrane receptors for toxins (van Heyningen, 1974). The mode of BoNT binding to nerve terminals is still poorly understood (Montecucco et al., 2004), particularly in comparison to other steps such as intracellular cleavage of SNARE substrates (Jahn and Scheller, 2006). The binding of BoNTs A and B to murine motoneurons was initially studied quantitatively by Black and Dolly (1986). Using iodinated BoNTs, they demonstrated that the toxins bound specifically to unmyelinated regions of the nerve terminals of mouse hemidiaphragms. Binding only occurred at the presynaptic membrane and was not detected on other cell types including muscle, blood vessels, connective tissue, Schwann cells or noradrenergic terminals. Binding was found to be temperature-dependent and was considerably reduced at 4°C compared to 22°C. Transfer of radioactivity across the nerve plasma membrane was detected within 20 minutes and the extent of internalization reached a maximum after

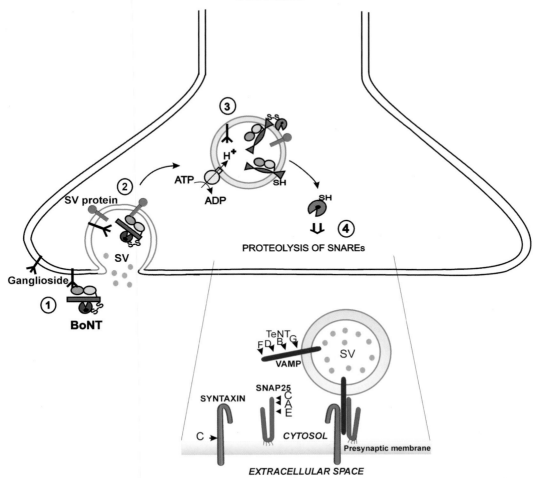

Fig. 11.3. Portrayal of the molecular mechanism of BoNTs at nerve terminals acting on the SNARE apparatus. See text for details.

90 minutes. Lowering the temperature and inhibitors of ATP production such as DNP abolished transfer. It was shown that the larger 97 kDa subunit inhibited binding, indicating that the receptor region was located on the HC. TeNT competed for binding but internalization was not affected in the presence of TeNT; 150–500 binding sites per μm² of membrane were estimated. These seminal findings showed that BoNT bound specifically in a saturable manner to presynaptic membranes at specialized target sites and that at least two distinguishable and sequential steps of binding and internalization are involved in BoNT intoxication.

A double receptor concept for BoNTs has been presented to explain specificity and avidity to the nerve terminals (Montecucco, 1986). Primary receptors are polysialogangliosides, generally of the GD1b and GT1b series, and certain proteins at the nerve terminus (Dong et al., 2003, 2006; Montecucco et al., 2004; Rummel

et al., 2004a, b). Phospholipids, and possibly lipid rafts, have been considered as primary molecules involved in binding for certain serotypes, particularly for BoNT/D (Tsukamoto et al., 2005; Geny and Popoff, 2006). Much progress has been made in recent years in identifying protein receptors for BoNTs. Recently, using gain-of-function and loss-of-function as well as other genetic, molecular and morphological approaches has led to strong evidence implicating protein receptors for BoNT/ A (Rummel et al., 2004a, 2007; Dong et al., 2006; Mahrhold et al., 2006), BoNT/B (Nishiki et al., 1994, 1996; Dong et al., 2003; Jin et al., 2006; Baldwin and Barbieri, 2007; Rummel et al., 2007), /C, /D and /G (Rummel et al., 2004a, 2007; Dong et al., 2007) entry into neuronal cell lines. Molecular structures have recently been achieved showing the interaction of BoNT/B with polysialogangliosides and synaptotagmin II (Chai et al., 2006; Jin et al., 2006).

Synaptic vesicle (SV) proteins participate with their luminal domains to the neurospecific binding of BoNT/A, /B and /G and this is probably true for the other BoNTs (Verderio et al., 2006). BoNT/B and BoNT/G interact with the luminal domain of the SV proteins synaptotagmin I (Syt-I) and Syt-II. BoNT/B has a higher affinity for Syt-II (Nishiki et al., 1996; Dong et al., 2003), whereas BoNT/G interacts preferentially with Syt-I (Rummel et al., 2004a; Dong et al., 2007). The crystal structures of BoNT/B in complex with the luminal domain of Syt-II (Chai et al., 2006; Jin et al., 2006) shows that HCC accommodates the α-helical segment 45–59 of Syt-II in a cleft adjacent to the polysialoganglioside-binding site of the toxin. Mutations in the synaptotagmin-binding cleft and in the polysialoganglioside-binding pocket greatly reduce the toxicity of BoNT/B and /G and double mutants at the two binding sites abolish neurotoxicity (Rummel et al., 2007; Dong et al., 2007).

SV2 is a membrane protein found associated with secretory vesicles of neural and endocrine cells of vertebrates (Scranton et al., 1993; Custer et al., 2006). It exists in three isoforms, SV2A, SV2B and SV2C, which differ in distribution in neuronal and endocrine tissues (Bajjalieh et al., 1992, 1993, 1994). Recently, the three isoforms of SV2 have been shown to serve as specific protein receptors for BoNT/A. The primary receptor for BoNT/A is SV2C, although SV2A and SV2B can also act as receptors (Dong et al., 2006; Mahrhold et al., 2006). The distribution of SV2 in neuronal and endocrine tissue has not been clearly delineated, but its location as well as that of other protein receptors will dictate the distribution of the toxins. The differential distribution of synaptic vesicle proteins in various neuronal tissues leads to the potential of using different serotypes of BoNTs for the treatment of peripheral and central nervous system diseases by targeting neuronal cell populations (Verderio et al., 2006). The NMJ also contains several proteins modified by glycosylation such as agrin, neural cell adhesion molecule, dystroglycan and SV2 (Kröger and Schröder, 2002; Martin, 2003) and the overall structure and organization of the NMJ contributes to binding of BoNTs by mechanisms that have not yet been elucidated.

An intriguing aspect of receptor binding for BoNT/A, /B and /G is that it depends on vesicle recycling and that their internalization within the nerve terminals is mediated by the synaptic vesicles themselves acting as sort of "Trojan horses" for the neurotoxins (Dong et al., 2006; Verderio et al., 2006). This mechanism favors toxin attack on the most active terminals. Theoretically a toxin-penetrated terminal will shut down exocytosis, allowing toxin molecules to enter actively exocytosing terminals yet to be poisoned. It is presently thought that synaptic vesicle recycling is involved in the uptake of most, if not all, serotypes.

11.12.3. Trafficking and internalization of BoNT-LCs into the neuronal cytosol

During or following internalization, both the H and L chains of BoNT/A, /B, /E and TeNT are phosphorylated by the Src family of tyrosine kinases (Ferrier-Montiel et al., 1996). Phosphorylation enhances thermal stability and increases catalytic activity of BoNTs, possibly by transitioning the structure to a more helical and compact form (Encinar et al., 1998). The primary stabilizing and thermal effects appear to be on the L chains (Blanes-Mira et al., 2001; Ibañez et al., 2004), suggesting that the phosphorylated L chains may be the dominant physiological form within the nerve terminals. Since phosphorylation and dephosphorylation have been implicated in regulation of synaptic transmission (Lee, 2006) it also seems possible that BoNT may act as an integral or surrogate component in the regulation of synaptogenesis.

An inherent property of bacterial protein toxins with intracellular targets is their ability to insert into and translocate across membranes (Montecucco et al., 1988; London, 1992; Parker and Pattus, 1993; Montecucco and Schiavo, 1995; Lesieur et al., 1997; Neale, 2003; Ménétrey et al., 2005). Once in the intracellular acidic compartment, the H chain is believed to form a channel in lipid bilayers through which the L chain enters into the cytosol following acidification of the vesicle lumen (Schiavo et al., 2000; Koriazova and Montal, 2003; Fischer and Montal, 2007b). Membrane translocation is the least understood step of the cellular mechanism of action of BoNTs. It has been proposed that the H chain acts as a transmembrane chaperone for the light chain to ensure a translocation competent conformation during its transit from the endosome (Koriazova and Montal, 2003; Fischer and Montal, 2007b). The mechanisms of trafficking and localization of LCs in the cytosol appear to differ according to the serotype and structure (Aikawa et al., 2006; Lawrence et al., 2007). Critical to entry of the catalytically active L chain of BoNTs into the neuronal cytosol is acidification of the lumen, which is thought to trigger a structural change of the toxin and initiation of membrane insertion (Montecucco et al., 1988; Koriazova and Montal, 2003; Puhar et al., 2004). To reach the cytosol the L chain must cross the hydrophobic barrier of the vesicle membrane. The pH gradient across the membrane is instrumental in such a movement (Simpson et al., 1994). In fact, the internal acidity causes a conformational change from a water-soluble "neutral" structure to an "acid" structure, with the surface exposure of hydrophobic patches which mediate the interaction of the H and L chains with the hydrocarbon core of the lipid bilayer (Montecucco et al., 1988, 1989; Puhar et al., 2004). The release of the L chain requires reduction of the interchain disulfide bond and an intact S-S bond is an absolute requirement for toxicity and membrane translocation (Schiavo et al., 1990; Fischer and Montal, 2007a).

Once internalized the LCs may locate to different compartments in neuronal cells. LC/A locates to the plasma membrane and LC/E to the cytoplasm within PC12 cells (Fernández-Salas et al., 2004). Mutations in the LC revealed amino acid sequences at the N terminus as well as a dileucine domain in the C terminus that affected localization. The location of the LCs was postulated as one factor affecting the duration of action of the toxins, which can be several months to a year for LC/A, while generally only a few weeks for LC/E. Certain other factors likely contribute to the duration of action and recovery from cellular intoxication including processing and degradation (Keller et al., 1999; Adler et al., 2001; Keller, 2006), as well as regeneration of a productive SNARE apparatus (Raciborska and Charlton, 1999; Meunier et al., 2003; Bajohrs et al., 2004). There is evidence that the long duration of action of BoNT/A and BoNT/C (Eleopra et al., 1997, 2004) is significantly contributed by the presence of a SNAP-25 molecule deprived of only a few C-terminal residues which act as a strong dominant negative in the assembly of the SNARE supercomplex which mediates the binding of the synaptic vesicle to the presynaptic membrane (Montecucco et al., 2005). Further elucidation of the mechanism of translocation and intracellular activities could lead to novel treatments for botulism and targeted drug delivery to neuronal cells.

11.12.4. Intracellular mechanisms of BoNT-LCs

The intracellular activities of BoNT-LCs in nerve terminals remained enigmatic until the 1990s. The determination of the nucleotide and amino acid sequences of BoNTs and TeNT (Fairweather and Lyness, 1986; Binz et al., 1990; Niemann, 1991) revealed that the light chain contains a zinc-binding motif and this led to the demonstration that BoNTs and TeNTs have zinc metalloprotease activity (Schiavo et al., 1992a, b, 1993a, b; Montecucco et al., 1993). They were demonstrated to act on specific isoforms of the SNARE proteins SNAP-25 synaptobrevin and syntaxin (Schiavo et al., 1992b, 1993a, b, 1995, 2000; Blasi et al., 1993a, b; Montecucco

and Schiavo, 1995), which are integral for trafficking of synaptic vesicles and their fusion with the plasma membrane.

The BoNT-LCs are a unique group of proteases that recognize 9-residue SNARE motifs within the natural substrates (Montecucco and Schiavo, 1993, 1995; Rossetto et al., 1994; Schiavo et al., 2000); the recognition is structurally based and contributes to the high specificity of the toxins for recognizing and cleaving their substrates. The interactions of the catalytic domain of BoNT with the neuronal substrates have been studied for all seven serotypes. TeNT, BoNT/B, /D, /F and /G cleave the vesicle-associated membrane protein VAMP, at different single peptide bonds; BoNT/C cleaves both syntaxin and SNAP-25, two proteins of the presynaptic membrane; whilst BoNT/A and /E cleave SNAP-25 at different sites within the COOH-terminus (Montecucco and Schiavo, 1995; Schiavo et al., 2000). Proteolysis of SNARE proteins prevents the formation of an active membrane fusion complex (Schiavo et al., 2000).

The findings that BoNT-LCs enzymatically cleaved SNARE proteins through recognition of the SNARE motif provided an explanation to morphological studies which showed, in some cases, accumulation of synaptic vesicles at the plasma membrane in BoNT poisoned nerves (Fig. 11.3). This clearly demonstrated that a primary mechanism of BoNTs in blocking exocytosis is to block exocytosis by disruption of SNARE trafficking and neurotransmitter release. However, other functions likely exist for these intriguing proteins. A summary of the current understanding of the cellular mechanism of action of the BoNTs at nerve terminals is illustrated in Fig. 11.4.

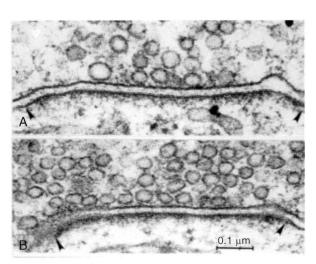

Fig. 11.4. Representation of blockade of vesicle fusion with the presynaptic membrane by BoNT action. (A) Control; (B) BoNT-treated.

11.13. Synaptic and postsynaptic effects

The synaptic and postsynaptic pathophysiology of BoNTs and secondary actions on muscle have been much less studied than presynaptic activities at nerve terminals. The onset, duration of paralysis, time for recovery and effects in distal neuromuscular regions is highly dependent on the serotype of BoNT, muscle activity, muscle stimulation and other factors (Hughes and Whaler, 1962; Eleopra et al., 1997, 2004, 2006; Sloop et al., 1997; Hesse et al., 1998; Davletov et al., 2005). The toxin's efficacy also depends strongly on the serotype and its method of preparation and composition (Schantz and Johnson, 1992; Mclellan et al., 1996; Eleopra et al., 1997; Sampaio et al., 2004; Rosales et al., 2006). In humans, muscle paralysis generally reaches its highest severity in 4–8 days depending on the serotype and dose of toxin, plateaus for several weeks to months and then muscle function gradually recovers (Sloop et al., 1997; Eleopra et al., 1998, 2006; Billante et al., 2002; Foran et al., 2003; Rosales et al., 2006). These studies demonstrated that local therapeutic injection into humans of BoNT/A, /B, /C and /E cause paralysis for durations of ~3–6, 3, 2–4 and 1–2 months, respectively.

The pathophysiology of synaptic and postsynaptic effects from BoNT has been most thoroughly studied in animal models. Local injections or application of the toxin to tissue preparations are well known to cause denervation and associated events including motor paralysis, spread of AChR-sensitive areas, neuronal sprouting, muscle fiber atrophy and some other changes in muscle morphology and composition (Thesleff, 1960, 1976, 1991; Drachman and Johnston, 1975; Pestronk et al., 1976; Alderson, 1993; Hassan et al., 1995; Dodd et al., 2005). In animal models, two primary morphological changes are observed at the NMJ following BoNT treatment. In proximal muscles, motor axon sprouting is prominent, which probably results from a signal related to denervation (Duchen, 1972; Pestronk and Drachman, 1978; Brown et al., 1981; Alderson, 1993; English, 2003). In more distal muscles, expansion of the endplate region is more evident, although both changes may occur in each muscle as observed in humans (Alderson, 1993). In animal models, particularly rat hemidiaphragm preparations, muscle activity increases uptake of BoNTs into the terminal nerve endings (Hughes and Whaler, 1962). Periodic electrical stimulation in patients being treated with BoNT for blepharospasm and hemifacial spasm increased the neuromuscular blockade (Eleopra et al., 1997). Reduction of the CMAP was also greater for the stimulated muscles. These results indicate that muscle activity can enhance the clinical effects of the

toxin. Although quantal and spontaneous release of neurotransmitter is blocked nearly completely by BoNT, the nerve terminals and neuromuscular junctions do not degenerate (Duchen and Strich, 1968; Duchen, 1971, 1972; Holland and Brown, 1981; Gomez and Queiroz, 1982; Yee and Pestronk, 1987). Paralysis by BoNT has also revealed trophic secretions at the NMJ (Thesleff, 1993), supporting exchange of pre- and postsynaptic information following the functional denervation.

Botulinum-treated muscles are supersensitive to ACh activation (Thesleff, 1960). Other than sprouting, the ultrastructure of nerve terminals in botulinum-intoxicated frog and cat muscles is not altered even after periods of 3–4 weeks' treatment (Thesleff, 1960). The muscle preparations did not show any miniature endplate potentials (mepps) or responses to nerve stimulation. In cat tenuissimus muscle neuromuscular blockade by a single application of botulinum toxin reached its maximum after 5 days and then remained at a constant level for several months (Thesleff, 1976). At high concentrations of toxin, spontaneous mepps were usually absent and nerve stimulation evoked no endplate potentials (epps). With lower quantities of toxin, the mepp frequency was about 100 times less than in normal muscle. Nerve stimulation was either ineffective or evoked tiny epps (Thesleff, 1960). The rate of recovery from the blocked state of the neuromuscular junction increased with age (Gutmann and Habnzlíková, 1972).

Elegant studies by Drachman (1964, 1971) demonstrated the utility of botulinum toxin for studying the nervous system. Injection of large intravenous doses of BoNT/A-complex to 7- and 12-day chick embryos resulted in skeletal muscle atrophy and only slight structural defects in heart and liver (Drachman, 1964, 1971). The significance and utility of the chick model has been reviewed (Drachman and Coulombre, 1962; Drachman, 1971; Johnson, 1999). The administration of enormous BoNT doses is possible in chick embryos because their respiratory gas exchange is by passive diffusion across the chorioalloantoic membrane (Drachman, 1964). Drachman administered doses which would kill 20 000 or more hatched chickens at 7 and 12 days. The embryos injected with BoNT/A-complex showed multiple joint contractures on hatching (arthrogryposis congenita multiplex) due to the immobility during embryonic development (Drachman, 1964) and had a slightly shortened upper beak. All skeletal muscles were markedly shrunken and fatty, an appearance most evident in the chick embryos injected on prenatal day 7. Heart and liver weights were reduced this was about 27% and 17%, respectively, whereas in body (and limb) muscle this was about 45% and 80%, respectively. Degenerative and fatty changes were more prominent in muscles of embryo injected on day 7, consistent with age-dependent susceptibility of the neuromuscular system to BoNT. The observed histologic changes are like those of physical denervation and atrophy, but on a greater scale in the less mature animals (Adams et al., 1960; MacIntosh et al., 2006). The results were interpreted to show a "trophic" influence of neurally released acetylcholine on skeletal muscle form and function (Drachman, 1964).

Physical denervation produces a physical separation of nerve and muscle membranes at the synapse within 4–5 days (Thesleff, 1976). Chemical denervation by BoNT is rapidly followed by copious sprouting of the motor nerve terminals as well as by some nodal sprouting (Duchen, 1971, 1972; Duchen and Strich, 1971; Brown et al., 1981; Alderson, 1993; English, 2003). In the experimental studies, terminal nerve sprouts appeared erratically on the surface of the muscle fibers and it is not clear whether these sprouts are attracted to the functionally denervated endplates; perhaps more likely, are seeking muscle sites for establishing new synaptic contacts. It is clear that nerve terminal sprouting is governed by the Schwann cells activated by the lack of supply of acetylcholine (Son and Thompson, 1995). In BoNT/A denervated muscle, uncharacterized biochemical changes were also detected (Gutmann, 1962; Watson, 2006). Determinants of sprout growth possibly include electrical stimulation, when applied, and pre- and postsynaptic secretion of neurotrophic growth factors, cytokines and proteases, including the ciliary neurotrophic factor and insulin-like growth factors I and II (Brown et al., 1981; Thoenen, 1995; English, 2003). The age of the animal also affects the propensity of sprout formation (Gutmann and Habnzlíková, 1972). In BoNT-treated muscle, the immature sprouts temporarily establish neuromuscular transmission (de Paiva et al., 1999; English, 2003). However, these immature connections tend not to reach full maturity nor establish permanent motor endplates; instead, in a second phase of reinnervation the original motor endplate becomes reactivated and the superfluous sprouts are eliminated (de Paiva et al., 1999).

The remodeling process occurs with alterations in neural plasticity (de Paiva et al., 1999; Sanes and Lichtman, 2001; Kummer et al., 2006). Sprouting and repair is also associated with intriguing physiological activities (Brown et al., 1981; de Paiva et al., 1999; English, 2003). Sprouts induced by BoNT denervation exhibit enhanced uptake and retrograde transport of adenoviral particles and increased uptake of exogenously introduced genes (Millecamps et al., 2001, 2002; Federici and Boulis, 2006), pointing to possible novel approaches for gene therapy of neuronal diseases, such as amyotrophic lateral sclerosis (ALS). Drachman and colleagues found that botulinum toxin and denervation increased sensitivity of skeletal muscle to Coxsackie A2 virus infection (Andrew et al., 1984).

The stability and regeneration of functional NMJ and myogenesis also depends on the half-life of acetylcholine receptors. In normally innervated muscle, a relatively long half-life of ~12 days is observed (Avila et al., 1989). Denervation leads to a much more rapid turnover of AChRs after a lag period. Avila et al. (1989) examined the effects of presynaptic and postsynaptic denervation on the stability on AChRs in soleus and flexor digitorum brevis muscles by repeated injection of BoNT/A complex and by continuous application of α-bungarotoxin in the soleus. Treatment with BoNT caused accelerated turnover of AChRs, like that after surgical denervation, but with a lag phase, while exposure to α-bungarotoxin led to AChR loss with the same time course as that observed after surgical denervation. These experiments indicated that neurotransmission regulates the stability of AChRs at the NMJ (Avila et al., 1989).

Muscle and nerve biopsies have been performed to assess the pathology of BoNT-induced functional denervation (Maselli et al., 1997; Keet et al., 2005). Animals exposed to BoNT display varying degrees of muscle atrophy depending on the dose applied (Drachman, 1971; Duchen, 1971; Capra et al., 1991; Hassan et al., 1995). Use of acetylcholinesterase staining and muscle fiber alterations have been employed to evaluate the potency of BoNT preparations and to study diffusion characteristics of the toxin (Borodic et al., 1994). The affected muscle fibers are abnormal in size, with most fibers atrophic and shrunken, and may also have a basophilic sarcoplasm, altered nuclei and nucleoli and shifts in myosin composition (Rosales et al., 1996; Dodd et al., 2005; Keet et al., 2005).

The molecular pathways of myogenesis, myofiber remodeling and muscle activity restoration following BoNT exposure are in the early stages of investigation. Extraocular muscles are highly sensitive to BoNT, probably due to their specialized innervation and muscle composition and topography, as well as supersensitivity to certain myasthenic diseases (Porter and Baker, 1996; Ruff, 2002; Buttner-Ennever et al., 2003; Conti-Fine et al., 2006). BoNT/A injection in the superior rectus muscles of rabbits resulted in a significant increase in the number of bromodeoxyuridine-positive nuclei and satellite cells. MyoD expression in satellite cells and myonuclei was also significantly increased following injection (Ugalde et al., 2005). Several genes were upregulated in skeletal muscle tissue in response to BoNT treatment. Transcription of the AChR α-subunit is enhanced, though not as rapidly as in surgically denervated muscles (Lipsky et al., 1989). In juvenile (1-month-old) rats, the expression of mRNA was determined following injection of BoNT/A-complex into the gastrocnemius muscle (Ma et al., 2005; Shen et al., 2005, 2006). mRNA was extracted from muscle extracts and real-time PCR and gene microarrays were used to identify genes involved in remodeling and stabilization of the NMJ and muscle functional recovery. Key genes that were upregulated included those encoding nAChR subunits, SNAP-25, GAP-43, plasminogen activator and members of the MyoD family (Tian et al., 1995; Ma et al., 2005; Shen et al., 2005). In an extensive study, Shen et al. (2006) examined more than 28 000 rat genes and observed that ~9000 genes were expressed in gastrocnemius muscle. Among these, 105 genes were up-regulated and 59 genes were down-regulated significantly in gastrocnemius muscle extracts in BoNT-treated muscle. As expected, the genes were expressed in a temporal order, suggesting that a sequence of cellular events is involved in the recovery process. Shen et al. (2006) suggested that recovery occurred in two major stages, which they designated as aneural and neural, and that IFG-1 was integral in the signaling process. Extensive proteomic studies are being performed on the systematic analysis of genes required for synapse structure and function (Sieburth et al., 2005) and this approach should yield valuable insights into the genetic regulation of neuromuscular function in response to denervation or other perturbations.

In therapeutic applications, BoNT affects classes of muscle tissue differently. When BoNT/A is injected into smooth detrusor muscle of the bladder and certain other smooth muscle systems, such as the esophagus, its effects last 6–9 months (occasionally up to 12 months) (Grosse et al., 2005; Schurch, 2006), compared to 3–6 months observed in striated muscles. The longer duration suggests that BoNT may act by different mechanisms in the lower urinary tract including the bladder, proximal urethra and external urethral sphincter (Smith et al., 2003). The reason for this is unclear, but lack of axonal sprouting and delayed innervation could be important factors (Schurch, 2006); a different rate of replacing the BoNT/A-cleaved SNAP-25 in different types of neurons may also play an important role in determining the duration of the effects. Additional mechanisms could include long-lasting atrophy or inactivation of smooth muscle, while in striated muscle repeated and long courses of injection do not appear to cause permanent muscle atrophy or weakening (Borodic et al., 1994).

Smith et al. (2003) suggested that autonomic nerves and parasympathetic and sympathetic nerves in the urethra may have different sensitivity to BoNT/A. A rat model was used to investigate the release of ^{14}C-choline and ^{3}H-norepinephrine at various frequencies of nerve stimulation (2, 4 and 20 Hz) in the urinary tract system. The fractional release of ACh in BoNT/A-treated animals was significantly inhibited at a higher frequency of stimulation (20 Hz), but not at lower frequencies (2 Hz) 5 days after injection. However, ACh release increased to SHAM-injected values 30 days after toxin injection. Although no significant differences were observed in the fractional release of norepinephrine from injected bladders, norepinephrine release was inhibited in the urethra for at least 30 days (Smith et al., 2003). These results indicated that BoNT/A injected into the bladder could depress the release of neurotransmitters in a frequency and time-dependent manner. No significant changes were observed in nerve density. Due to the heightened effect at high frequencies of stimulation, Smith et al. (2003) suggested that BoNT may affect intracellular signaling mechanisms involving protein kinase C. Furthermore, protein kinase C phosphorylation of SNAP-25 affects phorbol-12-myristate-13-acetate stimulation of norepinephrine release from PC12 cells. It has also been shown that BoNT/A depressed the facilitation of evoked release of norepinephrine and serotonin release by the protein kinase C activator 4-β-phorbol-12,13-dibutyrate in rabbit hippocampal slices (Nakov et al., 1989). These results indicate that BoNT may participate in signaling pathways, but further studies are needed to evaluate the toxin's involvement.

Distal temporal neuromuscular effects have been observed following injection of BoNT. Increased jitter was initially reported following periorbital treatment for blepharospasm (Sanders et al., 1986). Most other studies have evaluated distal effects on treatment of cervical dystonia, in which relatively high levels of BoNT/A are generally injected (e.g., 100–500 U) (Olsney et al., 1988). Modest increases in the magnitude of jitter and mean fiber density were observed (Lange et al., 1987; Olsney et al., 1988). Single-fiber EMG studies on distal muscles including biceps brachii to measure jitter and fiber density changes have been investigated. In most studies, patients did not develop weakness or decrement of muscle response to nerve stimulation in muscles distant from the injection site. Significant presynaptic blockage measured electrophysiogically were not observed. These data support the notion that relatively high doses can be well tolerated in clinical practice.

11.14. Central effects of botulinum neurotoxins

For many years there has been considerable debate about whether physiological concentrations of BoNT can enter the CNS (e.g., Koenig, 1971; Boroff and Chen, 1975; Habermann and Dreyer, 1986; de Groot et al., 2002; Abbruzzese and Berardelli, 2006). This is an intriguing area of study since BoNT injections have been tried to alleviate CNS-related syndromes including pain, epilepsy, migraine, visual function and psychological disorders such as depression (Aoki, 2003; Benecke et al., 2003; Lang, 2003; Luvisetto et al., 2003, 2004, 2006; Ashkenazi and Silberstein, 2004; Costantin et al., 2005; Johnson et al., 2006; Caleo et al., 2007). BoNTs have been shown to affect synaptic activity of central neurons in tissue preparations at high doses or after direct intracranial injection (Boroff and Chen, 1975; Habermann and Dreyer, 1986; Ashton and Dolly, 1988; Habermann, 1989). Presumably because of its large size of 150 kDa, BoNT is not able to permeate the blood–brain barrier or to be retrogradely transmitted to the CNS at physiological concentrations (Simpson, 2000). However, limited clinical observations in humans and animals suggest that BoNT affects the central nervous systems at physiologically relevant doses (Koenig, 1971; Habermann and Dreyer, 1986; Luvisetto et al., 2003, 2004; Abbruzzese and Berardelli, 2006; Bozzi et al., 2006). It is currently unclear if BoNT affects cortical excitability and plasticity in humans (Abbruzzese and Berardelli, 2006). The ability of BoNT to affect brain function remains controversial and needs further study. If BoNT entered the CNS and brain at physiological levels or elicited indirect effects from the periphery, this might open important therapeutic opportunities.

11.15. Possible role of BoNT in neuronal plasticity and learning

Motor systems throughout life within an organism have a dynamic capacity for adaptive remodeling and plasticity changes (Sanes and Donoghue, 2000; Franchi, 2002). For several years, certain physicians have reported that treatment of children for cerebral palsy with BoNT sometimes leads to positive adaptation of muscle function over time. Motor cortex reorganization has been proposed to occur following injection of BoNT/A into various muscles (Franchi, 2002). Adaptive changes in motor control have been observed after localized injections of BTX, suggesting remodeling of cortical activity. This has been postulated to occur in musicians who have developed and maintained high levels of skills in muscular activity and motor control (Peschel and Altenmuller, 2004; Watson, 2006). Musicians are also prone to suffer from focal dystonia. In patients with upper limb dystonia, patients treated with BoNT/A were found to transiently alter the excitability of the inhibitory and excitatory intracortical circuit activity, which was postulated to originate through peripheral mechanisms (Gilio

et al., 2000). Besides relieving spasticity, functional improvement by BoNT could involve synaptic plasticity of the muscle afferents (Krishnan, 2005). It was reported that BoNT generates synaptic plasticity in spinal α-motoneurons and facilitates relearning by Hebbian and Contrastive Hebbian modes. It is postulated that BoNT can be used as a tool for relearning of motor activity in various neural disorders (Krishnan, 2005).

11.16. Emergency information

The seriousness of botulism led to the establishment of a National Botulism Laboratory at the Centers for Disease Control and Prevention in the United States and similar laboratories in certain other countries. In suspected cases of botulism, the CDC can be contacted at www.cdc.gov and the emergency 24-hour phone number for state health departments is 770-4888-7100. Medical care providers who suspect botulism in patients should immediately call their state health department's emergency 24-hour telephone number. The state health department can arrange for clinical consultation and, if indicated, release of botulinum neurotoxin. State health departments can be located by consulting the local telephone operator or law enforcement agency, the telephone directory under "government listings" or the Internet at http://www.cdc.gov/other.htm#states or http://www.astho.org/state.html (Hatheway and Dang, 1994).

Acknowledgments

EAJ acknowledges support from the Pacific Southwest Regional Center of Excellence (grant U54 AI065359) and the Great Lakes Regional Center of Excellence (U54 AI57153), the University of Wisconsin – Madison, and sponsors of the Food Research Institute; and that in CM's laboratory by a Telethon grant and the Armenise-HMS Foundation. The authors are grateful to members of their laboratories over the years and to collaborators and mentors on various projects involving neurotoxigenic clostridia and botulinum neurotoxin.

References

Abbruzzese G, Berardelli A (2006). Neurophysiological effects of botulinum toxin type A. Neurotox Res 9: 109–114.

Abgueguen P, Delbos V, Chennebault JM, et al. (2003). Nine cases of foodborne botulism type B in France and literature review. Eur J Clin Microbiol Infect Dis 22: 749–752.

Adams CE (1960). Embryonic mortality induced experimentally in the rabbit. Nature 188: 332–333.

Adler M, Keller JE, Sheridan RE, et al. (2001). Persistence of botulinum neurotoxin A demonstrated by sequential administration of serotypes A and E in rat EDL muscle. Toxicon 39: 233–243.

Ahsan CR, Hajnóczky, Maksymowych, et al. (2005). Visualization of binding and transcytosis of botulinum toxin by human intestinal cells. J Pharmacol Exp Therapeut 315: 1028–1035.

Aikawa Y, Lynch KL, Boswell KL, et al. (2006). A second SNARE role for exocytic SNAP25 in endosome fusion. Molec Biol Cell 17: 2113–2124.

Alderson K (1993). Motor nerve terminal morphology following botulinum A toxin injection in humans. In: BR DasGupta (Ed.), Botulinum and Tetanus Neurotoxins. Plenum Press, New York, pp. 53–62.

Anderson TD, Shah UK, Schreiner MS, et al. (2002). Airway complications of infant botulism: ten year experience with 60 cases. Otolaryngol Head Neck Surg 126: 234–239.

Andrew CG, Drachman DB, Pestronk A, et al. (1984). Susceptibility of skeletal muscle to cosackie A2 virus infection. Effects of botulinum toxin and denervation. Science 223: 714–716.

Antharavally B, Tepp W, DasGupta BR (1998). Status of cys residues in the covalent structure of botulinum neurotoxins A, B, and E. J Prot Chem 17: 187–196.

Aoki KR (2002). Botulinum neurotoxin serotypes A and B preparations have different safety margins in preclinical models of muscle weakening efficacy and systemic safety. Toxicon 40: 923–928.

Aoki KR (2003). Evidence for antinociceptive activity of botulinum toxin type A in pain management. Headache 43(Suppl. 1): S9–S15.

Arndt JW, Chai Q, Christian T, et al. (2006a). Structure of botulinum neurotoxin type D light chain at 1.65 ansgstrom resolution: repercussions for VAMP-2 substrate specificity. Biochemistry 45: 3255–3262.

Arndt JW, Jacobson MJ, Abole EE, et al. (2006b). A structural perspective of the sequence variability within botulinum neurotoxin subtypes A1–A4. J Molec Biol 362: 733–742.

Arnon SS (2004). Infant botulism. In: RD Feigen, JD Cherry (Eds.), Textbook of Pediatric Infectious Diseases. 5th ed. WB Saunders, Philadelphia, pp. 1758–1766.

Arnon SS, Werner SB, Faber HK, et al. (1979). Infant botulism in 1931—discovery of a misclassified case. Am J Dis Child 133: 580–582.

Arnon SS, Damus K, Chin J (1981). Infant botulism: epidemiology and relation to sudden infant death syndrome. Epidemiol Rev 3: 45–66.

Arnon SS, Schechter R, Inglesby TW, et al. (2005). Botulinum toxin as a biological weapon. Medical and public health management. JAMA 285: 1059–1070.

Arnon SS, Schechter R, Maslanka SE, et al. (2006). Human immune globulin in for the treatment of infant botulism. N Engl J Med 354: 462–471.

Arntzen FJ, van den Heever J, Perovic O (2004). Fatal type A botulism in South Africa, 2002. Trans R Soc Trop Med Hyg 98: 290–295.

Ashkenazi A, Silberstein SD (2004). Botulinum toxin and other approaches to migraine therapy. Annu Rev Med 55: 505–518.

Ashton AC, Dolly JO (1988). Characterization of the inhibitory activity of botulinum neurotoxin type A on the release of several transmitters from rat cerebrocortical synaptosomes. J Neurochem 50: 1808–1816.

Avila OL, Drachman DB, Pestronk A (1989). Neurotransmission regulates stability of acetylcholine receptors at the neuromuscular junction. J Neurosci 9: 2902–2906.

Bajjalieh SM, Peterson K, Shinghal R, et al. (1992). SV2, a brain synaptic vesicle protein homologous to bacterial transporters. Science 257: 1271–1273.

Bajjalieh SM, Peterson K, Linial M, et al. (1993). Brain contains 2 forms of synaptic vesicle protein-2. Proc Natl Acad Sci U S A 90: 2150–2154.

Bajjalieh SM, Frantz GD, Weimann JM, et al. (1994). Differential expression of synaptic vesicle protein-2 (SV2) isoforms. J Neurosci 14: 5223–5235.

Bajohrs M, Rickman C, Binz T, et al. (2004). A molecular basis underlying differences in the toxicity of botulinum serotypes A and E. EMBO Rep 5: 1090–1095.

Bakheit AM, Ward CD, McLellan DL (1997). Generalised botulism-like syndrome after intramuscular injections of botulinum toxin type A: a report of two cases. J Neurol Neurosurg Psychiatry 62: 198.

Baldwin MR, Barbieri JT (2007). Association of botulinum neurotoxin serotypes A and B with synaptic vesicle protein complexes. Biochemistry 46: 3200–3210.

Barclay ML, Begg EJ (1994). Aminoglycoside toxicity and relation to dose regimen. Adverse Drug React Toxicol Rev 13: 207–234.

Bartlett JC (1986). Infant botulism in adults. N Engl J Med 315: 254–255.

Bartram U, Singer D (2004). Infant botulism and sudden infant death syndrome. Klin Padiatr 216: 26–30.

Benecke R, Dressler D, Kunesch E, et al. (2003). Botulinum toxin in the treatment of muscle pain. Schmerz 17: 450–458.

Bhatia KP, Munchau A, Thompson PD, et al. (1999). Generalized muscular weakness after botulinum toxin injections for dystonia: a report of three cases. J Neurol Neurosurg Psychiatry 67: 90–93.

Bigalke H, Rummel A (2005). Medical aspects of toxic weapons. Toxicol 214: 210–220.

Billante CR, Zealear DL, Billante M, et al. (2002). Comparison of neuromusculur blockade and recovery with botulinum neurotoxins A and F. Muscle Nerve 26: 395–403.

Binz T, Kurazano H, Wille M, et al. (1990). The complete sequence of botulinum neurotoxin type-A and comparison with other clostridial neurotoxins. J Biol Chem 265: 9153–9158.

Black RE, Gunn RA (1980). Hypersensitivity reactions associated with botulinal antitoxin. Am J Med 69: 567–570.

Black JD, Dolly JO (1986). Interaction of 125I-labeled botulinum neurotoxins with nerve terminals. Autoradiographic evidence for its uptake into motor nerves by acceptor-mediated endocytosis. J Cell Biol 103: 535–544.

Blanes-Mira C, Ibañez Fernández-Ballester G, et al. (2001). Thermal stabilization of the catalytic domain of botulinum neurotoxin E by phosphorylation of a single tyrosine residue. Biochemistry 40: 2234–2242.

Blasi J, Chapman ER, Link E, et al. (1993a). Botulinum neurotoxin-A selectively cleaves the synaptic protein SNAP-25. Nature 365: 160–163.

Blasi J, Chapman ER, Yamasaki S, et al. (1993b). Botulinum neurotoxin C1 blocks neurotransmitter release by means of cleaving HPC-1/syntaxin. EMBO J 12: 4821–4828.

Blasi J, Binz T, Yamasaki S, et al. (1994). Inhibition of neurotransmitter release by clostridial neurotoxins correlates with specific proteolysis of synaptosomal proteins. J Physiol (Paris) 88: 235–241.

Böhnel H, Gessler F (2005). Botulinum toxins—cause of botulism and systemic diseases? Veter Res Commun 29: 313–345.

Böhnel H, Behrens S, Loch P, et al. (2001). Is there a link between infant botulism and sudden infant death? Bacteriological results obtained in Central Germany. Eur J Pediatr 160: 623–628.

Bonventre PF (1979). Absorption of botulinal toxin from gastrointestinal tract. Rev Infect Dis 1: 663–667.

Borodic G (2007). Botulinum toxin: immunologic considerations with long-term repeated use, with emphasis on cosmetic applications. Facial Plastic Surg Clin North Amer 15: 11–16.

Borodic GE, Ferrante RJ, Pearce LB, et al. (1994). Pharmacology and histology of the therapeutic application of botulinum neurotoxin. In: J Jankovic, M Hallett (Eds.), Therapy with Botulinum Toxin. Marcel Dekker, Inc., New York, pp. 119–157.

Borodic G, Johnson E, Goodnough M, et al. (1996). Botulinum toxin therapy, immunologic resistance, and problems with available materials. Neurology 46: 26–29.

Boroff DA, Chen GS (1975). On the question of permeability of the blood brain barrier to botulinum toxin. Int Arch Allergy Appl Immunol 48: 495–504.

Boroff DA, del Castillo J, Evory WH, et al. (1974). Observations on the action of type A botulinum toxin on the frog neuromuscular junctions. J Physiol 240: 227–253.

Boyer A, Girault C, Bauer F, et al. (2001). Two cases of foodborne botulism type E and review of epidemiology in France. Eur J Clin Microbiol Infect Dis 20: 192–195.

Bozzi Y, Costantin L, Antonucci F, et al. (2006). Action of botulinum neurotoxins in the central nervous system: antiepileptic effects. Neurotox Res 9: 197–203.

Brin MF, Hallett M, Jankovic J (Eds.) (2002). Scientific and therapeutic aspects of botulinum toxin. Lippincott Williams and Wilkins, New York.

Brooks VB (1953). Motor nerve filament block by botulinum toxin. Science 117: 334–335.

Brooks VB (1954). The action of botulinum toxin on motor-nerve filaments. J Physiol (London) 123: 501–515.

Brown MC, Holland RL, Hopkins WG (1981). Motor nerve sprouting. Annu Rev Neurosci 4: 17–42.

Burgen ASV, Dickens F, Zatman LJ (1949). The action of botulinum toxin on the neuromuscular junction. J Physiol (Lon) 109: 10–24.

Buttner-Enneyer JA, Eberhorn A, Horn ADE (2003). Motor and sensory innervation of extraocular eye muscles. Ann N Y Acad Sci 1004: 40–49.

Byard RW, Moore L, Bourne AJ, et al. (1992). Clostridium botulinum and sudden infant death syndrome—a 10 year prospective study. J Paediatr Child Health 28: 156–157.

Caleo M, Restani L, Gianfranceschi L, et al. (2007). Transient synaptic silencing of developing striate cortex has persistent effects on visual function and plasticity. J Neurosci 27: 4530–4540.

Campos-Neto A, Mengel JO, Oliveira-Silva DA, et al. (1995). Potent stimulation of murine B cells to proliferate and to secrete immunoglobulins by a lipoteichoic acid-like molecule produced by Clostridium botulinum C and D. Braz J Med Biol Res 28: 575–584.

Capra NF, Bernanke JM, Porter JD (1991). Ultrastructural changes in the masseter muscle of Macaca fasciluaris resulting from intramuscular injections of botulinum toxin type A. Arch Oral Biol 36: 827–836.

Caya JG, Rashmi A, Miller JE (2004). Clostridium botulinum and the clinical laboratorian. A detailed review of botulism, including biological warfare ramifications of botulinum toxin. Arch Pathol Lab Med 128: 653–662.

Centers for Disease Control and Prevention (CDC) (1998). Botulism in the United States 1899–1996: Handbook for Epidemiologists, Clinicians, and Laboratory Workers. Centers for Disease Control and Prevention, Atlanta, GA. www.cdc.gov/ncidod/dbmd/diseaseinfo/files/botulinism.pdf (accessed March 2008).

Centers for Disease Control and Prevention (CDC) (2006). CDC Botulism. Available online at: http://www.bt.cdc.gov/agent/botulism, accessed March 2008.

Chai Q, Arndt JW, Dong M, et al. (2006). Structural basis of cell surface receptor recognition by botulinum neurotoxin B. Nature 444: 1096–1100.

Chang GY, Ganguly G (2003). Early antitoxin treatment in wound botulism results in better outcome. Eur Neurol 49: 151–153.

Chang KJ, Bennett V, Cuatrecasas P (1975). Membrane receptors as general markers for plasma membrane isolation procedures. The use of ^{125}I-labeled wheat germ agglutinin, insulin, and cholera toxin. J Biol Chem 250: 488–500.

Chang VH, Robinson LR (2000). Serum positive botulism with neuropathic features. Arch Phys Med Rehabil 81: 122–126.

Cherington M (1990). Botulism. Semin Neurol 10: 27–31.

Cherington M (1998). Clinical spectrum of botulism. Muscle Nerve 21: 701–710.

Cherington M (2004). Botulism: update and review. Seminar Neurol 24: 155–163.

Chertow DS, Tan ET, Maslanka SE, et al. (2006). Botulism in 4 adults following injections with an unlicensed, highly concentrated botulinum preparation. J Am Med Assoc 296: 2476–2479.

Chia JK, Clark JK, Ryan CA, et al. (1986). Botulism in an adult associated with foodborne intestinal infection with Clostridium botulinum. N Engl J Med 315: 239–241.

Claus D, Druschky A, Ergbuth F (1995). Botulinum toxin—influence on respiratory heart-rate variation. Mov Disord 10: 574–579.

Cohen RE, Anderson DL (1986). Botulism: emotional impact on patient and family. J Psychom Res 30: 321–326.

Colebatch JG, Wolff AH, Gilbert RJ, et al. (1989). Slow recovery from severe foodborne botulism. Lancet 2: 1216–1217.

Colice GL (1987). Prolonged intubation versus tracheostomy in the adult. J Intens Care Med 2: 85–102.

Conti-Fine BM, Milani M, Kaminski HJ (2006). Myasthenia gravis: past, present, future. J Clin Invest 116: 2843–2854.

Costantin L, Bozzi Y, Richichi C, et al. (2005). Antiepileptic effects of botulinum neurotoxin E. J Neurosci 25: 1943–1951.

Couesnon A, Pereira Y, Popoff MR (2008). Receptor-mediated transcytosis of botulinum neurotoxin A through intestinal cell monolayers. Cell Microbiol 10: 375–387.

Crawford TO (2003). Infantile botulism. In: HR Jones, Jr, DC DeVito, BT Barnes (Eds.), A Clinician's Approach Neuromuscular Diorders of Infancy, Childhood, and Adolescence. Butterworth Heinemann, Elsevier Science, Philadelphia, PA, pp. 547–554.

Custer KL, Austin NS, Sullivan JM, et al. (2006). Synaptic vesicle protein 2 enhances release probability at quiescent synapses. J Neurosci 26: 1303–1313.

Dack GM (1926). Behavior of botulinum toxin in alimentary tract of rats and guinea pigs. J Infect Dis 38: 174–181.

Dack GM, Wood WL (1928). Serum therapy for botulism in monkeys. J Infect Dis 42: 209–212.

DasGupta BR (1989). The structure of botulinum neurotoxin. In: LL Simpson (Ed.), Botulinum Toxin and Tetanus Toxin. Academic Press, San Diego, pp. 53–67.

DasGupta BR (2006). Botulinum neurotoxins: perspective on their existence and as polyproteins harboring viral proteases. J Gen Appl Microbiol 52: 1–8.

DasGupta BR, Dekleva ML (1990). Botulinum neurotoxin type A—sequence of amino acids at the N-terminus and around the nicking site. Biochimie 72: 661–664.

DasGupta BR, Rasmussen S (1983). Purification and amino acid composition of type E botulinum neurotoxin. Toxicon 21: 535.

DasGupta BR, Sathyamoorthy V (1984). Purification and amino acid composition of type A botulinum neurotoxin. Toxicon 22: 415–424.

DasGupta BR, Antharavally BS, Tepp W, et al. (2005). Botulinum neurotoxin types A, B, and E: fragmentations by autoproteolysis and other mechanisms including O-phenantrholine—dithiothreitol, and association of the dinucleotides NAD(+)/NADH with the heavy chain of the three neurotoxins. Protein J 24: 337–368.

Davis JB (1951). Clostridium botulinum in a fatal wound infection. JAMA 146: 646.

Davletov B, Bajohrs M, Binz T (2005). Beyond BOTOX: advantages and limitations of individual botulinum neurotoxins. Trends Neurosci 28: 446–452.

de Groot M, Schubert M, Rothe B, et al. (2002). Central effects of botulinum toxin type A. Klin Neurophysiol 33: 207–212.

de Paiva A, Poulain B, Lawrence GW, et al. (1993). A role for interchain disulfide or its participating thiols in the internalization of botulinum neurotoxin A revealed by a toxin derivative that binds to ecto-acceptors and inhibits transmitter release intracellularly. J Biol Chem 28: 20838–20844.

de Paiva A, Meunier FA, Molgó J, et al. (1999). Functional repair of motor endplates after botulinum neurotoxin type A poisoning: biphasic switch of synaptic activity between nerve sprouts and their parent terminals. Proc Natl Acad Sci U S A 96: 3200–3205.

Dessain SK, Adekar SP, Carpenter KA, et al. (2004). High efficiency creation of human monoclonal antibody-producing hybridomas. J Immunol Meth 291: 109–122.

Devriese PP, Devriese LA (2001). Historical aspects of botulinum toxin. Neurology 57: 1144.

Dezfulian M (1989). Animal models of botulism. In: LL Simpson (Ed.), Botulinum Neurotoxin and Tetanus Toxin. Academic Press, Inc., San Diego, CA, pp. 335–350.

Dickson EC (1918). Botulism. A clinical and experimental study. Monograph of the Rockefeller Institute, No. 8, New York, pp. 1–117.

Dineen SS, Bradshaw M, Johnson EA (2003). Neurotoxin gene clusters in Clostridium botulinum type A strains: sequence comparison and evolutionary implications. Curr Microbiol 46: 345–352.

Dineen SS, Bradshaw M, Karasek C, et al. (2004). Nucleotide sequence and transcriptional analysis of the type A2 neurotoxin gene cluster in Clostridium botulinum. FEMS Microbiol Lett 235: 9–16.

Dodd SL, Selsby J, Payne A, et al. (2005). Botulinum neurotoxin type A causes shift in myosin heavy chain composition in muscle. Toxicon 46: 196–203.

Dolman EC (1964). Botulism as a world health problem. In: KH Lewis, K Cassel (Eds.), Botulism. US Pub Health Serv, Washington, DC, pp. 5–32.

Dong M, Richards DA, Goodnough MC, et al. (2003). Synaptotagmins I and II mediate entry of botulinum neurotoxin B into cells. J Cell Biol 162: 1293–1303.

Dong M, Yeh F, Tepp WH, et al. (2006). SV2 is the protein receptor for botulinum neurotoxin A. Science 312: 592–596.

Dong M, Tepp WH, Liu H, et al. (2007). Mechanism of botulinism neurotoxin B and G entry into hippocampal neurons. J Cell Biol 31: 1511–1522.

Drachman DB (1964). Atrophy of skeletal muscle in chick embryos treated with botulinum toxin. Science 145: 719–721.

Drachman DB (1971). Botulinum toxin as a tool for research on the nervous system. In: LL Simpson (Ed.), Neuropoisons. Their Pathophysiological Actions, Vol. 1. Poisons of Animal Origin. Plenum, New York, pp. 325–347.

Drachman DB, Coulombre AJ (1962). Method for continuous infusion of fluids into the chorioallantoic circulation of the chick embryo. Science. 138: 144–145.

Drachman DB, Johnston DM (1983). Neurotrophic regulation of dynamic properties of skeletal muscle—effects of botulinum toxin and denervation. J Physiol (Lon) 252: 657–667.

Dressler D, Rothwell JC (2000). Electromyographic quantification of the paralysing effect of botulinum toxin in the sternocleidomastoid muscle. Eur Neurol 43: 13–16.

Dressler D, Benecke R (2003). Autonomic side effects of botulinum toxin type B treatment of cervical dystonia and hyperhydrosis. Eur Neurol 49: 34–38.

Dressler D, Saberi FA (2005). Botulinum toxin: mechanisms of action. Eur Neurol 53: 3–9.

Duchen LW (1971). An electron microscopic study of the changes induced by botulinum toxin in the motor end-plates of slow and fast skeletal muscle fibres of the mouse. J Neurol Sci 14: 47–60.

Duchen LW (1972). Motor nerve growth induced by botulinum toxin as a regenerative phenomenon. Proc R Soc Med 65: 10–11.

Duchen LW, Strich SJ (1968). The effects of botulinum toxin on the pattern of innervation of skeletal muscle in the mouse. Q J Exp Physiol Cogn Med Sci 53: 84–89.

Duchen LW, Strich SJ (1971). An electron microscopy study of the changes induced by botulinum toxin in the motor end-plates of skeletal muscle in the mouse. Q J Exp Physiol 53: 84–89.

Duffey P, Brown C (2006). Iatrogenic botulism in an amateur weight-lifter. Movement Disord 21: 1056.

Dumitru D, Amato AA, Zwarts M (Eds.) (2002). Electrodiagnostic Medicine, 2nd edn. Hanley and Belfus, Philadelphia.

Eklund MW (Ed.) (1995). Avian Botulism. Charles C. Thomas, Springfield, Illinois.

Eleopra R, Tugnoli V, de Grandis D (1997). The variability in the clinical effect induced by botulinum toxin type A: the role of muscle activity in humans. Movement Disord 12: 89–94.

Eleopra R, Tugnoli V, Rossetto O, et al. (1998). Different time courses in recovery after poisoning with botulinum neurotoxin serotypes A and E in humans. Neurosci Lett 256: 135–138.

Eleopra R, Tugnoli V, Quatrale R, et al. (2004). Different types of botulinum toxin in humans. Movement Disord 19(Suppl. 8): S53–S59.

Eleopra R, Tugnoli V, Quatrale R, et al. (2006). Clinical use of non-A botulinum toxins: botulinum toxin type C and botulinum type F. Neurotox Res 9: 127–131.

Elston HR, Wang M, Loo LK (1991). Arm abscesses caused by *Clostridium botulinum*. J Clin Microbiol 29: 2678–2679.

Encinar JA, Fernández A, Ferragut JA, et al. (1998). Structural stabilization of botulinum neurotoxins by tyrosine phosphorylation. FEBS Lett 429: 78–82.

English AW (2003). Cytokines, growth factors and sprouting at the neuromuscular junction. J Neurocytol 32: 943–960.

Erbguth FJ (2004). Historical notes on botulism, *Clostridium botulinum*, botulinum toxin, and the idea of the therapeutic use of the toxin. Movement Disord 19(Suppl. 8): S2–S6.

Erbguth F, Claus D, Engelhardt A, et al. (1993). Systemic effect of local botulinum toxin injections unmasks subclinical Lambert–Eaton syndrome. J Neurol Neurosurg Psychiatry 62: 198.

Fairweather NF, Lyness VA (1986). The complete nucleotide sequence of tetanus toxin. Nucl Acids Res 14: 7809–7812.

Federici T, Boulis NM (2006). Gene-based treatment of motor neuron diseases. Muscle Nerve 33: 302–323.

Fernández-Salas E, Steward LE, Ho H, et al. (2004). Plasma membrane localization signals in the light chain of botulinum neurotoxin. Proc Natl Acad Sci U S A 101: 3208–3213.

Ferrier-Montiel AV, Canaves JM, DasGupta BR, et al. (1996). Tyrosine phosphorylation modulates the activity of clostridial neurotoxins. J Biol Chem 271: 18322–18325.

Fischer D, Freislederer A, Jorch G (2004). Sudden death of twins: botulism because of contamination by pap vegetables. Klin Pediatr 216: 31–35.

Fischer A, Montal M (2007a). Crucial role of the disulfide bridge between botulinum neurotoxin light and heavy chains in protease translocation across membranes. J Biol Chem 282: 29604–29611.

Fischer A, Montal M (2007b). Single molecule detection of intermediates during botulinum neurotoxin translocation across membranes. Proc Natl Acad Sci U S A 104: 10447–10452.

Foran PG, Mohammed N, Lisk GO, et al. (2003). Evaluation of the therapeutic usefulness of botulinum neurotoxins B, C1, E and F compared with the long lasting type A. Basis for distinct durations of inhibition of exocytosis in central neurons. J Biol Chem 278: 1363–1371.

Fox CK, Keet CA, Strober JB (2005). Recent advances in infant botulism. Pediatr Neurol 32: 149–154.

Franchi G (2002). Time course of motor cortex reorganization following botulinum toxin injection into the vibrissal pad of the adult rat. Eur J Neurosci 16: 1333–1348.

Franciosa G, Aureli P, Schecter R (2003). In: MD Milliotis, JW Bier (Eds.), International Handbook of Foodborne Pathogens. Marcel Dekker, Inc., New York and Basel.

Francisco AMO, Arnon SS (2007). Clinical mimics of infant botulism. Pediatrics 119: 826–828.

Franz DR, Pitt LM, Clayton MA, et al. (1993). Efficacy of prophylactic and therapeutic administration of antitoxin for inhalational botulism. In: BR DasGupta (Ed.), Botulinum and Tetanus Neurotoxins. Neurotransmission and Biomedical Aspects. Plenum Press, New York, pp. 473–476.

Fujinaga Y (2006). Transport of bacterial toxins into target cells: pathways followed by cholera toxin and botulinum progenitor toxin. J Biochem (Tokyo) 140: 155–160.

Gangarosa EJ, Donadio JA, Armstrong RW, et al. (1971). Botulism in the United States, 1899–1969. Am J Epidemiol 93: 93–101.

Gartlan MG, Hofman HT (1993). Crystalline preparation of botulinum toxin type A (Botox): degradation in potency with storage. Otolaryngol Head Neck Surg 108: 135–140.

Geny B, Popoff MR (2006). Bacterial protein toxins and lipids: role in toxin targeting and activity. Biol Cell 98: 633–651.

Gilio F, Curra A, Lorenzano C, et al. (2000). Effects of botulinum toxin type A on intracortical inhibition in patients with dystonia. Ann Neurol 48: 20–26.

Gill DM (1982). Bacterial toxins: a table of lethal amounts. Microbiol Rev 46: 86–94.

Giménez DF, Giménez JA (1993). Serological subtypes of botulinal neurotoxins. In: BR DasGupta (Ed.), Botulism and Tetanus Neurotoxins: Neurotransmission and Biomedical Aspects. Plenum Press, New York, pp. 421–432.

Gioltzoglou T, Cordivari C, Lee PJ, et al. (2005). Problems with botulinum toxin treatment in mitochondrial cytopathy: case report and review of the literature. J Neurol Neurosurg Psychiatry 76: 1594–1596.

Gomez S, Queiroz LS (1982). The effects of black widow spider venom on the innervation of muscles paralyzed by botulinum toxin. Q J Exp Physiol Cog Med Sci 67: 495–506.

Goode GB, Shearn DL (1982). Botulism: a case associated with sensory abnormalities. Arch Neurol 39: 55.

Gordon RJ, Lowy FD (2005). Curent concepts—bacterial infections in drug users. N Engl J Med 353: 1945–1954.

Griffin PM, Hatheway CL, Rosenbaum R, et al. (1997). Endogenous antibody production to botulinum toxin in an adult with intestinal colonization botulism and underlying Crohn's disease. J Infect Dis 175: 633–637.

Grosse J, Kramer G, Stohrer M (2005). Success of repeated injections of botulinum A toxin in patients with severe neurogenic detrusor overactivity and incontinence. Eur Urol 47: 653–659.

Gupta A, Sumner CJ, Castor M, et al. (2005). Adult botulism type F in the United States, 1981–2002. Neurology 65: 1694–1700.

Gutierrez AR, Bonensteiner J, Gutmann L (1994). Electrodiagnosis of infantile botulism. J Child Neurol 9: 362–366.

Gutmann E (1962). Denervation and disuse atrophy in cross-striated muscle. Rev Can Biol 21: 353–365.

Gutmann E, Habnzlíková E (1972). Age Changes in the Neuromuscular Junction. Scientechnica Ltd., Bristol, UK.

Habermann E (1989). Clostridial neurotoxins and central nervous effects: functional studies on isolated preparations. In: LL Simpson (Ed.), Botulinum Neurotoxin and Tetanus Toxin. Academic Press, San Diego, CA, pp. 255–279.

Habermann E, Dreyer F (1986). Clostridial neurotoxins: handling and action at the cellular and molecular level. Curr Top Microbiol Immunol 129: 93–179.

Hanson MA, Stevens RC (2002). Structural views of botulinum neurotoxin in numerous functional states. In: MF Bain, J Jankovic, M Hallett (Eds.), Scientific and Therapeutic Aspects of Botulinum Toxin. Lippincott Williams & Wilkins, Philadelphia, pp. 9–27.

Hassan SM, Jennekens FGI, Veldman H (1995). Botulinum toxin-induced myopathy in the rat. Brain 118: 533–545.

Hatheway CL (1988). Botulism. In: WH Hausler, A Balows, M Ohashi, et al. (Eds.), Laboratory Diagnosis of Infectious Diseases. Vol. 1. Springer-Verlag, New York, pp. 111–133.

Hatheway CL (1993). Clostridium botulinum and other clostridia that produce botulinum neurotoxin. In: AHS Hauschild, KL Dodds (Eds.), Clostridium Botulinum: Ecology and Control in Foods. Marcel Dekker, New York, pp. 3–20.

Hatheway CL (1995). Botulism: the present status of the disease. Curr Top Microbiol Immunol 195: 55–75.

Hatheway CL, Dang C (1994). Immunogenicity of the neurotoxins of Clostridium botulinum. In: J Jankovic, M Hallett (Eds.), Therapy with Botulinum Toxin. Marcel Dekker, Inc., New York, pp. 93–107.

Hatheway CL, Johnson EA (1998). Clostridium: the spore-bearing anaerobes. In: L Collier, A Balows, M Sussman (Eds.), Topley & Wilson's Microbiology and Infections. 9th ed. Vol. 2. Systematic Bacteriology. Arnold, London, pp. 731–782.

Hatheway CL, Snydjer JD, Seals JE, et al. (1984). Antitoxin levels in botulism patients treated with trivalent equine botulism antitoxin to type A, type B, and type E. J Infect Dis 150: 407–412.

Hauschild AHS, Dodds KL (Eds.) (1993). Clostridium Botulinum: Ecology and Control in Foods. Marcel Dekker, New York, pp. 3–20.

Heckly RJ, Hildebrand GJ, Lamanna C (1960). On the size of the toxic particle passing the intestinal barrier in botulism. J Exp Med 111: 745–759.

Hesse S, Reiter F, Konrad M, et al. (1998). Botulinum toxin type A and short term electrical stimulation in the treatment of upper limb flexor spasticity after stroke: a randomized, double-blind, placebo-controlled trial. Clin Rehabil 12: 381–388.

Heuser J (1976). Morphology of synaptic vesicle discharge and reformation at the frog neuromuscular junction. In: S Thesleff (Ed.), Motor Innervation of Muscle. Academic Press, London, pp. 51–115.

Hikes DC, Manoli A (1981). Wound botulism. J Trauma 21: 68–71.

Hoch DH, Romero-Mira M, Ehrlich BE, et al. (1985). Channels formed by botulinum, tetanus, and diphtheria toxins in planar lipid bilayers: relevance to translocation of proteins across membranes. Proc Natl Acad Sci U S A 82: 1692–1696.

Hoffman RE, Pincomb BJ, Skuls MR (1982). Type F infant botulism. Am J Dis Child 136: 270–271.

Holland RL, Brown MC (1981). Nerve growth in botulinum toxin poisoned muscles. Neuroscience 6: 1167–1179.

Holmes GL, Moshé SL, Royden Jones H, Jr. (Eds.) (2006). Clinical Neurophysiology of Infancy, Childhood, and Adolescence. Elsevier, Inc., Philadelphia, PA.

Holzer E (1962). Botulism dürch inhalation. Med Klin 41: 1735–1740.

Horowitz MA, Hatheway CL, Dowell VR, Jr. (1976). Laboratory diagnosis of botulism complicated by pyridostigmine treatment of the patient—a method for selectively removing interfering substances from clinical samples. Am J Clin Pathol 66: 97–107.

Howard JF (1990). Adverse effects on neuromuscular transmission. Semin Neurol 10: 89–102.

Hughes JM, Blumenthal JR, Merson MH, et al. (1981). Clinical features of types A and B food-borne botulism. Ann Intern Med 95: 442–445.

Hughes R, Whaler BC (1962). Influence of nerve-ending activity and of drugs on the rate of paralysis of rat diaphragm preparations of Cl. botulinum type A toxin. J Physiol 160: 221–233.

Ibañez C, Blanes-Mira C, Fernández-Ballester G, et al. (2004). Modulation of botulinum neurotoxin A catalytic domain stability by tyrosine phosphorylation. FEBS Lett 578: 121–127.

Inoue K, Fujinaga Y, Watanabe T, et al. (1996). Molecular composition of *Clostridium botulinum* type A progenitor toxins. Infect Immun 64: 1589–1594.

Iwase T, Iwase C (2006). Systemic effect of local and small-dose botulinum toxin injection to unmask subclinical myasthenia gravis. Graefe's Arch Clin Exp Ophthalmol 244: 415–416.

Jahn R, Scheller RH (2006). SNAREs—engines for membrane fusion. Nature Rev Molec Cell Biol 7: 631–643.

Jankovic J, Hallett M (Eds.) (1994). Therapy With Botulinum Toxin. Marcel Dekker, Inc., New York, pp. 93–107.

Jenzer G, Mumenthaler M, Ludin HP, et al. (1975). Autonomic dysfunction in botulism B: a clinical report. Neurology 25: 150–153.

Jin R, Rummel A, Binz T, et al. (2006). Botulinum neurotoxin B recognizes its protein receptor with high affinity and specificity. Nature 444: 1092–1095.

Johnson EA (1999). Clostridial toxins as therapeutic agents: benefits of nature's most toxic proteins. Annu Rev Microbiol 53: 551–575.

Johnson EA (2005a). Clostridial neurotoxins. In: P Dürre (Ed.), Handbook on Clostridia. CRC Press, Boca Raton, FL, pp. 491–525.

Johnson EA (2005b). Bacteriophages encoding botulinum and diphtheria toxins. In: MK Waldor, DI Friedman, S Adhya (Eds.), Phages: Their Role in Bacterial Pathogenesis and Biotechnology. ASM Press, Washington, DC, pp. 280–296.

Johnson EA (2005c). *Clostridium botulinum* and Clostridium tetani. In: SP Borrellio, PR Murray, G Funke (Eds.), Topley & Wilson's Microbiology and Microbial Infections, 10th ed. Vol. 2. Bacteriology. Hodder Arnold, London, pp. 1035–1088.

Johnson EA (2006). Neurotoxigenic clostridia. In: VA Fischetti, RP Novick, JJ Feretti, et al. (Eds.), Gram-Positive Pathogens. 2nd ed. ASM Press, Washington, DC, pp. 688–702.

Johnson EA (2007). *Clostridium botulinum*. In: MP Doyle, LR Beuchat (Eds.), Food Microbiology. Fundamentals and Frontiers. 3rd ed. ASM Press, Washington, DC, pp. 401–421.

Johnson EA, Bradshaw M (2001). *Clostridium botulinum* and its neurotoxins: a metabolic and cellular perspective. Toxicon 39: 1703–1722.

Johnson EA, Goodnough MC (1998). Botulism. In: L Collier, A Balows, M Sussman (Eds.), Topley & Wilson's Microbiology and Microbial Infections. 98th ed. Vol. 2. Systematic Bacteriology. Arnold, London, pp. 723–741.

Johnson EA, Borodic GE, Acquadro MA (2006). Medical applications of botulinum neurotoxins. In: JE Alouf, MR Popoff (Eds.), Comprehensive Sourcebook of Bacterial Protein Toxins. 3rd ed. Elsevier, Inc., Philadelphia, PA, pp. 959–975.

Jones HR, Darras BT (2000). Acute care pediatric electromyography. Muscle Nerve Suppl 9: S53–S62.

Kaminski H (Ed.) (2003). Myasthenia Gravis and Related Disorders (Electronic Resource). Humana Press, Totowa, NJ.

Katz B (1966). Nerve Muscle, Synapse. McGraw Hill, New York.

Keet CA, Fox CK, Margeta M, et al. (2005). Infant botulism, type F, presenting at 54 hours of life. Pediatr Neurol 32: 193–196.

Keller JE (2006). Recovery from botulinum neurotoxin poisoning in vivo. Neuroscience 139: 629–637.

Keller JE, Neale EA, Oyler G, et al. (1999). Persistence of botulinum neurotoxin action in cultured spinal cord cells. FEBS Lett 456: 137–142.

Kelly H, Brussen KA, Lawrence A, et al. (2006). Polioviruses and other enteroviruses isolated from faecal samples of patients with acute flaccid paralysis in Australia, 1996–2004. J Paediatr Child Health 42: 370–376.

Kempner W (1897). Welterer Beitrag Zur Lehre von der Fleischvergiftung, Das Antitoxin des Botulismus. Z Hyg Infectionskr 26: 481–500.

Kerner C (1820). Neue Boebachtungen über die in Württenberg so häufig verfallenden tödtchen Vengiftungen durch den gennus geraucherter Würste, Tubingen, Osiander.

Kobayashi H, Fujisawa K, Saito Y, et al. (2003). A botulism case of a 12-year-old girl caused by intestinal colonization of *Clostridium botulinum* type Ab. Jpn J Infect Dis 56: 73–74.

Koenig MG (1971). The clinical aspects of botulism. In: LL Simpson (Ed.), Neuropoisons. Their Pathophysiological Actions, Vol. 1. Poisons of Animal Origin. Plenum Press, New York and London, pp. 283–301.

Koriazova LK, Montal M (2003). Translocation of botulinum neurotoxin light chain protease through the heavy chain channel. Nat Struct Biol 10: 13–18.

Krishnan RV (2005). Botulinum toxin: from spasticity reliever to neuromotor re-learning tool. Int J Neurosci 115: 1451–1467.

Kröger S, Schröder JE (2002). Agrin in the developing CNS: new roles for a synapse organizer. News Physiol Sci 17: 207–212.

Kummer TT, Misgeld T, Sanes JR (2006). Assembly of the postsynaptic membrane at the neuromuscular junction: paradigm lost. Curr Opin Neurol 16: 74–82.

Lacy DB, Stevens RC (1999). Sequence homology and structural analysis of the clostridial neurotoxins. J Molec Biol 291: 1091–1104.

Lacy DB, Tepp W, Cohen AC, et al. (1998). Crystal structure of botulinum neurotoxin type A and implications for toxicity. Nature Struct Biol 5: 898–902.

Lamanna C (1959). The most poisonous poison. Science 130: 763–772.

Lamanna C, Hillowalla RA, Alling CC (1967). Buccal exposure to botulinal toxin. J Infect Dis 117: 327–331.

Lang AM (2003). Botulinum toxin type A therapy in chronic pain disorders. Arch Phys Med Rehabil 84(Suppl. 1): S69–S73.

Lange DJ, Brin MF, Warner CL, et al. (1987). Distance effect of local injection of botulinum toxin. Muscle Nerve 10: 552–555.

Lawrence G, Wang J, KwoChion CKN, et al. (2007). Two protein trafficking processes at motor nerve endings unveiled by botulinum neurotoxin E. J Pharmacol Exp Therap 320: 410–418.

LeClaire RD, Pitt MLM (2005). Biological weapons defense. Effect levels. In: LE Lindler, FJ Lebeda, GW Korch

(Eds.), Infectious Diseases: Biological Weapons Defense: Infectious Diseases and Counterterrorism. Humana Press, Inc., Totowa, NJ, pp. 41–61.

Lee HK (2006). Synaptic plasticity and phosphorylation. Pharmacol Therapeut 112: 810–832.

Lesieur C, Vécsey-Semjén C, Abrami L, et al. (1997). Membrane insertion: the strategies of toxins (Review). Mol Memb Biol 14: 45064.

L'Hommedieu C, Stough R, Brown L, et al. (1979). Potentiation of neuromuscular weakness in infant botulism by aminoglycosides. J Pediatr 95: 1065–1070.

Li LYJ, Kelkar P, Exconde RE, et al. (1999). Adult onset "infant" botulism: an unusual cause of weakness in the intensive care unit. Neurol 53: 891.

Lindström M, Nevas M, Kurki J, et al. (2004). Type C botulism due to toxic feed affecting 52,000 farmed foxes and minks in Finland. J Clin Microbiol 42: 4718–4725.

Lipsky NG, Drachman DB, Pestronk A, et al. (1989). Neural regulation of messenger RNA for the alpha subunit of acetylcholine receptors. Role of neuromuscular transmission. Exp Neurol 105: 171–176.

Lonberg N (2005). Human antibodies from transgenic animals. Nature Biotechnol 23: 1117–1125.

London E (1992). How bacterial toxins enter cells: the role of partial unfolding in membrane translocation. Molec Microbiol 6: 3277–3282.

Long SS, Gajewski JL, Brown LW, et al. (1985). Clinical, laboratory and environmental features of infant botulism in Southeastern Pennsylvania. Pediatrics 75: 935–941.

Luvisetto S, Rossetto O, Montecucco C, et al. (2003). Toxicity of botulinum neurotoxins in central nervous system of mice. Toxicon 41: 475–481.

Luvisetto S, Marinelli S, Rossetto O, et al. (2004). Central injection of botulinum neurotoxins: behavioural effects in mice. Behav Pharmacol 15: 233–240.

Luvisetto S, Marinelli S, Lucchetti F, et al. (2006). Botulinum neurotoxins and formalin-induced pain: central vs. peripheral effects in mice. Brain Res 1082: 124–131.

Ma J, Shen J, Lee CA, et al. (2005). Gene expression following botulinum toxin A injection: a study in rats. J Orthopaed Res 23: 302–309.

MacDonald KL, Cohen ML, Blake PA (1986). The changing epidemiology of adult botulism in the United States. Am J Epidemiol 124: 794–799.

MacIntosh BR, Gardiner PF, McComas AJ (Eds.) (2006). Skeletal Muscle. Form and Function. 2nd ed. Human Kinetics, Champaign, IL.

Mackle IJ, Halcomb E, Parr MJ (2001). Severe adult botulism. Anaesth Intensive Care 29: 297–300.

Mahrhold S, Rummel A, Bigalke H, et al. (2006). The synaptic vesicle protein 2C mediates the uptake of botulinum neurotoxin A into phrenic nerves. FEBS Lett 580: 2011–2014.

Maksymowych AB, Simpson LL (2004). Structural features of the botulinum neurotoxin molecule that govern binding and transcytosis across polarized human intestinal epithelial cells. J Pharmacol Exp Ther 310: 633–641.

Maksymowych AB, Reinhard M, Malizio CJ, et al. (1999). Pure botulinum neurotoxin is absorbed from the stomach and small intestine and produces peripheral neuromuscular blockade. Infect Immun 67: 4708–4712.

Malizio CJ, Goodnough MC, Johnson EA (2000). Purification of botulinum type A neurotoxin. Meth Molec Biol 145: 27–39.

Mann JM, Martin S, Hoffmann R, et al. (1981). Patient recovery from type A botulism: morbidity assessment following a large outbreak. Am J Public Health 71: 266–269.

Martin PT (2003). Glycobiology of the neuromuscular junction. J Neurocytol 32: 915–929.

Marx JL (1978). Botulism in infants: a cause of sudden death? Science 201: 799–801.

Maselli RA, Ellis W, Mandler RN, et al. (1997). Cluster of wound botulism in California: clinical, electrophysiologic, and pathologic study. Muscle Nerve 20: 1284–1295.

Mayers CN, Holley JL, Brooks T (2001). Antitoxin therapy for botulinum intoxication. Rev Med Microbiol 12: 29–37.

McCroskey LM, Hatheway CL (1988). Laboratory findings in four cases of adult botulism suggest colonization of the intestinal tract. J Clin Microbiol 26: 1052–1054.

McLauchlin J, Grant KA, Little CL (2006). Food-borne botulism in the United Kingdom. J Public Health 28: 337–342.

McLellan K, Das RE, Ekong TA, et al. (1996). Therapeutic botulinum type A toxin: factors affecting potency. Toxicon 34: 975–985.

Meichsner M, Reichel G (2005). Effect of botulinum toxin A and B on vegetative cardiac innervation. Fortschr Neurol Psych 73: 409–414.

Ménétrey J, Gillet D, Ménez A (2005). Structural features common to intracellularly acting toxins from bacteria. Toxicon 45: 129–137.

Merriggioli MN, Howard JE, Jr., Harper CM (2004). Neuromuscular Junction Disorders. Diagnosis and Treatment. Marcel Dekker, Inc., New York and Basel.

Merson MH, Dowell VR (1973). Epidemiologic, clinical and laboratory aspects of wound botulism. N Engl J Med 289: 1005–1010.

Meunier FA, Lisk G, Sesardic D, et al. (2003). Dynamics of motor nerve terminal remodeling unveiled using SNARE-cleaving botulinum toxins: the extent and duration are dictated by the sites of SNAP-25 truncation. Molec Cell Neurosci 22: 454–466.

Meyer KF (1956). The status of botulism as a world health problem. Bull World Health Org 15281–15298.

Mezaki T, Kaji R, Kohara N, et al. (1996). Development of generalized weakness in a patient with amyotrophic lateral sclerosis after focal botulinum toxin injection. Neurol 46: 845–846.

Midura TF, Arnon SS (1976). Infant botulism—identification of Clostridium botulinum and its toxin in feces. Lancet 2: 934–936.

Millecamps S, Nicolle D, Ceballos-Picot I, et al. (2001). Synaptic sprouting increases the uptake capacities of motoneurons in amyotrophic lateral mice. Proc Natl Acad Sci U S A 98: 7582–7587.

Millecamps S, Mallet J, Barkats M (2002). Adenoviral retrograde gene transfer in motoneurons is greatly enhanced by prior intramuscular inoculation with botulinum toxin. Hum Gene Ther 13: 225–232.

Mitchell WG, Tseng-Ong L (2005). Catastrophic presentation of infant botulism may obscure or delay diagnosis. Pediatrics 116: E436–E438.

Montecucco C (1986). How do tetanus and botulinum neurotoxins bind to neuronal membranes? Trends Biochem Sci 11: 314–317.

Montecucco C, Schiavo G (1993). Tetanus and botulism neurotoxins: a new group of zinc proteases. Trends Biochem. Sci 18: 324–327.

Montecucco C, Schiavo G (1995). Structure and function of tetanus and botulinum neurotoxins. Q Rev Biophys 28: 423–472.

Montecucco C, Schiavo G, Gao Z, et al. (1988). Interaction of botulinum and tetanus toxins with the lipid bilayer surface. Biochem J 251: 379–383.

Montecucco C, Schiavo G, DasGupta BR (1989). Effect of pH on the interaction of botulinum neurotoxin A, neurotoxin B, and neurotoxin E with liposomes. Biochem J 259: 47–53.

Montecucco C, Papine E, Schiavo G (1994). Bacterial protein toxins penetrate cells via a 4-step mechanism. FEBS Lett 346: 92–98.

Montecucco C, Rosetto O, Schiavo G (2004). Presynaptic receptor arrays for clostridial neurotoxins. Trends Microbiol 12: 442–446.

Montecucco C, Schiavo G, Pantano S (2005). SNARE complexes and neuroexocytosis: how many, how close? Trends Biochem Sci 30: 367–372.

Moore P, Naumann M (Eds.) (2003). Handbook of Botulinum Toxin Treatment, 2nd ed. Blackwell Publishing, Malden, MA.

Morton HE (1961). The toxicity of Clostridium botulinum type A toxin for various species of animals, including man. The Institute for Cooperative Research, University of Pennsylvania, Philadelphia.

Nakov R, Habermann E, Hertting G, et al. (1989). Effects of botulinum toxin on presynaptic modulation of evoked transmitter release. Eur J Pharmacol 164: 45–53.

Neale EA (2003). Moving across membranes. Nat Struct Biol 10: 2–3.

Nevas M, Lindström M, Virtanen A, et al. (2005). Infant botulism acquired from household dust presenting as sudden infant death syndrome. J Clin Microbiol 43: 511–513.

Niemann H (1991). Molecular biology of clostridial neurotoxins. In: JE Alouf, JH Freer (Eds.), A Sourcebook of Bacterial Protein Toxins. Academic Press Ltd., London, pp. 303–348.

Nishikawa A, Uotsu N, Arimitsu H, et al. (2004). The receptor and transporter for internalization of Clostridium botulinum type C progenitor toxin into HT-29 cells. Biochem Biophys Res Commun 319: 327–333.

Nishiki T, Kamata Y, Nemoto Y, et al. (1994). Identification of protein receptor for Clostridium botulinum type B neurotoxin in rat brain synaptosomes. J Biol Chem 269: 10498–10503.

Nishiki T, Tokuyama Y, Kamata Y, et al. (1996). The high-affinity binding of Clostridium botulinum type B neurotoxin to synaptotagmin II associated with gangliosides GT1b/GD1a. FEBS Lett 378: 253–257.

Nishiura H (2007). Incubation period as a clinical predictor of botulism: analysis of previous Izushi-borne outbreaks in Hokkaido, Japan from 1951 to 1965. Epidemiol Infect 135: 126–130.

Ohishi I, Sugii S, Sakaguchi G (1977). Oral toxicities of Clostridium botulinum toxins in response to molecular size. Infect Immun 16: 107–109.

Olsney RK, Aminoff MJ, Gelb DJ, et al. (1988). Neuromuscular effects distant from the site of botulinum toxin injection. Neurol 38: 1780–1783.

Paik NJ, Seo K, Eun HC (2006). Reduced potency after refrigerated storage of botulinum toxin A: human extensor digitorum brevis muscle study. Mov Disord 21: 1759–1763.

Paisley JW, Lauer BA, Arnon SS (1995). A second case of infant botulism caused by Clostridium baratii. Pediatr Infect Dis 14: 912–914.

Park J-P, Simpson LL (2003). Inhalational poisoning by botulinum toxin and inhalational vaccination with its heavy chain component. Infect Immun 71: 1147–1154.

Parker MW, Pattus F (1993). Rendering a membrane soluble in water: a common packing motif in bacterial protein toxins. TIBS 39: 1–395.

Pellett S, Tepp WH, Clancy CM, et al. (2007). A neuronal cell-based botulinum neurotoxin assay for highly sensitive and specific detection of neutralizing serum antibodies. FEBS Lett 581: 4803–4808.

Peschel T, Altenmuller E (2004). Altered movement-related brain potentials in musicians suffering from action induced focal dystonia. Klin Neurophysiologie 35: 96–103.

Pestronk A, Drachman DB (1978). Motor nerve sprouting and acetylcholine receptors. Science 199: 1223–1225.

Pestronk A, Drachman DB, Griffin JW (1976). Effect of botulinum toxin on trophic regulation of acetylcholine receptors. Nature 264: 787–789.

Pickett J, Berg B, Chaplin E, et al. (1976). Syndrome of botulism in infancy—clinical and electrophysiological study. N Engl J Med 295: 770–772.

Pitt MLM, LeClaire RD (2005). Pathogenesis by aerosol. In: LE Lindler, FJ Lebeda, GW Korch (Eds.), Infectious Diseases: Biological Weapons Defense: Infectious Diseases and Counterterrorism. Humana Press, Inc., Totowa, NJ, pp. 65–78.

Pittinger C, Adamson R (1972). Antibiotic blockade of neuromuscular function. Ann Rev Pharmacol 12: 169.

Popoff MR (1995). Ecology of neurotoxigenic strains of clostridia. In: C Montecucco (Ed.), Clostridial Neurotoxins. 195. Curr Top Microbiol Immunol, Springer, Berlin, pp. 1–29.

Porter JD, Baker RS (1996). Muscles of a different "color": the unusual properties of the extraocular muscles may predispose them in neurogenic and myogenic disease. Neurol 46: 30–37.

Puhar A, Johnson EA, Rosetto O, et al. (2004). Comparison of pH-induced conformational change of different clostridial neurotoxins. Biochem Biophys Res Commun 319: 66–71.

Raciborska DA, Charlton MP (1999). Retention of cleaved synaptosome-associated protein of 25 kDa (SNAP-25) in neuromuscular junctions: a new hypothesis to explain persistence of botulinum A poisoning. Can J Physiol 77: 679–688.

Ravichandran E, Gong Y, Al Saleem FH, et al. (2006). An initial assessment of the systemic pharmacokinetics of botulinum toxin. J Pharmacol Exp Ther 318: 1343–1351.

Reller ME, Douce RW, Maslanka SE, et al. (2006). Wound botulism acquired in the Amazonian rain forest of Ecuador. Am J Trop Med Hyg 74: 628–631.

Rosales RL, Arimura K, Takenaga S, et al. (1996). Extrafusal and intrafusal muscle effects in experimental botulinum toxin A injection. Muscle Nerve 19: 488–496.

Rosales RL, Bigalke H, Dressler D (2006). Pharmacology of botulinum toxin: differences between type A preparations. Eur J Neurol 13(Suppl. 1): 2–10.

Rossetto O, Schiavo G, Polverino de Laureto P, et al. (1992). Surface topography of histidine residues of tetanus toxin probed by immobilized metal ion affinity chromatography. Biochem J 285: 9–12.

Rossetto O, Schiavo G, Montecucco C, et al. (1994). SNARE motif and neurotoxins. Nature 372: 415–416.

Ruff RL (2002). More than meets the eye: extraocular muscle is very distinct from extremity skeletal muscle. Muscle Nerve 25: 311–313.

Rummel A, Karnath T, Henke T, et al. (2004a). Synaptotagmins I and II act as nerve cell receptors for botulinum neurotoxin G. J Biol Chem 279: 30865–30870.

Rummel A, Mahrhold S, Bigalke H, et al. (2004b). The Hcc-domain of botulinum neurotoxin A and B exhibit a singular ganglioside binding site displaying serotype specific carbohydrate interaction. Mol Microbiol 51: 631–643.

Rummel A, Eichner T, Weil T, et al. (2007). Identification of the protein receptor binding site of botulinum neurotoxins B and G proves the double-receptor concept. Proc Natl Acad Sci U S A 104: 359–364.

Sakaguchi G (1983). Clostridium botulinum toxins. Pharmacol Ther 19: 165–194.

Sakaguchi G, Kosaki S, Ohishi S (1984). Structure and function of botulinum toxins. In: JE Alouf (Ed.), Bacterial Protein Toxins. Academic Press, London, pp. 435–443.

Sampaio C, Cost J, Ferreira JJ (2004). Clinical comparison of marketed formulations of botulinum toxin. Movement Disord 19(Suppl. 8): S129–S136.

Sanders DB, Massey EW, Buckley EG (1986). Botulinum toxin for blepharospasm: single fiber EMG studies. Neurology 36: 545–547.

Sandrock CE, Murin S (2001). Clinical predictors of respiratory failure and long-term outcome in black tar heroin-associated wound botulism. Chest 120: 562–566.

Sanes JN, Donoghue JP (2000). Plasticity and primary motor cortex. Annu Rev Neurosci 23: 393–415.

Sanes JR, Lichtman JW (2001). Induction, assembly, maturation and maintenance of a postsynaptic apparatus. Nat Rev Neurosci 2: 791–805.

Santos JI, Swensen P, Glasgow LA (1981). Potentiation of Clostridium botulinum toxin by aminoglycoside antibiotics— clinical and laboratory observations. Pediatrics 68: 50–54.

Schantz EJ, Johnson EA (1992). Properties and use of botulinum neurotoxin and other microbial neurotoxins in medicine. Microbiol Rev 56: 80–99.

Schechter R, Peterson B, McGee J, et al. (1999). Clostridium difficile colitis associated with infant botulism: near-fatal case analogous to Hirschsprung's enterocolitis. Clin Infect Dis 29: 367–374.

Schiavo G, Papini E, Genna G, et al. (1990). An intact interchain disulfide bond is required for the neurotoxicity of tetanus toxin. Infect Immun 58: 4136–4141.

Schiavo G, Benfenati F, Poulain B, et al. (1992a). Tetanus and botulinum-B neurotoxins block neurotransmitter release by proteolytic cleavage of synaptobrevin. Nature 92: 832–835.

Schiavo G, Poulain B, Rosetto O, et al. (1992b). Tetanus toxin is a zinc protein and its inhibition of neurotransmitter release depends on zinc. EMBO J 11: 3577–3583.

Schiavo G, Rosetto O, Catsicas S, et al. (1993a). Identification of the nerve terminal targets of botulinum neurotoxin serotypes A, D, and E. J Biol Chem 268: 23784–23787.

Schiavo G, Santucci A, DasGupta BR, et al. (1993b). Botulinum neurotoxins serotype A and serotype E cleave SNAP-25 at distinct COOH terminal peptide bonds. FEBS Lett 335: 99–103.

Schiavo G, Shone CC, Bennett MK, et al. (1995). Botulinum neurotoxin type C cleaves a single Lys-Ala bond within the carboxyl-terminal region of syntaxins. J Biol Chem 270: 10566–10570.

Schiavo G, Matteoli M, Montecucco C (2000). Neurotoxins affecting neuroexocytosis. Physiol Rev 80: 717–766.

Schneider HJ, Fisk R (1939). Botulism: demonstration of toxin in blood and tissues. J Am Med Assoc 113: 2299–2300.

Schurch B (2006). Botulinum toxin for the management of bladder dysfunction. Drugs 66: 1301–1318.

Scott AB (1989). Clostridial toxins as therapeutic agents. In: LL Simpson (Ed.), Botulinum Toxin and Tetanus Neurotoxin. Academic Press, Inc., San Diego, pp. 399–412.

Scott AB, Suzuki D (1988). Systemic toxicity of botulinum toxin by intramuscular injection in the monkey. Movement Disord 3: 333–335.

Scranton TW, Wwata M, Carlson SS (1993). The SV2 protein of synaptic vesicles is a keratan sulfate proteoglycan. J Neurochem 61: 29–44.

Sebald M, Saimot G (1973). Circulating toxin, an aid in the diagnosis of type B botulism in man. Ann Microbiol (Paris) 124: 61–69.

Sellin LC, Kauffman JA, DasGupta BR (1983a). Comparison of the effects of botulinum neurotoxin types A and E at the rat neuromuscular junction. Med Biol 61: 120–125.

Sellin LC, Thesleff S, DasGupta BR (1983b). Different effects of types A and B botulinum toxin on neurotransmitter release at the rat neuromuscular junction. Acta Physiol Scand 119: 127–133.

Setlow P, Johnson EA (2007). Spores and their significance. In: MP Doyle, LR Beuchat (Eds.), Food Microbiology. Fundamentals and Frontiers. 3rd ed. ASM Press, Washington, DC, pp. 35–67.

Shapiro RL, Hatheway C, Swerdlow DL (1998). Botulism in the United States: a clinical and epidemiologic review. Ann Intern Med 129: 221–228.

Shen J, Ma J, Elsaida GA, et al. (2005). Gene expression of myogenic regulatory factors following intramuscular injection of botulinum A toxin in juvenile rats. Neurosci Lett 381: 207–210.

Shen J, Ma J, Lee C, et al. (2006). How muscles recover from paresis and atrophy after intramuscular injection of botulinum toxin A: study in juvenile rats. J Orthopaed Res 24: 1128–1135.

Shen WPV, Felsing N, Land D, et al. (1994). Development of infant botulism in a 3-year-old female with neuroblastoma following autologous bone-marrow transplantation. Potential use of human botulism immune globulin. Bone Marrow Transplant 13: 345–347.

Sheth RD, Lotz BP, Hecox KE, et al. (1999). Infantile botulism: pitfalls in electrodiagnosis. J Child Neurol 14: 156–158.

Sieburth D, Ch'ng Q, Dybbs M, et al. (2005). Systematic analysis of genes required for synapse structure and function. Nature 436: 510–517.

Simpson LL (2000). Identification of the characteristics that underlie botulinum toxin potency: implications for designing novel drugs. Biochimie 82: 943–953.

Simpson LL, Coffield JA, Bakry N (1994). Inhibition of vacuolar adenosine triphosphatase antagonizes the effects of clostridial neurotoxins but not phospholipase A2 neurotoxins. J Pharmacol Exp Ther 269: 256–262.

Sloop R, Cole A, Escutin E (1997). Human response to botulinum toxin injection: type B compared with type A. Neurology 49: 189–194.

Smith CP, Franks ME, NcNeil BK, et al. (2003). Effect of botulinum toxin A on the autonomic nervous system of the rat lower urinary tract. J Urol 169: 1896–1900.

Smith LDS (1977). Botulism. The Organism, Its Toxins, the Disease Charles C. Thomas, Springfield, Illinois.

Smith LDS, Sugiyama H (1988). Botulism. The Organism, Its Toxins, the Disease. Charles C Thomas, Springfield, Illinois.

Smith TJ, Lou J, Geren I, et al. (2005). Sequence variation with botulinum neurotoxin serotypes impacts antibody binding and neutralization. Infect Immun 73: 5450–5457.

Sobel J (2005). Botulism. Clin Infect Dis 41: 1167–1173.

Sobel J, Tucker T, Sulka A, et al. (2004). Foodborne botulism in the United States, 1990–2000. Emerg Infect Dis 10: 1606–1611.

Solomon HM, Johnson EA, Bernard DT, et al. (2001). Clostridium botulinum and its toxins. In: FP Downes, K Ito (Eds.), Compendium for the Microbiological Examination of Foods. 4th ed. American Public Health Association, Washington, DC, pp. 317–324.

Son YJ, Thompson WJ (1995). Schwann cell processes guide regeneration of peripheral axons. Neuron 14: 125–132.

St. Louis ME, Peck SH, Bowering D, et al. (1988). Botulism from chopped garlic: delayed recognition of a major outbreak. Ann Intern Med 108: 363–368.

Sugii S, Ohishi I, Sakaguchi G (1977). Correlation between oral toxicity and in vitro stability of Clostridium botulinum type-A and type-B toxins of different molecular sizes. Infect Immun 16: 910–914.

Sugiyama H (1979). Animal models for the study of infant botulism. Rev Infect Dis 1: 683–688.

Sugiyama H (1980). Clostridium botulinum neurotoxin. Microbiol Rev 44: 419–448.

Sugiyama H, Mills DC (1978). Intraintestinal toxin in infant mice challenged intragastrically with Clostridium botulinum spores. Infect Immun 21: 59–63.

Swaminathan S, Eswaramoorthy S (2000). Structural analysis of the catalytic and binding sites of Clostridium botulinum neurotoxin B. Nat Struct Biol 7: 1751–1759.

Swaminathan S, Eswaramoorthy S (2002). Crystal structure of Clostridium botulinum serotype B. In: MF Brin, J Jankovic, M Hallett (Eds.), Scientific and Therapeutic Aspects of Botulinum Toxin. Lippincott Williams & Wilkins, Philadelphia, pp. 29–40.

Swoboda KJ, Jones HR, Jr. (2006). The floppy infant. In: GL Holmes, SL Moshé, HR Jones, Jr. (Eds.), Clinical Neurophysiology of Infancy, Childhood, and Adolescence. Elsevier, Inc., Philadelphia, PA, pp. 505–518.

Tabita K, Sakaguchi S, Kozaki S, et al. (1991). Distinction between Clostridium botulinum type A strains associated with foodborne botulism and those with infant botulism in Japan. FEMS Microbiol Lett 79: 251–256.

Tacket CO, Rogawski CO (1989). Botulism. In: LL Simpson (Ed.), Botulinum Neurotoxin and Tetanus Toxin. Academic Press, Inc., San Diego, pp. 351–378.

Tacket CO, Shandera WX, Mann JM, et al. (1984). Equine antitoxin use and other factors that predict outcome in type-A foodborne botulism. Am J Med 76: 794–798.

Tang-Liu DDS, Aoki KR, Dolly JO, et al. (2003). Intramuscular injection of 125I-botulinum neurotoxin complex versus 125I-botulinum-free neurotoxin: time course of tissue distribution. Toxicon 42: 461–469.

Tanzi MG, Gabay MP (2002). Association between honey consumption and infant botulism. Pharmacotherapy 22: 1479–1483.

Tarsy D, Bhattacharya N, Borodic G (2000). Myasthenia gravis after botulinum toxin for Meige syndrome. Movement Disord 15: 736–738.

Terranova W, Breman JG, Locey RP, et al. (1978). Botulism type B: epidemiologic aspects of an extensive outbreak. Am J Epidemiol 108: 150–156.

Thesleff S (1960). Supersensitivity of skeletal muscle produced by botulinum toxin. J Physiol 151: 598–607.

Thesleff S (Ed.) (1976). Motor Innervation of Muscle. Academic Press, London.

Thesleff S (1991). Highlights from 40 years' research on the neuromuscular junction. Physiol Res 40: 381–394.

Thesleff S (1993). Paralysis by botulinum neurotoxins uncovers trophic secretions at the neuromuscular junction. In: BR DasGupta (Ed.), Botulinum and Tetanus Neurotoxins. Plenum Press, New York, pp. 45–52.

Thobois S, Broussolle Toureille L, et al. (2001). Severe dysphagia after botulinum toxin injection for cervical dystonia in multiple system atrophy. Movement Disord 16: 764–765.

Thoenen H (1995). Neurotrophins and neuronal plasticity. Science 270: 593–598.

Tian W-H, Festoff BW, Blot S, et al. (1995). Synaptic transmission blockade increases plasminogen activator activity in mouse skeletal muscle poisoned with botulinum toxin type A. Synapse 20: 20–32.

Tintner R, Gross R, Winzer UF, et al. (2005). Autonomic function after botulinum toxin type A or B: a double-blind, randomized trial. Neurology 65: 765–767.

Tseng-Ong L, Mitchell WG (2005). Catastrophic presentation of infant botulism may obscure or delay diagnosis. Pediatrics 116: 436–438.

Tsuboi M, Furukawa Y, Kuroguchi F, et al. (2002). Botulinum neurotoxin A blocks cholinergic ganglionic neurotransmission in the dog heart. Jpn J Pharmacol 89: 249–254.

Tsukamoto K, Kohda T, Mukamoto M, et al. (2005). Binding of *Clostridium botulinum* type C and D neurotoxins to ganglioside and phospholipid. J Biol Chem 280: 35164–35171.

Tuite PJ, Lang AE (1996). Severe and prolonged dysphagia complicating botulinum toxin A injections for dystonia in Machado-Joseph disease. Neurology 46: 846.

Ugalde I, Christiansen SP, McLoon LK (2005). Botulinum toxin treatment of extraocular muscles in rabbits results in increased myofiber remodeling. Invest Ophthamol Visual Sci 46: 4114–4120.

Ungchusak K, Chunsuttiwat S, Braden C, et al. (2007). The need for global planned mobilization of essential medicine: lessons from a massive Thai botulism outbreak. Bull World Health Org 85: 238–240.

United States Public Health Service (USPHS) (1979). Botulism in the United States, 1899–1977: Handbook for Epidemiologists, Clinicians and Laboratory Workers. Centers for Disease Control, Atlanta, GA.

Uotso N, Nishikawa A, Watanabe T, et al. (2006). Cell internalization and traffic pathway of *Clostridium botulinum* type C neurotoxin into HT-29 cells. Biochim Biophys Acta 1763: 120–128.

van Ermengem EP (1897a). Contribution à l'étude des Intoxications Alimentaires. Recherches sur des accidents à caractéres botuliniques par du jammbon. Travaux du Laboratorie d'Hygiène et de Bactériologie, Université de Gan, J. van In & Cie Lierre/H. Engelcke, Gand, pp. 5–269. Extrat des Archives de Pharmacodynamie, Vol III.

van Ermengem EP (1897b). Ueber einen neuen anaëroben Bacilus und seine Beziehungen zum Botulismus. Zeitschrift für Hygiene und Infektionskrankheitein (Leipzig) 26: 1056.

van Ermengem EP (1979). Classics in infectious disease. A new anaerobic bacillus and its relation to botulism. Rev Infect Dis 1: 701–719.

van Heyningen S (1974). Gangliosides as membrane receptors for tetanus toxin, cholera toxin and serotonin. Nature 249: 415–417.

Varma JK, Katsitadze G, Moiscrafishvili M, et al. (2004). Signs and symptoms predictive of death in patients with foodborne botulism—Republic of Georgia, 1980–2002. Clin Infect Dis 39: 357–362.

Verderio C, Rossetto O, Grumelli C, et al. (2006). Entering neurons: botulinum toxins and synaptic vesicle recycling. EMBP Rep 7: 995–999.

Villar RG, Shapiro RL, Busto S, et al. (1999). Outbreak of type A botulism and development of a botulism surveillance and antitoxin release program in Argentina. JAMA 281: 1334–1338.

Wang YC, Burr DH, Korthals GJ, et al. (1984). Acute toxicity of aminoglycoside antibiotics as an aid in detecting botulism. Appl Environ Microbiol 48: 951–955.

Watson AHD (2006). What can studying musicians tell us about motor control of the hand? J Anatomy 208: 527–542.

Weber JT, Goodpasture HC, Alexander H, et al. (1993). Wound botulism in a patient with a tooth abscess—case report and review. Clin Infect Dis 16: 635–639.

Wenzel R, Jones D, Borrego JA (2007). Comparing two botulinum toxin type A formulations using manufacturers' product summaries. J Clin Pharm Ther 32: 387–402.

Werner SB, Passaro D, McGee J, et al. (2000). Wound botulism in California, 1951–1998: recent epidemic in heroin injectors. Clin Infect Dis 31: 1018–1024.

Wilcox PG, Morrison NJ, Pardy RL (1990). Recovery of ventilatory and upper airway muscles and excercise performance after type A botulism. Chest 98: 620–626.

Woodruff BA, Griffin PM, McCroskey LM, et al. (1992). Clinical and laboratory comparison of botulism from types A, B, and E in the United States, 1975–1988. J Infect Dis 166: 1281–1286.

Wright GP (1955). The neurotoxins of *Clostridium botulinum* and Clostridium tetani. Pharmacol Rev 7: 413–465.

Yee WC, Pestronk A (1987). Mechanisms of postsynaptic plasticity: remodeling of the junctional acetylcholine receptor cluster induced by motor nerve terminal outgrowth. J Neurosci 7: 2019–2024.

Yoneda S, Shimazawa M, Kato M, et al. (2005). Comparison of the therapeutic indexes of different molecular forms of botulinum toxin type A. Eur J Pharmacol 508: 223–229.

Yule AM, Barker IK, Austin JW, et al. (2006). Toxicity of *Clostridium botulinum* type E neurotoxin to Great Lakes fish: implications for infant botulism. J Wildlife Dis 42: 479–493.

Handbook of Clinical Neurology, Vol. 91 (3rd series)
Neuromuscular junction disorders
A.G. Engel, Editor

Chapter 12

Neurotoxicology of neuromuscular transmission

JAMES F. HOWARD, JR. [1]* AND DONALD B. SANDERS [2]

[1]*Laboratory for Myasthenia Gravis Research, Department of Neurology, The University
of North Carolina at Chapel Hill, Chapel Hill, NC, USA*

[2]*Duke University Medical School, Durham, NC, USA*

12.1. Introduction

The neuromuscular junction (NMJ) is uniquely sensitive to the effects of neurotoxins. Unlike the brain, spinal cord and nerve, which are protected by the blood–brain and blood–nerve barriers, there are no barriers to protect the NMJ from the deleterious effects of circulating toxins. Neurotoxins directed to the NMJ come from many sources. Many occur as natural substances of plants or animals, others are prescribed pharmaceutical compounds and still others are environmental hazards or weapons of terror. Nearly all of these agents reduce the safety factor of neuromuscular transmission (NMT) by interfering with either the presynaptic or postsynaptic elements of the NMJ, or both. The clinical features of the toxicity produced by these agents are quite varied as many have toxic effects on other parts of the central, peripheral or autonomic nervous systems. Many have other systemic effects as well. While feared for their potential morbidity and mortality, many of these neurotoxins have led to major advances in our understanding of the molecular mechanisms of normal and pathological NMT pharmacology and physiology. For example, recognition that α-bungarotoxin binds to the acetylcholine receptor (AChR) led to development of the assay for antibodies against the AChR, a major advance in the diagnosis and treatment of myasthenia gravis (MG) (Fambrough et al., 1973).

Worldwide, the most common neuromuscular junction toxicity results from envenomation. Of more concern to the clinician are the effects of pharmacologic agents that produce weakness in patients with disordered NMT. All forms of NMJ neurotoxicity are characterized by progressive, typically symmetrical muscle weakness. Muscles of eye movement or the eyelids are most often involved, as are the muscles of neck flexion and the pectoral and pelvic girdles. More severe toxicity may affect bulbar or respiratory muscles, or both. Cognition and sensation are usually spared unless other parts of the nervous system are also involved. Muscle stretch reflexes are often preserved or only minimally diminished, particularly during the early phases of the illness, but may be lost if muscle weakness is severe.

12.2. Pharmacological blockade of neuromuscular transmission

Drugs that produce worsening of neuromuscular function can be put into four categories (Table 12.1). First are drugs that have a direct effect on NMT in otherwise normal individuals; second are drugs that disturb the immune system and result in the development of MG; third are drugs that unmask subclinical MG or worsen muscle strength in patients with disorders of NMT (e.g., MG, Lambert–Eaton Syndrome (LES), botulism); and fourth drugs that delay recovery of strength, particularly respiratory function, following general anesthesia during which neuromuscular blocking agents have usually been used.

Altered drug clearance due to renal or hepatic disease, concomitant drug administration, electrolyte disturbances or direct toxicity may predispose patients to neuromuscular weakness in the first situation. An example would be the patient with chronic renal failure

---

*Correspondence to: James F. Howard, Jr., MD, Laboratory for Myasthenia Gravis Research, Department of Neurology, 3114 Bioinformatics Bldg., CB#7025, The University of North Carolina at Chapel Hill, Chapel Hill, NC 27599-7025, USA. E-mail: howardj@neurology.unc.edu.

Table 12.1

Mechanisms of Pharmacological Blockade at the Neuromuscular Junction

1. Direct deleterious effects on synaptic transmission in an otherwise normal individual
2. Drug-induced disturbance of the immune system with the resulting development of Myasthenia Gravis
3. Unmasking of subclinical disease or the worsening of muscle strength in patients with disorders of neuromuscular transmission
4. Delayed recovery of strength, particularly respiratory function, following general anesthesia during which neuromuscular blocking agents may or may not have been used

undergoing a surgical procedure during which a neuro-muscular blocking agent and an aminoglycoside antibiotic are given. The most common example of the second situation is the induction of MG by d-penicillamine (D-P). In the third situation, persistence of neuromuscular dysfunction after a drug has been discontinued implies that subclinical disease had been unmasked by the drug. This is seen when previously asymptomatic patients given D-P develop weakness that does not resolve following discontinuation of the drug.

The adverse effects of drugs on synaptic transmission may be classified in three ways (Table 12.2). They may act presynaptically, reducing acetylcholine (ACh) release by a local anesthetic-like effect on the nerve terminal, by impairing calcium influx into the nerve terminal or by reducing the synthesis of ACh in the nerve terminal, similar to the effect of hemicholinium. They may act postsynaptically, producing a curare-like blockade of ACh receptors or potentiating the effects of depolarizing or non-depolarizing neuromuscular blocking agents. And some drugs have both pre- and postsynaptic effects. Other than several reviews of adverse effects of various drugs on patients with MG or other diseases of NMT (Argov and Mastaglia, 1979a; Swift, 1981; Kaeser, 1984; Howard, 1991) much of the literature on this subject is anecdotal, often involving individual case reports. Only a few in vitro studies have examined the effect of selected drugs on neuromuscular transmission in animal or human nerve-muscle preparations. The adverse effects of these potentially neurotoxic medications must be

Table 12.2

Mechanisms of Arthropod Blockade of Synaptic Transmission

1. Facilitation of ACh release with subsequent exhaustion of neurotransmitter
2. Facilitation of ACh release without subsequent exhaustion of neurotransmitter
3. Depletion of ACh release with subsequent exhaustion of neurotransmitter

taken into consideration when deciding which drugs to use in patients with MG or related conditions. For most drugs the actual incidence of adverse effects is unknown because we do not know how many at-risk patients have used each drug without complication. Also, in vitro and animal studies may suggest an adverse drug effect that does not correlate with clinically significant side effects. While it is most desirable for these patients to avoid all drugs that may adversely affect NMT, in certain instances they must be used for the management of other illness. In such situations a thorough knowledge by the physician of the deleterious side effects can minimize the potential danger. When possible it is wise to use the drug within each class that has been shown clinically or at least experimentally to have the least effect on NMT.

There are no drugs that are absolutely contraindicated in patients with MG and LES, with the possible exceptions of d-penicillamine, perhaps botulinum toxin and interferon alpha. There are, however, many drugs that can make the weakness of these patients worse or prolong the duration of action of muscle relaxants.

Drugs that perturb NMT produce varying degrees of ptosis, ocular, facial, bulbar, respiratory and generalized muscle weakness, similar to MG. Treatment includes discontinuing the offending drug and, when necessary, reversing the neuromuscular blockade with intravenous calcium or potassium or cholinesterase inhibitors. The most frequently encountered such problems in our experience result from administration of antibiotics (aminoglycoside and macrolides) and β-adrenergic blocking agents to patients with MG.

This summary will review the adverse effects of major drug classes on NMT. The references section includes the anecdotal experiences of others.

12.2.1. Analgesics

The narcotic analgesics, in therapeutic concentrations, do not appear to directly depress neuromuscular transmission in myasthenic muscle (Kim et al., 1979; Sanders et al., 1981). We routinely use morphine sulfate for analgesia after thymectomy, without adverse effects on muscle strength. They should be used with caution in patients with reduced breathing capacity because these agents depress respiratory drive. Cholinesterase inhibitors may potentiate the analgesic effects of morphine, hydromorphone, codeine and opium alkaloids (Slaughter, 1950).

12.2.2. Anesthetics, general

No controlled studies specifically address the advantages or disadvantages of general anesthesia in patients with disordered NMT. There may be a potentiation of the effects of neuromuscular blocking agents in patients with MG due to the reduction in the safety factor of NMT. This may be attributed to rapid desensitization of the myasthenic endplate ACh receptors and the rapid development of phase II block or the reduction in the number of available receptors (Baraka et al., 1971, 1993, 1999). Treating the myasthenic patient with, for example, corticosteroids or plasma exchange, or both, to a state of marked improvement or remission prior to surgery obviates much of the concern about prolonged post-operative ventilatory failure (Howard and Sanders, 1983; Sanders and Howard, 1991). Intubation and induction with ethrane and nitrous oxide avoids the use of neuromuscular blocking agents and only rarely do MG patients so-treated require post-operative ventilation; most can be extubated after awakening fully in the operating room or the recovery room. The reader is referred to an old but comprehensive review of this topic (Foldes and McNall, 1962).

A single study reports subclinical MG that was unmasked by the inhalation anesthetic, methoxyflurane (Foldes and McNall, 1962; Elder et al., 1971). Studies have shown that inhalation anesthetics alter ionic conductance and the post-junctional sensitivity to ACh and shorten receptor channel open time following activation by ACh (Gage and Hamill, 1976).

12.2.3. Anesthetics, local

Local anesthetics per se do not cause neuromuscular weakness in otherwise normal individuals. However, intravenously administered lidocaine, procaine and similar local anesthetic agents can potentiate the effects of neuromuscular blocking agents. Local anesthetics appear to have both pre- and postsynaptic effects, impairing the propagation of the nerve action potential in the nerve terminal, thus reducing ACh release and reducing the sensitivity of the post-junctional membrane to ACh (Hirst and Wood, 1971; Matthews and Quilliam, 2000). Procaine has been reported to produce an acute myasthenic crisis, although this has been contested by others (Katz and Gissen, 1969). We have seen an acute myasthenic worsening in a young woman following injection of large amounts of lidocaine for a brachial plexus block (Howard JF, personal observation).

12.2.4. Antibiotics

In 1941 it was demonstrated that tyrothricin, one of the first antibiotics, produced respiratory weakness in animals (Pridgen, 1956). The earliest report of antibiotic-induced neuromuscular blockade in man was in 1956: four patients without prior evidence of neuromuscular disease developed apnea (which resulted in death in two) after receiving intraperitoneal neomycin sulfate. To date there are several hundred reports of purported neuromuscular weakness from antibiotics. Some patients were otherwise normal, others were receiving neuromuscular blocking agents or drugs with known effects on the NMJ, others had MG and others had diseases that alter the pharmacokinetics of the drug (Bodley and Brett, 1962; McQuillen et al., 1968; Pittinger et al., 1970; Albiero, 1978a; Burkett et al., 1979).

The aminoglycoside antibiotics are well recognized for producing neuromuscular weakness irrespective of the route of administration (Pittinger et al., 1970). The weakness is related to dose and serum levels and can be reversed in part by cholinesterase inhibitors, calcium infusion and aminopyridines (Singh et al., 1978a, b, c; Maeno and Enomoto, 1980). Aminoglycosides may have pre- or postsynaptic effects, or both, at the NMJ. For example, tobramycin has a predominantly presynaptic action, inhibiting ACh release, whereas netilmicin acts predominantly postsynaptically, blocking ACh binding to the receptor similar to curare (Dretchen et al., 1972; Waterman and Smith, 1977; Caputy et al., 1981). Specific neuromuscular blocking effects have been demonstrated for amikacin, gentamicin, kanamycin, neomycin, netilmicin, streptomycin and tobramycin (Elmqvist and Josefsson, 1962; Dretchen et al., 1973; Albiero, 1978b; De Rosayro and Healy, 1978; Singh et al., 1978c; Paradelis et al., 1980; Torda, 1980). Neomycin is the most toxic of these, tobramycin the least (Caputy et al., 1981).

Only gentamicin, kanamycin, neomycin, tobramycin and streptomycin have been implicated in producing muscle weakness in non-myasthenic patients (Kaeser, 1984). Exacerbation of weakness by aminoglycoside antibiotics in MG was first reported in 1964 (Hokkanen, 1964). The degree of weakness varied from minimal to ventilatory failure. Similar effects have also been reported in infant botulism (L'Hommedieu et al., 1979).

Macrolide and ketolide antibiotics also are reported to acutely exacerbate myasthenic weakness in children and adults. These include the macrolides erythromycin and azithromycin (May and Calvert, 1990; Absher and Bale, 1991; Cadisch et al., 1996). Repetitive nerve stimulation studies in normal volunteers receiving erythromycin demonstrated a facilitatory response suggestive of a presynaptic neuromuscular block (Herishanu and Taustein, 1971), but there have been no microphysiologic studies to demonstrate the mechanism of action. Abrupt worsening in MG has also been reported with the ketolide, telithromycin (Anonymous, 2004; Moreno et al., 2003; Nieman et al., 2003).

Polypeptide and monobasic amino-acid antibiotics, penicillins, sulfonamides, tetracyclines and fluoroquinolones also have known or theoretical adverse effects on NMT. Some of these have been reported to cause transient worsening of myasthenic weakness or to potentiate the weakness of neuromuscular blocking agents.

The precise mechanism by which these antibiotics impair neuromuscular transmission is not fully known. There is some data to suggest that the macrolides and penicillins induced a combination of open channel and competitive block of nAChR channel currents (Schlesinger et al., 2004). This block of AChR current occurred with therapeutic concentrations of erythromycin; other drugs required much higher concentrations.

Lincomycin and clindamycin, monobasic amino acid antibiotics, have structures that differ slightly from the aminoglycosides, but they differ considerably in their effects on NMT (Fogdall and Miller, 1974; Samuelson et al., 1975). Both have pre- and postjunctional effects and produce neuromuscular block that is not readily reversible with cholinesterase inhibitors (Rubbo et al., 1977). The neuromuscular blocking effects of lincomycin are actually worsened by cholinesterase inhibitors but are reversed by increasing the calcium concentration or by aminopyridines (Booij et al., 1978). Clindamycin appears to block muscle contractility directly, as well as having a local anesthetic action (Wright and Collier, 1976a). Vancomycin may potentiate the neuromuscular blockade of succinylcholine (Albrecht and Lanier, 1993).

Polymyxin B, colistimethate and colistin have also been reported to produce neuromuscular weakness, particularly in patients with renal disease or when used in combination with other antibiotics or neuromuscular blocking agents (Parisi and Kaplan, 1965; Gold and Richardson, 1966; Pohlmann, 1966; Lindesmith et al., 1968; Pittinger and Adamson, 1972; McQuillen and Engbaek, 1975). These drugs have mixed effects, reducing ACh release and, to a lesser degree, blocking the post-junctional AChR (Wright and Collier, 1976b; Viswanath and Jenkins, 1978; Durant and Lambert, 1981). Acute ventilatory failure has been reported in a myasthenic patient given a single intramuscular injection of colistimethate (Decker and Fincham, 1971). Colistin is also reported to acutely exacerbate the strength of myasthenic patients (Herishanu, 1969).

Tetracycline analogs oxytetracycline and rolitetracycline have also been reported to exacerbate MG, though the mechanism is unclear (Gibbels, 1967; Wullen et al., 1967). It has been suggested that magnesium in the diluent reduced ACh release from the nerve terminal (Wullen et al., 1967). Others have reported no adverse reactions or alteration of NMT in nerve-muscle preparations from tetracycline (Hokkanen, 1964; Caputy et al., 1981).

It has been suggested that ampicillin may aggravate the strength of patients with MG or worsen the decrement of repetitive nerve stimulation in rabbits with experimental autoimmune myasthenia gravis (EAMG) (Argov et al., 1986). Abnormal NMT has been demonstrated by single fiber electromyography (SFEMG) in healthy volunteers receiving ampicillin (Sanders and Howard, 1986; Girlanda et al., 1989). The mechanism of action is not known and bath application to nerve-muscle preparations has not shown an effect on NMT (Argov et al., 1986).

A few case reports suggest that the quinolone antibiotics ciprofloxacillin, perfloxacin and norfloxacin may worsen myasthenic weakness acutely (Moore et al., 1988; Rauser et al., 1990; Vial et al., 1995). In our experience, some MG patients tolerate ciprofloxacillin without difficulty and others experience substantial worsening. The mechanism of action is not known.

12.2.5. Anticonvulsants

Diphenylhydantoin (DPH) depresses both pre- and postsynaptic mechanisms of NMT in vitro (Norris et al., 1964; Yaari et al., 1977, 1979). Symptomatic MG has been reported in previously asymptomatic patients receiving phenytoin, mephenytoin, trimethadione and gabapentin (Norris et al., 1964; Regli and Guggenheim, 1965; Peterson, 1966; Booker et al., 1970; Brumlik and Jacobs, 1974). Reversal of weakness following discontinuation of the drug in some cases suggests a direct neuromuscular blocking effect. Phenytoin reduces quantal release from the nerve terminal and simultaneously increases spontaneous neurotransmitter release, miniature endplate potentials (MEPPs). This could be due to reduction in the nerve action potential amplitude or interference with influx of calcium and its intracellular sequestration in the nerve terminal. Phenytoin also acts postsynaptically; reducing the MEPP amplitude, presumably by desensitizing the endplate (Yaari et al., 1979). We have seen no acute worsening of strength in our few MG patients who have required phenytoin therapy for seizures.

Aggravation of myasthenic strength by barbiturates has also been reported (Osserman and Genkins, 1971). Barbiturates and ethosuximide produce a postsynaptic neuromuscular block, whereas carbamazepine has predominantly presynaptic effects (Thesleff, 1956; Alderdice and Trommer, 1980). A decremental response to high frequency repetitive nerve stimulation has been reported in children who had received an overdose of carbamazepine (Zaidat et al., 1999). There have been no reports of adverse neuromuscular reactions with ethosuximide.

Patients receiving trimethadone may develop systemic lupus erythematosus and nephrotic syndrome and have autoantibodies against skeletal muscle, nuclear antigens and thymic tissue (Rallison et al., 1961; Talamo and Crawford, 1963; Peterson, 1966; Booker et al., 1970). These observations have led to the suggestion that this drug may also induce an autoimmune reaction against the neuromuscular junction.

12.2.6. Cardiovascular drugs

After antibiotics, cardiovascular drugs produce most of the adverse drug reactions in patients with neuromuscular disorders. Quinine, a close analog of quinidine, was actually used as a diagnostic test for MG in the past because of its known neuromuscular blocking action (Harvey and Whitehill, 1937; Eaton, 1943).

12.2.6.1. Beta-adrenergic blocking agents

The β-adrenergic blocking agents oxprenolol, propranolol, practolol and timolol have all been implicated in causing worsening of strength in patients with MG (Herishanu and Rosenberg, 1975; Hughes and Zacharias, 1976; Shaivitz, 1979; Coppeto, 1984; Verkijk, 1985). Several cases have been reported of transient diplopia in patients receiving one of several ophthalmic β-blockers (Weber, 1982). Exacerbation of ocular weakness may occur even with β-blockers topically applied on the eye (see ophthalmic drugs). We have seen abrupt worsening of weakness in several MG patients after parenteral or ophthalmic-applied β-blockers; other patients have had onset of myasthenic symptoms shortly after beginning one of these drugs. Studies examining the effects of various β-blockers on muscle twitch tension demonstrate a reduction in twitch tension following the application of these drugs (Turker and Kiran, 1965; Wislicki and Rosenblum, 1967; Usubiaga, 1968; Davis, 1970; Lilleheil and Roed, 1971; Patel et al., 1974; Harry et al., 1975; Chiarandini, 1980). Repetitive nerve stimulation studies have not shown ill-effects of β-blockers given intravenously to MG patients (Jonkers et al., 1996). However, microphysiologic studies show a dose-dependent reduction in the efficacy of NMT in normal rat skeletal muscle and human myasthenic muscle bathed in atenolol, labetolol, metoprolol, nadolol, propranolol or timolol (Howard JF, unpublished observations) (Howard et al., 1987). Different β-blockers have reproducibly different pre- and postsynaptic effects. The reduction in MEPP amplitude caused by all of these drugs suggests a postsynaptic site of action. Additional presynaptic effects are suggested by the relatively large reductions in endplate potential (EPP) amplitude compared to MEPP amplitude, alterations in MEPP frequency caused by all except timolol and reduction in quantal content caused by metoprolol and propranolol. Of the drugs examined, propranolol has the greatest effect on NMT; atenolol has the least.

The molecular mechanisms of β-blocker-induced neuromuscular blockade have yet to be elucidated. One possibility is that activation of the β-adrenergic receptors blocked by these drugs is important for NMT. Enzymes responsible for the synthesis of catecholamines are present in human and rat nerve terminals (Chan-Palay et al., 1982) and it has been suggested that β-receptor stimulation plays an important role in NMT (Bowman, 1981). Adrenaline modulates the Na+/K+ pump and this effect can be blocked by propranolol (Kaibara et al., 1985). Pump activity may control endplate depolarization by ACh agonists through its electrogenic effects and control ACh receptor sensitivity by regulating the phosphorylation state of the receptor (Ayrapetyan et al., 1985; Creese et al., 1987). β-adrenergic receptors also appear to be involved in the modulation of transmitter release from mammalian motor nerve terminals; noradrenaline and isoprenaline enhance neurally evoked transmitter output and this is blocked by propranolol and atenolol (Wessler and Anschutz, 1988). Other mechanisms of action for these drugs could include competitive curare-like effects, channel blockade, reduction of single channel conductance and general anesthetic effects (Colquhoun, 1986). That β-blockers have qualitatively different concentration-dependent effects on MEPP frequency and that not all drugs have the same qualitative effects on MEPP and EPP time courses suggest that at least some of their effects are not related to β-receptor blockade. Of course, β-blocker specific and more general effects of these drugs could contribute to both the quantitative and qualitative concentration-dependent effects that have been described.

12.2.6.2. Bretylium

Bretylium is a quaternary ammonium compound used in the past for refractory ventricular arrhythmias. In high concentrations it is reported to cause significant weakness in normal muscles and to significantly potentiate the neuromuscular block of competitive neuromuscular blocking agents (Campbell and Montuschi, 1960; Bowman, 1981).

12.2.6.3. Calcium channel blockers

The effects of calcium channel blockers on myocardial muscle have been extensively characterized, but their effects on skeletal muscle are less well understood. Studies to date have produced conflicting results: some have demonstrated postsynaptic curare-like effects, others have shown presynaptic inhibition of ACh release or both pre- and postsynaptic effects (Van der Kloot and Kita, 1975; Chiarandini and Bentley, 1978; Bikhazi et al., 1982, 1983; Ribera and Nastuk, 1989). Oral administration of calcium channel blockers to cardiac patients without neuromuscular disease did not produce any evidence of altered NMT by SFEMG (Adams et al., 1984). There is one report of a patient with Duchenne muscular dystrophy who had an acute exacerbation of weakness with respiratory failure following intravenous administration of verapamil (Zalman et al., 1983). It was postulated that even minimal alteration of synaptic efficacy was enough to produce acute decompensation in this patient with end-stage muscle disease. Acute respiratory failure after beginning oral verapamil has been seen in a patient with LES (Krendel and Hopkins, 1986) and in a patient with moderately severe, generalized myasthenia (Howard, JF, unpublished observations). Elderly myasthenic patients have experienced worsening of strength after receiving felodipine and nifedipine for hypertension (Pina Latorre et al., 1998). Low doses of verapamil or its timed-release preparation have been used without problems in patients with MG (Howard, JF, unpublished observations; Phillips, JT, personal communication) (Jonkers et al., 1996).

12.2.6.4. Cholesterol lowering agents

Several published works suggest that the statin cholesterol lowering agents may be causal in the exacerbation of myasthenic weakness (O'Riordan et al., 1994; Parmar et al., 2002; Engel, 2003; Cartwright et al., 2004; Purvin et al., 2006). The mechanism for this worsening is not clear but several postulates have been proposed. It is well recognized that HMG-CoA reductase therapy may produce a myopathy (Evans and Rees, 2002; Huynh et al., 2002; Jacobson, 2006; Law and Rudnicka, 2006). Is it possible the myasthenic worsening could be due to a co-existing disorder of the muscle membrane? Statins have immunomodulatory properties, with the ability to induce production of the Th2 cytokines interleukin (IL)-4, IL-5 and IL-10 (Youssef et al., 2002). Animal and human studies

suggest that these Th2 cytokines play a role in the development of MG (Milani et al., 2003). Therefore, it is possible that, by up-regulation of Th2, cytokine production could lead to worsening MG. Statins have been postulated to cause mitochondrial dysfunction by depleting endogenous coenzyme Q10 (Hargreaves and Heales, 2002). Statin-induced mitochondrial failure in the nerve terminal has been proposed as a mechanism to impair neuromuscular transmission given the high content of mitochondria in the nerve terminal (Cartwright et al., 2004). There is no evidence to suggest that HMG-CoA reductase is known to directly interfere with neuromuscular transmission (Wierzbicki et al., 2003).

12.2.6.5. Procainamide

Procainamide is reported to produce acute worsening of strength in patients with MG (Drachman and Skom, 1965; Kornfeld et al., 1976). The rapid onset of neuromuscular block and rapid resolution of symptoms following discontinuation suggest that this drug has a direct toxic effect on synaptic transmission. The postulated mechanism of action is primarily at the presynaptic membrane with impaired formation or release of ACh, or both, though it is known to have postsynaptic blocking effects as well.

12.2.6.6. Propafenone

Two case reports suggest that the anti-arrhythmic P-glycoprotein inhibitor, propafenone, may cause acute exacerbations of myasthenic weakness (Fierro et al., 1987; Lecky et al., 1991). Like the effects of procainamide, the rapid onset of worsening and resolution following the discontinuation of the drug implicates a direct toxic effect on neuromuscular transmission.

12.2.6.7. Quinine and quinidine

Quinine increases AChR channel open time and blocks these channels when closed. Myasthenic patients may develop markedly increased weakness within hours to days of starting quinine for muscle cramps; therefore it should not be used, or used only with extreme caution, in disorders having a reduced safety margin of NMT (Pascuzzi, R, personal communication). The literature suggests that ingestion of even small amounts of quinine, as in a gin and tonic, may acutely worsen myasthenic weakness; however, this has not been substantiated by objective reports (Engel et al., 1974; Donaldson, 1978; Patten, 1978).

Quinidine, the stereoisomer of quinine, has been reported to exacerbate weakness in MG (Weisman, 1949; Shy et al., 1985) and to unmask previously unrecognized cases of this disease (Kornfeld et al., 1976; Stoffer and Chandler, 1980; Shy et al., 1985). Quinidine has both pre- and postsynaptic effects, impairing either the formation or release of ACh and, in larger doses, blocking the interaction of ACh with its receptor, like curare (Miller et al., 1968). Quinidine can also potentiate the weakness produced by non-depolarizing and depolarizing neuromuscular blocking agents (Grogono, 1963; Way et al., 1967).

Quinolone derivatives reduce quantal content of the endplate potential and decrease the amplitude and decay time constant of MEPPs and miniature endplate currents at concentrations close to those used clinically (Sieb et al., 1996). At high concentrations MEPPs are undetectable and the effects are not reversed by neostigmine.

12.2.6.8. Trimethaphan

Trimethaphan is a ganglionic blocking agent used in hypertensive emergencies, dissecting aortic aneurysms, cerebral aneurysm surgery and for decreasing cardiac overload in patients with myocardial infarction. It has been reported to cause acute respiratory paralysis, probably due to a curare-like action at the neuromuscular junction (Dale and Schroeder, 1976). It has also been reported to potentiate the neuromuscular block in patients receiving both non-depolarizing and depolarizing neuromuscular blocking agents (Wilson et al., 1976; Poulton et al., 1979; Nakamura et al., 1980).

12.2.7. Hormones

12.2.7.1. Estrogen and progesterone

Estrogen therapy has been reported to acutely worsen the strength of a patient with MG, though the details of this case are open to question (Vacca and Knight, 1957). Parenteral progesterone has been reported to aggravate the strength of myasthenic women after a delay of 3–5 days (Frenkel and Ehrlich, 1964), but the mechanism of action has yet to be elucidated. There are no data to suggest that oral birth control use increases the incidence or worsens the strength of MG (Bickerstaff, 1975). There is one case report of a levonorgestrel implant that precipitated signs and symptoms of myasthenia gravis that improved with its removal (Brittain and Lange, 1995). This article states that an additional 34 cases of myasthenic worsening had been reported to the US Food and Drug Administration through 1995. Details of these individual cases are not known.

12.2.7.2. Thyroid hormone

The relationship of the thyroid gland to MG is well recognized (Drachman, 1962). The older literature states that thyroid hormone and anti-thyroid medications can aggravate the strength of patients with myasthenia, perhaps by

reducing the release of ACh. This is not felt to be a problem with current modes of therapy (Thorner, 1939; McEachern and Parnell, 1948; MacLean and Wilson, 1954; Perez et al., 1995).

12.2.8. Immune modulators

Patients treated with interferon alpha develop a variety of autoantibodies and autoimmune diseases, including MG, or may have an acute worsening of their myasthenic weakness (Batocchi et al., 1995; Gu et al., 1995; Perez et al., 1995; Quilichini et al., 1995; Konishi, 1996; Lensch et al., 1996; Mase et al., 1996; Piccolo et al., 1996; Rohde et al., 1996; Uyama et al., 1996; Bora et al., 1997; Gurtubay et al., 1999; Borgia et al., 2001; Dionisiotis et al., 2004; Kreutzer et al., 2004). Interferon-induced MG was first reported in 1995: a 66-year-old man developed sero-positive generalized MG 6 months after starting interferon alpha therapy for leukemia (Perez et al., 1995). Subsequent reports describe patients who developed MG 6–9 months after beginning interferon alpha-2b treatment for malignancy (Batocchi et al., 1995; Lensch et al., 1996) or chronic active hepatitis C (Konishi, 1996). In one case MG symptoms persisted for at least 7 months after stopping the drug (Mase et al., 1996; Piccolo et al., 1996). Fulminant myasthenic crisis has also been described after interferon alpha therapy (Konishi, 1996). Recent reports have also suggested that MG may occur independently in association with hepatitis C, bringing into question the role of interferon in these patients (Uyama et al., 1996; Bora et al., 1997; Eddy et al., 1999; Gurtubay et al., 1999).

Expression of interferon gamma at motor endplates of transgenic mice produces abnormal NMJ function and generalized weakness that improves with cholinesterase inhibitors. Sera from these mice and from human MG patients recognize an 87-kD target antigen. This suggests that the expression of interferon gamma in these mice provokes an autoimmune humoral response similar to that in human MG (Gu et al., 1995).

12.2.9. Magnesium

Hypermagnesemia is an uncommon clinical complication from the use of magnesium-containing drugs (Krendel, 1990). Magnesium (Mg^{++}) is contained in some antacids and laxatives. Magnesium sulfate ($MgSO_4$) is used in the treatment of pre-eclampsia and eclampsia, for hemodynamic control during anesthesia and the early postoperative period and in patients depleted of Mg^{++}, such as chronic alcoholism (Fuchs-Buder and Tassonyi, 1996). The serum Mg^{++} concentration is normally maintained at 1.5–2.5 mEq/L (2–3 mg/dL) by exchange with tissue stores in bone, liver, muscle and brain, and by renal excretion. Renal failure predisposes to hypermagnesemia and is reason to avoid magnesium-containing antacids and laxatives (Randall et al., 1964; Castlebaum et al., 1989). Elevated serum Mg^{++} due to oral magnesium-containing compounds is very uncommon if renal function is normal (Mordes and Wacker, 1978; Lemcke and Fucks, 1984). Excessive use of enemas containing Mg^{++} may produce hypermagnesemia, but this is usually in patients with underlying gastrointestinal (GI) tract disease (Mordes and Wacker, 1978; Collins and Russell, 2002). Hypermagnesemia commonly results from administration of high doses of parenteral $MgSO_4$ for treatment of eclampsia, at times resulting in serious side effects to the mother or the newborn (Flowers, 1965; Lipsitz, 1971; Pritchard, 1979). The clinical manifestations of hypermagnesemia correlate with serum Mg^{++} levels (Fishman, 1965; Somjen et al., 1966; Mordes and Wacker, 1978). Muscle stretch reflexes become reduced when the serum Mg^{++} level exceeds 5 mEq/L; levels of 9–10 mEq/L are associated with absent reflexes and muscle weakness. During treatment of pre-eclampsia, muscle stretch reflexes are monitored and Mg^{++} administration is discontinued if the reflexes disappear (Pritchard, 1979). Fatal respiratory failure can occur at levels greater than 10 mEq/L (Flowers, 1965; Pritchard, 1979). Serum levels greater than 14 mEq/L can induce acute cardiac arrhythmia, including heart block and arrest. Symptoms of autonomic dysfunction in hypermagnesemia include dry mouth, dilated pupils, urinary retention, hypotension and flushing and are thought to result from presynaptic blockade at autonomic ganglia (Hutter and Kostial, 1953). Mental function is usually not directly affected, even when weakness is severe (Somjen et al., 1966), but consciousness may be indirectly impaired from hypoxia, hypercarbia or hypotension. The muscles of ocular motility tend to be spared and the clinical findings of hypermagnesemia resemble those of LES rather than MG (Swift, 1979).

Magnesium inhibits release of ACh by competitively blocking calcium entry at the motor nerve terminal (Del Castillo and Engback, 1954). There may also be a milder postsynaptic effect. Magnesium also potentiates the action of neuromuscular blocking agents and this must be considered in women undergoing cesarean section after receiving Mg^{++} for preeclampsia (Ghoneim and Long, 1970; De Silva, 1973). Patients with underlying junctional disorders are more sensitive to Mg^{++}-induced weakness. Patients with MG and LES may become weaker after receiving Mg^{++}, even when serum Mg^{++} levels are normal or only slightly elevated (George and Han, 1962; Gutmann and Takamori, 1973; Strieb, 1973; Cohen et al., 1976). Reports exist of the uncovering of previously unrecognized MG following treatment

of preeclampsia with magnesium salts (Howard JF, unpublished observation) (Bashuk and Krendel, 1990). Increased MG symptoms most often occur when Mg^{++} is administered parenterally, but on occasion is seen with oral use (Strieb, 1973). Therefore, parenteral Mg^{++} administration should be avoided and oral Mg^{++} preparations should be used with caution in patients with known disorders of synaptic transmission, such as MG, LES and botulism.

Train-of-four (TOF) recordings suggest that clinically used doses of $MgSO_4$ produce significant changes in NMT as manifested by loss of the treppe phenomenon and diminished response to nerve stimulation (Ross and Baker, 1996). Doses of 60 mg/kg augment the neuromuscular block produced by vecuronium (Fuchs-Buder and Tassonyi, 1996). Patients given Mg^{++} within one hour after recovering from vecuronium block may have rapid and profound recurarization as measured by electromyography and TOF studies.

Treatment of hypermagnesemia depends on the severity of clinical symptoms. Discontinuation of Mg^{++} is the first step; if the patient is significantly weak, administration of intravenous calcium gluconate, 1 gram over 3 minutes, can produce rapid, albeit temporary, improvement if renal function is normal. If hypermagnesemia is more severe or if there are life-threatening side effects such as cardiac arrhythmia or renal failure, hemodialysis is indicated (Alfrey et al., 1970). Patients with MG or LES respond poorly to calcium and may respond better to cholinesterase inhibitors (Cohen et al., 1976).

12.2.10. Neuromuscular blocking drugs

Muscle relaxants are categorized as depolarizing or nondepolarizing agents depending upon their effects on the muscle membrane potential. The actions of these drugs are modified by factors such as the degree of neuromuscular blockade, underlying diseases, acid-base state and electrolyte imbalance (Miller, 1979). Competitive, nondepolarizing neuromuscular blocking agents have a much greater effect in patients with MG and LES than in normal individuals and even small amounts produce a greater and more prolonged period of neuromuscular blockade. Depolarizing agents such as succinylcholine must also be used with caution in these patients: because MG muscle is more resistant to depolarizing agents, higher doses may be used, resulting in prolonged blockade (Foldes and McNall, 1962). MG and LES may first be recognized when prolonged postoperative paralysis follows administration of neuromuscular blocking agents during surgery (Anderson et al., 1953; Elder et al., 1971).

The pharmacologic effects of these neuromuscular blocking agents are potentiated by many of the drugs previously discussed, including antibiotics, general anesthetics, local anesthetics and anti-arrhythmic drugs. Although newer synthetic neuromuscular blocking agents have a much shorter duration of action, prolonged muscle weakness has been reported in myasthenic patients receiving these drugs. The same concerns and guidelines apply when they are used in MG or LES. Benzing et al. (1990) report a child with a terminal motor axonopathy and presynaptic conduction block who developed severe, generalized muscle weakness which persisted for 6 weeks, after receiving muscle relaxants for 1 week while requiring ventilator support.

Prolonged apnea and muscle weakness in patients given depolarizing neuromuscular blocking agents may also occur when plasma cholinesterase levels are reduced, either by plasma exchange or as a result of genetic abnormalities of plasma cholinesterase (Evans et al., 1980; Viby-Mogensen, 1981).

12.2.11. Ophthalmic drugs

Eye drops containing β-adrenergic blocking agents (timolol maleate, betaxolol hydrochloride) have been associated temporally with exacerbation of MG (Shaivitz, 1979; Coppeto, 1984; Verkijk, 1985) (Howard, JF, unpublished observations). The mechanism of neuromuscular blockade is as described above (see Section 12.2.6.1). Ecothiophate, a long acting cholinesterase inhibitor used in the treatment of open angle glaucoma, has been reported to produce generalized muscle weakness and fatigue that resolved following discontinuation of the drug (Alexander, 1981). The mechanism of weakness was not determined, but long acting cholinesterase inhibitors could produce cholinergic weakness by their additive effects in MG patients receiving cholinesterase inhibitors. They might also potentiate the weakness induced by depolarizing neuromuscular blocking agents (Gesztes, 1966).

12.2.12. Psychotropic drugs

12.2.12.1. Phenothiazines

Chlorpromazine was reported to produce an acute exacerbation of muscle weakness in a myasthenic schizophrenic patient in 1963 (McQuillen et al., 1963), confirming previous studies showing that this drug produces a postsynaptic block of NMT. Other reports have suggested that chlorpromazine has presynaptic effects as well (Argov and Mastaglia, 1979b). Phenothiazines (chlorpromazine and promazine) antagonize applied ACh and may prolong the effects of succinylcholine. There have been anecdotal reports of prolonged neuromuscular blockade in patients given depolarizing neuromuscular blocking drugs while receiving promazine (Regan and Aldrete, 1967) or phenelzine (Bodley et al., 1969).

12.2.12.2. Lithium

Chronic lithium carbonate administration has been reported to produce varying degrees of muscle weakness. Some reports have postulated that lithium accumulates inside the presynaptic nerve terminal where it competes with calcium, resulting in inhibition of ACh synthesis and reduced quantal release (Havdala et al., 1979). Others have demonstrated a reduction in the number of ACh receptors in denervated muscle, suggesting that lithium selectively increases the rate of receptor degradation without altering receptor synthesis (Pestronk and Drachman, 1980). There are several reports of prolonged neuromuscular blockade in patients chronically receiving lithium and neuromuscular blocking agents (Borden et al., 1974; Hill et al., 1977). Fatigable weakness responsive to cholinesterase inhibitors and electrophysiologic abnormalities consistent with MG have been reported after lithium (Neil et al., 1976). Ptosis and weakness developing within 48 hours after beginning lithium has been reported in a patient who did not respond to cholinesterase inhibitors and had no decremental response with repetitive nerve stimulation (Granacher, 1977). Acute worsening of the decremental response to repetitive nerve stimulation has been observed in a patient recovering from botulism who was given lithium (Howard, JF, unpublished observations).

12.2.12.3. Others

Amitriptyline, amphetamines, droperidol, haloperidol, imipramine, paraldehyde and trichloroethanol have all been identified as being capable of interfering with synaptic transmission in experimental studies (Argov and Mastaglia, 1979b).

12.2.13. Recreational drugs

Several cases of MG exacerbation following recreational use of cocaine have been reported (Berciano et al., 1991; Daras et al., 1996; Venkatesh et al., 1996). These attacks frequently include respiratory insufficiency requiring ventilatory support (Daras et al., 1996; Venkatesh et al., 1996) and improve with therapeutic apheresis (Venkatesh et al., 1996) (Sanders, DB, unpublished observations) or high dose intravenous immunoglobulin (Venkatesh et al., 1996). Myasthenic exacerbations have been associated with elevated serum creatine kinase in some patients (Daras et al., 1996).

Cocaine reduces the skeletal muscle response to repetitive nerve stimulation in mice by decreasing the muscle and nerve excitability, but without an apparent effect on NMT (Venkatesh et al., 1996). Cocaine inhibits nicotinic AChR in cultured muscle cells (Krivoshein and Hess, 2004).

12.2.14. Rheumatologic drugs

12.2.14.1. Chloroquine

Chloroquine is used primarily as an antimalarial drug, but in higher doses is also used in the treatment of rheumatoid arthritis, discoid lupus erythematosus and porphyria cutanea. It may produce a number of neurological side effects among which are myopathies and disorders of NMT. The reported mechanisms of action for the latter have been both presynaptic, with a reduction in EPP amplitude resulting from a decrease in the amplitude of nerve action potentials and ACh release, and postsynaptic, with competitive post-junctional blockade (Jui-Yen, 1971; Vartanian and Chinyanga, 1972). It has also been reported that chloroquine directly suppresses muscle membrane excitability. There is some evidence to suggest that chloroquine may alter immune regulation and produce a clinical syndrome of MG similar to that reported with d-penicillamine. Two cases are reported, one with rheumatoid arthritis and the other with systemic lupus erythematosus, who developed clinical, physiological and pharmacological findings typical of MG following prolonged treatment with chloroquine. Antibodies to the AChR were present and subsequently slowly disappeared after discontinuation of the drug, as did the clinical and electrophysiological abnormalities (Schumm et al., 1981; Sghirlanzoni et al., 1988). Persistent MG following the intermittent use of anti-malarials has also been reported (De Bleecker et al., 1991), as has transient development of a post-junctional disorder of NMT following 1 week of chloroquine therapy (Robberecht et al., 1989). In the latter case, AChR antibodies were not found and rapid resolution of symptoms suggested that the weakness resulted from a direct toxic effect at the neuromuscular junction rather than a derangement of immune function. Direct and immunologic effects on NMT as hypothesized for chloroquine are also seen with the hydantoin drugs.

12.2.14.2. D-penicillamine

D-penicillamine (D-P) is used in the treatment of rheumatoid arthritis (RA), Wilson's disease and cystinuria. A number of autoimmune diseases have been reported in patients receiving D-P, including immune complex nephritis, pemphigus, polymyositis, systemic lupus erythematosus and, most frequently, MG (Schraeder, 1972; Ansell, 1974; Balint et al., 1975; Bucknall et al., 1975; Czlonkowska, 1975; Hewitt et al., 1975; Cucher and Goldman, 1976; Dische et al.,

1976; Petersen et al., 1978). Myasthenia gravis begins only after prolonged D-P therapy in most patients and is less frequent in patients receiving D-P for Wilson's disease than for RA (Komal-Kumar et al., 2004). The myasthenia induced by D-P is usually mild and may be restricted to the ocular muscles. In many patients the symptoms are not recognized and it may be difficult to demonstrate mild weakness of the limbs in the presence of severe arthritis. The diagnosis can be confirmed by the response to cholinesterase inhibitors, EMG abnormalities and elevated serum antibodies to the acetylcholine receptors (AChR-Abs) (Masters et al., 1977; Russell and Lindstrom, 1978; Vincent et al., 1978). In our experience, repetitive stimulation studies are abnormal less often than is SFEMG, reflecting the relatively mild degree of neuromuscular abnormality present in most of these patients. Microphysiologic studies have shown reduced MEPP amplitude as in acquired MG (Vincent et al., 1978).

In normal rats, D-P given in doses equivalent to the human therapeutic dose produces no neuromuscular abnormality (Aldrich et al., 1979). In guinea pigs, chronic administration of doses more than 10 times the therapeutic level produced a mild degree of neuromuscular block (Burres et al., 1979). These studies provide no evidence that D-P produces a direct, clinically significant effect on NMT. It is more likely that D-P induces MG by stimulating or enhancing an immunologic reaction against the neuromuscular junction.

Myasthenia that begins while the patient is receiving D-P remits within a year after the drug is discontinued in 70% of patients (Albers et al., 1980). As the myasthenia improves, the AChR antibody level falls and the electromyographic abnormalities improve or disappear altogether (Russell and Lindstrom, 1978; Vincent et al., 1978; Albers et al., 1980) (Sanders DB, Howard JF, unpublished observations). When MG persists after D-P is discontinued, as is rarely the case, it is likely that a subclinical myasthenic state existed prior to treatment with D-P.

Tiopronine and pyrithioxine have also been reported to induce MG after prolonged administration (Kirjner et al., 1980; Menkes et al., 1988). Antibodies to the AChR were demonstrated and the time course of resolution was prolonged. This suggests the effects of these drugs are not due to direct toxicity to the neuromuscular junction but rather an alteration of immune function occurs, as with D-P.

12.2.15. Miscellaneous

D,L-carnitine, but not L-carnitine, has been reported to acutely worsen the strength of patients with MG undergoing dialysis (Bazzato et al., 1979, 1981). The precise mechanism of neuromuscular blockade is not known but is postulated to be a presynaptic block similar to that produced by hemicholinium or a postsynaptic block by the accumulation of acylcarnitine esters (De Grandis et al., 1980).

Diuretics have been suspected of aggravating weakness in MG, probably by potassium wasting (Jenkins et al., 1970). It has been long recognized that myasthenic patients are sensitive to hypokalemia or even low normal levels of serum potassium.

Emetine, originally used as an amebicide and the principal ingredient of ipecac, has been reported to produce acute neuromuscular weakness in non-myasthenic patients (Brown, 1935). Experimental studies suggest that emetine produces inhibition of indirectly elicited action potentials that is not reversed by cholinesterase inhibitors (Ng, 1966).

Acute crisis has been reported in MG patients given enemas preparatory to radiographic procedures. This has not been confirmed by others (Russell, 1984) but could be due to removal of cholinesterase inhibitors from the GI tract or the effect of magnesium in the enema solutions (see above).

Intravenous infusion of iodinated contrast agents has been reported to acutely worsen MG (Canal and Franceschi, 1983; Chagnac et al., 1985), although this was not confirmed in a retrospective study (Frank et al., 1987). There is one report that a patient with LES developed transient, severe respiratory insufficiency following the intravenous infusion of iodinated contrast material (Van den Bergh et al., 1986). The postulated mechanism of action is acute hypocalcemia due to direct binding by the contrast agent.

Intravenous infusion of sodium lactate is reported to worsen the strength, including respiratory function, in patients with MG (Engel et al., 1974). The postulated mechanism is transient hypocalcemia, resulting in impaired neurotransmitter release from the nerve terminal.

There is a single report of myasthenic weakness occurring following administration of tetanus antitoxin (Ionescu-Drinea et al., 1973).

Trihexiphenidyl has been reported to have unmasked and worsened the weakness of a single patient with MG. In this report it is stated that the AChR-Ab level paralleled the degree of weakness (Ueno et al., 1987).

Botulinum neurotoxin, when used therapeutically for focal dystonia, has unmasked subclinical LES (Erbguth et al., 1993). Worsening of weakness or crisis has also been reported in MG following injections of botulinum toxin (Emmerson, 1994; Borodic, 1998; Tarsy et al., 2000; Martinez-Matos et al., 2003). A known defect of

NMT is considered to be a relative contraindication to the use of botulinum toxin, although others have reported its successful use in patients with MG (Goncalves et al., 1999; Fasano et al., 2005).

Numerous drugs, including the following, produce or worsen neuromuscular block in laboratory studies, but to date there are no known reports of clinical adverse neuromuscular reactions to them. Amantadine reduces the post-junctional sensitivity to inotophoretically applied ACh by interacting with the ionic channel of the AChR (Tsai et al., 1978). Ironically, azathioprine, which is used as treatment for MG, has been shown to potentiate the neuromuscular block of succinylcholine in cat nerve-muscle preparations, but to antagonize the neuromuscular block of curare (Dretchen and Morgenroth, 1976). As with theophylline, azathioprine inhibits the action of phosphodiesterase, the enzyme that hydrolyses cyclic AMP (cAMP). The increased concentration of cAMP increases neurotransmitter release. We have seen no untoward neuromuscular blocking effects in myasthenic patients receiving these drugs. Diphenhydramine has been shown to potentiate the neuromuscular block of barbiturates and neuromuscular blocking agents and to reduce the amount of neurotransmitter released from the neuromuscular junction (Abdel-Aziz and Bakry, 1973).

12.3. Clostridial neurotoxins

The clostridial neurotoxins are gram-positive, anaerobic, spore-forming bacteria found ubiquitously in the environment. The neurotoxins of clostridial organisms produce botulism and tetanus by the inhibition of neurotransmitter release via their metalloproteolytic activity directed against SNARE proteins, although the site of action and clinical picture of each is quite different (Montecucco and Schiavo, 1994; Schiavo et al., 2000). Clostridial neurotoxins are the most toxic substances to humans known. In most cases, exposure to the neurotoxin of *Clostridium* species results from food poisoning, wound infections or a colonizing intestinal infection. Humans are usually exposed to the neurotoxin of *Clostridium tetani* from wound infections. Immunization provides effective protection against tetanus toxin, but tetanus remains a serious public health problem in developing countries.

12.3.1. Botulism

Botulism was first reported in patients who had eaten improperly smoked sausage, in 1820 by Julius Kerner, who later showed that the symptoms could be reproduced by ingestion of an extract from the sausage (Kerner, 1820). Emile van Ermengen of Ghent identified the toxin of botulism by isolating an anaerobic bacterium from ham and reproducing the disease in animals by injecting the toxin produced by the bacteria (Van Ermengen, 1897). The term botulism is derived from the Latin word *botulus*, meaning sausage. The reader is referred to Chapter 11 for a more detailed discussion of this entity.

The vast majority of cases of botulism are caused by toxins produced by *Clostridium botulinum. C. botulinum* is ubiquitous in soil and survives under anaerobic and alkaline conditions. All forms of the toxin block ACh release at the presynaptic motor nerve terminal and parasympathetic and sympathetic ganglia (Burgen et al., 1949).

12.3.1.1. Clinical features

Clinical botulism occurs in five forms: classic or food-borne botulism, infantile botulism, wound botulism, hidden botulism and iatrogenic botulism. Most cases of food-borne botulism are caused by types A, B or E, all three of which may cause death. Type E botulism results from the ingestion of contaminated seafood. Disorders of neuromuscular transmission (LES and myasthenic crisis) have been worsened or unmasked following therapeutic botulinum toxin injection (Erbguth et al., 1993; Borodic, 1998).

12.3.1.2. Bioterrorism

The potential for intentional poisoning with botulinum toxin has become a major concern in the 21st century. In 1996 at least 17 countries were suspected to have or to be developing biological agents in their offensive weapons programs (Cole, 1996). This number has more than doubled since ratification in 1972 of the *Convention on the Prohibition of the Development, Production and Stockpiling of Bacteriological (Biological) and Toxin Weapons and on Their Destruction* treaty (Kadlec et al., 1997). Four of the countries listed by the US government as "state sponsors of terrorism" (Iran, Iraq, North Korea and Syria) have developed, or are believed to be developing, botulinum toxin as a weapon of mass destruction (Bermudez, 2001). With the economic difficulties in Russia after the demise of the Soviet Union, some of the thousands of scientists formerly employed by its bioweapons program have been recruited by nations attempting to develop biological weapons (Smithson, 1999). The increased interest in botulism as a weapon of terror is in part due to the relative ease with which the toxin can be produced and its high lethality in small quantities— the LD_{50} is estimated to be 0.001 µg/kg (Franz, 1997). Dissemination of large quantities of the toxin by aerosols could produce mass casualties.

Development and use of botulinum toxin as a biological weapon began in the 1940s (Smart, 1997). The head of the Japanese biological warfare group admitted to feeding cultures of *C. botulinum* to prisoners with lethal effect during that country's occupation of Manchuria in the 1930s (Hill, 1947). The United States biological weapons program first produced botulinum toxin during World War II due to concerns that Germany had weaponized botulinum toxin (Bryden, 1989). RISE, a terrorist group of the early 1970s, reportedly planned to introduce botulinum toxin into the Chicago water supply (Carus, 1999). Iraq revealed to the United Nations that during the Persian Gulf War, 19 000 liters of concentrated botulinum toxin was prepared, of which 11 200 liters were loaded into specially designed SCUD missile warheads (Ekeus, 1996; Zilinskas, 1997). This is more than three times the quantity necessary to annihilate the entire human race. Further, Aum Shinrikyo, the apocalyptic cult that used sarin in the 1995 terrorist attack on the Tokyo subway system, had produced and stockpiled quantities of botulinum toxin and other biological agents (Kadlec et al., 1999). Despite being one of the signatories of the 1972 *Biological and Toxin Weapons Convention*, the then Soviet Union subsequently produced botulinum toxin for use as a weapon. Botulinum toxin was one of several agents tested at the Soviet site Aralsk-7 on Vozrozhdeniye Island in the Aral Sea (Patocka and Splino, 2002).

12.3.1.3. Differential diagnosis

The differential diagnosis of botulism includes other disorders of NMT, i.e., MG and LES (Table 12.3). Botulism is suggested by the combination of a descending pattern of weakness in association with autonomic dysfunction. Diurnal variability will often distinguish these disorders from botulism. The Landry–Guillain–Barré (LGB) syndrome, tick paralysis, the Miller–Fisher variant of LGB syndrome (MFV) and diphtheritic neuropathy are also in the differential. The latter two entities are often the most difficult to distinguish from botulism. The pattern of descending weakness helps distinguish botulism from the classical form of LGB, which usually presents with ascending weakness. The MFV, with ocular and bulbar abnormalities, may present a more difficult diagnostic challenge. The preservation of deep tendon reflexes would suggest botulism rather than LGB and MFV (Cherington, 2002). The pharyngeal-cervical brachial-variant of LGB has clinical features similar to botulism but in contrast to botulism most of these patients have serum antibodies to GQ1b. Infants with suspected botulism must be assessed for the myriad other causes of

Table 12.3

Differential diagnosis of botulism

Disease entity	Characteristic features
Botulism	Initial oculobulbar then rapid descending pattern of weakness; autonomic involvement
Landry–Guillain–Barré (LGB) syndrome	Rapid ascending pattern of weakness; loss of muscle stretch reflexes, elevated CSF protein
Myasthenia gravis	Variable weakness of ocular, limb and bulbar muscle groups; preserved reflexes
Lambert–Eaton syndrome	Variable weakness (often less than MG); absent or diminished reflexes, autonomic involvement
Tick paralysis	Ascending pattern of weakness; typically children
Diphtheritic neuropathy	Tonsilar exudates; peripheral neuropathy (late)
Poliomyelitis	Acute, rapid, asymmetrical weakness; CSF pleocytosis with elevated protein
Miller–Fisher variant of LGB	See Landry–Guillain–Barré syndrome; ataxia

CSF, cerebrospinal fluid.

hypotonia, as well as poliomyelitis and spinal muscular atrophy. In many cases, the rapid course of progression will be the defining feature. The diagnosis of wound botulism should be considered whenever a patient with a wound develops bulbar signs and a rapidly evolving descending pattern of weakness. In drug addicts, an infected injection site may not be obvious without careful examination.

12.3.2. Tetanus

The word tetanus is derived from the Greek *tetanos*, which comes from the term *teinein*, meaning to stretch. Hippocrates described tetanus in the 5th century B.C., but modern understanding of tetanus began in 1884 when Carle and Rattone produced tetanus in animals by injecting them with pus from a patient who died of the disease (Carle and Rattone, 1884; Major, 1965). In the same year, Nicolaier produced tetanus in animals by injecting them with samples of soil. Kitasato isolated *C. tetani* from a patient in 1889 and demonstrated that it produced disease when injected into animals. He further showed that the toxin could be neutralized by specific antibodies. In 1897, Nocard demonstrated the protective effect of antitoxin, and passive immunization in humans was used during World War I. Descombey developed tetanus toxoid in 1924 and the effectiveness of active immunization was demonstrated during World War II (Major, 1965).

Tetanus is caused by the neurotoxin tetanospasmin, which is produced by *C. tetani*, a gram-positive, spore-forming, motile, obligate anaerobic bacterium. The organism has a distinctive drumstick-like appearance. Tetanospasmin blocks the inhibitory spinal reflex arc, allowing excitatory reflexes to predominate (Montecucco and Schiavo, 1994). This results in increased

muscle tone and the spasms that are the cardinal manifestations of the disease. Tetanus is predominantly seen in neonates and children in developing countries with inadequate immunization programs (Anonymous, 1998a; Montecucco and Schiavo, 1994; Cook et al., 2001; Oladiran et al., 2002). In developed countries, tetanus is most often encountered in patients over 50 years of age, often after a minor injury acquired outdoors, and in drug addicts (Anonymous, 1998b; Cherubin and Sapira, 1993; Izurieta et al., 1997).

12.3.2.1. Pathogenesis

Clostridium tetani is ubiquitous worldwide. The spores are relatively resistant to drying and various disinfectants (e.g., phenol, formaldehyde and chloramine) require more than 15 hours to kill the spores. The spores can be killed by autoclaving, aqueous iodine and 2% glutaraldehyde at pH 7.5–8.5. *C. tetani* spores are found in animal and human feces and in domestic dust and can survive for decades, especially in manure-rich soil. Spores germinate into the vegetative form under appropriate anaerobic conditions, particularly in wounds associated with necrosis. Two exotoxins, tetanolysin and tetanospasmin, are elaborated by the vegetative form. Tetanolysin is not thought to be involved in the pathogenesis of tetanus, but its function is not really known. Tetanospasmin, a zinc metalloprotease, is formed under plasmid control as a single 1315 amino acid polypeptide chain that is cleaved by bacterial protease to form a heterodimer consisting of a 100 kd heavy chain and a 50 kd light chain joined by a disulfide bond (Rossetto et al., 1995). Biophysical studies indicate that the toxin is similar to other 3-dimensional toxins (e.g., diphtheria toxin) and is folded into three functionally distinct domains that play important roles in cell intoxication (Choe et al.,

1992). The carboxyl terminal of the H-chain is primarily responsible for neuro-specific binding. The amino terminal of the same chain is responsible for cell penetration and the L-domain is responsible for the blockade of neurotransmitter exocytosis (Montecucco and Schiavo, 1994). The exotoxin is very sensitive to heat and cannot survive when exposed to oxygen.

Cell intoxication occurs in four steps: cell binding, internalization, membrane translocation and targeted cell dysfunction (Mellanby and Green, 1981). When tetanospasmin is released in infected wounds, the C-fragment binds to specific axonal membrane gangliosides (GDIb and GT) predominantly at the terminals of alpha motor and, to a lesser extent, autonomic neurons. The toxin is then internalized into the lumen of synaptic vesicles after vesicle reuptake. It is translocated from the endosomes to the cytosol where it is then transported by retrograde transsynaptic axonal transport to the cell bodies of inhibitory interneurons in the spinal cord and brain stem. The light-chain fragment causes proteolytic cleavage of the synaptosomal-associated protein complexes, particularly the synaptobrevin vesicle-associated membrane protein, and prevents neurotransmitter release (glycine in the spinal cord and γ-aminobutyric acid in the brain). This disinhibition produces uncontrolled excessive efferent discharge of motor and autonomic neurons resulting in muscle rigidity, spasms and autonomic dysfunction. The amino acid structures of botulinum toxin and tetanospasmin are partially homologous. The estimated human lethal dose of tetanospasmin is less than 2.5 ng/kg, making it one of the more potent neurotoxins known.

12.3.2.2. Clinical features

Tetanus occurs in three forms: localized, generalized and cephalic. The incubation period is usually 7–8 days after injury but varies from 3–21 days. Clinical manifestations may appear as early as 24 hours or may be delayed for several months (Brown, 1968). The incubation period is directly related to the distance of the wound from the central nervous system (CNS). Injuries to the head and neck are associated with significantly shorter incubation periods than injuries to the lower extremities. The incubation time is a prognosticator of ultimate outcome—the shorter the incubation period, the greater the likelihood of death. In developed countries tetanus is a disease of older individuals and typically follows a small puncture wound. It is a disease of infants and children in underdeveloped countries primarily due to the lack of effective immunization. Death from tetanus exceeds several hundreds of thousands each year, with the greatest number occurring in countries where anti-tetanus vaccination is not mandatory (Galazka and Gasse, 1995).

12.3.2.2.1. Localized tetanus

Localized tetanus is uncommon in humans and is generally mild (Millard, 1954). It accounted for 13% of cases in one report, but otherwise has not been well characterized in the literature (Izurieta et al., 1997). Localized tetanus produces painful muscle spasms in a restricted area close to the site of injury. Death occurs in less than 1% of cases. Muscle spasms may persist for several weeks to a few months before subsiding spontaneously.

12.3.2.2.2. Generalized tetanus

Generalized tetanus is the most common form and typically starts with spasms of the muscles of mastication, producing trismus or "lockjaw." This is quickly followed by spasms of other muscles of the head and neck, then involvement of the axial muscles, shoulders, hips and limbs. Symptoms abate in the reverse order. Abdominal involvement produces a rigid abdomen and sustained contraction of the facial muscles produces the classic grimace called *risus sardonicus*. Sustained contraction of paraspinal muscles produces the characteristic opisthotonus position, a finding that occurs early in the disease, perhaps due to the short length of nerves innervating these muscles. Death may result from asphyxia due to laryngospasm. Auditory or tactile stimuli often produce paroxysmal, generalized, repetitive spasms (tentanospasms) that become exhausting to the patient.

Autonomic dysfunction may occur, particularly in the more severe cases. Cardiac and vasomotor instability and thermoregulatory disturbances are common. Labile or sustained hypertension, hyperpyrexia, excessive sweating and tachycardia and other arrhythmias may occur. Severe cardiac instability may lead to cardiac arrest and death.

Neonatal tetanus is a form of generalized tetanus occurring in newborn infants (Anonymous, 2000; Izurieta et al., 1997). It occurs in the absence of passive immunity. While rare in the United States, it is estimated to cause more than 200 000 deaths per year worldwide in developing countries (Anonymous, 1994; Stanfield and Galazka, 1987; Lawn et al., 2006). The route of entry is usually through an unhealed umbilical stump that has been cut with a non-sterile instrument or contaminated by animal dung. Symptoms occur 3–14 days after birth during which development and feeding are normal. Antitetanic serum and sedation are the basis of supportive treatment once symptoms appear. More than 95% of infants will die of neonatal tetanus without specific therapy. Even with specific therapy, and depending on the intensity of supportive care, lethality rates are still between 25 and 90% (Stanfield and Galazka, 1984; Wassilak et al., 1999).

12.3.2.2.3. Cephalic tetanus

Cephalic tetanus is rare (Bagratuni, 1952). It occurs following localized infections about the head and neck, typically in the distribution of the facial nerve. It is characterized by unilateral facial paralysis, trismus, nuchal rigidity, pharyngeal spasms causing dysphagia, frequent laryngeal spasms and facial stiffness on the unaffected side. Death may result from asphyxia. Glossopharyngeal, vagus and, rarely, the oculomotor nerves may be involved. The incubation period is short. Cephalic tetanus may progress to generalized tetanus.

12.3.2.3. Differential diagnosis

The differential diagnosis of tetanus depends on the clinical pattern of presentation (Table 12.4). In patients with trismus, the differential includes dental caries, peritonsilar and retropharyngeal abscesses, tonsillitis, parotid gland abnormalities and temporomandibular dysfunction (Carrillo, 1966; Clark, 1970; Kanesada and Mogi, 1981; van Loosen and van der, 1987; Epperly and Wood, 1990; de Boer et al., 1995; Friedman et al., 1997; Szuhay and Tewfik, 1998). Less commonly, trismus may be seen with meningitis and encephalitis (Vic-Dupont et al., 1969; Sandyk and Brennan, 1982; Tokuoka et al., 1997). Trismus does not occur in hypocalcemic tetany and, in this disorder, the trunk is often spared and the patient will exhibit Trousseau and Chvostek signs. The stiffperson syndrome evolves more insidiously, only rarely involves facial muscles and is frequently associated with antibodies to glutamic acid decarboxylase. However, other features of stiffperson syndrome resemble tetanus, with axial stiffness and spasms provoked by a variety of stimuli (Moersch and Woltman, 1956; Thompson, 1993; Meinck et al., 1995). Electrodiagnostic features also help to differentiate between the two.

12.3.2.4. Laboratory diagnosis

There are no laboratory findings characteristic of tetanus. The diagnosis is entirely clinical and does not depend upon bacteriologic confirmation. Clues to the diagnosis include a wound or recent history of a wound, no clear history of tetanus toxoid immunization and headache, low grade fever, irritability and restlessness. However, the absence of a wound should not preclude considering the diagnosis and tetanus has been reported in those who have been previously immunized (Shimoni et al., 1999). *C. tetani* is recovered from the wound in only 30% of cases and is not infrequently isolated from patients who do not have tetanus. Routine blood and CSF studies are normal. Electrodiagnostic studies demonstrate bursts of motor unit potentials, similar to voluntary contraction, during spasms. Characteristically, there is a shortening or absence of the silent period after supramaximal nerve stimulation (Fernandez et al., 1983; Steinegger et al., 1996; Warren et al., 1999; Poncelet, 2000).

12.3.2.5. Management

The primary treatment for tetanus is directed at elimination of the source of toxin by cleaning and thoroughly debriding the wound, antibiotics and neutralization of circulating unbound toxin. Human tetanus immunoglobulin should be given immediately at the time of diagnosis to prevent further spread of the toxin. Tetanus antitoxin does not cross the blood–brain barrier and has no effect on toxin already bound to neurons. Intrathecal antitoxin administration has yet to be of proven benefit. Modern critical care units have decreased the fatality rates significantly (Saady and Torda, 1973; Trujillo et al., 1980; Olsen and Hiller, 1987; Udwadia et al., 1987). Tracheostomy and ventilatory support are often necessary when there is laryngeal spasm. Sedatives, muscle relaxants

Table 12.4

Differential diagnosis of tetanus

Disease entity	Characteristic features
Tetanus	Initial oculobulbar then rapid descending pattern of weakness; autonomic involvement
Retropharyngeal or dental abscess	Pseudo-trismus, localized findings to the jaw; fever
Meningitis	CSF pleocytosis with elevated protein
Encephalitis	Sensorial clouding; CSF pleocytosis with elevated protein
Rabies	Trismus is not present, usually incubation period is longer; CSF pleocytosis
Hypocalcemic tetany	
Phenothiazine-induced dystonia	Known exposure to drug; multifocal dystonic posturing
Epilepsy	Witnessed seizure, incontinence, post-ictal state
Strychnine poisoning	Trismus appears late; low serum calcium

CSF, cerebrospinal fluid.

and a quiet environment reduce rigidity and control spasms. Typically, diazepam is used in doses of 0.5–1.0 mg/kg per day given either as an infusion or in divided doses. An alternative is the intravenous infusion of midazolam (Ernst et al., 1997). Larger doses of these agents may cause respiratory depression. Baclofen, given intravenously, has the advantage of treating spasms and preserving voluntary movement and respiration (Boots et al., 2000; Engrand and Benhamou, 2001; Reddy, 2002). Dantrolene and propofol have been used with variable results (Reddy, 2002). Neuromuscular blockade may be necessary when spasms are refractory to other measures.

The management of the autonomic disturbance can be difficult (Corbett et al., 1969, 1973; Tsueda et al., 1973; Bhagwanjee et al., 1999). Hypotension can be treated with fluid load and, if needed, inotropic support. Hypertensive episodes can be treated with short acting β-blockers, such as intravenous esmolol or labetolol (Wesley et al., 1983). However, the use of β-blockers is not without risk, particularly in patients whose blood pressure and heart rate vary widely and are likely to develop hypotension or bradycardia (Reddy, 2002).

The key to the treatment of tetanus is its prevention. Tetanus immunization, usually combined with diphtheria and petussis, is recommended for all children over the age of 6 years who have no contraindication to vaccination. Three doses are administered usually at 6–8 week intervals and a fourth dose is given at least 6 months after the third. Booster injections should be given upon entry to school (aged 5–6) and every 10 years thereafter. Individuals with simple wounds should receive a booster injection if they have not been immunized within 10 years or if the vaccination history is not known. If the wound is severe the recommendations are the same except that the acceptable interval since last immunization is shortened to 5 years.

12.3.3. Envenomation

Most biological toxins of animal origin affect the cholinergic system and either facilitate the release of neurotransmitter from the presynaptic nerve terminal or block the ACh receptor. In general, bites from snakes, scorpions and ticks are more common during summer months. In contrast, marine toxins may be encountered at any time as they are usually acquired through ingestion and less often by injection or penetration. Specific animal envenomations occur in defined geographic areas. For example, tick paralysis occurs predominantly in states west of the Rocky Mountains, the western provinces of Canada and Australia. The geography of snake envenomation is species-specific. Cobras are found in Asia and Africa,

kraits in Southeast Asia, mambas in Africa, coral snakes in North America and sea snakes in the Pacific near Australia and New Guinea.

12.3.3.1. Arthropods

Arthropod venoms have been known since antiquity when they were used to incapacitate prey or as a defense against predators (Maretic, 1978). The few arthropod venoms that are toxic to the NMJ act by one of three mechanisms. In the first there is an initial augmentation of ACh release followed by depletion of neurotransmitter. The second enhances ACh release without subsequent presynaptic neurotransmitter depletion. The third blocks ACh release. Untreated arthropod envenomation is fatal in 12–25% of cases, but with the improvement in critical care facilities in the last few decades these intoxications are rarely fatal (Temple, 1912; Rose, 1954).

12.3.3.1.1. Spider bites

Only a few spider venoms affect the neuromuscular junction. The funnel web spider and the redback spider of Australia are the most dangerous members of this group. In North America, only the bite of the black widow spider is of concern. The usual victim of a black widow spider bite is a small male child, perhaps because of their inquisitiveness in exploring nooks and crannies.

Latrotoxins in the venoms of spider genus *Latrodectus* (black widow spider) produce a marked facilitation in neurotransmitter release at all neurosecretory synapses including the neuromuscular junction by depolarizing the presynaptic nerve terminal and increasing Ca^{++} influx into the nerve terminal (Rosenthal, 1989; Hurlbut et al., 1990; Henkel and Sankaranarayanan, 1999). This depletes the neurotransmitter stores in the nerve terminal, resulting in a blockade of synaptic transmission. This toxin exerts its effects on the nerve terminal by several mechanisms. The toxin binds to neurexin and thereby activates the presynaptic protein complex of neurexin, syntaxin, synaptotagmin and the N-type calcium channel to facilitate massive ACh release (Ushkaryov et al., 1992). Neurotransmitter release in nerve-muscle preparations, as measured by MEPP frequency, increases several hundred-fold within a few minutes (Longenecker et al., 1970). There is a subsequent depletion of synaptic vesicles and disruption of the highly organized active zone region of the presynaptic nerve terminal, thus inhibiting the docking of synaptic vesicles to the terminal membrane and preventing effective recycling of vesicular membranes (Clark et al., 1970, 1972; Pumplin and Reese, 1977; Gorio et al., 1978; Ceccarelli et al., 1979; Gorio and Mauro, 1979; Howard, 1980).

Symptoms begin within minutes after a black widow spider bite and reflect the massive release of neurotransmitter from peripheral, autonomic and central synapses (Gilbert and Stewart, 1935). Severe muscle rigidity and cramps are followed by generalized muscle weakness due to the depolarizing neuromuscular blockade. Death from cardiovascular collapse may occur in the elderly or in young children, but otherwise black widow spider bites are rarely fatal. Treatment is primarily supportive. Calcium gluconate may help alleviate severe muscle cramps and rigidity (Miller, 1992). Magnesium salts may reduce neurotransmitter release if given soon after the bite (Gilbert and Stewart, 1935). Equine-serum antivenom is very effective and rapidly reverses the neurotoxic effects (D'Amour et al., 1936).

12.3.3.1.2. Tick paralysis

Tick paralysis is a worldwide disorder that was first described at the turn of the 20th century in North America and Australia, although there is vague reference to an earlier case in 1824 (Cleland, 1912; Temple, 1912; Todd, 1912; Gregson, 1973). It is one of several neuromuscular disorders that may result from tick venom exposure. Tick paralysis results from a neurotoxin produced by one of more than 60 tick species (Gothe et al., 1979; Anonymous, 1996). In North America, the *Dermacentor andersoni*, *D. variabilis*, *D. occidentalis*, *Amblyomma americanum* and *A. maculatum* species are toxic. The toxic species in Europe and in the Pacific are *Ixodes ricinus* and *I. cornuatus*, respectively, and in Australia, *I. holocyclus*. Tick paralysis is more common in states west of the Rocky Mountains and in British Columbia and Alberta (Weingart, 1967).

The symptoms of tick paralysis follow a stereotyped course. Within 5–6 days of tick attachment, there is a prodrome of paresthesiae, headache, malaise, nausea and vomiting which parallels the feeding pattern of the tick. Over the next 24–48 hours paralysis begins symmetrically in the lower extremities and ascends to the trunk and arms. In most instances when a tick is found, it is fully engorged. Weakness from the Australian tick is more severe and much slower to resolve than paralysis produced by the most common North America ticks (*Dermacentor* and *Amblyomma* species). In these Australian patients there is often a worsening of symptoms 24–48 hours following the removal of the tick (Brown and Hamilton, 1998). Sensation is preserved but muscle stretch reflexes are often diminished or absent, findings that suggest the LGB syndrome (Table 12.5), a common misdiagnosis (Felz et al., 2000). There is no demonstrable response to cholinesterase inhibitors (Cherington and Synder, 1968; Swift and Ignacio, 1975). There is some indication of an association between the proximity of the site of attachment to the brain and the severity of the disease. Resolution of symptoms depends in part on how quickly the tick is removed, suggesting a dose-dependent relationship. In paralyses due to the *Dermacentor* species, improvement often begins within hours of removing the tick and continues over several days. More prolonged weakness has been reported (Donat and Donat, 1981). Anti-toxin may be of benefit in some cases, but the high frequency of acute allergic reactions limits its widespread use (Grattan-Smith et al., 1997). Death may occur due to respiratory failure from severe bulbar and respiratory muscle weakness and the clinical picture may be clouded by central nervous system findings (Weingart, 1967; Lagos and Thies, 1969).

Children are affected more often than adults. This may be due in part to their play habits or their lower body mass relative to the amount of toxin acquired. The tick is usually attached to the head or neck. Some studies suggest that girls are affected more often because their long hair hides the tick, allowing more prolonged feeding (Dworkin et al., 1999; Felz et al., 2000). Identification of the tick bite is often delayed, leading to confusion with the LGB syndrome, MG, spinal cord disease, periodic paralysis,

Table 12.5

Comparative features of ascending paralysis

Clinical and laboratory features	Tick paralysis	Landry–Guillain–Barré syndrome
Rate of progression	Hours to days	Days to 1–2 weeks
Sensory loss	Absent	Mild
Muscle stretch reflexes	Diminished or absent	Diminished or absent
Time to recovery	<24 h after tick removal	Weeks to months
CSF white blood cell count	<10 per mm^2	<10 per mm^2
CSF protein	Normal	Elevated

CSF, cerebrospinal fluid.

diphtheria, heavy-metal intoxication, insecticide poisoning, porphyria and hysteria (Jones, 1995; Felz et al., 2000). Careful, systematic inspection of the scalp, neck and perineum, often with a fine-toothed comb, may be necessary to locate the tick. In many instances the tick is found by the nurse, the house officer, the mortician or the pathologist at the time of autopsy (Stanbury and Huyck, 1945; Rose, 1954; Felz et al., 2000).

Radiolabeled monoclonal antibodies have demonstrated the toxin in tick salivary glands (Crause et al., 1994). The most potent toxin is from the Australian tick, *Ixodes holocyclus*. Characteristics of the toxin from most species of tick are not known and the mechanism by which the toxin produces weakness remains controversial. Holocyclotoxin, isolated from the salivary glands of female ticks, causes a temperature-dependent block of neurally evoked release of ACh from the nerve terminal (Stone and Aylward, 1992). Others also have suggested a postsynaptic block of NMT (Rose and Gregson, 1959). Paralysis produced by the *Dermacentor* species is understood less well. Some studies suggest an abnormality due to impaired depolarization of the nerve terminal with secondary impairment of ACh release (Stone, 1988; Gothe and Neitz, 1991). Electrodiagnostic studies in patients with tick paralysis have demonstrated prolonged distal motor latencies, slowed nerve conduction velocities and reduced CMAP amplitudes (Esplin et al., 1960; DeBusk and O'Connor, 1972; Haller and Fabara, 1972; Gothe et al., 1979; Hawrylewicz et al., 2002).

12.3.3.2. Scorpion bites

Scorpion neurotoxins contain peptides that cause a number of neurological effects, the most significant of which affect Na^+ and K^+ channel function. Some, however, affect the neuromuscular junction by enhancing presynaptic depolarization, resulting in release of neurotransmitter from synaptic vesicles (Warnick et al., 1976). Increased excretion of catecholamines has been demonstrated after scorpion stings; this may be a primary effect of the venom or the result of a secondary sympathetic adrenergic surge (Henriques et al., 1968; Gueron and Weizmann, 1969; Murdock, 1971; Moss et al., 1973). Treatment is non-specific and focuses on maintaining respiratory and cardiac as well as coagulation function. Antivenom does not appear to be effective (Sofer et al., 1994; Belghith et al., 1999).

12.3.3.3. Snake bites

Venomous snakes fall into four major groups: *Viperidae* (true vipers), *Crotalidae* (rattlesnakes and pit vipers), *Elapidae* (American coral snakes, cobras, kraits, mambas) and *Hydrophiodae* (sea snakes). Neuromuscular blockade results primarily from the venom of *Elapidae* and *Hydrophiodae* species (Lee, 1970; Vital-Brazil, 1972; Campbell, 1975). One *Crotalidae* species, *C. durissus terrificus*, a South American rattlesnake, produces a very potent neuromuscular blocking venom. Venoms from other rattlesnakes and pit vipers act through hematological and cardiovascular mechanisms. Venom is produced and stored in salivary glands and inoculation occurs through fangs or modified premaxillary teeth (Campbell, 1975).

An in-depth discussion of the pharmacology of snake toxins is beyond the scope of this chapter. These toxins may act either presynaptically or postsynaptically. β-neurotoxins (β-bungarotoxin, notexin and taipoxin) act presynaptically to inhibit the release of ACh from the motor nerve terminal. Often, there is an initial augmentation of release followed by depletion of neurotransmitter. Presynaptic toxins tend to be more potent than the α-neurotoxins, which act postsynaptically by producing a curare-mimetic, nondepolarizing neuromuscular block that is variably reversible. Most venoms are a mixture of both types of neurotoxins, although one may predominate in a given venom. For example, the venom of the Thai cobra is composed primarily of a single postsynaptic neurotoxin (Karlsson et al., 1971), whereas Bungarus multicinctus venom contains β-bungarotoxin, four other presynaptic toxins, α-bungarotoxin and two other postsynaptic toxins (Lee et al., 1972). The venoms of the *Hydrophiodae* species are more toxic than those of land snakes and the amount of toxin injected per bite is less (Barme, 1963; Tu and Tu, 1970). The postsynaptic α-neurotoxins, like curare, bind to the nicotinic ACh receptor of muscle. They have a slower onset of action and a longer-lasting effect and are 15–40 times more potent than d-tubocurarine (Karlsson, 1979). There are numerous subforms of β-neurotoxin. Most have a phospholipase component that is essential for their toxic activity. All suppress the release of ACh from the nerve terminal, but via several different mechanisms. Toxins from different species potentiate each other, suggesting that they occupy different binding sites at the neuromuscular junction (Chang and Su, 1980). Taipoxin from the Australian and Papua New Guinean taipan snake is unique. In addition to producing a potent presynaptic blockade of synaptic transmission, it also has a direct toxic effect on muscle that produces rapid muscle necrosis and degeneration. Different species vary in their susceptibility to snake toxins. For example, the venom of the Australian mulga snake is fatal in man, produces ptosis in monkeys and has no apparent neuromuscular blocking effect in rabbits (Kellaway, 1932; Rowlands et al., 1969).

The clinical course of snake envenomation follows a variable pattern. After envenomation by a pit viper or cobra, there is local pain, but pain is often absent after bites by other *Elapidae* and *Hydrophiodae*. Swelling typically occurs within 1 hour following bites by *Viperidae*, *Crotalidae* or the cobra, but is not seen following bites by other *Elapidae* (mambas, kraits, coral snakes) and *Hydrophiodae*. There is then a preparalytic stage with headache, vomiting, loss of consciousness, paresthesias, hematuria or hemoptysis (Bouquier et al., 1974). These symptoms are not common after envenomation by cobras or mambas. The time between snake bite and paralytic signs and symptoms varies from 0.5–19 hours (Mitrakul et al., 1984). The first signs of neuromuscular toxicity are usually ptosis and ophthalmoparesis, although these are absent following the bite of the South American rattlesnake. Facial and bulbar weakness then develops over hours (Reid, 1964). Limb, diaphragmatic and intercostal muscle weakness follows and may progress for up to 2–3 days (Campbell, 1975; Warrell et al., 1976). Without appropriate treatment, cardiovascular collapse, seizures and coma ensue. There is no sensory abnormality other than around the bite itself. Other systemic effects result from coagulation deficits. Cerebral and subarachnoid hemorrhage have been reported after bites from many snake species and are the leading cause of death following viper bites in several parts of the world (Kerrigan, 1991; Ouyang et al., 1992).

Treatment of snake bites includes antivenoms, which are most effective against venoms that do not contain significant amounts of phospholipase, a component of presynaptic neurotoxins (Reid, 1964, 1975; Theakston et al., 1990). Antivenoms are used to shorten the duration of weakness. If the type of snake is known, high-titer specific monovalent antivenom is given. However, often the type of snake is not known and a polyvalent antivenom must be used. Respiratory, cardiovascular and hematological support measures may be required. Supportive measures are the mainstay of treatment for most coral snake bites. Intensive care treatment and airway maintenance are similar to that used in MG. Cholinesterase inhibitors have been recommended when there is a predominantly postsynaptic abnormality; electrodiagnostic testing may be useful in determining whether these agents are likely to be effective (Kumar and Usgaonkar, 1968; Pettigrew and Glass, 1985).

12.3.3.4. Marine toxins

The rapid rise in marine pollution has spurred a renewed interest in marine toxins. Previously these toxins were only of interest to physiologists and pharmacologists who used them as tools for the investigation of biological systems. Examples of marine neurotoxins date to biblical times (The Holy Bible, Exodus 7:20–21). The reader is referred to Southcott's (1975) excellent review of this subject. Marine neurotoxins that affect the neuromuscular junction are rare and come primarily from poisonous fish, a few mollusks and dinoflagellates. Unlike poisoning from arthropods and snakes, most marine toxins are ingested. Unique to some marine toxins is an increase in the concentration of toxin through successive predatory transvection up the food chain.

Dinoflagellates are single-celled, biflagellated, algae-like organisms. Diatoms are similar to dinoflagellates, but are not flagellated and are encased by a silica shell. Toxins produced by these organisms have a variety of systemic and neurological effects. Marine intoxications affecting the neuromuscular junction are rare. They include paralytic shellfish poisoning (PSP), which results from neurotoxins produced by less than 1% of the 2000–3000 species of known dinoflagellates and diatoms (Steidinger and Steinfield, 1984). These toxins are rapidly absorbed from the GI tract and produce symptoms within 30 minutes of ingestion. Characteristically, there is an initial burning sensation or paresthesiae of the face and mouth, which spread quickly to the neck and limbs. These sensory symptoms slowly abate and are replaced by numbness, ataxia and, in severe cases, progressive generalized weakness and respiratory failure. Overall, the mortality from PSP approaches 10%. Rapid notification of public health authorities is essential, because timely investigation may identify the source of the contaminated seafood and prevent additional illnesses. Environmental monitoring and, if necessary, the seasonal quarantine of a harvest can be employed to reduce the risk of exposure (Lehane, 2001; Sobel and Painter, 2005). Most neurotoxins from dinoflagellates and diatoms block sodium channels (e.g., saxitoxin and tetrodotoxin). Brevetoxin, a milder neurotoxin that causes the non-lethal neurotoxic shellfish poisoning (NSP), depolarizes cholinergic systems by opening sodium channels, which indirectly alters NMT (de Carvalho et al., 1998).

Conotoxins, a diverse group of toxins from predatory cone snails, inject their venom through a small harpoon-like dart (Olivera et al., 1985). It is only the fish predatory species (*Conus geographus*, *C. textile*, *C. marmoreus* and *C. omaria*) of this mollusk that are dangerous to man (Kohn, 1958, 1963; Cruz and White, 1995). The effects of these toxins vary among species and within a single species. Several have direct effects on the neuromuscular junction. The α-conotoxins block the binding of ACh to the ligand binding site similarly to the snake α-neurotoxins described earlier (Gray et al., 1981; McIntosh et al., 1982; Hopkins et al., 1995). The ω-conotoxins block the voltage-gated calcium channel of the presynaptic nerve terminal (McCleskey et al., 1987). ω-conotoxins have played an important role in our understanding of the Lambert–Eaton syndrome and are used in the voltage-gated calcium channel antibody assay for that condition (De Aizpurua et al., 1988; Adams et al., 1999). Injection of ω-conotoxin is followed by intense local pain, then malaise and headache and, within 30 minutes, a progressive generalized weakness. Respiratory failure often occurs within 1–2 hours. Most cone snail bites are preventable. These snails should be handled carefully with forceps and thick gloves. The proboscis protrudes from the small end of the shell but is flexible and long enough to sting the holder at the other end. Live cone snails should never be placed in a pocket as the dart can penetrate cloth (Southcott, 1975). Treatment is directed toward respiratory and cardiovascular support. There is no antivenom available. There is no published information about the potential efficacy of cholinesterase inhibitors. More than 60% of reported cone snail stings have been fatal (Yoshiba, 1984; Cruz and White, 1995).

The most venomous fish is the stonefish, *Synanceja horrida*, *S. traachynis* and *S. verrucosa*, found in the Indo-Pacific oceans and Red Sea, and the genus *Inimicus* found off the coast of Japan (Halstead, 1970). The toxin, stonustoxin, is inflicted by injection through 13 dorsal spines when the victim steps on the small fish buried in the sand. Neuromuscular blockade occurs as the result of induced neurotransmitter release and depletion of ACh stores, similar to that of other presynaptic toxins (Kreger et al., 1993; Gwee et al., 1994). Envenomation produces immediate excruciating pain that may last for 1–2 days. Severe edema occurs due to the actions of hyaluronidase, which promotes the rapid spread of venom through the tissue (Southcott, 1975). Tissue necrosis may also occur. In addition to gastrointestinal, autonomic and cognitive difficulties, the victim may experience generalized muscle weakness due to the mechanism noted above. Death occurs from cardiotoxicity. Treatment is supportive; a specific antitoxin may be helpful in some cases.

12.3.3.5. Plant toxins

Plant neurotoxins rarely affect the NMJ of humans; they are more likely to affect animals. Their neurotoxicity depends on the potency, concentration and interaction with other toxins or substrates in the victim. Many plant toxins are alkaloids. Coniine, the neurotoxin from the herb *Conium maculatum* (poison hemlock), produces a rapidly ascending paralysis which is often fatal. Socrates is said to have died from hemlock poisoning

(Davies and Davies, 1994). Sensory abnormalities are common and prominent (Hardin and Arena, 1974). The mechanisms of action of this piperidine alkaloid neurotoxin are not completely understood. There is evidence that the toxin acts at least in part like curare (Panter and Keeler, 1989).

12.4. Occupational neurotoxins

12.4.1. Heavy metals

Heavy metal intoxication is a rare cause of clinical neuromuscular toxicity. Numerous polyvalent cations affect NMT but these effects are seen mainly in physiology and pharmacology laboratories where they have been used as tools to study the basic mechanisms of synaptic transmission. These include barium, erbium, cadmium, cobalt, gadolinium, lanthium, manganese, nickel, praseodymium, triethyltin and zinc (Benoit and Mambrini, 1970; Kajimoto and Kirpekar, 1972; Balnave and Gage, 1973; Kita and van der kloot, 1973; Weakly, 1973; Alnaes and Rahaminoff, 1975; Forshaw, 1977; Silinsky, 1977, 1978; Metral et al., 1978; Allen et al., 1980; Cooper and Manalis, 1984; Molgo et al., 1991). Nearly all of these have multiple effects on synaptic transmission but they predominantly block the release of ACh from the presynaptic nerve terminal. All of them also facilitate the spontaneous quantal release of neurotransmitter. Mechanisms by which they exert these effects include blocking the flux of Ca^{++} through voltage-gated calcium channels and disrupting intracellular stores of Ca^{++} (Cooper and Manalis, 2001).

Interest in heavy metal intoxication increased after the 1971 contamination of grain with a methylmercury fungicide in Iraq. Despite appropriate warnings, the grain was fed to animals, ground for flour and used for making bread (Rustam and Hamdi, 1974). Symptoms began within 1 month of consumption and ultimately affected more than 6500 people, 8% fatally (Bakir et al., 1973). Patients experienced ataxia, fatigue, generalized muscle weakness and occasionally optic atrophy. Although one of the expected abnormalities following mercurial poisoning is peripheral neuropathy (based on the Minamata experience), extensive electrodiagnostic examinations of the affected population did not demonstrate this (LeQuense et al., 1974; Igata, 1986). Repetitive nerve stimulation studies demonstrated a decremental response that was partially reversible by cholinesterase inhibitors (Rustam et al., 1975). Similar abnormalities have been demonstrated in experimental animals (Atchinson and Narahashi, 1982).

There are reports that gadolinium acutely worsened the strength of myasthenic patients (Molgo et al., 1991; Nordenbo and Somnier, 1992).

12.5. Summary

One can readily appreciate the wide range of neurotoxic compounds whose end-organ is the neuromuscular junction. While some of these toxins are of passing or historical interest, the inadvertent use of potentially neuromuscular junction toxic drugs is a matter of concern. Health care personnel must carefully assess each patient's potential complications and risk of adverse events before prescribing these agents to someone whose neuromuscular transmission is perturbed.

References

Abdel-Aziz A, Bakry N (1973). The action and interaction of diphenhydramine (Benadryl) hydrochloride at the neuromuscular junction. Eur J Pharmacol 22: 169–174.

Absher JR, Bale JF, Jr. (1991). Aggravation of myasthenia gravis by erythromycin. J Pediatr 1191: 155–156.

Adams DJ, Alewood PF, Craik DJ, et al. (1999). Conotoxins and their potential pharmaceutical applications. Drug Dev Res 46: 219–234.

Adams RJ, Rivner MH, Salazar J, et al. (1984). Effects of oral calcium antagonists on neuromuscular transmission. Neurology 34(Suppl 1): 132–133.

Albers JW, Hodach RJ, Kimmel DW, et al. (1980). Penicillamine-associated myasthenia gravis. Neurology (Minneapolis) 30: 1246–1250.

Albiero L (1978a). Comparison of neuromuscular effects and acute toxicity of some aminoglycoside antibiotics. Arch Int Pharm Ther 233: 343.

Albiero L (1978b). The neuromuscular blocking activity of a new aminoglycoside antibiotic netilmicin sulphate (SCH 20569). Eur J Pharmacol 50: 1–7.

Albrecht RF, Lanier WL (1993). Potentiation of succinylcholine-induced phase II block by vancomycin. Anesth Analg 77: 1300–1302.

Alderdice MT, Trommer BA (1980). Differential effects of the anticonvulsants phenobarbital, ethosuximide and carbamazepine on neuromuscular transmission. J Pharmacol Exp Therapeut 215: 92–96.

Aldrich MS, Kim YI, Sanders DB (1979). Effects of D-penicillamine on neuromuscular transmission in rats. Muscle Nerve 2: 180–185.

Alexander WD (1981). Systemic effects with eye drops. BMJ 282: 1359.

Alfrey AC, Terman DS, Brettschneider L, et al. (1970). Hypermagnesemia after renal homotransplantation. Ann Intern Med 73: 367–371.

Allen JE, Gage PW, Leaver DD, et al. (1980). Triethyltin decreases evoked transmitter release at the mouse neuromuscular junction. Chem Biol Interact 31: 227–231.

Alnaes E, Rahaminoff R (1975). Dual action of praseodymium (Pr3+) on transmitter release at the frog neuromuscular synapse. Nature 247: 478–479.

Anderson HJ, Churchill-Davidson HC, Richardson AT (1953). Bronchial neoplasm with myasthenia. Prolonged apnea after administration of succinylcholine. Lancet 1: 1291–1293.

Anonymous (1994). Progress towards the global elimination of neonatal tetanus, 1989–1993. MMWR 43: 885–887.

Anonymous (1998a). Neonatal tetanus—Montana, 1998. MMWR 47: 928–930.

Anonymous (1998b). Tetanus among injecting-drug users—California, 1997. MMWR 47: 149–151.

Anonymous (2000). Case definitions. Neonatal tetanus. Epidemiol Bull 21: 11.

Anonymous (2004). Telithromycin and myasthenia. Prescrire Int 13: 21.

Anonymous (1996). Tick paralysis—Washington, 1995. From the Centers for Disease Control and Prevention. JAMA 275: 1470.

Ansell BM (1974). Other case reports and discussion of adverse reactions to penicillamine. Postgrad Med J 50: 78–80.

Argov Z, Mastaglia FL (1979a). Disorders of neuromuscular transmission caused by drugs. N Engl J Med 301: 409–413.

Argov Z, Mastaglia FL (1979b). Drug therapy: disorders of neuromuscular transmission caused by drugs. N Engl J Med 301: 409–413.

Argov Z, Brenner T, Abramsky O (1986). Ampicillin may aggravate clinical and experimental myasthenia gravis. Arch Neurol 43: 255–256.

Atchinson WD, Narahashi T (1982). Methylmercury induced depression of neuromuscular transmission in the rat. Neurotoxicology 3: 37–50.

Ayrapetyan SN, Arvaov VL, Maginyan SB, et al. (1985). Further study of the correlation between Na-pump activity and membrane chemosensitivity. Cell Mol Neurobiol 5: 231–243.

Bagratuni L (1952). Cephalic tetanus. With report of a case. BMJ 1: 461–463.

Bakir F, Damluji SF, Amin-Saki L, et al. (1973). Methylmercury poisoning in Iraq. Science 181: 230–241.

Balint G, Szobor A, Temesvari P (1975). Myasthenia gravis developed under D-penicillamine treatment. Scand J Rheumatol Sup: 12–21.

Balnave RJ, Gage PW (1973). The inhibitory effect of manganese on transmitter release at the neuromuscular junction of the toad. Br J Pharmacol 47: 339–352.

Baraka A, Afifi A, Muallem M, et al. (1971). Neuromuscular effects of halothane, suxamethonium and tubocurarine in a myasthenic undergoing thymectomy. Br J Anaesth 43: 91–95.

Baraka A, Baroody M, Yazbeck V (1993). Repeated doses of suxamethonium in the myasthenic patient. Anaesthesia 48: 782–784.

Baraka A, Siddik S, Kawkabani N (1999). Cisatracurium in a myasthenic patient undergoing thymectomy. Can J Anaesth 46: 779–782.

Barme M (1963). Venomous sea snakes of Vietnam and their venoms. In: HL Keegan, W MacFarlane (Eds.), Venomous and Poisonous Animals and Noxious Plants of the Pacific Region. MacMillan and Company, Oxford, pp. 373–378.

Bashuk RG, Krendel DA (1990). Myasthenia gravis presenting as weakness after magnesium administration. Muscle Nerve 13: 708–712.

Batocchi AP, Evoli A, Servidei S, et al. (1995). Myasthenia gravis during interferon alfa therapy. Neurology 45: 382–383.

Bazzato G, Mezzina C, Ciman M, et al. (1979). Myasthenia-like syndrome associated with carnitine in patients on long-term hemodialysis. Lancet i: 1041–1042.

Bazzato G, Coli U, Landini S, et al. (1981). Myasthenia-like syndrome after D,L- but not L-carnitine. Lancet i: 1209.

Belghith M, Boussarsar M, Haguiga H, et al. (1999). Efficacy of serotherapy in scorpion sting: a matched-pair study. J Toxicol Clin Toxicol 37: 51–57.

Benoit PR, Mambrini J (1970). Modification of transmitter release by ions which prolong the presynaptic action potential. J Physiol (Lon) 210: 681–695.

Benzing G, III, Iannaccone ST, Bove KE, et al. (1990). Prolonged myasthenic syndrome after one week of muscle relaxants. Pediatr Neurol 6: 190–196.

Berciano J, Oterino A, Rebollo M, et al. (1991). Myasthenia gravis unmasked by cocaine abuse [letter]. N Engl J Med 325: 892.

Bermudez JS (2001). The Armed Forces of North Korea. I.B. Tauris, London.

Bhagwanjee S, Bosenberg AT, Muckart DJ (1999). Management of sympathetic overactivity in tetanus with epidural bupivacaine and sufentanil: experience with 11 patients. Crit Care Med 27: 1721–1725.

Bickerstaff ER (1975). Neurological Complication of Oral Contraceptives. 1st ed. Oxford University Press, London.

Bikhazi GB, Leung I, Foldes FF (1982). Interaction of neuromuscular blocking agents with calcium channel blockers. Anesthesiology 57: A268.

Bikhazi GB, Leung I, Foldes FF (1983). Ca-channel blockers increase potency of neuromuscular blocking agents in vivo. Anesthesiology 59: A269.

Bodley PO, Brett JE (1962). Post-operative respiratory inadequacy and the part played by antibiotics. Anaesthenia 17: 438–443.

Bodley PO, Halwax K, Potts L (1969). Low serum pseudo-cholinesterase levels complicating treatment with phenelzine. BMJ 3: 510–512.

Booij LHD, Miller RD, Crul JF (1978). Neostigmine and 4-aminopyridine antagonism of lincomycin-pancuronium neuromuscular blockade in man. Anesth Analg 57: 316–321.

Booker HE, Chun RWM, Sanguino M (1970). Myasthenia gravis syndrome associated with trimethadione. J Am Med Assoc 212: 2262–2263.

Boots RJ, Lipman J, O'Callaghan J, et al. (2000). The treatment of tetanus with intrathecal baclofen. Anaesth Intensive Care 28: 438–442.

Bora I, Karli N, Bakar M, et al. (1997). Myasthenia gravis following IFN-alpha-2a treatment. Eur Neurol 38: 68.

Borden H, Clark MT, Katz H (1974). The use of pancuronium bromide in patients receiving lithium carbonate. Can Anaesth Soc J 21: 79–82.

Borgia G, Reynaud L, Gentile I, et al. (2001). Myasthenia gravis during low-dose IFN-alpha therapy for chronic hepatitis C. J Interferon Cytokine Res 21: 469–470.

Borodic G (1998). Myasthenic crisis after botulinum toxin. Lancet 352: 1832.

Bouquier JJ, Guibert J, Dupont C, et al. (1974). Les piqures de vipere chez l'enfant. Arch Fr Pediatr 31: 285–296.

Bowman WC (1981). Effects of adrenergic activators and inhibitors on the skeletal muscle. In: L Szekeres (Ed.), Handbook of Experimental Pharmacology. Springer-Verlag, Berlin, pp. 47–128.

Brittain J, Lange LS (1995). Myasthenia gravis and levonorgestrel implant. Lancet 346: 1556.

Brown AF, Hamilton DL (1998). Tick bite anaphylaxis in Australia. J Accid Emerg Med 15: 111–113.

Brown H (1968). Tetanus. J Am Med Assoc 204: 614–616.

Brown PW (1935). Results and dangers in the treatment of amebiasis. JAMA 105: 1319–1325.

Brumlik J, Jacobs RS (1974). Myasthenia gravis associated with diphenylhydantoin therapy for epilepsy. Can J Neurol Sci 1: 127–129.

Bryden J (1989). Deadly Allies: Canada's Secret War, 1937–1947, 1st ed. McClelland & Stewart, Toronto.

Bucknall RC, Dixon A, Glick EN, et al. (1975). Myasthenia gravis associated with penicillamine treatment for rheumatoid arthritis. BMJ 1: 600–602.

Burgen ASV, Dickens F, Zatman LJ (1949). The action of botulinum toxin on the neuro-muscular junction. J Physiol (Lon) 109: 10–24.

Burkett L, et al. (1979). Mutual potentiation of the neuro-muscular effects of antibiotics and relaxants. Anesth Analg 58: 107–115.

Burres SA, Richman DP, Crayton JW, et al. (1979). Penicillamine-induced myasthenic responses in the guinea pig. Muscle Nerve 2: 186–190.

Cadisch R, Streit E, Hartmann K (1996). [Exacerbation of pseudoparalytic myasthenia gravis following azithromycin (Zithromax)]. Schweiz Med Wochenschr 126: 308–310.

Campbell CH (1975). The effects of snake venoms and their neurotoxins on the nervous system of man and animals. Contemp Neurol Ser 12: 259–293.

Campbell EDR, Montuschi E (1960). Muscle weakness caused by bretylium tosylate. Lancet ii: 789.

Canal N, Franceschi M (1983). Myasthenic crisis precipitated by iothalamic acid. Lancet 1: 1288.

Caputy AJ, Kim YI, Sanders DB (1981). The neuromuscular blocking effects of therapeutic concentrations of various antibiotics on normal rat skeletal muscle: a quantitative comparison. J Pharmacol Exp Therapeut 217: 369–378.

Carle A, Rattone G (1884). Studio experimentale sull'eziologia del tetano. Girón Accad Med Torino 32: 174–179.

Carrillo AM (1966). A peculiar and unusual case of trismus. ADM 23: 267–268.

Cartwright MS, Jeffery DR, Nuss GR, et al. (2004). Statin-associated exacerbation of myasthenia gravis. Neurology 63: 2188.

Carus WS (1999). Unlawful acquisition and use of biological agents. In: J Lederberg (Ed.), Biological Weapons: Limiting the Threat. The MIT Press, Cambridge, pp. 211–230.

Castlebaum AR, Donofrio PD, Walker FO, et al. (1989). Laxative abuse causing hypermagnesemia quadriparesis and neuromuscular junction defect. Neurology 39: 746–747.

Ceccarelli B, Grohovaz F, Hurlbut WP (1979). Freeze-fracture studies of frog neuromuscular junctions during intense release of neurotransmitter. I. Effects of black widow spider venom and Ca2+-free solutions on the structure of the active zone. J Cell Biol 81: 163–177.

Chagnac Y, Hadani M, Goldhammer Y (1985). Myasthenic crisis after intravenous administration of iodinated contrast agent. Neurology 35: 1219–1220.

Chang CC, Su MJ (1980). Mutual potentiation a nerve terminals, between toxins from snake venoms that contain phospholipase A activity: β-bungarotoxin, crotoxin, taipoxin. Toxicon 18: 641–648.

Chan-Palay V, Engel AG, Wu JY, et al. (1982). Coexistence in human and primate neuromuscular junctions of enzymes synthesising acetylcholine, catecholamine, taurine and τ-aminobutyric acid. Proc Natl Acad Sci U S A 79: 7027–7030.

Cherington M (2002). Botulism. In: B Katirji, et al. (Eds.), Neuromuscular Disorders in Clinical Practice. 1st ed. Butterworth Heinemann, Boston, pp. 942–952.

Cherington M, Synder RD (1968). Tick paralysis. Neurophysiologic studies. N Engl J Med 278: 95–97.

Cherubin CE, Sapira JD (1993). The medical complications of drug addiction and the medical assessment of the intravenous drug user: 25 years later. Ann Intern Med 119: 1017–1028.

Chiarandini DJ (1980). Curare-like effect of propranolol on rat extraocular muscles. Br J Pharmacol 69: 13–19.

Chiarandini DJ, Bentley PJ (1978). The effects of verapamil on excitation-contraction coupling in frog sartorius muscle. J Pharmacol Exp Ther 205: 49–57.

Choe S, Bennett MJ, Fujii G, et al. (1992). The crystal structure of diphtheria toxin. Nature 357: 216–222.

Clark AW, Mauro A, Longenecker HE, et al. (1970). Effects of black widow spider venom on the frog neuromuscular junction. Effects on the fine structure of the frog neuromuscular junction. Nature 225: 703–705.

Clark AW, Hurlbut WP, Mauro A (1972). Changes in the fine structure of the neuromuscular junction of the frog caused by black widow spider venom. J Cell Biol 52: 1–14.

Clark DC (1970). Prolonged trismus in chronic abscess of the pterygomandibular space. J Oral Surg 28: 424–431.

Cleland JB (1912). Injuries and diseases of man in Australia attributable to animals (except insects). Australas Med Gaz 32: 295–299.

Cohen BA, London RS, Goldstein PJ (1976). Myasthenia gravis and preeclampsia. Obstet Gynecol 48: 35S–37S.

Cole LA (1996). The specter of biological weapons. Sci Am 275: 60–65.

Collins EN, Russell PW (2002). Fatal magnesium poisoning. Cleve Clin Q 16: 162–166.

Colquhoun D (1986). On the principles of postsynaptic action of neuromuscular blocking agents. In: DA Kharkevich (Ed.), New Neuromuscular Blocking Agents, Handbook of Experimental Pharmacology. Springer-Verlag, Berlin, pp. 59–113.

Cook TM, Protheroe RT, Handel JM (2001). Tetanus: a review of the literature. Br J Anaesth 87: 477–487.

Cooper GP, Manalis RS (1984). Cadmium: effects on transmitter release at the frog neuromuscular junction. Eur J Pharmacol 99: 251–256.

Cooper GP, Manalis RS (2001). Influence of heavy metals on synaptic transmission. Neurotoxicology 4: 69–84.

Coppeto JR (1984). Timolol-associated myasthenia gravis. Am J Ophthalmol 98: 244–245.

Corbett JL, Kerr JH, Prys-Roberts C, et al. (1969). Cardiovascular disturbances in severe tetanus due to overactivity of the sympathetic nervous system. Anaesthesia 24: 198–212.

Corbett JL, Spalding JM, Harris PJ (1973). Hypotension in tetanus. BMJ 3: 423–428.

Crause JC, van Wyngaardt S, Gothe R, et al. (1994). A shared epitope found in the major paralysis inducing tick species of Africa. Exp Appl Acarol 18: 51–59.

Creese R, Head SD, Jenkinson DF (1987). The role of the sodium pump during prolonged end-plate currents in guinea-pig diaphragm. J Physiol 384: 377–403.

Cruz LJ, White J (1995). Clinical toxicology of Conus snail stings. In: J Meier, J White (Eds.), CRC Handbook on Clinical Toxicology of Animal Venoms and Poisons. CRC Press, Boca Raton, pp. 117–128.

Cucher BG, Goldman AL (1976). D-penicillamine-induced polymyositis in rheumatoid arthritis. Ann Intern Med 85: 615–616.

Czlonkowska A (1975). Myasthenia syndrome during penicillamine treatment. BMJ 2: 726–772.

Dale RC, Schroeder ET (1976). Respiratory paralysis during treatment of hypertension with trimethaphan camsylate. Arch Intern Med 136: 816–818.

D'Amour EF, Becker FE, Van Riper W (1936). The black widow spider. Q Rev Biol 11: 123–160.

Daras M, Samkoff LM, Koppel BS (1996). Exacerbation of myasthenia gravis associated with cocaine use. Neurology 46: 271–272.

Davies ML, Davies TA (1994). Hemlock: murder before the Lord. Med Sci Law 34: 331–333.

Davis WG (1970). A comparison of the local anesthetic-, "quinidine-like"- and adrenergic β-blocking-activities of five β-receptor antagonists. J Pharm Pharmacol 22: 284–290.

De Aizpurua HJ, Lambert EH, Griesmann GE, et al. (1988). Antagonism of voltage-gated calcium channels in small cell carcinomas of patients with and without Lambert–Eaton myasthenic syndrome by autoantibodies omega-conotoxin and adenosine. Cancer Res 48: 4719–4724.

De Bleecker J, De Reuck J, Quatacker J, et al. (1991). Persisting chloroquine-induced myasthenia? Acta Clin Belg 46: 401–406.

de Boer MP, Raghoebar GM, Stegenga B, et al. (1995). Complications after mandibular third molar extraction. Quintessence Int 26: 779–784.

de Carvalho M, Jacinto J, Ramos N, et al. (1998). Paralytic shellfish poisoning: clinical and electrophysiological observations. J Neurol 245: 551–554.

De Grandis D, Mezzina C, Fiaschi A, et al. (1980). Myasthenia due to carnitine treatment. J Neurol Sci 46: 365–371.

De Rosayro M, Healy TEJ (1978). Tobramycin and neuromuscular transmission in the rat isolated phrenic nerve-diaphragm preparation. Br J Anaesth 50: 251.

De Silva AJC (1973). Magnesium intoxication: an uncommon cause of prolonged curarization. Br J Anaesth 45: 1228–1229.

DeBusk FL, O'Connor S (1972). Tick toxicosis. Pediatrics 50: 328–329.

Decker DA, Fincham RW (1971). Respiratory arrest in myasthenia gravis with colistimethate therapy. Arch Neurol 25: 141–144.

Del Castillo J, Engback L (1954). The nature of the neuromuscular block produced by magnesium. J Physiol 124: 370–384.

Dionisiotis J, Zoukos Y, Thomaides T (2004). Development of myasthenia gravis in two patients with multiple sclerosis following interferon beta treatment. J Neurol Neurosurg Psychiatry 75: 1079.

Dische FE, Swinson DR, Hamilton EB (1976). Immunopathology of penicillamine-induced glomerular disease. J Rheumatol 3: 145–154.

Donaldson JO (1978). Neurology of Pregnancy. 1st ed. W.B. Saunders, Philadelphia.

Donat JR, Donat JF (1981). Tick paralysis with persistent weakness and electromyographic abnormalities. Arch Neurol 38: 59–61.

Drachman DA, Skom JH (1965). Procainamide—a hazard in myasthenia gravis. Arch Neurol 13: 316–320.

Drachman DB (1962). Myasthenia gravis and the thyroid gland. N Engl J Med 266: 330–333.

Dretchen KL, Morgenroth VH (1976). Azathioprine: effects on neuromuscular transmission. Anesthesiology 45: 604–609.

Dretchen KL, Gergis SD, Sokoll MD, et al. (1972). Effect of various antibiotics on neuromuscular transmission. Eur J Pharmacol 18: 201–203.

Dretchen KL, Sokoll MD, Gergis SD (1973). Relative effects of streptomycin on motor nerve terminal endplate. Eur J Pharmacol 22: 10–16.

Durant NN, Lambert JJ (1981). The action of polymyxin B at the frog neuromuscular junction. Br J Pharm 72: 41–47.

Dworkin MS, Shoemaker PC, Anderson DE (1999). Tick paralysis: 33 human cases in Washington State, 1946–1996. Clin Infect Dis 29: 1435–1439.

Eaton LM (1943). Diagnostic tests for myasthenia gravis with prostigmine and quinine. Proc Staff Meet Mayo Clinic 18: 230–236.

Eddy S, Wim R, Peter VE, et al. (1999). Myasthenia gravis: another autoimmune disease associated with hepatitis C virus infection. Dig Dis Sci 44: 186–189.

Ekeus R (1996). Memorandum to the Biological Weapons Convention Fourth Review Conference. United Nations Special Commission (UNSCOM), New York.

Elder BF, Beal H, DeWald W, et al. (1971). Exacerbation of subclinical myasthenia by occupational exposure to an anesthetic. Anesth Analg 50: 383–387.

Elmqvist D, Josefsson JO (1962). The nature of the neuromuscular block produced by neomycin. Acta Physiol Scand 54: 105–110.

Emmerson J (1994). Botulinum toxin for spasmodic torticollis in a patient with myasthenia gravis. Mov Disord 9: 367.

Engel WK (2003). Reversible ocular myasthenia gravis or mitochondrial myopathy from statins? Lancet 361: 85–86.

Engel WK, Festoff BW, Patten BM, et al. (1974). Myasthenia gravis. Ann Intern Med 81: 225–246.

Engrand N, Benhamou D (2001). About intrathecal baclofen in tetanus. Anaesth Intensive Care 29: 306–307.

Epperly TD, Wood TC (1990). New trends in the management of peritonsillar abscess. Am Fam Physician 42: 102–112.

Erbguth F, Claus D, Engelhardt A, et al. (1993). Systemic effect of local botulinum toxin injections unmasks subclinical Lambert–Eaton myasthenic syndrome. J Neurol Neurosurg Psychiatry 56: 1235–1236.

Ernst ME, Klepser ME, Fouts M, et al. (1997). Tetanus: pathophysiology and management. Ann Pharmacother 31: 1507–1513.

Esplin DW, Phillip CB, Hughes LE (1960). Impairment of muscle stretch reflexes in tick paralysis. Science 132: 958–959.

Evans M, Rees A (2002). Effects of HMG-coa reductase inhibitors on skeletal muscle: are all statins the same? Drug Saf 25: 649–663.

Evans RT, MacDonald R, Robinson A (1980). Suxamethonium apnoea associated with plasmapheresis. Anaesthesia 35: 198–201.

Fambrough DM, Drachman DB, Satymurti S (1973). Neuromuscular function in myasthenia gravis: decreased acetylcholine receptors. Science 182: 293–295.

Fasano A, Bentivoglio AR, Ialongo T, et al. (2005). Treatment with botulinum toxin in a patient with myasthenia gravis and cervical dystonia. Neurology 64: 2155–2156.

Felz MW, Smith CD, Swift TR (2000). A six-year-old girl with tick paralysis [see comments]. N Engl J Med 342: 90–94.

Fernandez JM, Ferrandiz M, Larrea L, et al. (1983). Cephalic tetanus studied with single fibre EMG. J Neurol Neurosurg Psychiatry 46: 862–866.

Fierro B, Castiglione MG, Salemi G, et al. (1987). Myasthenia-like syndrome induced by cardiovascular agents. Report of a case. Ital J Neurol Sci 8: 167–169.

Fishman RA (1965). Neurological aspects of magnesium metabolism. Arch Neurol 12: 562–596.

Flowers CJ (1965). Magnesium in obstetrics. Am J Obstet Gynecol 91: 763–776.

Fogdall RP, Miller RD (1974). Prolongation of a pancuronium-induced neuromuscular blockade by clindamycin. Anesthesiology 41: 407–408.

Foldes FF, McNall PG (1962). Myasthenia gravis: a guide for anesthesiologists. Anesthesiology 23: 837–872.

Forshaw PJ (1977). The inhibitory effect of cadmium on neuromuscular transmission in the rat. Eur J Pharmacol 42: 371–377.

Frank JH, Cooper GW, Black WC, et al. (1987). Iodinated contrast agents in myasthenia gravis. Neurology 37: 1400–1402.

Franz DR (1997). Defense against toxin weapons. In: FR Sidell, ET Takafuji, DR Franz (Eds.), Medical Aspects of Chemical and Biological Warfare. Borden Institute, Walter Reed Army Medical Center, Washington, pp. 603–620.

Frenkel M, Ehrlich EN (1964). The influence of progesterone and mineralocorticoids upon myasthenia gravis. Ann Intern Med 60: 971–981.

Friedman NR, Mitchell RB, Pereira KD, et al. (1997). Peritonsillar abscess in early childhood. Presentation and management. Arch Otolaryngol Head Neck Surg 123: 630–632.

Fuchs-Buder T, Tassonyi E (1996). Magnesium sulphate enhances residual neuromuscular block induced by vecuronium. Br J Anaesth 76: 565–566.

Gage PW, Hamill OP (1976). Effects of several inhalation anesthetics on the kinetics of post-synaptic conductance in mouse diaphragm. Br J Pharmacol 57: 263–272.

Galazka A, Gasse F (1995). The present status of tetanus and tetanus vaccination. Curr Top Microbiol 195: 31–53.

George WK, Han CL (1962). Calcium and magnesium administration in myasthenia gravis. Lancet ii: 561.

Gesztes T (1966). Prolonged apnoea after suxamethonium injection associated with eye drops containing anticholinesterase agent: a case report. Br J Anaesth 38: 408–409.

Ghoneim MM, Long JP (1970). The interaction between magnesium and other neuromuscular blocking agents. Anesthesiology 32: 23–27.

Gibbels E (1967). Weitere Beobachtungen zur Nebenwirkung intravenoser Reverin-Gaben Bei Myasthenia gravis pseudoparalytica. Dtsch Med Wochenschr 92: 1153–1154.

Gilbert WW, Stewart CM (1935). Effective treatment of arachiodism by calcium salts. Am J Med Sci 189: 532–536.

Girlanda P, Venuto C, Mangiapane R (1989). Effect of ampicillin on neuromuscular transmission in healthy men: a single-fiber electromyographic study. Eur Neurol 29: 36–38.

Gold GN, Richardson AP (1966). An unusual case of neuromuscular blockade seen with therapeutic blood levels of colistin methanesulfonate (Coly-Mycin). Am J Med 41: 316–321.

Goncalves MR, Barbosa ER, Zambon AA, et al. (1999). Treatment of cervical dystonia with botulinum toxin in a patient with myasthenia gravis. Arq Neuropsiquiatr 57: 683–685.

Gorio A, Mauro A (1979). Reversibility and mode of action of Black Widow spider venom on the vertebrate neuromuscular junction. J Gen Physiol 73: 245–263.

Gorio A, Rubin LL, Mauro A (1978). Double mode of action of black widow spider venom on frog neuromuscular junction. J Neurocytol 7: 193–202.

Gothe R, Neitz AWH (1991). Tick paralyses: pathogenesis and etiology. Adv Dis Vector Res 8: 177–204.

Gothe R, Kunze K, Hoogstraal H (1979). The mechanisms of pathogenicity in the tick paralyses. J Med Entomol 16: 357–369.

Granacher RP, Jr. (1977). Neuromuscular problems associated with lithium. Am J Psychiatry 134: 702.

Grattan-Smith PJ, Morris JG, Johnston HM, et al. (1997). Clinical and neurophysiological features of tick paralysis. Brain 120: 1975–1987.

Gray WR, Luque A, Olivera BM, et al. (1981). Peptide toxins from Conus geographus venom. J Biol Chem 256: 4734–4740.

Gregson JD (1973). Tick Paralysis—An Appraisal of Natural and Experimental Data. Canada Department of Agriculture, Ottawa.

Grogono AW (1963). Anaesthesia for atrial defibrillation. Effect of quinidine on muscular relaxation. Lancet ii: 1039–1040.

Gu D, Wogensen L, Calcutt NA, et al. (1995). Myasthenia gravis-like syndrome induced by expression of interferon gamma in the neuromuscular junction. J Exp Med 181: 547–557.

Gueron M, Weizmann S (1969). Catecholamine excretion in scorpion sting. Isr J Med Sci 5: 855–857.

Gurtubay IG, Morales G, Arechaga O, et al. (1999). Development of myasthenia gravis after interferon alpha therapy. Electromyogra Clin Neurophysiol 39: 75–78.

Gutmann L, Takamori M (1973). Effect of Mg++ on neuromuscular transmission in the Eaton–Lambert syndrome. Neurology 23: 977–980.

Gwee MC, Gopalakrishnakone P, Yuen R, et al. (1994). A review of stonefish venoms and toxins. Pharmacol Ther 64: 509–528.

Haller JS, Fabara JA (1972). Tick paralysis. Case report with emphasis on neurological toxicity. Am J Dis Child 124: 915–917.

Halstead BW (1970). Poisonous and Venomous Marine Animals of the World. US Government Printing Office, Washington, DC.

Hardin JW, Arena JW (1974). Human Poisoning from Native and Cultivated Plants. 1st ed. Duke University Press, Durham, NC.

Hargreaves IP, Heales S (2002). Statins and myopathy. Lancet 359: 711–712.

Harry JD, Linden RJ, Snow HM (1975). The effects of three β-adrenoceptor blocking drugs on isolated preparations of skeletal and cardiac muscle. Br J Pharmacol 52: 275–281.

Harvey AM, Whitehill MR (1937). Quinine as an adjuvant to prostigmine in the diagnosis of myasthenia gravis. Bull Johns Hopkins Hosp 61: 216–217.

Havdala HS, Borison RL, Diamond BI (1979). Potential hazards and applications of lithium in anesthesiology. Anesthesiology 50: 534–537.

Hawrylewicz E, Gowdy B, Ehrlich R (2002). Microorganisms under simulated Martian environment. Nature 193: 497.

Henkel AW, Sankaranarayanan S (1999). Mechanisms of α-latrotoxin action. Cess Tissue Res 296: 229–233.

Henriques MC, Gazzinelli G, Diniz CR, et al. (1968). Effect of the venom of the scorpion Tityus serrulatus on adrenal gland catecholamines. Toxicon 5: 175–179.

Herishanu Y (1969). The effect of streptomycin and colistin on myasthenic patients. Confin Neurol 31: 370–373.

Herishanu Y, Rosenberg P (1975). Beta-blockers and myasthenia gravis. Ann Intern Med 83: 834–835.

Herishanu Y, Taustein I (1971). The electromyographic changes induced by antibiotics: a preliminary study. Confin Neurol 33: 41–45.

Hewitt J, Benveniste M, Lessana-Leibowitch M (1975). Pemphigus induced by d-penicillamine. BMJ 3: 371.

Hill EV (1947). Botulism. Summary Report on B.W. Investigations. Memorandum to Alden C. Waitt, Chief Chemical Corps, United States Army. Washington, United States Army, Ref Type: Sound Recording.

Hill GE, Wong KC, Hodges MR (1977). Lithium carbonate and neuromuscular blocking agents. Anesthesiology 45: 122–126.

Hirst GDS, Wood DR (1971). On the neuromuscular paralysis produced by procaine. Br J Pharm 41: 94–104.

Hokkanen E (1964). The aggravating effect of some antibiotics on the neuromuscular blockade in myasthenia gravis. Acta Neurol Scand 40: 346–352.

Hopkins C, Grilley M, Miller C, et al. (1995). A new family of Conus peptides targeted to the nicotinic acetylcholine receptor. J Biol Chem 270: 22361–22367.

Howard BD (1980). Effects and mechanisms of polypeptide neurotoxins that act presynaptically. Annu Rev Pharmacol 20: 307–336.

Howard JF (1991). Adverse drug interactions in disorders of neuromuscular transmission. J Neurol Orthop Med Surg 12: 26–34.

Howard JF, Sanders DB (1983). The management of patients with myasthenia gravis. In: EX Albuquerque, AT Eldefrawi (Eds.), Myasthenia Gravis. 1st ed. Chapman and Hall Ltd., London, pp. 457–489.

Howard JF, Johnson BR, Quint SR (1987). The effects of beta-adrenergic antagonists on neuromuscular transmission in rat skeletal muscle. Soc Neurosci Abst 13: 147.

Hughes RO, Zacharias FJ (1976). Myasthenic syndrome during treatment with practolol. BMJ 1: 460–461.

Hurlbut WP, Iezzi N, Fesce R, et al. (1990). Correlation between quantal secretion and vesicle loss at the frog neuromuscular junction. J Physiol 424: 501–526.

Hutter OF, Kostial K (1953). Effect of magnesium ions upon the release of acetylcholine. J Physiol 120: 53P.

Huynh T, Cordato D, Yang F, et al. (2002). HMG coa reductase-inhibitor-related myopathy and the influence of drug interactions. Intern Med J 32: 486–490.

Igata A (1986). Neurological aspects of methylmercury poisoning in Minamata. In: T Tsubaki, H Takahashi (Eds.), Recent Advances in Minamata Disease Studies. Kodansha, Tokyo, pp. 41–57.

Ionescu-Drinea M, Vioculescu V, Serbanescu G, et al. (1973). Association of myasthenic and neuritic symptoms following administration of antitetanic serum. Rev Roum Neurol 10: 239–243.

Izurieta HS, Sutter RW, Strebel PM, et al. (1997). Tetanus surveillance—United States, 1991–1994. MMWR CDC Surveill Summ 46: 15–25.

Jacobson TA (2006). Statin safety: lessons from new drug applications for marketed statins. Am J Cardiol 97: S44–S51.

Jenkins RB, Witorsch P, Smythe NPD (1970). Aspects of treatment of crisis in myasthenia gravis. South Med J 46: 365–371.

Jones HR, Jr. (1995). Guillain-Barre syndrome in children. Curr Opin Pediatr 7: 663–668.

Jonkers I, Swerup C, Pirskanen R, et al. (1996). Acute effects of intravenous injection of beta-adrenoreceptor- and calcium channel antagonists and agonists in myasthenia gravis. Muscle Nerve 19: 959–965.

Jui-Yen T (1971). Clinical and experimental studies on mechanisms of neuromuscular blockade by chloroquine diorotate. Jpn J Anesth 50: 491–503.

Kadlec RP, Zelicoff AP, Vrtis AM (1997). Biological weapons control. Prospects and implications for the future. JAMA 278: 351–356.

Kadlec RP, Zelicoff AP, Vrtis AM (1999). Biological weapons control: prospects and implications for the future. In: J Lederberg (Ed.), Biological Weapons: Limiting the Threat. The MIT Press, Cambridge, pp. 95–112.

Kaeser HE (1984). Drug-induced myasthenic syndromes. Acta Neurol Scand Suppl 100: 39–47.

Kaibara K, Akasu T, Tokimasa T, et al. (1985). Beta-adrenergic modulation of the Na+-K+ pump in frog skeletal muscles. Pflugers Arch 405: 24–28.

Kajimoto N, Kirpekar SM (1972). Effects of manganese and lanthanum on spontaneous release of acetylcholine at frog motor nerve terminals. Nature 235: 29–30.

Kanesada K, Mogi G (1981). Bilateral peritonsillar abscesses. Auris Nasus Larynx 8: 35–39.

Karlsson E (1979). Chemistry of protein toxins in snake venoms. In: CY Lee (Ed.), Snake Venoms. Springer-Verlag, New York, pp. 159–212.

Karlsson E, Arnberg H, Eaker D (1971). Isolation of the principal neurotoxin of two *Naja naja* subspecies. Eur J Biochem 21: 1–16.

Katz RL, Gissen AJ (1969). Effects of intravenous and intra-arterial procaine and lidocaine on neuromuscular transmission in man. Acta Anaesthesiol Scand 36: 103–113.

Kellaway CH (1932). The peripheral action of the Australian snake venoms. 2. The curari-like action in mammals. Aust J Exp Biol Med Sci 10: 181–194.

Kerner CAJ (1820). Neue Beobachtungen uber die in Wurttemberg so haufig vorfallenden todtlichen Vergiftungen durch in den Genuss geraucherter Wurste. Osiander, Tubingen.

Kerrigan KR (1991). Venomous snake bites in Eastern Ecuador. Am J Trop Med Hygiene 44: 93–99.

Kim YI, Howard JF, Sanders DB (1979). Depressant effects of morphine and meperidine on neuromuscular transmission in rat and human myasthenic muscles. Soc Neurosci Abst 5: 482.

Kirjner M, Lebourges J, Camus JP (1980). Myasthenie indulte par la pyrithioxine au cours du traitement d'une polyarthrite rhumatoide. Nouv Presse Med 9: 3098.

Kita H, Van der Kloot W (1973). Action of Co and Ni at the frog neuromuscular junction. Nature 245: 52–53.

Kohn AJ (1958). Recent cases of human injury due to venomous marine snails of the genus *Conus*. Hawaii Med J 17: 528–532.

Kohn AJ (1963). Venomous marine snails of the genus Conus. In: HC Keegan, WV McFarlane (Eds.), Venomous and Poisonous Animals and Noxious Plants of the Pacific Region. Permagon Press, Oxford, pp. 1–456.

Komal Kumar RN, Patil SA, Taly AB, et al. (2004). Effect of D-penicillamine on neuromuscular junction in patients with Wilson disease. Neurology 63: 935–936.

Konishi T (1996). A case of myasthenia gravis which developed myasthenic crisis after alpha-interferon therapy for chronic hepatitis C. Rinsho Shinkeigaku—Clin Neurol 36: 980–985.

Kornfeld P, Horowitz SH, Genkins G, et al. (1976). Myasthenia gravis unmasked by antiarrhythmic agents. Mt Sinai J Med 43: 10–14.

Kreger AS, Molgo J, Comella JX, et al. (1993). Effects of stonefish (*Synanceia trachynis*) venom on murine and frog neuromuscular junctions. Toxicon 31: 307–317.

Krendel DA (1990). Hypermagnesemia and neuromuscular transmission. Semin Neurol 10: 42–45.

Krendel DA, Hopkins LC (1986). Adverse effect of verapamil in a patient with the Lambert–Eaton syndrome. Muscle Nerve 9: 519–522.

Kreutzer K, Bonnekoh B, Franke I, et al. (2004). Sarcoidosis, myasthenia gravis and anterior ischaemic optic neuropathy: severe side effects of adjuvant interferon-alpha-therapy in malignant melanoma? J Dtsch Dermatol Ges 2: 689–694.

Krivoshein AV, Hess GP (2004). Mechanism-based approach to the successful prevention of cocaine inhibition of the neuronal (alpha3beta4) nicotinic acetylcholine receptor. Biochemistry 43: 481–489.

Kumar S, Usgaonkar RS (1968). Myasthenia gravis like picture resulting from snake bite. J Indian Med Assoc 50: 428–429.

Lagos JC, Thies RE (1969). Tick paralysis without muscle weakness. Arch Neurol 21: 471–474.

Law M, Rudnicka AR (2006). Statin safety: a systematic review. Am J Cardiol 97: S52–S60.

Lawn JE, Wilczynska-Ketende K, Cousens SN (2006). Estimating the causes of 4 million neonatal deaths in the year 2000. Int J Epidemiol 35: 706–718.

Lecky BR, Weir D, Chong E (1991). Exacerbation of myasthenia by propafenone. J Neurol Neurosurg Psychiatry 54: 377.

Lee CY (1970). Elapid neurotoxins and their mode of action. Clin Toxicol 3: 457–472.

Lee CY, Chang SL, Kau ST, et al. (1972). Chromatographic separation of the venon of *Bungarus multicinctus* and characteristics of its components. J Chromatogr 72: 71–82.

Lehane L (2001). Paralytic shellfish poisoning: a potential public health problem. Med J Aust 175: 29–31.

Lemcke B, Fucks C (1984). Magnesium load induced by ingestion of magnesium-containing antacids. Contrib Nephrol 38: 185–194.

Lensch E, Faust J, Nix WA, et al. (1996). Myasthenia gravis after interferon-alpha treatment. Muscle Nerve 19: 927–928.

LeQuense P, Damluji SF, Berlin M (1974). Electrophysiological studies of peripheral nerves in patients with organic mercury poisoning. J Neurol Neurosurg Psychiatry 37: 333–339.

L'Hommedieu C, Stough R, Brown L, et al. (1979). Potentiation of neuromuscular weakness in infant botulism by aminoglycosides. J Pediatr 95: 1065–1070.

Lilleheil G, Roed A (1971). Antitetanic effect of propranolol on mammalian motor-nerve and skeletal muscle and combined action of propranolol and neostigmine on the neuromuscular transmission. Arch Int Pharmacodyn 194: 129–140.

Lindesmith LA, Baines RD, Bigelow DB, et al. (1968). Reversible respiratory paralysis associated with polymyxin therapy. Ann Intern Med 68: 318–327.

Lipsitz PJ (1971). The clinical and biochemical effects of excess magnesium in the newborn. Pediatrics 47: 501–509.

Longenecker HE, Hurlbut WP, Mauro A, et al. (1970). Effects of black widow spider venom on the frog neuromuscular junction. Effects on end-plate potential, miniature end-plate potential and nerve terminal spike. Nature 225: 701–703.

MacLean B, Wilson JAC (1954). See-saw relationship between hyperthyroidism and myasthenia gravis. Lancet i: 950–953.

Maeno T, Enomoto K (1980). Reversal of streptomycin induced blockade of neuromuscular transmission by 4-aminopyridine. Proc Jap Acad 56: 486–491.

Major RH (1965). Classic Descriptions of Disease. 1st ed. Charles C. Thomas, Springfield.

Maretic Z (1978). Epidemiology of envenomation. In: S Bettini (Ed.), Arthropod Venoms. Springer Verlag, Berlin, pp. 185–212.

Martinez-Matos JA, Gascon J, Calopa M, et al. (2003). Myasthenia gravis unmasked by botulinum toxin. Neurologia 18: 234–235.

Mase G, Zorzon M, Biasutti E, et al. (1996). Development of myasthenia gravis during interferon-alpha treatment for anti-HCV positive chronic hepatitis [letter]. J Neurol Neurosurg Psychiatry 60: 348–349.

Masters CL, et al. (1977). Penicillamine-associated myasthenia gravis, antiacetylcholine receptor and antistriational antibodies. Am J Med 63: 689–694.

Matthews EK, Quilliam JP (2000). Effects of central depressant drugs upon acetylcholine release. Br J Pharmacol 22: 415–440.

May EF, Calvert PC (1990). Aggravation of myasthenia gravis by erythromycin. Ann Neurol 28: 577–579.

McCleskey EW, Fox AP, Feldman D, et al. (1987). Calcium channel blockade by a peptide from *Conus*: specificity and mechanism. Proc Natl Acad Sci U S A 84: 4327–4331.

McEachern D, Parnell JL (1948). Relationship of hyperthyroidism to myasthenia gravis. J Clin Endocrinol 8: 842–850.

McIntosh M, Cruz LJ, Hunkapiller MW, et al. (1982). Isolation and structure of a peptide toxin from the marine snail *Conus magnus*. Arch Biochem Biophys 218: 329–334.

McQuillen MP, Engbaek L (1975). Mechanism of colistin-induced neuromuscular depression. Arch Neurol 32: 235.

McQuillen MP, Gross M, Johns RJ (1963). Chlorpromazine-induced weakness in myasthenia gravis. Arch Neurol 8: 402–415.

McQuillen MP, Cantor HE, O'Rourke JR (1968). Myasthenic syndrome associated with antibiotics. Arch Neurol 18: 402–415.

Meinck HM, Ricker K, Hulser PJ, et al. (1995). Stiff man syndrome: neurophysiological findings in eight patients. J Neurol 242: 134–142.

Mellanby J, Green J (1981). How does tetanus toxin act? Neuroscience 6: 281–300.

Menkes CJ, Job-Deslandre C, Bauer-Vinassac D, et al. (1988). Myasthenia caused by tiopronin during treatment of rheumatoid polyarthritis (letter). Presse Med 17: 1156–1157.

Milani M, Ostlie N, Wang W, et al. (2003). T cells and cytokines in the pathogenesis of acquired myasthenia gravis. Ann N Y Acad Sci 998: 284–307.

Millard AH (1954). Local tetanus. Lancet 2: 844–846.

Miller RD (1979). Recent developments with muscle relaxants and their antagonists. Can Anaesth Soc J 26: 83.

Miller RD, Way WL, Katzung BG (1968). The neuromuscular effects of quinidine. Proc Soc Exp Biol Med 129: 215–218.

Miller TA (1992). Bite of the black widow spider. Am Fam Physician 45: 181–187.

Mitrakul C, Dhamkrong-At A, Futrakul P, et al. (1984). Clinical features of neurotoxic snake bite and response to antivenom in 47 children. Am J Trop Med Hygiene 33: 1258–1266.

Moersch FP, Woltman HW (1956). Progressive fluctuating muscular rigidity and spasms ("stiff-man" syndrome): report of a case and some observations in 13 other cases. Mayo Clin Proc 31: 421–427.

Molgo J, del Pozo E, Banos JE, et al. (1991). Changes in quantal transmitter release caused by gadolinium ions at the frog neuromuscular junction. Br J Pharmacol 104: 133–138.

Montecucco C, Schiavo G (1994). Mechanism of action of tetanus and botulinum neurotoxins. Mol Microbiol 13: 1–8.

Moore B, Safani M, Keesey J (1988). Possible exacerbation of myasthenia gravis by ciprofloxacin [letter]. Lancet 1: 882.

Mordes JP, Wacker WEC (1978). Excess magnesium. Pharmacol Rev 29: 273–300.

Moreno Alvarez PJ, Madurga SM (2003). Telithromycin and exacerbation in myasthenia gravis. Farm Hosp 27: 199–200.

Moss J, Kazic T, Henry DP, et al. (1973). Scorpion venom-induced discharge of catecholamines accompanied by hypertension. Brain Res 54: 381–385.

Murdock LL (1971). Catecholamines in arthropods: a review [Review]. Comparative Gen Pharmacol 2: 254–274.

Nakamura K, Koide M, Imanaga T, et al. (1980). Prolonged neuromuscular blockade following trimetaphan infusion. Anaesthesia 35: 1202–1207.

Neil JF, Himmelhoch JM, Licata SM (1976). Emergence of myasthenia gravis during treatment with lithium carbonate. Arch Gen Psychiatry 33: 1090–1092.

Ng KKF (1966). Blockade of adrenergic and cholinergic transmissions by emetine. Br J Pharmacol Chemother 28: 228–237.

Nieman RB, Sharma K, Edelberg H, et al. (2003). Telithromycin and myasthenia gravis. Clin Infect Dis 37: 1579.

Nordenbo AM, Somnier FE (1992). Acute deterioration of myasthenia gravis after intravenous administration of gadolinium-DTPA. Lancet 340: 1168.

Norris F, Colella J, McFarlin D (1964). Effect of diphenylhydantoin on neuromuscular synapse. Neurology (Minneapolis) 14: 869–876.

Oladiran I, Meier DE, Ojelade AA, et al. (2002). Tetanus: continuing problem in the developing world. World J Surg 26: 1282–1285.

Olivera BM, Gray WR, Zeikus R, et al. (1985). Peptide neruotoxins from fish-hunting cone snails. Science 230: 1338–1343.

Olsen KM, Hiller FC (1987). Management of tetanus. Clin Pharm 6: 570–574.

O'Riordan J, Javed M, Doherty C, et al. (1994). Worsening of myasthenia gravis on treatment with imipenem/cilastatin. J Neurol Neurosurg Psychiatry 57: 383.

Osserman KE, Genkins G (1971). Studies in myasthenia gravis: review of a 20-year experience in over 1200 patients. Mt. Sinai J Med 38: 497–537.

Ouyang C, Teng C-M, Huang T-F (1992). Characterization of snake venom components acting on blood coagulation and platelet function. Toxicon 30: 945–966.

Panter KE, Keeler RF (1989). Piperidine alkaloids of poison hemlock (*Conium maculatum*). In: LP Cheeke (Ed.), Alkaloids, Toxicants of Plant Origin, Vol 1. CRC Press, Boca Raton, pp. 109–130.

Paradelis AG, Triantaphyllidis C, Giala MM (1980). Neuromuscular blocking activity of aminoglycoside antibiotics. Methods Find Exp Clin Pharmacol 2: 45–51.

Parisi AF, Kaplan MH (1965). Apnea during treatment with sodium colistimethate. J Am Med Assoc 194: 298–299.

Parmar B, Francis PJ, Ragge NK (2002). Statins, fibrates, and ocular myasthenia. Lancet 360: 717.

Patel VK, Jindal MN, Kelkar VV (1974). In vivo study of mechanism of propranolol-induced blockade of neuromuscular transmission. Indian J Physiol Pharmacol 18: 126–128.

Patocka J, Splino M (2002). Botulinum toxin: from poison to medicinal agent. ASA Newsl 02–1: 14–23.

Patten BM (1978). Myasthenia gravis: review of diagnosis and management. Muscle Nerve 1: 190–205.

Perez A, Perella M, Pastor E, et al. (1995). Myasthenia gravis induced by alpha-interferon therapy. Am J Hematol 49: 365–366.

Pestronk A, Drachman DB (1980). Lithium reduces the number of acetylcholine receptors in skeletal muscle. Science 210: 342–343.

Petersen J, Halberg P, Hojgaard K, et al. (1978). Penicillamine-induced polymyositis-dermatomyositis. Scand J Rheumatol 7: 113–117.

Peterson H (1966). Association of trimethadione therapy and myasthenia gravis. N Engl J Med 274: 506–507.

Pettigrew LC, Glass JP (1985). Neurologic complications of coral snake bite. Neurology 35: 589–592.

Piccolo G, Franciotta D, Versino M, et al. (1996). Myasthenia gravis in a patient with chronic active hepatitis C during interferon-alpha treatment [letter]. J Neurol Neurosurg Psychiatry 60: 348.

Pina Latorre MA, Cobeta JC, Rodilla F, et al. (1998). Influence of calcium antagonist drugs in myasthenia gravis in the elderly. J Clin Pharm Ther 23: 399–401.

Pittinger C, Adamson R (1972). Antibiotic blockade of neuromuscular function. Annu Rev Pharmacol 12: 109–184.

Pittinger CB, Eryasa Y, Adamson R (1970). Antibiotic-induced paralysis. Anesth Analg 49: 487.

Pohlmann G (1966). Respiratory arrest associated with intravenous administration of polymyxin B sulfate. J Am Med Assoc 196: 181–183.

Poncelet AN (2000). Blink reflexes and the silent period in tetanus. Muscle Nerve 23: 1435–1438.

Poulton TJ, James FM, Lockridge O (1979). Prolonged apnea following trimethaphan and succinylcholine. Anesthesiology 50: 54–56.

Pridgen JE (1956). Respiratory arrest thought due to intraperitoneal neomycin. Surgery 40: 571–574.

Pritchard JA (1979). The use of magnesium sulfate in preeclampsia/eclampsia. J Reprod Med The 23: 107–114.

Pumplin DW, Reese TS (1977). Action of brown widow spider venom and botulinum toxin on the frog neuromuscular junction examined with the freeze-fracture technique. J Physiol 273: 443–457.

Purvin V, Kawasaki A, Smith KH, et al. (2006). Statin-associated myasthenia gravis: report of 4 cases and review of the literature. Medicine (Baltimore) 85: 82–85.

Quilichini R, Mazzerbo F, Baume D, et al. (1995). Myasthenia during interferon alpha therapy. Presse Med 24: 1178.

Rallison ML, Carlisle JW, Less RE, et al. (1961). Lupus erythematosus and Stevens-Johnson syndrome: occurrence as reactions to anticonvulsant medications. Am J Dis Child 101: 725–738.

Randall RE, Cohen MD, Spray CC, et al. (1964). Hypermagnesemia in renal failure. Ann Intern Med 61: 73–88.

Rauser EH, Ariano RE, Anderson BA (1990). Exacerbation of myasthenia gravis by norfloxacin [letter]. DICP 24: 207–208.

Reddy VG (2002). Pharmacotherapy of tetanus—a review. Middle East J Anesthesiol 16: 419–442.

Regan AG, Aldrete JA (1967). Prolonged apnea after administration of promazine hydrochloride following succinylcholine infusion. Anesth Analg 46: 315–318.

Regli F, Guggenheim P (1965). Myasthenisches syndrom als seltene komplikation unter hydantoin. Nervenarzt 36: 315–318.

Reid HA (1964). Cobra-bites. BMJ 2: 540–545.

Reid HA (1975). Antivenom in sea-snake bite poisoning. Lancet i: 622–623.

Ribera AB, Nastuk WL (1989). The actions of verapamil at the neuromuscular junction. Comp Biochem Physiol C: Comp Pharmacol Toxicol 93C: 137–141.

Robberecht W, Bednarik J, Bourgeois P, et al. (1989). Myasthenic syndrome caused by direct effect of chloroquine on neuromuscular junction. Arch Neurol 46: 464–468.

Rohde D, Sliwka U, Schweizer K, et al. (1996). Oculo-bulbar myasthenia gravis induced by cytokine treatment of a patient with metastasized renal cell carcinoma. Eur J Clin Pharmacol 50: 471–473.

Rose I (1954). A review of tick paralysis. Can Med Assoc J 70: 175–176.

Rose I, Gregson JD (1959). Evidence of neuromuscular block in tick paralysis. Nature 178: 95–96.

Rosenthal L (1989). Alpah-lathrotoxin and related toxins. Pharmacol Ther 42: 115–134.

Ross RM, Baker T (1996). An effect of magnesium on neuromuscular function in parturients. J Clin Anesth 8: 202–204.

Rossetto O, Deloye F, Poulain B, et al. (1995). The metalloproteinase activity of tetanus and botulism neurotoxins. J Physiol Paris 89: 43–50.

Rowlands JB, Mastaglia FL, Kakulas BA, et al. (1969). Clinical and pathological aspects of a fatal case of mulga (Pseudechis australis) snakebite. Med J Aust 1: 226–230.

Rubbo JT, Gergis SD, Sokoll MD (1977). Comparative neuromuscular effects of lincomycin and clindamycin. Anesth Analg 56: 329–332.

Russell AS, Lindstrom JM (1978). Penicillamine-induced myasthenia gravis associated with antibodies to acetylcholine receptor. Neurology 28: 847–849.

Russell JGB (1984). Enemas and myasthenia gravis. Br J Radiol 57: 655.

Rustam H, Hamdi T (1974). Methylmercury poisoning in Iraq: a neurological study. Brain 97: 499–510.

Rustam H, von Burg R, Amin-Saki L, et al. (1975). Evidence of a neuromuscular disorder in methylmercury poisoning. Arch Environ Health 30: 190–195.

Saady A, Torda TA (1973). Tetanus: principles of management and review of 37 cases. Anaesth Intensive Care 1: 226–231.

Samuelson RJ, Giesecke AH, Jr., Kallus FT, et al. (1975). Lincomycin-curare interaction. Anesth Analg 54: 103–105.

Sanders DB, Howard JF (1986). AAEE minimonograph #25: single-fiber electromyography in myasthenia gravis. Muscle Nerve 9: 809–819.

Sanders DB, Howard JF (1991). Disorders of neuromuscular transmission. In: WG Bradley, et al. (Eds.), Neurology in Clinical Practice. 1st ed. Butterworth, Boston, pp. 1819–1842.

Sanders DB, Kim YI, Howard JF, et al. (1981). Intercostal muscle biopsy studies in myasthenia gravis: clinical correlations and the direct effects of drugs and myasthenic serum. Ann N Y Acad Sci 377: 544–566.

Sandyk R, Brennan MJ (1982). Tuberculous meningitis presenting with trismus. J Neurol Neurosurg Psychiatry 45: 1070.

Schiavo G, Matteoli M, Montecucco C (2000). Neurotoxins affecting neuroexocytosis. Physiol Rev 80: 717–766.

Schlesinger F, Krampfl K, Haeseler G, et al. (2004). Competitive and open channel block of recombinant nachr channels by different antibiotics. Neuromuscul Disord 14: 307–312.

Schraeder PL (1972). Polymyositis and penicillamine. Arch Neurol 27: 456–457.

Schumm F, Wietholter H, Fateh-Moghadam A (1981). Myasthenie-syndrom unter chloroquin-therapie. Deutscha Medizinische Wochenschrit 25: 1745–1747.

Sghirlanzoni A, Mantegazza R, Mora M, et al. (1988). Chloroquine myopathy and myasthenia-like syndrome. Muscle Nerve 11: 114–119.

Shaivitz SA (1979). Timolol and myasthenia gravis. JAMA 242: 1611–1612.

Shimoni Z, Dobrousin A, Cohen J, et al. (1999). Tetanus in an immunised patient. BMJ 319: 1049.

Shy ME, Lange DJ, Howard JF, et al. (1985). Quinidine exacerbating myasthenia gravis: a case report and intracellular recordings. Ann Neurol 18: 120.

Sieb JP, Milone M, Engel AG (1996). Effects of the quinoline derivative quinine, quinidine and chloroquine in neuromuscular transmission. Brain Res 712: 179–189.

Silinsky EM (1977). Can barium support the release of acetylcholine by nerve impulses? Br J Pharmacol 59: 215–217.

Silinsky EM (1978). On the role of barium in supporting the asynchronous release of acetylcholine quanta by motor nerve impulses. J Physiol (Lon) 274: 157–171.

Singh YN, Harvey AL, Marshall IG (1978a). Antibiotic-induced paralysis of the mouse phrenic nerve-hemidiaphragm preparation, and reversibility by calcium and by neostigmine. Anesthesiology 48: 418–424.

Singh YN, Marshall IG, Harvey AL (1978b). Reversal of antibiotic-induced muscle paralysis by 3,4-diaminopyridine. J Pharm Pharmacol 30: 249.

Singh YN, Marshall IG, Harvey AL (1978c). Some effects of the aminoglycoside antibiotic amikacin on neuromuscular and autonomic transmission. Br J Anaesth 50: 109.

Slaughter D (1950). Neostigmine and opiate analgesia. Arch Int Pharmacodyn 83: 143–148.

Smart JK (1997). History of chemical and biological warfare: an American perspective. In: FR Sidell, ET Takafuji, DR Franz (Eds.), Textbook of Military Medicine. Medical Aspects of Chemical and Biological Warfare, 3. Office of the Surgeon General, Washington, DC, pp. 9–86.

Smithson AE (1999). Toxic Archipelago: Preventing Proliferation from the Former Soviet Chemical and Biological Weapons Complexes. Henry L. Stimson Center, Washington, DC, p. 32.

Sobel J, Painter J (2005). Illnesses caused by marine toxins. Clin Infect Dis 41: 1290–1296.

Sofer S, Shahak E, Gueron M (1994). Scorpion envenomation and antivenom therapy. Pediatrics 124: 973–978.

Somjen G, Hilmy M, Stephen CR (1966). Failure to anesthetize human subjects by intravenous administration of magnesium sulfate. J Pharmacol Exp Ther 154: 652–659.

Southcott RV (1975). The neurologic effects of noxious marine creatures. In: RW Hornabrook (Ed.), Topics on Tropical Neurology. F.A. Davis Company, Philadelphia, pp. 165–258.

Stanbury JB, Huyck JH (1945). Tick paralysis: critical review. Medicine 24: 219–242.

Stanfield JP, Galazka A (1984). Neonatal tetanus in the world today. Bull World Health Organ 62: 647–669.

Stanfield JP, Galazka A (1987). Neonatal tetanus: an under-reported scourge. Nurs RSA 2: 3747.

Steidinger KA, Steinfield HJ (1984). Toxic marine dinoflagellates. In: DL Spector (Ed.), Dinoflagellates. Academic Press, New York, pp. 201–206.

Steinegger T, Wiederkehr M, Ludin HP, et al. (1996). Electromyography as a diagnostic aid in tetanus. Schweiz Med Wochenschr 126: 379–385.

Stoffer SS, Chandler JH (1980). Quinidine-induced exacerbation of myasthenia gravis in patient with myasthenia gravis. Arch Intern Med 140: 283–284.

Stone BF (1988). Tick paralysis, particularly involving Ixodes holocyclus and other *Ixodes* species. In: KF Harris (Ed.), Advances in Disease Vector Research 5. Springer-Verlag, New York, pp. 61–85.

Stone BF, Aylward JH (1992). Holocyclotoxin—the paralysing toxin of the Australian paralysis tick Ixodus holocyclus: chemical and immunological characterization. Toxicon 30: 552–553.

Strieb EW (1973). Adverse effects of magnesium salt cathartics in a patient with the myasthenic syndrome. Ann Neurol 2: 175–176.

Swift TR (1979). Weakness from magnesium containing cathartics. Muscle Nerve 2: 295–298.

Swift TR (1981). Disorders of neuromuscular transmission other than myasthenia gravis. Muscle Nerve 4: 334–353.

Swift TR, Ignacio OJ (1975). Tick paralysis: electrophysiologic studies. Neurology 25: 1130–1133.

Szuhay G, Tewfik TL (1998). Peritonsillar abscess or cellulitis? A clinical comparative paediatric study. J Otolaryngol 27: 206–212.

Talamo RC, Crawford JD (1963). Trimethadione nephrosis treated with cortisone and nitrogen mustard. N Engl J Med 269: 15–18.

Tarsy D, Bhattacharyya N, Borodic G (2000). Myasthenia gravis after botulinum toxin A for Meige syndrome. Mov Disord 15: 736–738.

Temple IU (1912). Acute ascending paralysis, or tick paralysis. Med Sentinel 20: 507–514.

Theakston RDG, Phillips RE, Warrell DA, et al. (1990). Envenoming by the common krait (*Bungarus caeruleus*) and Sri Lankan cobra (*Naja naja naja*): efficacy and complications with Haffkine antivenom. Trans R Soc Trop Med Hygiene 84: 301–308.

Thesleff S (1956). The effect of anesthetic agents on skeletal muscle membrane. Acta Physiol Scand 37: 335–349.

The Holy Bible, Exodus 7: 20–21, (1989). Thomas Nelson Publishers, Nashville, p 54.

Thompson PD (1993). Stiff muscles. J Neurol Neurosurg Psychiatry 56: 121–124.

Thorner MW (1939). Relation of myasthenia gravis to hyperthyroidism. Arch Intern Med 64: 330–335.

Todd JL (1912). Tick bite in British Columbia. Can Med Assoc J 2: 1118–1119.

Tokuoka K, Hamano H, Ohta T, et al. (1997). An adult case of purulent meningitis secondary to retropharyngeal and deep neck abscess after treatment of odontogenic infection. Rinsho Shinkeigaku 37: 417–419.

Torda T (1980). The nature of gentamicin-induced neuromuscular block. Br J Anaesth 52: 325.

Trujillo MJ, Castillo A, Espana JV, et al. (1980). Tetanus in the adult: intensive care and management experience with 233 cases. Crit Care Med 8: 419–423.

Tsai MC, Mansour NA, Eldefrawi AT, et al. (1978). Mechanism of action of amantadine on neuromuscular transmission. Mol Pharmacol 14: 787–803.

Tsueda K, Jean-Francois J, Richter RW (1973). Cardiac standstill in tetanus: review of seven consecutive cases. Int Surg 58: 599–603.

Tu AT, Tu T (1970). Sea snakes from southeast Asia and Far East and their venoms. In: BW Halstead (Ed.), Poisonous and Venomous Marine Animals of the World. US Government Printing Office, Washington, DC, pp. 885–903.

Turker K, Kiran B (1965). Action of pronethalol on neuromuscular activity. Arch Int Pharmacodyn 155: 356–364.

Udwadia FE, Lall A, Udwadia ZF, et al. (1987). Tetanus and its complications: intensive care and management experience in 150 Indian patients. Epidemiol Infect 99: 675–684.

Ueno S, Takahashi M, Kajiyama K, et al. (1987). Parkinson's disease and myasthenia gravis: adverse effect of trihexyphenidyl on neuromuscular transmission. Neurology 37: 832–833.

Ushkaryov YA, Petrenko AG, Geppert M, et al. (1992). Neurexins: synaptic cell surface proteins related to the α-lathrotoxin receptor and laminin. Science 257: 50–56.

Usubiaga J (1968). Neuromuscular effects of beta-adrenergic blockers and their interaction with skeletal muscle relaxants. Anesthesiology 29: 484–492.

Uyama E, Fujiki N, Uchino M (1996). Exacerbation of myasthenia gravis during interferon-alpha treatment [letter]. J Neurol Sci 144: 221–222.

Vacca JB, Knight WA (1957). Estrogen therapy in myasthenia gravis: report of two cases. Mo Med 54: 337–340.

Van den Bergh P, Kelly JJ, Carter B, et al. (1986). Intravascular contrast media and neuromuscular junction disorders. Ann Neurol 19: 206–207.

Van der Kloot W, Kita H (1975). The effects of verapamil on muscle action potentials in the frog and crayfish and on neuromuscular transmission in the crayfish. Comp Biochem Physiol 50C: 121–125.

Van Ermengen E (1897). Ueber einen neuen anaeroben Bacillus und seine Beziehungen zum Botulismus. Zeitschrift fur Hygeine und Infektionskrankheiten 26: 1–56.

van Loosen J, van der DF (1987). Trismus as a symptom. Ned Tijdschr Geneeskd 131: 683.

Vartanian GA, Chinyanga HM (1972). The mechanism of acute neuromuscular weakness induced by chloroquine. Can J Physiol Pharmacol 50: 1099–1103.

Venkatesh S, Rao A, Gupta R (1996). Exacerbation of myasthenia gravis with cocaine use [letter]. Muscle Nerve 19: 1364.

Verkijk A (1985). Worsening of myasthenia gravis with timolol maleate eyedrops. Ann Neurol 17: 211–212.

Vial T, Chauplannaz G, Brunel P, et al. (1995). Exacerbation of myasthenia gravis by pefloxacin. [French]. Rev Neurol (Paris) 151: 286–287.

Viby-Mogensen J (1981). Succinylcholine neuromuscular blockade in subjects homozygous for atypical plasma cholinesterase. Anesthesiology 55: 429–434.

Vic-Dupont V, Emile J, Bazin C, et al. (1969). Neuro-meningeal listeriosis in adults. Apropos of 15 cases. Presse Med 77: 155–158.

Vincent A, Newsom-Davis J, Martin V (1978). Antiacetylcholine receptor antibodies in D-penicillamine-associated myasthenia gravis. Lancet 1: 1254.

Viswanath DV, Jenkins HJ (1978). Neuromuscular block of the polymyxin group of antibiotics. J Pharm Sci 67: 1275.

Vital-Brazil O (1972). Venoms: their inhibitory action on neuromuscular transmission. In: J Cheymol (Ed.), Neuromuscular Blocking and Stimulating Agents. Permagon Press, New York, pp. 145–167.

Warnick JE, Albuquerque EX, Diniz CR (1976). Electrophysiological observations on the action of the purified scorpion venom, Tityus-toxin, on nerve and skeletal muscle of the rat. J Pharmacol Exp Ther 198: 155–167.

Warrell DA, Barnes HJ, Piburn MF (1976). Neurotoxic effects of bites by the Egyptian cobra (Naja haje) in Nigeria. Trans R Soc Trop Med Hygiene 70: 78–79.

Warren JD, Kimber TE, Thompson PD (1999). The silent period after magnetic brain stimulation in generalized tetanus. Muscle Nerve 22: 1590–1592.

Wassilak SGF, Orenstein WA, Sutter RW (1999). Tetanus toxoid. In: S Plotkin, W Orenstein (Eds.), Vaccines. 3rd ed. WB Saunders Company, Philadelphia, pp. 441–474.

Waterman PM, Smith RB (1977). Tobramycin-curare interaction. Anesth Analg 56: 587–588.

Way WL, Katzung BG, Larson CP (1967). Recurarization with quinidine. JAMA 200: 153–154.

Weakly JN (1973). The action of cobalt ions on neuromuscular transmission in the frog. J Physiol (Lon) 234: 597–612.

Weber JCP (1982). Beta-adrenoreceptor antagonists and diplopia. Lancet ii: 826–827.

Weingart JL (1967). Tick paralysis. Minn Med 50: 383–386.

Weisman SJ (1949). Masked myasthenia gravis. J Am Med Assoc 141: 917–918.

Wesley AG, Hariparsad D, Pather M, et al. (1983). Labetalol in tetanus. The treatment of sympathetic nervous system overactivity. Anaesthesia 38: 243–249.

Wessler I, Anschutz S (1988). β-adrenergic stimulation enhances transmitter output from rat phrenic nerve. Br J Pharmacol 94: 669–674.

Wierzbicki AS, Poston R, Ferro A (2003). The lipid and non-lipid effects of statins. Pharmacol Ther 99: 95–112.

Wilson SL, Miller RN, Wright C, et al. (1976). Prolonged neuromuscular blockade associated with trimethaphan: a case report. Anesth Analg Curr Res 35: 1202–1207.

Wislicki L, Rosenblum I (1967). Effects of propranolol on the action of neuromuscular blocking drugs. Br J Anaethesia 39: 939–942.

Wright JM, Collier B (1976a). Characterization of the neuromuscular block produced by clindamycin and lincomycin. Can J Physiol Pharmacol 54: 937–944.

Wright JM, Collier B (1976b). The site of the neuromuscular block produced by polymyxin B and rolitetracycline. Can J Physiol Pharmacol 54: 926–936.

Wullen F, Kast G, Bruck A (1967). Uber Nebenwirkungen bei Tetracyclin-Verabreichung an Myastheniker. Deutsche Medizinische Wochenschrift 92: 667–669.

Yaari Y, Pincus JH, Argov Z (1977). Depression of synaptic transmission by diphenylhydantoin. Ann Neurol 1: 334–338.

Yaari Y, Pincus JH, Argov Z (1979). Phenytoin and transmitter release at the neuromuscular junction of the frog. Brain Res 160: 479–487.

Yoshiba S (1984). An estimation of the most dangerous species of cone shell, Conus (Gastridium) geographus Linne, 1758, venom's lethal dose in humans. Jap J Hygiene 39: 565–572.

Youssef S, Stuve O, Patarroyo JC, et al. (2002). The HMG-coa reductase inhibitor, atorvastatin, promotes a Th2 bias and reverses paralysis in central nervous system autoimmune disease. Nature 420: 78–84.

Zaidat OO, Kaminski HJ, Berenson F, et al. (1999). Neuromuscular transmission defect caused by carbamazepine. Muscle Nerve 22: 1293–1296.

Zalman F, Perloff JK, Durant NN, et al. (1983). Acute respiratory failure following intravenous verapamil in Duchennes's muscular dystrophy. Am Heart J 105: 510–511.

Zilinskas RA (1997). Iraq's biological weapons. The past as future? JAMA 278: 418–424.

Handbook of Clinical Neurology, Vol. 91 (3rd series)
Neuromuscular junction disorders
A.G. Engel, Editor

Chapter 13

Organophosphate and carbamate poisoning

JAN L. DE BLEECKER *

Neurology Department, University Hospital, Ghent, Belgium

Highly toxic acetylcholinesterase (AChE)-inhibiting organophosphates (OPs) and carbamates (CMs) are intensively used as pesticides throughout the world. In industrialized countries, their use is highly regulated and epidemic occupational poisoning is rare. In developing countries, the situation is often worse. A combination of high need of insecticides in tropical climates, poor knowledge of pesticide toxicity among farm workers, inadequate central regulations and legislation, and lack of adequate spraying infrastructure all lead to large numbers of accidental poisoning casualties annually (Rantanen et al., 2004). Due to poor medical and research infrastructure, this vast number of OP poisoned victims in developing countries has added little to the global understanding of human OP toxicology or the development of optimal treatment protocols. Indeed, most of these data still stem from small case series studied in highly equipped tertiary medical centers in the US and Europe (Buckley et al., 2004).

13.1. Classification and uses of OPs and CMs

13.1.1. Historical notes on OP development

The synthesis of an OP anticholinesterase agent was first reported in 1854 by Philippe de Clermont in his account given before the French Academy of Sciences (de Clermont, 1854, 1855). In the 1930s, Otto Bayer, the scientific leader of the German Company I.G. Farbenindustrie, appointed Gerhard Schrader to develop the field of OP insecticide production. The first commercial insecticide, i.e., Bladan, was available in 1940, and at the end of World War II, nearly 2000 OPs had been synthesized, among these the still popular pesticides paraoxon (E.600) and parathion (E.605). In these same years, the German Ministry of Defence supported investigations of highly toxic OP

agents for warfare. The first amounts of the nerve agents tabun and sarin were handed to the Ministry of Defence in 1937. The construction of a large factory for industrial production started in 1940 and the first industrial lot of tabun was manufactured as late as May 1943. During World War II, similar studies on warfare nerve gases were conducted in England (Kilby and Kilby, 1947).

13.1.2. Current classification and use of OPs

Since World War II, several thousand OPs have been synthesized for various purposes. Most OPs are currently used as pesticides, whereas others are used as paraciticides in veterinary medicine, warfare agents, or flame retardants. Different classes and types of OP exist, but they all share a phosphorus atom and a characteristic phosphoryl ($P = O$) or thiophosphoryl ($P = S$) bond (Table 13.1). Some classifications comprise 13 types of OPs (Table 13.1, adapted from Marrs, 1993). The complex classification of OPs is due to different side chains attached to the phosphorus atom and the position at which these side chains are attached. Some OPs possess anticholinesterase activity, whereas others possess little or no anticholinesterase activity or need desulfuration to the analogous oxon before acquiring anticholinesterase activity.

OP nerve agents include tabun (GA), sarin (GB), soman (GD), cyclosarin (GF), and VX. VX is the most toxic nerve agent. They all irreversibly inhibit AChE at its active site. Soldiers and military personnel can be exposed during war or accidentally, and the general population can be exposed by accidental leakage from military storage facilities or during terrorist attacks, such as the sarin poisoning in the Tokyo subway in 1995 (Suzuki et al., 1995).

---

*Correspondence to: Professor Jan L. De Bleecker, MD, PhD, Neurology Department, University Hospital, De Pintelaan 185, B-9000 Ghent, Belgium. E-mail: jan.debleecker@Ugent.be, Tel: 32-9-332-4539, Fax: 32-9-332-4971.

Table 13.1

General structure and various types of OPs

Type	Chemical structure	Examples
General structure of organophosphates	(O or S); $R_1-P(=)-R_2$ with OR below	
Phosphates	$RO-P(=O)-OR$ with OR below	Chlorfenvinphos, Dichlorvos, Monocrotophos, Tri-*o*-cresyl phosphate, Trichlorfon
Phosphonates	$RO-P(=O)-R$ with OR below	
Phosphinates	$R-P(=O)-R$ with OR below	Glufosinate
Phosphorothioates (S=)	$RO-P(=S)-OR$ with OR below	Bromophos, Diazinon, Fenthion, Parathion, Pirimiphos-methyl
Phosphonothioates (S=)	$RO-P(=S)-R$ with OR below	EPN, Leptophos
Phosphorothioates (S-substituted)	$RS-P(=O)-OR$ with OR below	Demeton-S-methyl, Ecothiopate
Phosphonothioates (S-substituted)	$RS-P(=O)-R$ with OR below	VX
Phosphorodithioates	$RS-P(=O)-SR$ with OR below or $RS-P(=S)-OR$ with OR below	Azinphos-ethyl, Azinphos-methyl, Dimethoate, Disulfoton, Malathion, Methidathion
Phosphorotrithioates	$RS-P(=O)-SR$ with SR below	DEF (tribufos)
Phosphoramidates	$RO-P(=O)-N(R)(R)$ with OR below	Fenamiphos

(Continued)

Table 13.1

(Continued)

Phosphoramidothioates	$\underset{\overset{\displaystyle \|}{OR}}{RO-\overset{\displaystyle S}{\overset{\|}{P}}-N{\overset{\displaystyle R}{\underset{\displaystyle R}{}}}}$ or $\underset{\overset{\displaystyle \|}{OR}}{RS-\overset{\displaystyle O}{\overset{\|}{P}}-N{\overset{\displaystyle R}{\underset{\displaystyle R}{}}}}$	Methamidophos Isofenphos
Phosphorofluoridates	$\underset{\overset{\displaystyle \|}{OR}}{RO-\overset{\displaystyle O}{\overset{\|}{P}}-F}$	Diisopropyl Phosphorofluoridate (DFP)
Phosphonofluoridates	$\underset{\overset{\displaystyle \|}{R}}{RO-\overset{\displaystyle O}{\overset{\|}{P}}-F}$	Cyclosarin Sarin Soman

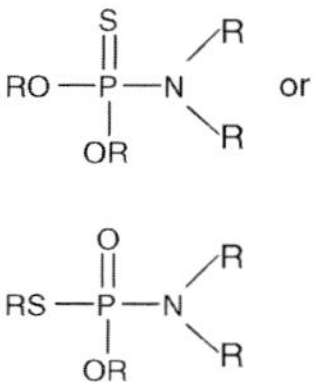

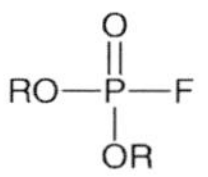

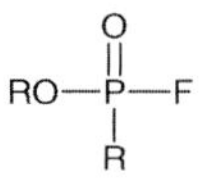

After Marrs, 1993.

Some OPs act as flame retardants when added to polymers, and are extensively used in textiles, packaging materials, polyurethane foam etc. These compounds do not pose a direct risk to humans because they do not possess anticholinesterase activity.

13.1.3. Carbamates

CMs are more recent compounds and structurally less complex than esters of carbamic acid (NH_3CO_2) (Fig. 13.1). They are mainly used as pesticides, with volumes larger than OP pesticides, but also in human and veterinary medicine and in prophylaxis of OP nerve agent poisoning. Thiocarbamates are used as fungicides or herbicides and have very low human toxicity.

13.1.4. Use of AChE inhibitors in human medicine

The most common use of AChE inhibitors is currently in Alzheimer's disease, aiming at preventing the

breakdown of acetylcholine (ACh) in brain regions critical for cognitive functions. Several molecules have been studied for this purpose: tacrine (an aminoacridine), donepezil (a benzylpiperidine), rivastigmine (a CM) and galantamine (a tertiary alkaloid). The action of the CM physostigmine was too short, and tacrine was withdrawn because of hepatotoxicity. For several years, the OP compound metrifonate was also studied, but was withdrawn because of respiratory side effects, and it is currently labeled as a mutagen and carcinogen. In clinical practice, second generation selective AChE inhibitors currently used in Alzheimer's disease include rivastigmine, a pseudo-irreversible inhibitor and a derivative of physostigmine, donepezil and galantamine. A number of other compounds with more brain-selective or more selective AChE than BuChE inhibitory activity (e.g., phenserine, ganstigmine) are under study. A first case of accidental rivastigmine poisoning in an 11-month-old child who chewed up her grandmother's prescription drug has been reported (Lai and Moen, 2005).

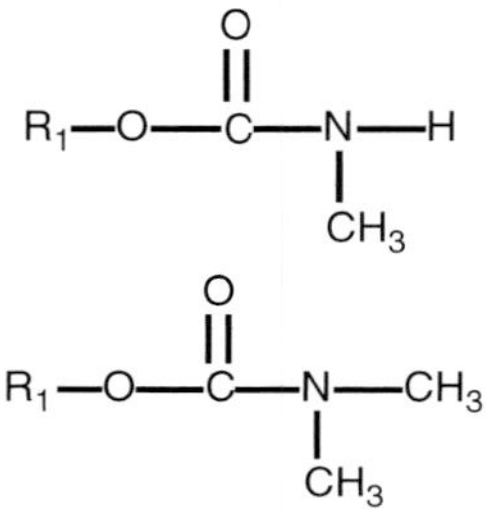

Postsynaptic disorders of neuromuscular transmission, most commonly autoimmune myasthenia gravis, are symptomatically treated with CM AChE inhibitors such as neostigmine, pyridostigmine and ambenonium. Edrophonium is sometimes used in the diagnostic work-up of suspected myasthenia. Physostigmine (eserine; CM) and ecothiopate (phospholine; OP) are used in glaucoma treatment. CMs such as neostigmine are used in urine bladder detrusor muscle weakness with voiding problems.

$$R_1-O-\overset{\overset{\displaystyle O}{\|}}{C}-\overset{\underset{\displaystyle CH_3}{|}}{N}-H$$

$$R_1-O-\overset{\overset{\displaystyle O}{\|}}{C}-\overset{\underset{\displaystyle CH_3}{|}}{N}-CH_3$$

Fig. 13.1. General structure of carbamate insecticides.

13.2. Epidemiology

More than 1.5 million tons of pesticides are manufactured each year. Most pesticides are hazardous. Pesticide poisoning results from occupational, accidental, and intentional exposure. Adults are principally affected, but children may be victims of accidental poisoning (Zwiener and Ginsburg, 1988). Comprehensive epidemiological studies on the global incidence of pesticide poisoning in general and OP and CM poisoning in particular are not available and therefore all estimates are somewhat contentious. Problems with recording and reporting of poisonings and health seeking behavior are only some of the factors. The World Health Organization (WHO) estimated the global annual incidence of unintentional pesticide poisonings in the range of 2.9 million acute poisonings and 220000 associated deaths (World Health Organization, 1990).

The epidemiological pattern of OP and CM poisoning shows considerable variation between developing and industrialized countries. Even between developing countries, major differences exist in the frequency and type of poisoning. Deliberate self-poisoning by pesticide ingestion is commonest in South East Asia and the Indian subcontinent (Eddleston et al., 2002a; Buckley et al., 2004). In 1998, these poisonings were amongst the three leading causes of hospital deaths in Sri Lanka (Senanayake, 1998), putting enormous pressure on the limited health resources in this country (Jeyaratnam et al., 1982). In contrast, the commonest cause of pesticide poisonings in Latin America is occupational exposure (Hena and Finkelman, 1993). In Western countries, severe OP and CM poisonings are mainly suicidal, but accidental or occupational exposures also occur. An estimated 3000 to 5000 cases of accidental poisonings occur annually in the US according to Environmental Protection Agency data (1995). The health impact of low-level occupational exposure, such as the exposure of sheep dippers in the UK, is still under debate (Forbat and Skehan, 1992; Stephens et al., 1995).

13.3. Cholinesterase inhibitors as warfare agents

An in-depth account of OP nerve agents is beyond the scope of this chapter. However, the 1995 Tokyo subway terrorist incident and the common occurrence of diffuse complaints in military personnel who have possibly been exposed to OP nerve agents or their prophylactic treatment have confronted non-military physicians with this subject (Newmark, 2004). The nerve agents are commonly divided into two groups,

the G agents (tabun, sarin, soman, cyclosarin) and the V agents (most common agent: VX). The G and V agents differ in physical properties such as volatility. Therefore the G agents are percutaneous and respiratory hazards, whereas the V agents, unless aerosolized, are contact poisons. The toxicity of nerve agents is essentially the same as for OP insecticides, but nerve agents inhibit AChE at much lower concentrations and are several orders of magnitude more acutely toxic (Weinbroum, 2005). Moreover, with soman, aging occurs so fast after inhibition that spontaneous reactivation does not occur and oximes are unable to reactivate AChE (see Sections 13.4.2 and 13.4.3).

The failure of reactivating post-exposure therapy has led to the development and testing of prophylactic or pre-treatment strategies. Pre-treatment was tried with oximes (Brimblecombe et al., 1970), and then, based on a number of animal experiments (Gordon et al., 1978; Anderson et al., 1991), with carbamates. Pre-treatment with carbamates acts by carbamylating the active site of AChE, largely the same way as OPs phosphorylate the active site. The carbamylated enzyme reactivates much more quickly than does the phosphorylated enzyme. Moreover, the carbamylated enzyme is temporarily unavailable for phosphorylation by the nerve agent. The proportion of carbamylated AChE should be sufficiently stable to be protective and not to inhibit military performance. Although the action of pyridostigmine, unlike that of physostigmine, is mostly peripheral, pyridostigmine has mainly been used in soldiers because it has a larger half-life than physostigmine (Inns and Marrs, 1992). The first large scale use of pyridostigmine bromide tablets has been in the Gulf War. Later, the use of this carbamate was suggested as a possible cause of the so-called Gulf War Syndrome (Haley et al., 1997a, b) (see Section 13.12).

13.4. Interaction of OPs and CMs with cholinesterases

13.4.1. Inhibition of cholinesterases by OPs and CMs

Cholinesterases are enzymes that preferentially hydrolyse choline esters. In vertebrates, two main cholinesterases are involved, i.e., acetylcholinesterase (AChE; EC 3.1.1.7) and butyrylcholinesterase (BuChE; EC 3.1.1.8). The difference between both is their relative substrate selectivity. AChE hydrolyses ACh faster than BuChE, and BuChE hydrolyses BuCh and propionylcholine faster than AChE. This difference is probably due to differences in the active acyl pocket structure (Harel et al., 1992; Cygler et al., 1993; Kovarik et al., 2003). AChE terminates the action of ACh at neuromuscular junctions and other cholinergic synapses, but the roles of BuChE are less well defined.

Most OPs and CMs exert their acute toxicity through inhibition of AChE with accumulation of excess ACh at nicotinic and muscarinic synapses. BuChE inhibition has not been shown to result in specific symptoms. BuChE is often considered an important means of detoxifying cholinesterase (ChE) inhibitors and is often used as a surrogate measure for AChE in other body compartments.

The ChEs are serine hydrolases that catalyze the breakdown of ACh through an acyl-transfer, where water is the acceptor molecule to which the substrate acyl moiety is transferred (Walsh, 1979). A serine oxygen of the active site gorge in ChEs carries out a nucleophilic attack on the electrophilic carbon of the carbonyl group of ACh, resulting in an acetylated enzyme intermediate and the release of choline (Fig. 13.2) (Froede

and Wilson, 1984; Quinn, 1987). De-acylation occurs when an hydroxyl ion from an attacking water molecule acts as a more effective nucleophilic agent, thereby releasing acetate (Walsh, 1979). The inhibition of AChE and BuChE by OPs and CMs can be viewed as a reaction very similar to that of the hydrolysis of ACh (Fig. 13.2).

The molecular interaction between OPs and AChE has been studied by a number of techniques and much is known of how OPs bind to and phosphorylate AChE (Ordentlich et al., 1996). The acyl pocket of the active gorge in AChE participates in the positioning of an OP molecule for the attack by the catalytic serine. Ordentlich (1996) interpreted this as the formation of some sort of Michaelis complex and found that this complex was very important in determining the reactivity of an OP towards AChE. Further work with the warfare agent VX has shown that the peripheral anionic site as well as other sites of the active gorge play important

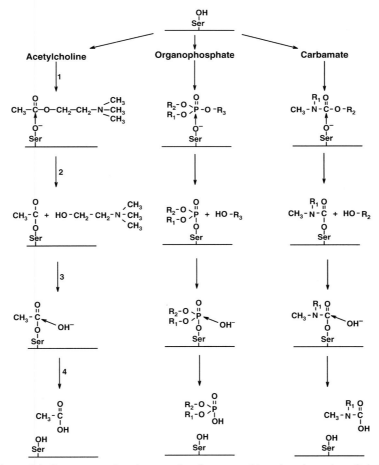

Fig. 13.2. Interaction of acetylcholine, organophosphates and carbamates with active site serine of cholinesterase. Step 1 represents the formation of a stable Michaelis complex and the initiation of the nucleophilic attack on the active site serine of AChE. Step 2 is the acetylation of this serine and the release of the leaving group. Step 3 represents the nucleophilic attack of a hydroxyl ion. Step 4 represents the subsequent regeneration of the active enzyme.

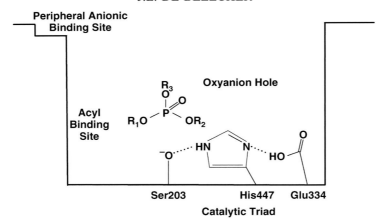

Fig. 13.3. Schematic representation of the active site gorge of AChE with entry of an OP compound. R_1 and R_2 are alkyl chains and R_3 represents the leaving group. The catalytic triad is formed by Ser203, His447, and Glu334. The acyl binding site (left) is probably important in positioning the OP molecule for the nucleophilic attack from the Ser203. (After Ordentlich et al., 1996 and Ordentlich et al., 2004.)

roles in the stereoselectivity towards enantiomers of VX (Ordentlich et al., 2004) (Fig. 13.3). The same authors (Ordentlich et al., 1998) suggested that the oxyanion hole subsite may polarize the $P = O$ bond (or $C = O$ bond in the case of CMs) during the formation of the Michaelis complex and therefore activate the phosphorus, thus promoting a nucleophilic attack by the active serine oxygen (Fig. 13.3). The serine is phosphorylated and the remaining half of the molecule, the so-called leaving group, dissociates from the enzyme (Soreq and Seidman, 2001). The phosphorylated enzyme intermediate is very stable and is only slowly destroyed by a water molecule attack. The presence of the phosphyl moiety covalently bound to the active serine prevents AChE from hydrolysing ACh, thereby leading to the accumulation of ACh in the synaptic cleft, causing the acute cholinergic crisis.

Most OP insecticides are actually relatively poor inhibitors of AChE and BuChE since they contain a P–S moiety. They are metabolically activated by cytochrome P450 to produce oxygen analogs, called oxons, which are very potent AChE inhibitors. It is generally assumed that the inhibition of AChE and BuChE following exposure to OP insecticides is mainly the result of the oxygen analog and not the parent compound.

The CMs are thought to inhibit AChE and BuChE in a similar way. CMs contain an electrophilic carbonyl carbon, which undergoes a nucleophilic attack by the active serine oxygen (Fig. 13.2). The resulting carbamylated enzyme intermediate inhibits AChE activity until a water molecule attacks the carbonyl carbon to reactivate the enzyme and produce a carbamic acid derivative. This rate of reactivation is considerably faster than that of phosphorylated AChE, although

not as rapid as reactivation of the acetylated intermediate that is formed normally after ACh binding.

13.4.2. Fate of inhibited cholinesterases

The phosphorylated enzyme (Fig. 13.4A) is subject to two reactions: spontaneous reactivation, discussed above (Fig. 13.4B), and the so-called aging process (Fig. 13.4C). Aging refers to the reaction that, after phosphorylation of serine at the active site of AChE or BuChE, a dealkylation of the phosphyl moiety can occur, resulting in the loss of an alkyl group. The remaining negatively charged monophosphylate ester of serine is resistant to spontaneous or oxime-mediated reactivation (Aldridge and Reiner, 1972; Worek et al., 1996; Worek et al., 1999). Aged ChE can only be regained through the synthesis of a new enzyme. The recovery of aged red blood cell AChE takes longer than that of aged plasma BuChE since the turnover of red blood cells is much slower than the turnover of plasma ChE (Mason, 2000; Mason et al., 2000). The rate and extent of aging is a function of the chemical structure of the phosphyl moiety and differs between OP insecticides and nerve agents (Talbot et al., 1988; Worek et al., 1999; Lockridge and Masson, 2000).

13.4.3. Reactivation of inhibited cholinesterases by oximes

Wilson and Ginsburg (1955) found that compounds more nucleophilic than water enhanced reactivation of phosphorylated AChE. A number of reactivators, termed oximes, have been synthesized and tried in OP poisoned victims. In the US, pralidoxime chloride

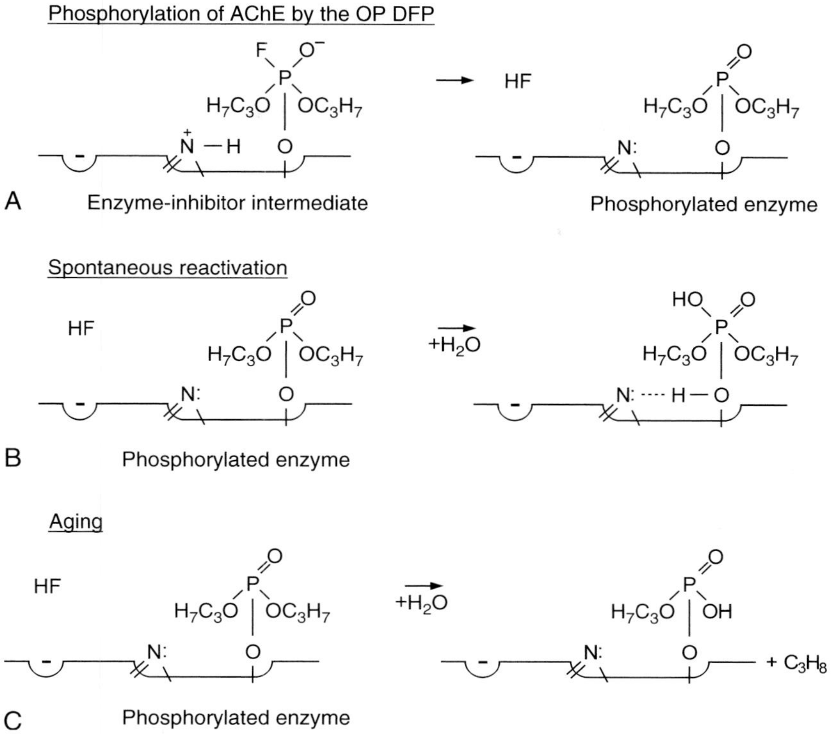

Phosphorylation of AChE by the OP DFP

A   Enzyme-inhibitor intermediate   Phosphorylated enzyme

Spontaneous reactivation

B   Phosphorylated enzyme

Aging

C   Phosphorylated enzyme

Fig. 13.4. Phosphorylation of AChE by OP and fate of the phosphorylated AChE. ACh and the OP inhibitor compete for AChE as their substrate. The phosphorylated AChE is subject to two reactions: spontaneous reactivation (B) and aging (C). Both reactions occur concurrently but at largely different rates with different OPs.

(PAMCl) is the only reactivator approved for medical use whereas obidoxime is also available in Europe and some other parts of the world. Other experimental reactivators, often tried in military context, include HI6, TMB4 and LüH6 (Rousseaux and Dua, 1989; Luo et al., 1999). All reactivators accelerate reactivation of phosphorylated AChE through a nucleophilic attack of the oxime on the phosphorus of the phosphorylated enzyme to give phosphorylated oxime and free enzyme (Fig. 13.4B). Oxime reactivation can only occur provided aging has not yet occurred. Also, certain phosphorylated oximes appear to be able to re-inhibit reactivated AChE, thereby reducing their efficacy in the treatment of OP intoxication. This unwanted new inhibition can be prevented by drugs, such as edrophonium, that compete with the phosphorylated oxime for the AChE active site (Luo et al., 1998, 1999; Kiderlen et al., 2000). Although the exact molecular interactions between the phosphorylated enzyme and oxime that lead to reactivation are not known, a number of studies using mutant forms of AChE have concluded that certain amino acid residues are most important, probably determining the best fitting position of the oxime in the active center of AChE (Ashon et al., 1995; Wong et al., 2000).

Pralidoxime is generally not used to treat CM insecticide poisoning since it enhances the toxicity of carbaryl (Harris et al., 1989). On the other hand, pralidoxime and HI6 reduced the lethality of the CM physostigmine in rats, providing the rationale for their combined use in pre-treatment protocols for nerve agent poisoning (Harris et al., 1989).

13.5. Electrophysiological aspects in peripheral neurotoxicity

Electrophysiological studies are generally assumed to be the best way to resolve the functional mechanism of OP and CM toxicity. Such studies mainly examine effects on the nerve action potential conduction and synaptic transmission. Daily administration of trichlorfon progressively shortens the duration and time to peak amplitude of the nerve action potential, increasing its rate of rise and shortening the relative refractory period (Averbook and Anderson, 1983). By contrast, acute exposure to trichlorfon and chronic administration of parathion does not change these action potential parameters. It has been suggested that changes in nerve excitability may be a sensitive indicator of incipient delayed neuropathy (see Section 13.10).

Synaptic transmission is much more vulnerable to the action of OP and CM drugs than action potential conduction. Defects stem either from the sustained presence of excess ACh in the synaptic cleft or from direct action of the drug on the acetylcholine receptor (AChR). From the late 1940s to the 1960s, many studies involving vertebrate and insect neuromuscular transmission have been reported. Using the frog phrenic nerve-diaphragm preparation, Eccles and McFarlane (1949) showed that the CMs physostigmine and neostigmine and the OP diisopropylphosphorofluoridate (DFP) increased the duration of endplate potential (EPP) and at high concentrations decreased its amplitude. This study established that these inhibitors cause a postsynaptic block. Pre- as well as postsynaptic changes were demonstrated in the rat nerve-diaphragm preparation in which paraoxon first increased the spontaneous miniature EPP (MEPP) frequency and half-decay time, but ultimately it blocked neuromuscular transmission (Laskowski and Dettbarn, 1979). Maselli and Soliven poisoned rats with DFP and observed muscle weakness. They demonstrated in vitro that DFP prolonged the half-decay time of the MEPPs and nerve-evoked EPPs, but had no effect on the MEPP amplitude and the quantal content of the EPPs (Maselli and Soliven, 1991). D-tubocurarine had an antagonistic effect. They concluded that sustained postsynaptic depolarization was responsible for the weakness observed in vivo. The question of a possible direct effect of DFP on the endplate remained unanswered.

Involvement of a direct action of CMs and OPs on the endplate was derived from focal recordings of miniature endplate currents (MEPCs) from frog sartorius muscle (Deana and Scuka, 1990). Neostigmine initially lengthened the decay phase of MEPCs and increased the amplitude of MEPCs probably due to AChE inhibition, but later it suppressed the amplitude and shortened the decay phase, suggesting a direct effect of the CM on the endplate.

Fade of tetanic contractions induced by high-frequency repetitive nerve stimulation was observed in phrenic nerve-diaphragm preparations of mice treated with neostigmine (Chang et al., 1986). The fade was caused by failure to elicit muscle action potentials due to endplate depolarization and a decrease in transmitter release. Both effects were attributed to excess ACh accumulation due to AChE inhibition.

Albuquerque and co-workers have conducted a vast number of experiments on the mechanism of action of various ChE inhibitors at the neuromuscular junction, and ultimately concluded that, in addition to effects through AChE inhibition, there were direct actions on the nicotinic AChRs (Albuquerque et al., 1984, 1985, 1986, 1987, 1988). This group of investigators

also provided evidence that the antidotal effect of oximes is not only due to carbamylation and reactivation of AChE but also to a direct effect on the nicotinic ACh receptors (Kawabuchi et al., 1988).

At the frog endplate (−)physostigmine at low concentration increased the peak amplitude of the EPC and prolonged the decay phase of EPC. At high concentrations, the EPC peak amplitude was decreased, the EPC decay was accelerated, and single-channel life time was shortened (Shaw et al., 1985).

DFP, tabun, VX and (−)physostigmine interacted with pre- and postsynaptic regions of the glutamatergic neuromuscular synapse of locust muscle (Idriss et al., 1986). These agents initiated spontaneous endplate potentials and muscle action potentials. This is a novel target of action of these anti-ChEs. In addition to (−)physostigmine, the (+)physostigmine enantiomer also protected against agonist lethality and the myopathy caused by sarin in rats, a protective effect most certainly not dependent on ChE inhibition but due to direct block of nicotinic ACh receptors (Albuquerque et al., 1988).

Whole-cell and single-channel patch-clamp studies were performed on the nicotinic AChRs in rat PC12 cells (Nagata et al., 1997). Neostigmine and carbaryl showed a biphasic effect (Fig. 13.5). At low concentration they greatly potentiated carbachol induced whole-cell currents and at high concentrations they suppressed the current. Single-channel experiments indicated that both carbaryl and neostigmine increased short closures or gaps during channel opening, decreased the mean open time and burst duration, but caused no change in single-channel conductance. These effects appear to be exerted by direct block of nicotinic AChRs.

Studies on the effects of receptor subunits have only been reported for the neuronal $\alpha 4 \beta 2$ nicotinic ACh receptor subunits (Smulders et al., 2004). Various OPs were found to interact directly with neuronal $\alpha 4 \beta 2$ nicotinic AChRs to inhibit the agonist induced response.

In summary, OPs and CMs stimulate and then suppress neuromuscular transmission. The effects are partly due to AChE inhibition and partly due to direct effects on nicotinic AChRs. The degree and time course of these effects is variable depending on the agent, dose, duration of administration and species of animal.

13.6. Electromyography in patients with OP and CM intoxication

Besser et al. (1989a) studied the EMG features at the neuromuscular junction in a number of OP poisoned patients and found distinctive and sensitive abnormalities. These consist of repetitive firing of single evoked

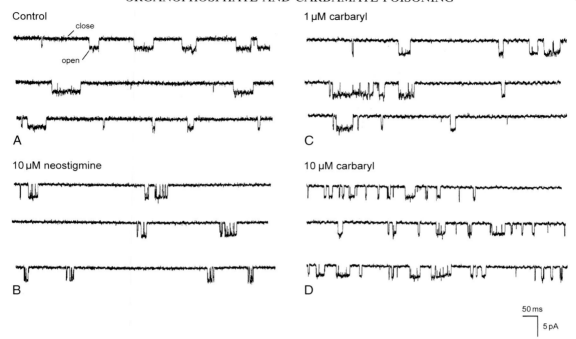

Fig. 13.5. Effects of neostigmine and carbaryl on ACh-induced single-channel currents. Rat clonal pheochromocytoma (PC12) cells expressing the nicotinic AChR channel were used. Single-channel currents induced by co-applications of ACh and neostigmine or carbaryl to cell-attached membrane patches. (A) Currents induced by 30 μM ACh occur in opening bursts interrupted by a few short closures. (B) Co-application of 30 μM ACh and 10 μM neostigmine. (C) Co-application of 30 μM ACh and 1 μM carbaryl. (D) Co-application of 30 μM ACh and 10 μM carbaryl. In panels B, C and D an increasing number of brief closures appear within the bursts, indicating a progressive short-lived noncompetitive block of the AChR. (From Nagata et al., 1997.)

compound muscle action potentials (CMAPs) (Fig. 13.6), and two distinctive abnormalities in response to repetitive nerve stimulation: the decrement and the decrement-increment phenomenon. Repetitive firing associated with the CMAP following single nerve stimulus was the earliest sign of endplate AChE inhibition, regardless of the severity of the intoxication (Van Dijk et al., 1996). The amplitude of the single CMAP remained unaltered even in severe stages of the poisoning. Repetitive nerve stimulation abnormalities were seen later in more severe stages of the poisoning. A decremental response on repetitive nerve stimulation was observed in very weak patients (Fig. 13.7). The decrement-increment preceded or followed the severe stage of the poisoning (Fig. 13.8). The decrement-increment phenomenon was proposed by these authors as a repetitive nerve stimulation pattern unique to OP intoxication. Based on studies on rat phrenic nerve-diaphragm preparations with AChE partially inactivated, they concluded that stimulus-induced antidromic backfiring in the phrenic nerve, a presynaptic event, was responsible for the decrement-increment phenomenon. Low concentrations of (+)tubocurarine abolished stimulus-induced antidromic backfiring and simultaneously prevented the decrement of the second CMAP

(Besser et al., 1992). This group concluded that neuromuscular transmission studies in their hands were superior to plasma BuChE levels and blood OP levels for determining the severity of the poisoning and for guiding therapeutic decisions such as removal from respiratory support (Besser et al., 1989b).

13.7. The acute cholinergic poisoning

13.7.1. Clinical presentation

The acute cholinergic syndrome is generally assumed to be the result of excess ACh accumulation at all cholinergic transmission sites. The symptoms are usually systematically subdivided into those resulting from muscarinic or nicotinic ACh receptor overstimulation and central nervous system (CNS) effects. Table 13.2 summarizes the typical signs and symptoms of acute AChE inhibitor poisoning in humans. The opposite cardiac effects of muscarinic and central nicotinic stimulation usually result in tachycardia when poisoning is moderate, while severely poisoned patients usually have bradycardia. Most life-threatening is respiratory depression, due to paralysis of CNS respiratory centers in combination with muscarinic bronchoconstriction and laryngospasm,

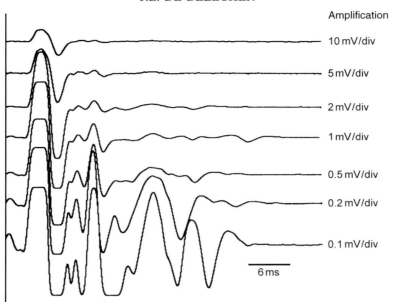

Fig. 13.6. Repetitive activity of the compound muscle action potential recorded at increasing amplification after a single nerve stimulation.

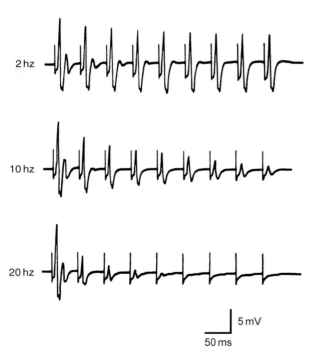

Fig. 13.7. Decrement of the CMAP and decreasing repetitive activity with increasing frequency of stimulation. (From Besser et al., 1989a.)

excessive tracheobronchial and salivary secretions, and nicotinic paralysis of the diaphragm and other respiratory muscles. CNS effects are mainly attributed to cholinergic over-stimulation. Convulsions may be life-threatening.

OPs vary in their potency to induce seizures, with some investigators ascribing the differences to different lipoid solubility of the various OPs, with lipoid-soluble OPs crossing the blood–brain barrier more readily (Frederikssons 1957, 1958; Firemark et al., 1964; Gupta et al., 1999). Others believe that this difference in seizure frequency is not entirely related to AChE inhibition but to direct effects of the OP on neuronal nicotinic AChRs. Rare CNS clinical manifestations include extrapyramidal symptoms (Senanayake and Sanmuganathan, 1995; Okumura et al., 2004; Brahmi et al., 2004), atypical ocular bobbing (Hata et al., 1986; De Bleecker et al., 1992d), and transient opsoclonus (De Bleecker, 1992).

The severity of the acute cholinergic poisoning depends on the OP or CM compound and the amount and duration of exposure. Even after a single oral intake, which is most often the case in suicide attempts, prolonged absorption of the poison may continue for several days, even with adequate gastric lavage (Willems, 1981). Toxicokinetics of the individual substances play an important role (Willems and Belpaire, 1991). Individual variations in toxicity with the same compound may be due to genetic causes, such as differences in paraoxonase function (Costa et al., 1990, 2003a,b, 2005; Gan et al., 1991; Bryk et al., 2005) and pharmacogenetic differences in AChE and BuChE (Prody et al., 1989; Loewenstein-Lichtenstein et al., 1995; Hasin et al., 2004; Bryk et al., 2005). Altered metabolism and excretion rates by the systemic effects of the actual poisoning with impaired cardiac, renal and liver function prolongs

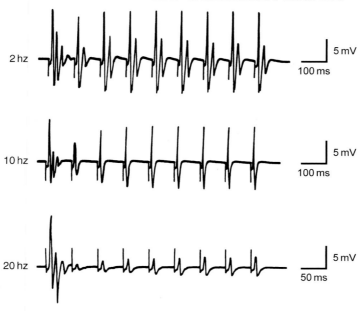

Fig. 13.8. Decrement-increment phenomenon recorded at different rates of repetitive nerve stimulation. Decrement of the CMAP is most pronounced at the second response and is larger with increasing rate of stimulation. Time calibration is for potentials only and not for interpotential interval. (From Besser et al., 1989a.)

Table 13.2

Signs and symptoms of acute cholinesterase inhibitor poisoning

Muscarinic	*Bronchial tree:* tightness of the chest, wheezing, dyspnea, increased secretions, cough, pulmonary edema, cyanosis
	Gastrointestinal system: nausea, vomiting, abdominal tightness and cramps, diarrhea, tenesmus, fecal incontinence
	Cardiovascular system: bradycardia, fall in blood pressure, arrhythmias, ventricular fibrillation, asystole
	Exocrine glands: increased sweating, salivation, lacrimation
	Urinary system: frequency, urinary incontinence
	Eyes: myosis, blurred vision, headache
	Cardiovascular system: pallor, tachycardia, high blood pressure
Nicotinic	*Striated muscle:* muscular twitching, fasciculations, cramps, weakness, respiratory failure
Central nervous system	Giddiness, anxiety, restlessness, emotional lability, excessive dreaming, insomnia, tremor, apathy, depression, drowsiness, confusion, ataxia, coma with areflexia, Cheyne–Stokes respiration, convulsions, depression of respiratory and circulatory centers

After Grob, 1963; Willems and Belpaire, 1991.

the clinical course in severely poisoned animals and patients (Maxwell et al., 1987; De Bleecker et al., 1992b; Betrosian et al., 1995).

13.7.2. Measurement of cholinesterase activity in acutely poisoned patients

The diagnosis is confirmed by measuring levels of AChE in red blood cells and of BuChE in plasma. Both enzymes can reliably be used as markers for enzyme inhibition in the central and peripheral nervous system. There are, however, differences in the kinetics of the inhibition of the two enzymes (Wilson et al., 1992) and large ranges of normal values. Erythrocyte AChE levels are invariably more specific than BuChE activity as a marker of OP poisoning, although some OPs (malathion, chlorpyrifos) depress plasma BuChE to a larger degree. Most information is therefore obtained if both red blood cell AChE and plasma BuChE can be obtained. In order to determine the activity of each enzyme separately, erythrocytes and plasma have to be separated, or selective substrates and/or inhibitors to assay only one enzyme have to be applied. Neither option is fully feasible at present. No substrates or inhibitors are known that are fully selective for either AChE or BuChE. Full separation of erythrocytes from plasma is difficult without losing some enzyme activity.

Many methods have been developed for measuring cholinesterase activities. Choline and thiocholine esters are good substrates of AChE and BuChE. ACh is the physiological substrate of AChE, and benzoylcholine is the suggested substrate for monitoring BuChE activity. The reader is referred to comprehensive reviews that cover a number of previous and current methods of assay (Ellman et al., 1961; Augustinsson, 1971; Whittaker, 1986; Evans, 1986; Wilson, 2001). Pitfalls when interpreting results of assays of AChE and BuChE activity include large inter-individual variations for BuChE, the presence of unreacted OP or CM in the blood sample, the presence of oxime in the blood sample of treated patients (Petroianu et al., 2004), and genetic variants in BuChE and to a probably lesser extent in AChE activity (Lockridge and Masson, 2000).

Red blood cell AChE levels do not perfectly reflect the inhibition in the nervous tissue, partly due to pharmacokinetic factors causing different access of the inhibitor to nervous or erythrocyte AChE. Furthermore, unlike nervous tissue, red blood cells lack the capability to synthesize new AChE protein, resulting in faster recovery of nervous tissue AChE due to de novo synthesis (Wehner et al., 1985).

13.8. The necrotizing myopathy

Ariëns et al. (1969) were the first to describe a myopathy in rats a few hours after IV injection of DFP, paraoxon, and tabun. The first lesions appeared 2 h after injection and included localized eosinophilia and swelling of the sarcoplasm, and loss of cross striations. The lesions quickly progressed towards myophagocytosis, followed by regeneration within a few days. The muscle fiber necrosis was more extensive when the muscles had been more active, with the diaphragm being the most affected muscle. Unilateral phrenic nerve neurotomy prevented the necrosis on that side of the diaphragm. Electrical stimulation, on the other hand, enhanced the necrosis. DFP poisoned rats treated with oximes within 2 h after injection showed no necrosis. D-tubocurarine in higher doses prevented necrosis. Fenichel and co-workers (1972) used paraoxon and noted similar changes in the examined

muscles. They drew attention to the early disappearance of the normal "lace" pattern on NADH-TR stain with accumulation of highly positive material in the subsarcolemmal area and rarefaction at the center of the affected fibers. Electron microscopy (EM) confirmed that the early change is disruption of myofilaments in the center of the muscle fiber with relative preservation of the subsarcolemmal zone. The deleterious effect was predominantly on type I fibers. Section of the sciatic nerve protected the ipsilateral gastrocnemius and soleus muscles from the myopathy. Hemicholinium also markedly reduced the number of necrotic muscle fibers.

Both Ariëns and Fenichel ascribed the necrotizing myopathy to ACh excess with overstimulation of the postsynaptic membrane. Fenichel and co-workers (1974a) strengthened this hypothesis by producing similar muscle lesions through guanidine administration, a drug enhancing ACh release from the nerve terminal. In a subsequent experiment, these authors demonstrated that hind leg immobilization was protective, but exercise did not aggravate the paraoxon induced myopathy (Fenichel et al., 1974b). There are large differences in susceptibility of various rat skeletal muscles, but muscles composed mainly of highly oxidative fibers are the most susceptible (De Bleecker et al., 1992e).

The first human case of OP induced necrotizing myopathy was described in 1975 by De Reuck and Willems. Lesions similar to those in rats were abundant in the diaphragm of a parathion poisoned man. Limb muscles were normal. The authors ascribed the predominant diaphragm involvement to the excessive use of this muscle. Similar necrotic changes were reported in several muscle biopsies of a worker chronically using several OP agents, most often diazinon (Ahlgren et al., 1979), and in several muscles after severe trichlornate poisoning (De Reuck et al., 1979). Another patient was reported as having intercostal muscle fiber necrosis 4 days after acute malathion and diazinon poisoning (Wecker et al., 1985).

Dettbarn's group carried out further studies on rats with paraoxon (Wecker et al., 1978b; De Bleecker et al., 1991) and largely confirmed the earlier findings. In vitro electrophysiologic studies with phrenic nerve-hemidiaphragm preparations showed enhanced MEPP frequency and spontaneous as well as impulse-related antidromic nerve activity along the phrenic nerve. Biochemical investigation disclosed an 86% AChE inhibition. They also demonstrated—using various time intervals between poisoning and oxime administration—that a critical time period of AChE inhibition was necessary for a full-blown myopathy to develop (Wecker et al., 1978a). In denervated hemidiaphragms necrotic muscle fibers were scarce. Although denervation on its own caused AChE loss, the remaining AChE in the denervated hemidiaphragm appeared less susceptible to inhibition by paraoxon than on the innervated side (de Clermont, 1855). Atropine and gentamicin attenuated the necrotizing myopathy in soman and paraoxon poisoning, probably through interaction with the presynaptic Ca^{2+} uptake mechanism (Leonard and Salpeter, 1979). In a study using daily low-dose paraoxon injections, it was noted that prolonged exposure to low doses of OP AChE inhibitors eventually also caused skeletal muscle fiber necrosis without apparent signs of cholinergic toxicity (Dettbarn, 1984).

Apart from paraoxon, other OP compounds such as soman (Dekleva et al., 1989), DFP (Ariëns et al., 1969; Gupta et al., 1986), and carbamate AChE inhibitors such as pyridostigmine (Hudson and Foster, 1984; Hudson et al., 1985) and neostigmine (de Clermont, 1854) have been reported to induce a similar myopathy in rats.

Meshul et al. (1985) described the ultrastructural lesions in rat neuromuscular junctions after acute sarin or soman, or chronic pyridostigmine treatment. They noted early swelling of membrane-bound organelles (mitochondria, sarcoplasmic reticulum, nuclear envelope) followed by dissolution of Z-disks and a pronounced expansion of nuclear chromatin. Apart from their principal occurrence at the endplate areas, it was not established that any of the EM findings were typical or specific for OP-induced myopathy.

In patients, no separate treatment regimens to prevent the necrotizing myopathy have been studied. In animals, a large variety of agents, such as postsynaptic blocking drugs, but also the nicotinic ganglion blocking agent hexamethonium, have been reported to be myoprotective (Table 13.3). Although protection of the endplate AChR appears to be the mechanism most frequently involved, the protective action of so widely different drugs suggests that the mechanisms underlying OP-induced myopathy may be multiple and that the hypothesis of acute ACh overflow due to endplate AChE inhibition may be an oversimplification of its pathogenesis (Albuquerque et al., 1985).

13.9. The intermediate syndrome

13.9.1. Introduction

In 1987, Senanayake and Karalliedde reported 10 patients who developed facial, proximal limb and respiratory muscle weakness. Because this occurred in the interval between the acute cholinergic crisis and the possible development of a delayed neuropathy

called organophosphate-induced delayed polyneuropathy, they termed this new entity the "Intermediate Syndrome" (IMS). The acute cholinergic crisis is due to inhibition of carboxylic esterases, of which AChE is clinically the most important (Grob, 1963), and the delayed neuropathy has been linked to inhibition of a separate esterase, termed the neuropathy target esterase (Johnson, 1975; Abou-Donia and Lapadula, 1990) (see Section 13.10). The pathogenesis of the IMS was unclear and the question arose whether or not the IMS bore a separate structure–activity relationship (De Bleecker et al., 1992d; Marrs, 1993).

13.9.2. Original description

Senanayake and Karalliedde observed 10 patients of Asian origin who were admitted with a well-defined cholinergic crisis. Following treatment with atropine and oximes in conventional doses, the initial outcome was favorable, but the patients went on to develop an IMS 1–4 days after the cholinergic poisoning (Senanayake and Karalliedde, 1987). The most threatening clinical symptom was the occurrence of sudden respiratory distress, often requiring re-intubation and positive-pressure ventilation. Various degrees of weakness of muscles innervated by several cranial nerves were present in eight patients. All subjects had weakness of neck flexors and of proximal limb muscles. In all but one patient, the tendon reflexes were absent or markedly decreased. There was no sensory impairment. Two patients died on the 3rd and 5th hospital day from respiratory failure, whereas one patient died on the 15th day because of a technical failure.

There was no distinct pattern in the development of the symptoms, but their regression followed a characteristic order in the seven survivors. Cranial nerve palsies—palatal, facial, and external ocular, in that order—were the first to recover, then followed improvement of respiratory function and proximal limb muscle strength. Neck flexors were the last to recover. The time to recovery ranged from 5 days to 18 days. One methamidophos poisoned patient developed delayed neuropathy. The causative organophosphate was identified in 9 subjects: fenthion (4), dimethoate (2), monocrotophos (2), and methamidophos (1). Cholinesterase assays were not available.

EMG showed normal motor and sensory nerve conduction velocities and normal needle myography. Tetanic stimulation of the abductor pollicis brevis muscle 24 h to 48 h after the onset of the IMS showed a marked fade at 20 Hz and 50 Hz. A train of four stimuli at 2 Hz produced no changes in the amplitude of the CMAPs.

Table 13.3

Drugs reported to protect from OP-induced necrotizing myopathy in animal models

Drug	Working mechanism	Reference
Hemicholinium	Inhibitor of ACh synthesis	Fenichel et al., 1972
d-Tubocurarin	Postsynaptic nicotinic receptor blocker	Ariëns et al., 1969; Clinton and Dettbarn, 1987
Atropine	Muscarinic receptor antagonist	Dettbarn 1984; Clinton and Dettbarn, 1987
Pralidoxime	AChE reactivating oxime	Ariëns et al., 1969; Dekleva et al., 1989
HI-6	AChE reactivating oxime and mild nicotinic ganglion blocker	Dekleva et al., 1989
Hexamethonium	Nicotinic ganglion blocker	Dekleva et al., 1989
Pyridostigmine	Reversible AChE inhibitor	Kawabuchi et al., 1989
EGTA	Intracellular calcium chelator	Leonard and Salpeter, 1979
Diltiazem	Calcium channel blocker	Meshul et al., 1990
Gentamicin	Aminoglycoside antibiotic	Dettbarn, 1984
Alpha-bungarotoxin	Inactivation of postsynaptic ACh receptors	Leonard and Salpeter, 1979
Diazepam	Facilitates GABA mediated neurotransmission in spinal cord and brain	Clinton and Dettbarn, 1987
Quinidine	Blocks voltage-dependent Na^+, K^+ and possibly Ca^{2+} channels	De Bleecker et al., 1998

Treatment was mainly symptomatic. Atropine did not seem to influence the course of the IMS. No definite mechanism of the IMS was identified, but the authors wondered whether the necrotizing myopathy was involved (De Reuck and Willems, 1975; Dettbarn, 1984; Wecker et al., 1986; Inns et al., 1990; De Bleecker et al., 1991, 1992e, 1998).

13.9.3. Previous reports

Several patients reported before the recognition of the IMS can retrospectively be related to this syndrome.

The largest cohort was presented by Wadia et al. (1974) for diazinon poisoning. These authors divided the signs and symptoms into type I (those present on admission) and type II (those appearing 24 h after onset of poisoning). Type I signs included impaired consciousness and fasciculations, and were responsive to atropine therapy. Type II signs were very much like the IMS and included proximal limb weakness, areflexia and cranial nerve palsies, and were not influenced by atropine. Some type I patients developed type II signs after an initial recovery. Thirty-six of 200 consecutive patients developed type II signs, and 15 died from respiratory paralysis.

In 1966, Clarman and Geldmacher-von Mallinckradt successfully managed a fenthion poisoned patient with relapse of respiratory paralysis a few hours after initial improvement. In another fenthion poisoned victim, sudden respiratory insufficiency necessitating artificial ventilation occurred 72 h after ingestion (Dean et al., 1967). This patient at the same time was restless, sweating, salivating, and had profuse fasciculations. He had considerable strength in all limbs and could lift his trunk from the bed. Combined atropine and oxime (PAM) treatment was successful in rapidly controlling the muscarinic signs; it took 7 days, however, before spontaneous breathing returned. The authors mentioned the disproportion between respiratory (intercostal, bulbar and diaphragm muscles) and non-respiratory muscle strength as the most striking feature in their patient. A Belgian group reported severe relapses of an initial cholinergic crisis 31 h, 72 h, 7 days, 12 days, 13 days and 16 days after ingestion of fenthion, despite atropine and oxime administration (Mahieu et al., 1982).

Relapse of cholinergic symptoms and unconsciousness has also been reported following dimethoate intoxication (Molphy and Rathus, 1964). A tractor driver with subacute dicrotophos poisoning, probably through both skin contact and inhalation, recovered from a moderate cholinergic crisis after atropine and pralidoxime treatment. He further improved when atropine dosage was tapered, but on the 7th day after the last exposure, he relapsed with prominent respiratory paralysis. The outcome was favorable (Perron and Johnson, 1969).

Gadoth and Fisher reported a patient with malathion ingestion who 20 h after a mild and apparently well-treated cholinergic crisis needed urgent re-intubation, with vomiting, muscle cramps, and diarrhea at the same time (Gadoth and Fisher, 1978). A progressive paresis emerged, and after 50 h a neurological evaluation revealed complete respiratory paralysis, bilateral ptosis, myosis and external ophthalmoplegia. Tendon reflexes were absent. Repeated doses of atropine and obidoxime were ineffective. The eventual outcome was favorable.

13.9.4. Further characterization of the IMS: author's observations

13.9.4.1. Experimental animal studies

We compared in Wistar rats the acutely toxic OP paraoxon with fenthion, one of the agents frequently involved in the human IMS. The clinical course was studied in relation to the development of muscle fiber necrosis, histochemically assessed AChE activity at the neuromuscular junction, biochemically assessed brain AChE activity, and EMG studies including repetitive nerve stimulation at various frequencies.

Marked differences in the clinical course of the cholinergic crisis were noted between paraoxon and fenthion poisoning, regardless of the route of administration (De Bleecker et al., 1994a). Paraoxon provoked an acute, severe and short-lasting cholinergic crisis lasting less than 24 h. In contrast, fenthion poisoning produced a gradual increase of cholinergic signs lasting several days. All surviving animals were symptom-free after one week. Fasciculations peaked within the first days of fenthion poisoning, and gradually decreased and ultimately disappeared when the rats got weaker. Single poisoning with these two OPs turned out to be a good model to compare acute and chronic types of poisoning in animals, but most clinical signs relevant to the human IMS cannot be ascertained in rodents.

Histochemically determined endplate AChE and spectrophotometrically determined brain AChE activity closely paralleled each other. In paraoxon poisoning, AChE inhibition was severe from 1h to 3 h after subcutaneous injection and gradually recovered within 24 h. In fenthion poisoned animals, a slowly progressive decline in AChE activity occurred with maximal inhibition after 8 days. At that time, most animals had no more weakness or fasciculations.

The necrotizing myopathy began shortly after the initiation of the cholinergic crisis with both OPs and involved a maximal number of muscle fibers after 24–48 h. The necrotizing myopathy did not get worse by a further decline in AChE activity in fenthion poisoned animals. It appeared to be a monophasic event related to the initial decline in endplate AChE activity. The severity of the myopathy was similar in paraoxon and fenthion poisoned rats with similar degrees of fasciculations.

Repetitive activity after single motor nerve stimulation and decrement after repetitive nerve stimulation were the major EMG findings in either type of poisoning (Fig. 13.9A) (Besser et al., 1989a,b, 1992; De Bleecker et al., 1994b; Van Dijk et al., 1996; Singh et al., 1998b). Repetitive activity is defined as at least one negative deflection occurring immediately after the initial biphasic CMAP (for a review see Bowman et al., 1986) (Fig. 13.9A, B). CMAP amplitude decrements provoked by repetitive nerve stimulation occurred only in weak rats with severe endplate AChE inhibition. The smallest amplitude occurred either at the second response followed by a gradual increase in the subsequent responses (decrement-increment phenomenon) (Fig. 13.9C), or the amplitude decreased progressively towards the last response (decrement phenomenon) (Fig. 13.9D). The decrement-increment phenomenon preceded the decrement phenomenon and occurred at a slightly less severe degree of AChE inhibition.

Conclusions from the animal studies were that:

1. The AChE inhibition by fenthion is very prolonged.
2. The necrotizing myopathy is determined by the initial decline in endplate AChE activity, and is not further aggravated by continued inhibition.
3. Decrement-increment and decrement responses to EMG are related to severe AChE inhibition and appear at a slightly different level of AChE inhibition.

The data argued against monophasic necrotizing myopathy being the cause of the IMS, and were suggestive of persistent AChE inhibition being involved. This hypothesis was tested on patients.

13.9.4.2. Observations in patients

Consecutive OP poisoned patients admitted to our institution were prospectively studied. The study included a standard neurological examination at frequent fixed time intervals, plasma BuChE and erythrocyte AChE activity, urinary OP metabolite excretion and EMG with repetitive nerve stimulation. Some patients underwent a muscle biopsy.

Eight out of 19 patients developed clinical signs and symptoms of the IMS. In some, short relapses of muscarinic symptoms were superimposed on the IMS. No clinical, electromyographic, biochemical or other differences were noted between patients with or without symptom-free intervals, or those with or without short relapses of muscarinic signs and symptoms. OPs such as fenthion ($n = 1$), dimethoate ($n = 1$) (De Bleecker et al., 1992a) and methyl-parathion ($n = 5$) (De Bleecker et al., 1992c) apparently carried a higher

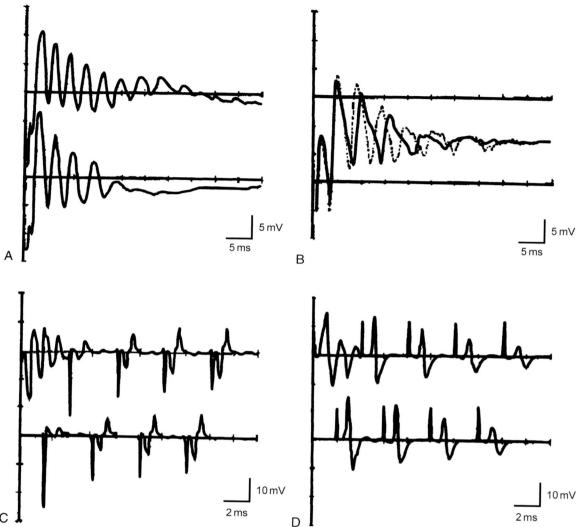

Fig. 13.9. Electromyographic findings in OP poisoned rats. (A) Response to two subsequent stimuli at 2 Hz administered 2.5 h after subcutaneous injection of paraoxon. Note prominent repetitive activity after the first stimulus (upper line). After the second stimulus, the repetitive activity is less marked. The initial CMAP amplitudes are normal. (B) Response to two subsequent nerve stimuli at 3 Hz administered 2.5 h after subcutaneous paraoxon poisoning. Repetitive action potentials at the second stimulus (full line) are less frequent, are delayed and have less steep slopes. Note slightly decreased CMAP amplitude at the second response. (C) Decrement-increment phenomenon in response to 50 Hz repetitive nerve stimulation 3 h after subcutaneous paraoxon injection. The odd responses are displayed on top, the even at the bottom. The second response has the smallest amplitude, with gradual but incomplete recovery in the subsequent responses. Note that the marked repetitive activity at the first response is entirely abrogated at the second response and does not recur. The sharp initial deflection preceding each CMAP represents the stimulation artifact. (D) Decrement phenomenon in response to 50 Hz repetitive nerve stimulation 9 days after subcutaneous injection of fenthion. Gradual decrease in amplitude and area towards the ninth response. The repetitive activity disappears completely at the second response.

risk. However, we also noted a prolonged IMS in a parathion poisoned man with severe renal and hepatic failure, indicating that the IMS is not restricted to a few OP agents (De Bleecker et al., 1992b). Table 13.4 lists the OPs frequently involved in IMS (cases cited here). Prospective studies on the relative incidence of

IMS with certain OPs are needed to avoid a number of biases inherent in case reports.

The clinical signs of the IMS were weakness in the territory of multiple cranial nerves (diplopia, dysphagia, facial diplegia), sudden respiratory distress necessitating re-intubation, neck and proximal limb muscle

Table 13.4

Causative organophosphates in the intermediate syndrome (total 82)

Fenthion	11
Dimethoate—omethoate	6 – 5
Parathion	8
Methyl-parathion	5
Malathion	4
Monocrotophos—dicrotophos	2 – 1
Methamidophos	1
Dichlorvos—Trichlorvos	1 – 1
Chlorpyrifos	1
Diazinon*	36

*The incidence of IMS per compound is skewed by the single report of 36 cases in an early study by Wadia et al., 1974.

weakness, and depression of the tendon reflexes. Fasciculations were not part of the IMS but coincided with the appearance of muscarinic signs. The duration of the IMS varied from a few days to several weeks. The outcome was good. No patients developed clinical or EMG features of delayed polyneuropathy (De Bleecker et al., 1993).

All patients had severe AChE inhibition during the entire period of the IMS. Metabolite excretion was also prolonged. Consecutive EMG findings in the evolution of the IMS were: decrement, decrement-increment, increment, and finally normal repetitive nerve stimulation studies. The EMG normalized before the last neurological symptom, i.e., fatigable external ocular muscle weakness had disappeared (De Bleecker et al., 1993).

In the four patients who underwent muscle biopsy, a few necrotic muscle fibers were noted, but these were too sparse to explain severe muscle weakness and were no more frequent in IMS than in non-IMS patients.

We concluded from the prospective patient study that:

1. The IMS is not rare, and although it is more likely to occur with certain OPs, it is not restricted to these agents. Toxicokinetic factors such as high lipid-solubility of certain OPs (Davies et al., 1975), but also impaired systemic functions (cardiovascular, hepatic, renal) (Betrosian et al., 1995) with prolongation of OP metabolism and excretion, can probably all contribute to the development of an IMS.
2. The syndrome invariably coincides with prolonged AChE inhibition and is not due to muscle fiber necrosis. No separate structure–activity relationship is involved.

3. When viewed together, the clinical and EMG features are best explained by combined pre- and postsynaptic impairment of neuromuscular transmission (De Wilde et al., 1991) (see also Section 13.9.5).
4. The IMS is not related to incipient delayed neuropathy.

13.9.5. Comparison with other human diseases with impaired neuromuscular transmission

The clinical, EMG, micro-electrophysiological and morphological features of a number of acquired or congenital human disorders of neuromuscular transmission have been well characterized. Comparison of the IMS with some of these entities is helpful in interpreting the observations made in IMS patients. Besides practical problems involved in studies of endplate-rich human intercostal muscle biopsies, the changing dynamics of the endplate AChE inhibition in the course of OP poisonings make the IMS less amenable to micro-electrophysiological studies than more stable disorders.

Table 13.5 summarizes the main clinical and EMG characteristics of some disorders of neuromuscular transmission. Myasthenia gravis is an autoimmune disorder with postsynaptic impairment of neuromuscular transmission due to complement-mediated destruction of the junctional folds and accelerated internalization of the AChR. In the Lambert–Eaton myasthenic syndrome, antibodies against the presynaptic voltage-sensitive calcium channel reduce release of ACh quanta from the motor nerve terminal. In botulinum toxin poisoning, the ACh release from the nerve terminal is reduced by impaired fusion of the synaptic vesicles with the presynaptic membrane. The distribution of the weakness and the obvious fatigability of some muscle groups in the IMS are very similar to those of myasthenia gravis. Areflexia or hyporeflexia, on the other hand, is more typical of presynaptic disorders. Likewise, the EMG findings of the IMS are a combination of those observed in pre- and postsynaptic disorders of neuromuscular transmission. In some IMS patients with severe weakness, persistent decrements at low stimulation frequencies were found, comparable to severe myasthenia gravis. In most patients, a decrement-increment phenomenon with the smallest amplitude at the second stimulus occurred at intermediate or high frequency stimulation only. This is similar to presynaptic disorders. However, reduced amplitude of the CMAP after a single nerve stimulus, the most typical and constant EMG feature of the Lambert–Eaton myasthenic syndrome, was never noted. The decrement-increment

Table 13.5

Main characteristics of some human disorders of neuromuscular transmission

	Myasthenia gravis	Lambert–Eaton myasthenic syndrome	Botulinum toxin poisoning	Intermediate syndrome	Congenital AChE deficiency
Site of defect	Postsynaptic	Presynaptic	Presynaptic	Pre- and postsynaptic	Pre- and postsynaptic
Clinical findings	Fatigable	Fatigable	Fatigable, descending	Fatigable	Fatigable
Distribution of muscle weakness	Extraocular, bulbar, facial, respiratory, proximal limb	Proximal limb	Extraocular, head and neck, trunk and proximal limb	Extraocular, bulbar, facial, neck, respiratory, proximal limb	Extraocular, bulbar, facial, neck, proximal limb
Tendon reflexes	Normal	Decreased	Decreased	Decreased	Decreased
Response to AChE inhibitors	Yes	Poor or absent	Absent	Absent or adverse	Absent
Electromyography					
CMAP amplitude	Normal	Small	Some small	Normal	Normal
Repetitive activity	No	No	No	Yes	Yes
Repetitive nerve stimulation	Decrement at low frequency	Increment at high frequency	Increment at high frequency	Decrement at low frequency; decrement-increment at intermediate and high frequency	Decrement at low and high frequency

phenomenon, with the smallest amplitude at the second muscle action potential, may well be typical of the IMS.

Taken together, the data in IMS are compatible with a combined pre- and postsynaptic disturbance of neuromuscular transmission, presumably to a different proportion during the evolution of the IMS.

A congenital myasthenic syndrome with synaptic AChE deficiency, resulting from a mutation in the collagenic tail subunit of asymmetric AChE, has been described by Engel et al. (Engel et al., 1977; Ohno et al., 1998). Clinically these patients resemble IMS patients to some extent. They have persistent fatigable weakness of external ocular, facial, palatal, masticatory, neck, and proximal limb muscles, and depressed tendon reflexes. EMG shows repetitive CMAPs after single nerve stimuli, and decrements at slow and rapid rates of repetitive nerve stimulation. Detailed microelectrophysiological and morphological studies have revealed combined pre- and postsynaptic abnormalities of neuromuscular transmission (Table 13.5).

13.9.6. Later reports

In the years following the initial description, the IMS has been diagnosed increasingly due to heightened awareness. He et al. (1998) found IMS in 21 of 272 cases (7.7%). The causative OPs were parathion, omethoate, dimethoate, dichlorvos and some pesticide mixtures. Persisting red blood cell AChE inhibition was a constant finding and decrements were noted in weak patients at 20 Hz or 30 Hz repetitive nerve stimulation. The fatality rate was 19%. Two cases were reported after malathion poisoning (Choi and Quinonez, 1998; Benslama and Moutaouakkil, 1998) and one case after chlorpyrifos ingestion (Guadarrama-Naveda, 2001). Karademir et al. (1990) observed IMS in a young female poisoned by trichlorfon and the CM proxyfur, and in a fenthion poisoned female, both with complete recovery. Two pregnant fenthion poisoned women were successfully managed by Karalliedde et al. (1988). An ethyl-parathion poisoned woman developed both IMS and delayed neuropathy (Nisse et al., 1998).

Other investigators undertook in vivo electrodiagnostic studies in experimental animals (Dongren et al., 1999) and in man (Baker and Sedgwick, 1996; Singh et al., 1998b). Baker and Sedgwick used single fiber EMG. In sarin poisoned healthy volunteers, they found small changes in single fiber EMG parameters at 3 h and 3 days after exposure to a small dose of sarin sufficient to cause a reduction in red blood cell AChE of 60%. These people had no clinical neuromuscular signs or symptoms (Baker and Sedgwick, 1996). They and others (Norman, 1990) considered

that a non-depolarizing block underlies the IMS, and concluded from their studies in volunteers that reversible sub-clinical changes indicating a non-depolarizing block could be found to a variable extent in all study persons and probably also in patients. Inter-individual differences in the safety factor of neuromuscular transmission; the degree and duration of endplate AChE inhibition; and conformational changes of the ACh receptors in the postsynaptic membrane due to the precedent cholinergic overstimulation may explain why not all OP poisoned patients with a similar severity of intoxication develop the IMS. Based on observations in a fenthion poisoned IMS patient, the same group proposed down-regulation of postsynaptic AChRs as a possible explanation for the clinical and electrophysiological abnormalities in that patient (Sedgwick and Senanayake, 1997). Different affinity of different OPs for nicotinic versus muscarinic cholinesterases or selective distribution of some OPs to muscle have also been proposed (Benson et al., 1992).

Studies in dimethoate or diazinon poisoned rats confirmed the higher sensitivity of single fiber EMG over repetitive nerve stimulation to detect subtle changes in neuromuscular transmission after OP poisoning (Dongren et al., 1999; de Blaquiere et al., 2000).

13.9.7. Therapeutic considerations

A definite therapeutic regimen that successfully treats or ideally prevents IMS is not yet available. A high index of suspicion allowing early diagnosis, and intensive care facilities for respiratory monitoring, tracheal intubation and artificial ventilation, when necessary, are the best guarantees for a favorable outcome.

Since prolonged AChE inhibition at the neuromuscular junction is involved in the pathogenesis of the IMS, the main aim is to prevent further inactivation and enhance reactivation of AChE. Benson et al. suggested that IMS may be an artifact of insufficient oxime therapy (Benson et al., 1992). The efficacy of oxime therapy to improve neuromuscular transmission in patients has been demonstrated by electrophysiological techniques (Benson et al., 1992). Early high-dose oxime administration in severely poisoned patients is therefore logical (Besser et al., 1995; Tush and Anstead, 1997; Thiermann et al., 1999), but does not always prevent the IMS from developing (Willems et al., 1992, 1993; Sudakin et al., 2000).

Glycopyrrolate, a quaternary ammonium compound, had a beneficial effect in a case of IMS due to malathion poisoning (Nisse et al., 1998). This predominantly antimuscarinic agent mitigated the bronchorrhea, but it is not likely to prevent or remove most IMS symptoms.

13.9.8. Diagnostic criteria

On the basis of my personal observations and cases reported from experienced centers worldwide we propose the following diagnostic guidelines:

1. Persistent acquired inhibition of red blood cell AChE through OP or CM poisoning.
2. Fatigable weakness of the extraocular, bulbar, facial, respiratory, neck flexor and proximal limb muscles. The weakness occurs 1–4 days after a cholinergic crisis, with or without a symptom-free interval. Fluctuation of muscarinic signs and symptoms does not exclude the diagnosis.
3. Absent or depressed tendon reflexes without other identifiable cause (e.g., pre-existent neuropathy).
4. The EMG abnormalities indicating pre- or postsynaptic impairment of neuromuscular transmission are not constant. Repetitive nerve stimulation may reveal a decrement, a decrement-increment or an abnormal increment. Single fiber EMG is likely to be more sensitive, but is less specific. Further studies are needed to determine the reliability of single fiber EMG studies.

13.10. Organophosphate induced delayed polyneuropathy

Organophosphate induced delayed polyneuropathy (OPIDP) is characterized by distal degeneration of motor and sensory axons in both the peripheral nerves and the spinal cord (Lotti et al., 1984; Lotti, 1992). Several species, including man, are susceptible to OPIDP to variable degrees (Johnson, 1975). The hen is the animal model of choice; rodents are relatively resistant to OPIDP (Veronesi, 1984; Moretto et al., 1992). The clinical and morphological signs of OPIDP in hens develop between 10 days and 15 days after the toxic exposure, but depending on the dose, they can develop even in 1 week. Young animals, including chicks, are much less susceptible than adult animals (Moretto et al., 1991). In humans, symptoms and signs develop more gradually.

13.10.1. Mechanism of OPIDP: neuropathy target esterase

Unlike OP or CM, OPIDP does not inhibit serine hydrolases such as AChE or BuChE. The putative target in OPIDP is a neural protein with esteratic activity termed neuropathy target esterase (NTE). Phosphorylation and subsequent aging of at least 70% of NTE is needed to provoke axonal degeneration (Johnson, 1990). OP insecticides are very different in their capability to inhibit NTE, varying from absent to strong inhibitory capacity. Some do also inhibit AChE, and induce a cholinergic crisis first. Other compounds, such as the triaryl phosphates, are potent NTE inhibitors, but do not inhibit AChE. Studies on the sensitivity of the target enzymes of a variety of OPs showed that the comparative inhibitory capacity of hen AChE and NTE in vitro correlates well with their relative effects in vivo. The hen model well predicts the development of OPIDP in humans, and is currently used in pre-marketing testing of suspected compounds (Lotti and Johnson, 1978). The risk of developing OPIDP from existing insecticides or other products is therefore small (Moretto, 1999). Neuropathic doses of currently used OP insecticides would cause a severe cholinergic syndrome before the possible later onset of OPIDP. Large amounts of poison would have to be ingested to cause OPIDP, and many cases of polyneuropathy diagnosed in the weeks after severe OP poisoning actually represent critical illness neuropathy or myopathy, rather than cases of OPIDP.

By contrast, triaryl phosphates, used as lubricants, hydraulic fluids or plasticizers, have no cholinergic toxicity. Currently used triaryl phosphates no longer contain tri-ortho-cresyl phosphate (TOCP), the original model compound for NTE inhibition (Cavanagh, 1964; Mackerer et al., 1999).

Some OPs and CMs covalently react with NTE but undergo no aging. These compounds produce no OPIDP. When given to rats, they even protect from OPIDP induced by a neuropathic OP provided that 30% of NTE active sites are occupied (Johnson, 1990; Lotti et al., 1993). The loss of NTE catalytic activity is therefore not the mechanism leading to axonal degeneration. Other hypotheses have been proposed, including loss of a non-esterase function of NTE essential for axonal function or a toxic gain-of-function of the phosphorylated and aged NTE (Glynn, 1999).

The molecular events leading to axonal degeneration remain unknown. A deficit in retrograde axonal transport has been shown in hens (Moretto et al., 1987). The retrograde axonal transport is selectively impaired within a few days after neuropathic OP poisoning and reaches its nadir before the onset of OPIDP. However, the cascade of events from NTE inhibition/aging to impaired retrograde axonal transport and axonal degeneration is not well understood.

13.10.2. Clinical findings of OPIDP in man

Thousands of victims of accidental triaryl phosphate, chiefly TOCP, ingestion have occurred worldwide (Senanayake, 1981; Inoue et al., 1988). Currently used triaryl phosphate mixtures contain little or no TOCP. Much less OPIDP cases have been ascribed to

OP insecticide poisoning (recently reviewed by Lotti and Moretto, 2005). Compounds reported to convincingly cause OPIDP in humans include chlorpyrifos (Lotti et al., 1986; Tracy and Gallagher, 1990), dichlorvos (Vasilescu and Florescu, 1980; Vasconcellos et al., 2002; Sevim et al., 2003), mipafox (Bidstrup et al., 1953), isofenfos (Moretto and Lotti, 1998), trichlorfon (Hierons and Johnson, 1978; Vasilescu and Florescu, 1980; Vasilescu et al., 1984), methamidophos (Senanayake and Johnson, 1982; McConnell et al., 1999; Aygun et al., 2003), trichlornate (Jedrzejowska et al., 1980; De Kort et al., 1986), and phosphamidon/mevinphos (Chuang et al., 2002). For a number of other OPs, claims of OPIDP were less convincing, e.g., parathion (de Jager et al., 1981), fenthion (Martinez-Chuecos et al., 1992; Aygun et al., 2003), and malathion (Dive et al., 1994).

A number of cases have been ascribed to the CMs carbaryl, carbofuran and metolcarb (Dickoff et al., 1987; Umehara et al., 1991; Yang et al., 2000). The ingested doses were very high and all patients first suffered a severe cholinergic crisis. Perhaps the effective initial antidotal and supportive treatment during the acute cholinergic crisis allowed a very high level of NTE inhibition in these subjects, similar to what has been observed in animals poisoned with repeated doses that allowed spontaneous AChE reactivation and survival, but caused almost complete NTE inhibition (Lotti et al., 1993).

Symptoms usually appear 2–3 weeks after a single exposure to a neurotoxic OP. The precise interval between exposure and symptoms can be difficult to ascertain in the case of triaryl phosphate poisoning due to the absence of initial cholinergic signs and symptoms. Cramping pain in the legs is followed by distal numbness and paresthesias. Progressive lower limb weakness then ensues and the ankle reflexes are lost. In severe cases, the arms may get affected as well. Patients have mainly flaccid weakness on clinical examination with bilateral foot drop and high stepping gait. Flaccid paralysis of the lower limbs has been seen in severe cases. Objective sensory deficits are less evident in most patients. Pyramidal signs occur later in severe cases, with development of a spastic-ataxic gait (Susser and Stein, 1957; Morgan and Petrovich, 1978). In less severe cases, the peripheral neuropathy may recover rather well, but the sequels of long tract spinal cord involvement rarely remit.

Nerve conduction studies initially show reduced CMAP amplitudes followed by increased distal latencies and slightly reduced conduction velocities. Needle EMG studies reveal an acute distal axonal neuropathy (Lotti et al., 1986; Sevim et al., 2003). Rat nerve biopsies (Jortner et al., 2005) and sural nerve biopsies in patients show distal axonal neuropathy (Shiraishi et al., 1983; Vasilescu et al., 1984; De Kort et al., 1986; Lotti et al.,

1986; Chuang et al., 2002). Using the teased-fiber technique in cat phrenic nerve, Boulding and Cavanagh (1979a, b) observed that the axonal degeneration, initially suspected to begin at the very distal end of the axon, was in fact non-terminal and focal. They suggested that the lesion was due to "chemical transection" inducing a focal distal, but not terminal, axonal lesion, which precipitated Wallerian degeneration. Neuromuscular junctions of TOCP treated cats were not affected at the light microscopic level (Prineas, 1969). Electron microscopic studies of TOCP treated cats and hens revealed osmiophilic bodies that contained degenerated mitochondria, synaptic vesicles and small electron-dense granules in the terminal axoplasmic expansion, but the pre- and postsynaptic membranes were normal. No studies of the endplate AChR were carried out at that time (Prineas, 1969; Abou-Donia, 1981). Examination of human spinal cords revealed degeneration of pyramidal tracts and posterior columns in the lumbosacral segments of the spinal cord (Aring, 1942; Susser and Stein, 1957), consistent with findings in TOCP poisoned hens (Fenthon, 1955; Cavanagh, 1964; Abou-Donia, 1979).

13.11. Noncholinesterase mechanisms of neurotoxicity

There is general agreement that the irreversible inhibition of AChE activity at cholinergic synapses explains the acute OP cholinergic toxicity (Taylor, 2001; Casida and Quistad, 2004). On the other hand, not all toxic effects of OP compounds can be attributed to AChE inhibition. Interaction of OPs with other proteins is proven and may explain inter-individual differences in sensitivity to OP toxicity. These proteins may themselves represent biomarkers of OP exposure and aid in the diagnosis. Some of these proteins may have a therapeutic potential as bioscavengers. The following observations point to additional sites of toxic action:

1. The dissociation between OPIDP induction, caused by inhibition of NTE above a 70% threshold, and the weak or even absent AChE inhibiting effects of some of these same OPs (see Section 13.10.1).
2. The biotinylated OP called FP-biotin causes no cholinergic signs when given to mice. At least 12 proteins are labeled in the mouse plasma, four of them identified as AChE, BuChE, carboxylesterase, and albumin (Peeples et al., 2005).
3. Different OP insecticides cause different degrees of cholinergic toxicity, despite similar levels of erythrocyte AChE inhibition. Toxicologists hypothesize that toxicologically relevant sites other than AChE explain

these observations (Chaudhuri et al., 1993; Pope, 1999; Richards et al., 1999).

4. The AChE knock-out mouse has no AChE activity in any tissue. Nevertheless, this mouse is very sensitive to OP toxicity, indicating non-AChE protein sites to explain this toxicity (Xie et al., 2000; Lockridge et al., 2005). Studies in AChE knock-out mice have shown that AChE$^{-/-}$, mice present the same cholinergic signs of toxicity after nerve agent VX poisoning than wild-type mice. However, wild-type, but not AChE$^{-/-}$, mice were protected by atropine pre-treatment (Duysen et al., 2001). Similar observations were made after exposure to the insecticide DFP (Li et al., 2000), all suggesting that mechanisms not mediated by AChE inhibition must also contribute to acute OP neurotoxicity. BuChE may functionally replace AChE in this knock-out model because the mouse has normal BuChE levels and BuChE is capable of hydrolizing ACh (Casida and Quistad, 2004; Cousin et al., 2005). In this view, BuChE would be the target for OP toxicity in these mice, but this has not been proven thus far.

5. Low doses of OPs cause distinct effects that depend on the compound involved. For example, a low dose of fenthion decreased motor activity in rats by 86%, whereas a low dose of parathion did not affect motor activity but depressed the tail-pinch response, suggesting that targets other than AChE are involved (Moser, 1995).

6. Low levels of chlorpyrifos administered to weanling rats impaired cognitive function without AChE inhibition and without downregulation of central cholinergic receptors (Jett et al., 2001). It was proposed that chlorpyrifos may affect the phosphorylation and function of nuclear transcription factors that govern cell differentiation (Aldridge et al., 2003).

The exact number and role of the proteins that react covalently with a given OP compound is unknown. It appears that the set of OP-reactive proteins is unique for each OP, but almost all OPs react with AChE and BuChE. The importance of a possible toxicological, biomarker and scavenger role of some of these non-esterase proteins remains to be elucidated.

13.12. Role of OPs and CMs in the Gulf War Syndrome

In 1991, Operation Desert Storm was an intense and short ground warfare by US-led coalition forces intent on liberating Kuwait from an Iraqi invasion. During the post-combat period, a number of Iraqi military posts and ammunition depots were destroyed. One such operation included the detonation of nerve gas stores at Khamisiyah, in which there was overwhelming exposure to OP chemical warfare agents. About 35–45% of troops who served in Desert Storm received the CM pyridostigmine bromide (PB), an antidote used for the prevention of soman poisoning. Reports of various health symptoms emerged in veterans shortly after the end of Operation Desert Storm and continue to appear after more than a decade. Complaints were often non-specific and included fatigue, sensory disturbances, musculoskeletal pain, and muscle weakness. The relationship of these multiple complaints now known as the Gulf War Syndrome (GWS) and the exposure to OPs or CMs is still a matter of fierce debate (Rose et al., 2004).

Troops were exposed to numerous potentially harmful factors: extreme temperatures; combat and chemical warfare stress; severe sand storms; insects and insecticides; petrochemicals; oil and ammunition combustion products; depleted uranium; anthrax; and other vaccines. It is therefore difficult to single out the role of PB treatment or OP exposure. Approximately one-half of the soldiers who took PB (30 mg tid; doses far below those used in myasthenia gravis treatment) reported anticholinesterase side effects such as headache, vision disturbances and abdominal cramping. Several epidemiological studies found an association between the side effects while taking PB pills and the likelihood of having GWS complaints later (Haley et al., 1997a). Others found an association between any combination of symptoms during PB intake, even if totally unspecific for PB side effects, and the likelihood of reporting unexplained illness after the war (Spencer et al., 2001). Because singular PB exposure has been rare, several authors have postulated, based on rat studies, interaction of several psychological and toxicological factors to explain the GWS (Abou-Donia et al., 1996, 2001; McCain et al., 1997).

Several studies have reported an increased incidence of amyotrophic lateral sclerosis (ALS) in Gulf War veterans (Haley, 2003; Horner et al., 2003). Haley found an increase from 0.93 cases/year in 1991 to 1.57 cases/year in 1998 in veterans younger than age 45. The absolute number of cases remains low, however, and no further rise in ALS incidence in Gulf War veterans has been observed. The small number of ALS cases precludes the possibility of showing a causal relation of these cases to PB or OP exposure (Rose, 2003). A recent prospective study found an increased risk of ALS in military personnel independent of the branch of service and the time served (Weisskopf et al., 2005). Studies of peripheral nerve involvement in Gulf War veterans have mostly been negative (Sharief et al., 2002; Davis et al., 2004).

More than 15 years after the Gulf War, the precise etiology of the vague complaints of a large number of veterans remains unexplained. The lack of objective exposure data, the confounding of multiple associated health risk factors as outlined above, and the variability in the subjective and objective clinical data will probably preclude a definite conclusion on a possible role of OP or CM chemicals. But in the wake of this GWS experience, additional advisory panels on the health risks of low-dose OP and CM exposure in warfare and measures to improve surveillance during military deployments have been put in place (Research Advisory Committee on Gulf War Veterans' Illnesses, 2004. Scientific progress in understanding Gulf War Veterans' illnesses: Report and recommendations. Available at www.ngwrc.org).

13.13. Therapeutic management of OP pesticide poisoning

13.13.1. Chemical and toxicodynamic factors influence onset and duration of poisoning

Most OP insecticides are lipophilic and are rapidly absorbed after ingestion or inhalation. Dermal absorption is usually slow but may be prolonged. Several factors including dose and time of exposure, the lipophilicity of the compound involved, and the presence of solvents or emulsifiers in the formulation can facilitate further absorption. Following absorption, the OPs accumulate in fat, liver, kidneys and salivary glands. Fat storage is very variable between different OPs. The phosphorothioates (P = S), such as parathion and diazinon, are much more lipophilic than phosphates (P = O). Extensive fat storage may result in prolonged recirculation of the AChE inhibitor, resulting in clinical cholinergic relapse after an initial recovery. Phosphates are biologically active, whereas phosphorothioates need to be transformed to their active oxon metabolite to become biologically active. This process of oxidative desulfuration is mediated by P450 isoforms and a number of other reactions. Clearly, a number of chemical and other parameters strongly determine the speed of onset and the duration of cholinergic features. These toxicodynamic factors also determine in part why oxime therapy is more effective for poisoning by some OPs than by others.

13.13.2. Diagnosis and assessment of severity of poisoning

In patients with a history of accidental or suicidal OP intake, cholinergic signs, and a typical odor of the breath, the diagnosis of cholinesterase inhibitor intoxication is easy to make. In some patients, coma may have developed, precluding history taking, or the patients may present with heart block or seizures. A high index of suspicion is the key to a fast diagnosis. Clinical features are more useful than laboratory parameters to determine severity of the intoxication and its initial prognosis.

The diagnosis is confirmed by measuring red blood cell AChE and plasma BuChE (see Section 13.7.2). Quantitative determination of the pesticide or its metabolite in body fluids is available for some OPs and in some laboratories, but is much slower and has little place in the early diagnosis and management of suspected OP poisoned patients.

13.13.3. General measures on admission

1. Removal of patient from the contaminated environment.
2. Decontamination.
3. Gastric lavage has no evidence-based proven value. A single dose of activated charcoal is often used within 1 h of ingestion.
4. Establish airway; remove secretions and vomit from mouth; intubate trachea when necessary.
5. Restore circulation and heart rate >50 beats per min. Establish venous access, support blood pressure with catecholamines. Treat arrhythmias.
6. Monitor level of consciousness. Treat convulsions with IV diazepam.

13.13.4. Atropine

Atropine competes with ACh for a common binding site on the muscarinic receptors. Apart from its antagonistic action at muscarinic binding sites, atropine has also been effective in the treatment of dystonia during the acute cholinergic phase (Smith, 1977; Joubert et al., 1984; Joubert and Joubert, 1988). The efficacy of atropine has been convincingly demonstrated in animals (Sanderson, 1961; Lekeux et al., 1986). Although clinical efficacy in patients is beyond doubt (Namba et al., 1971; DuToit et al., 1981; Bardin et al., 1987; Senanayake and Karalliedde, 1987; Zilker and Hibler, 1996), no controlled studies have been published.

Atropine sulphate, 2 mg IV (0.02–0.1 mg/kg in children), is administered as soon as possible in patients with increased secretions. Fast repeated dosing may be necessary in severely poisoned patients, sometimes up to a total dose of 100 mg. The dose is titrated according to bronchorrhea and bronchospasm. The degree of atropinization is determined by the amount of tracheobronchial secretions, pupil size and heart rate, with the quantity of secretions being the most reliable measure (DuToit et al., 1981; Bardin et al., 1987). The quaternary ammonium compound glycopyrrolate is an alternative anti-muscarinic agent when atropine is not tolerated (Nisse et al., 1998).

13.13.5. Oximes

The action of oximes is to reactivate AChE inhibited by OPs, before the phosphorylated complex undergoes aging (see also Section 13.4.3). Aged enzyme reactivates neither spontaneously nor by oxime treatment. BuChE is reactivated more slowly than AChE (Hobbiger, 1963; Worek et al., 1999). The pyridinium oximes PAM and obidoxime are most frequently used in civil medicine (Eyer, 2003). Traditionally, PAM salts have been used in English-speaking countries and France, and obidoxime has been the first choice in German-speaking countries. The Hagedorn oximes, e.g., HI-6, are used in warfare nerve agent (especially soman) protection (Kusic et al., 1991; Dawson, 1994). It is assumed that the beneficial effects of oximes are confined to peripheral nicotinic sites and that CNS effects are clinically insignificant (Bismuth et al., 1992). Therefore, the main benefit is for neuromuscular transmission, with little effect on parasympathetic symptoms and signs, such as bronchorrhea, rhinorrhea and bronchoconstriction, and there are no proven CNS effects (Singh et al., 1998a). Besser et al. (1995) studied six OP poisoned patients treated with obidoxime. Dramatic electrophysiologic improvement, assessed by single and repetitive nerve stimulation, was seen in the three patients who received the drug within the first 12 h of intoxication. These patients had less weakness, but their overall clinical status was not uniformly improved. Plasma BuChE activity did not predict the oxime effect on neuromuscular transmission. Oximes are contraindicated in patients with myasthenia gravis, as they may precipitate a myasthenic crisis (Bismuth et al., 1992). Apart from their main action as AChE reactivators, animal studies have provided evidence of other effects of oximes, including direct interaction with the nicotinic ACh receptor complex (van Helden et al., 1996). The mechanism of these alternative actions is not understood.

A number of dosing schemes are used in different centers. Based on some studies, 2-PAMCl or P2S 30 mg/kg is administered as an intravenous loading dose as soon as possible after exposure. An intravenous maintenance dose of 8–10 mg/kg/h is then continued until persistent and complete clinical neuromuscular recovery is achieved and the atropine has been stopped (Willems and Belpaire, 1992; Willems et al., 1993).

The clinical effectiveness of oxime therapy has been challenged (De Silva et al., 1992; Eddleston et al., 2002b). De Silva found the same 29% mortality rate in 21 patients treated with atropine alone and in 24 patients treated with 2-PAMCl and atropine. Adequate dosing of the oxime and the differential reactivating capacity of oximes in poisoning with different OPs may limit the conclusions drawn from this study. Animal studies have yielded convincing evidence that AChE inhibited by dimethoxy and diethoxy OPs can be reactivated by oximes (Food and Agriculture Organization/World Health Organization, 1993, 1994). Human case reports and small series are more difficult to interpret. Willems et al. (1993) found that ethyl-parathion and methyl-parathion poisoning could be treated effectively with 2-PAM and atropine provided that the concentration of pesticide circulating in plasma was low. In severe poisoning, even high doses of PAM gave no clinical benefit. A similar dose-related effect was found by Thiermann et al. (1997) in parathion poisoned patients treated with obidoxime and atropine. In dimethoate poisoning, omethoate-inhibited enzyme could not be reactivated by high dose PAM treatment (Willems et al., 1993). Differential reactivating capacity with different OPs, the severity of the poisoning, oxime dose regimens and treatment duration, and the time elapsed between the onset of the poisoning and the start of the oxime treatment are key factors limiting the interpretation of the human data (Buckley et al., 2005). Further studies are desperately needed to clarify these issues.

13.13.6. Anticonvulsants

Intravenous diazepam is the most studied and most widely used therapy for OP induced convulsions with midazolam as a more recent alternative (Karalliedde and Szinicz, 2001). The effect of diazepam on fasciculations is not clear. The effectiveness of midazolam on persistent soman induced seizures has been demonstrated in pigs (Capacio et al., 2005).

References

Abou-Donia MB (1979). Delayed neurotoxicity of phenyl-phosphonothioate esters. Science 205: 713–715.

Abou-Donia MB (1981). Organophosphorus ester-induced delayed neurotoxicity. Ann Rev Pharmacol Toxicol 21: 511–548.

Abou-Donia MB, Lapadula DM (1990). Mechanisms of organophosphorus ester-induced delayed neurotoxicity: type 1 and type 2. Ann Rev Pharmacol Toxicol 30: 405–440.

Abou-Donia MB, Wilmarth KR, Jensen KF, et al. (1996). Neurotoxicity resulting from coexposure to pyridostigmine bromide, DEET, and permethrin: implications of Gulf War chemical exposures. J Toxicol Environ Health 48: 35–56.

Abou-Donia MB, Goldstein LB, Jones KH, et al. (2001). Locomotor and sensorimotor performance deficit in rats following exposure to pyridostigmine bromide, DEET, and permethrin, alone and in combination. Toxicol Sci 60: 305–314.

Ahlgren JD, Manz HJ, Harvey JC (1979). Myopathy of chronic organophosphate poisoning. A clinical entity? South Med J 72: 555–563.

Albuquerque EX, Akaike A, Shaw K-P, et al. (1984). The interaction of anticholinesterase agents with the acetylcholine receptor–ionic channel complex. Fundam Appl Toxicol 4: S27–S33.

Albuquerque EX, Deshpande SS, Kawabuchi M, et al. (1985). Multiple actions of anticholinesterase agents on chemosensitive synapses: molecular basis for prophylaxis and treatment of organophosphate poisoning. Fundam Appl Toxicol 5: S182–S203.

Albuquerque EX, Allen CN, Aracava Y, et al. (1986). Activation and inhibition of the nicotinic receptor: actions of physostigmine, pyridostigmine and meproadifen. In: I Hanin (Ed.), Dynamics of Cholinergic Function. Plenum, New York, pp. 677–695.

Albuquerque EX, Aracava Y, Idriss M, et al. (1987). Activation and blockade of the nicotinic and glutamatergic synapses by reversible and irreversible cholinesterase inhibitors. In: NJ Dun and E Perlman (Eds.), Neurobiology of Acetylcholine. Plenum, New York, pp. 301–328.

Albuquerque EX, Alkondon M, Deshpande SS, et al. (1988). Molecular interactions of organophosphates (OPs), oximes and carbamates at nicotinic receptors. In: T Narahashi and E Chambers (Eds.), Insecticide Action: From Molecule to Organism. Plenum, New York, pp. 33–53.

Aldridge JE, Seidler FJ, Meyer A, et al. (2003). Serotonergic systems targeted by developmental exposure to chlorpyrifos: effects during different critical periods. Environ Health Perspect 111: 1736–1743.

Aldridge WN, Reiner E (1972). Enzyme Inhibitors as Substrates. Interactions of Esterases with Esters of Organophosphorus and Carbamic Acids. North Holland, New York.

Anderson DR, Harris LW, Lennox WJ, et al. (1991). Effects of subacute pretreatment with carbamate together with acute adjunct pretreatment against nerve agent exposure. Drug Chem Toxicol 14: 1–19.

Ariëns AT, Meeter E, Wolthuis OL, et al. (1969). Reversible necrosis at the end-plate region in striated muscles of the rat poisoned with cholinesterase inhibitors. Experientia 25: 57–59.

Aring CD (1942). The systemic nervous affinita of triorthocresylphosphate. Brain 65: 34–47.

Ashon Y, Radic Z, Tsigelny I, et al. (1995). Amino acid residues controlling reactivation of organophosphonyl conjugates of acetylcholinesterase by mono- and bisquaternary oximes. J Biol Chem 270: 6370–6380.

Augustinsson KB (1971). Determination of activity of cholinesterases. Methods Biochem Anal 19: 217–273.

Averbook BJ, Anderson RJ (1983). Electrophysiological changes associated with chronic administration of organophosphates. Arch Toxicol 52: 167–172.

Aygun D, Onar MK, Alintop BL (2003). The clinical and electrophysiological features of a delayed polyneuropathy developing subsequently after acute organophosphate poisoning and its correlation with the serum acetylcholinesterase. Electromyogr Clin Neurophysiol 43: 421–427.

Baker DJ, Sedgwick ME (1996). Single fibre electromyographic changes in man after organophosphate exposure. Hum Exp Toxicol 15: 369–375.

Bardin PG, Van Eeden SF, Joubert JR (1987). Intensive care management of acute organophosphate poisoning. A 7-year experience in the western Cape. S Afr Med J 72: 593–597.

Benslama A, Moutaouakkil S (1998). Syndrome intermédiaire lors d'une intoxication aigue par la malathion. Presse Méd 27: 713–715.

Benson B, Tolo D, McIntire M (1992). Is the intermediate syndrome in organophosphate poisoning the result of insufficient oxime therapy? Clin Toxicol 30: 347–349.

Besser R, Gutmann L, Dillmann U, et al. (1989a). End-plate dysfunction in acute organophosphate intoxication. Neurology 39: 561–567.

Besser R, Gutmann L, Weilemann LS (1989b). Inactivation of end-plate acetylcholinesterase during the course of organophosphate intoxications. Arch Toxicol 63: 412–415.

Besser R, Vogt T, Gutmann L, et al. (1992). Impaired neuromuscular transmission during partial inhibition of acetylcholinesterase: the role of stimulus-induced backfiring in the generation of the decrement-increment phenomenon. Muscle Nerve 15: 1072–1080.

Besser R, Weilemann LS, Gutmann L (1995). Efficacy of obidoxime in human organophosphorus poisoning: determination by neuromuscular transmission studies. Muscle Nerve 18: 15–22.

Betrosian A, Balla M, Kafiri G, et al. (1995). Multiple systems organ failure from organophosphate poisoning. Clin Toxicol 33: 257–260.

Bidstrup PL, Bonnell JA, Beckett AG (1953). Paralysis following poisoning by a new organic phosphorus insecticide (Mipafox): report on two cases. Br Med J 1: 1068–1072.

Bismuth C, Inns RH, Marrs TC (1992). Efficacy, toxicity and clinical use of oximes in anticholinesterase poisoning. In: B Ballantyne and TC Marrs (Eds.), Clinical and Experimental Toxicology of Organophosphates and Carbamates. Butterworth-Heinemann, Oxford, pp. 555–577.

Bouldin TW, Cavanagh JB (1979a). A fine-structural study of the early stages of axonal degeneration. Am J Pathol 94: 253–270.

Bouldin TW, Cavanagh JB (1979b). A teased-fiber study of the spatio-temporal spread of axonal degeneration. Am J Pathol 94: 241–251.

Bowman WC, Gibb AS, Harvey AC, et al. (1986). Prejunctional actions of cholinoceptor agonists, and of anticholinesterase drugs. In: DA Kharkevic (Ed.), New Neuromuscular Blocking Agents. Springer-Verlag, Berlin, Heidelberg, New York, pp. 141–170.

Brahmi N, Gueye PN, Thabet H, et al. (2004). Extrapyramidal syndrome as a delayed and reversible complication of acute dichlorvos organophosphate poisoning. Vet Hum Toxicol 46: 187–203.

Brimblecombe RW, Green DM, Stratton JA, et al. (1970). The protective actions of some anticholinesterase drugs in sarin poisoning. Br J Pharmacol 9: 822–830.

Bryk B, Moyal-Segal LB, Podoly E, et al. (2005). Inherited and acquired interactions between ACHE and PON1 polymorphisms modulate plasma acetylcholinesterase and paraoxonase activities. J Neurochem 92: 1216–1227.

Buckley NA, Roberts D, Eddleston M (2004). Overcoming apathy in research on organophosphate poisoning. Br Med J 329: 1231–1233.

Buckley NA, Eddleston M, Szinicz L (2005). Oximes for acute organophosphate pesticide poisoning. Cochrane Collaboration 2: 1–13.

Capacio BR, Byers CE, Merk KA, et al. (2005). Pharmacokinetic studies of intramuscular midazolam in guinea pigs challenged with soman. Drug Chem Toxicol 27: 95–110.

Casida JE, Quistad GB (2004). Organophosphate toxicology: safety aspects of nonacetylcholinesterase secondary targets. Chem Res Toxicol 17: 983–998.

Cavanagh JB (1964). The significance of the "dying-back" process in experimental and human neurological disease. Int Rev Exp Path 3: 219.

Chang CC, Hong SJ, Ko JL (1986). Mechanisms of the inhibition by neostigmine of tetanic contraction in the mouse diaphragm. Br J Pharmacol 87: 757–762.

Chaudhuri J, Chakraborti TK, Chanda S, et al. (1993). Differential modulation of organophosphate-sensitive muscarinic receptors in rat brain by parathion and chlorpyrifos. J Biochem Toxicol 8: 207–216.

Choi P-L, Quinonez L (1998). The use of glycopyrrolate in a case of intermediate syndrome following acute organophosphate poisoning. Can J Anaesth 45: 337–340.

Chuang CC, Lin TS, Tsai MC (2002). Delayed neuropathy and myelopathy after organophosphate intoxication. N Engl J Med 347: 1119–1121.

Clarman M, Geldmacher-von Mallinckradt M (1966). Über eine erfolgreich behandelte akute orale Vergiftung durch Fenthion und dessen Nachweis in Mageninhalt und Harn. Archiv Für Toxikol 22: 2–11.

Clinton ME, Dettbarn W (1987). Prevention of phospholine-induced myopathy with d-tubocurarine, atropine sulfate, diazepam, and creatine phosphate. J Toxicol Environ Health 21: 435–444.

Costa LG, McDonald BE, Murphy SD, et al. (1990). Serum paraoxonase and its influence on paraoxon and chlorpyrifos-oxon toxicity in rats. Toxicol Appl Pharmacol 103: 66–76.

Costa LG, Cole TB, Furlong CE (2003a). Polymorphisms of paraoxonase (PON1) and their significance in clinical toxicology of organophosphates. J Toxicol Clin Toxicol 41: 37–45.

Costa LG, Cole TB, Jarvik GP, et al. (2003b). Functional genomics of the paraoxonase (PON1) polymorphisms: effect on pesticide sensitivity, cardiovascular disease and drug metabolism. Annu Rev Med 54: 371–392.

Costa LG, Cole TB, Vitalone A, et al. (2005). Measurement of paraoxonase (PON1) status as potential biomarker of susceptibility to organophosphate toxicity. Clin Chem Acta 352: 37–47.

Cousin X, Strahle U, Chatonnet A (2005). Are there non-catalytic functions of acetylcholinesterases? Lessons from mutant animal models. Bioassays 27: 189–200.

Cygler M, Schrag JD, Sussman JL, et al. (1993). Relationship between sequence conservation and three-dimensional structure in a large family of esterases, lipases, and related enzymes. Protein Sci 2: 366–382.

Davies JE, Barquet A, Freed VH, et al. (1975). Human pesticide poisonings by a fat-soluble organophosphate insecticide. Arch Environ Health 30: 608–613.

Davis LE, Eisen A, Murphy FM, et al. (2004). Clinical and laboratory assessment of distal peripheral nerves in Gulf War veterans and spouses. Neurology 63: 1070–1077.

Dawson RM (1994). Review of oximes available for treatment of nerve agent poisoning. J Appl Toxicol 14: 317–331.

de Blaquiere GE, Waters L, Blain P, et al. (2000). Electrophysiological and biochemical effects of single and multiple doses of the organophosphate Diazinon in the mouse. Toxicol Appl Pharmacol 166: 81–91.

De Bleecker JL (1992). Transient opsoclonus in organophosphate poisoning. Acta Neurol Scand 86: 529–531.

De Bleecker J, Willems J, De Reuck J, et al. (1991). Histological and histochemical study of paraoxon myopathy in the rat. Acta Neurol Belg 91: 255–270.

De Bleecker J, Van Den Neucker K, Willems J (1992a). The intermediate syndrome in organophosphate poisoning: presentation of a case and review of the literature. Clin Toxicol 30: 321–329.

De Bleecker J, Vogelaers D, Ceuterick C, et al. (1992b). Intermediate syndrome due to prolonged parathion poisoning. Acta Neurol Scand 86: 421–424.

De Bleecker J, Willems J, Van Den Neucker K, et al. (1992c). Prolonged toxicity with intermediate syndrome after combined parathion and methyl parathion poisoning. Clin Toxicol 30: 333–345.

De Bleecker JL, De Reuck JL, Willems JL (1992d). Neurological aspects of organophosphate poisoning. Clin Neurol Neurosurg 94: 93–103.

De Bleecker JL, Van Den Abeele KG, De Reuck JL (1992e). Variable involvement of rat skeletal muscles in paraoxon-induced necrotizing myopathy. Res Commun Pathol Pharmacol 75: 309–322.

De Bleecker J, Van Den Neucker K, Colardyn F (1993). Intermediate syndrome in organophosphorus poisoning: a prospective study. Crit Care Med 21: 1706–1711.

De Bleecker J, Lison D, Van Den Abeele K, et al. (1994a). Acute and subacute organophosphate poisoning in the rat. Neurotoxicol 15: 341–348.

De Bleecker JL, Van Den Abeele KG, De Reuck JL (1994b). Electromyography in relation to end-plate acetylcholinesterase in rats poisoned by different organophosphates. Neurotoxicol 15: 331–340.

De Bleecker JL, Meire VI, Pappens S (1998). Quinidine prevents paraoxon-induced necrotizing myopathy in rats. Neurotoxicol 19: 833–838.

de Clermont Ph (1854). Note sur la préparation de quelques éthers (Séance du lundi 14 août 1854). C R 39: 338–340.

de Clermont Ph (1855). Mémoire sur les éthers phosphoriques. Ann Chim Phys 44: 330–336.

de Jager AE, van Weerden TW, Houthoff HJ, et al. (1981). Polyneuropathy after massive exposure to parathion. Neurology 31: 603–605.

De Kort WLAM, Savelkoul TFJ, Sindram JW, et al. (1986). "Delayed neurotoxicity" na intoxicatie met organofosforverbindingen. Ned Tijdschr Geneeskd 130: 1896–1898.

De Reuck J, Willems J (1975). Acute parathion poisoning: myopathic changes in the diaphragm. J Neurol 208: 309–314.

De Reuck J, Colardyn F, Willems J (1979). Fatal encephalopathy in acute poisoning with organophosphorus insecticides. A clinico-pathologic study of two cases. Clin Neurol Neurosurg 81: 247–254.

De Silva HJ, Wijewickrema R, Senanayake N (1992). Does pralidoxime affect outcome of management in acute organophosphorus poisoning? Lancet 339: 1136–1138.

De Wilde V, Vogelaers D, Colardyn F, et al. (1991). Postsynaptic neuromuscular dysfunction in organophosphate induced intermediate syndrome. Klin Wochenschr 69: 177–183.

Dean G, Coxon J, Brereton D (1967). Poisoning by an organophosphorus compound: a case report. S A Med J 41: 1017–1019.

Deana A, Scuka M (1990). Time course of neostigmine action on the endplate response. Neurosci Lett 118: 82–84.

Dekleva A, Sket D, Sketelj J, et al. (1989). Attenuation of soman-induced lesions of skeletal muscle by acetylcholinesterase reactivating and non-reactivating antidotes. Acta Neuropathol 79: 183–189.

Dettbarn W-D (1984). Pesticide induced muscle necrosis: mechanisms and prevention. Fund Appl Toxicol 4: S18–S26.

Dickoff DJ, Gerber O, Turovsky Z (1987). Delayed neurotoxicity after ingestion of carbamate pesticide. Neurology 37: 1229–1231.

Dive A, Mathieu R, Van Binst R, et al. (1994). Unusual manifestations after malathion poisoning. Hum Exp Toxicol 13: 271–274.

Dongren Y, Tao L, Fengsheng H (1999). Electroneurophysiological studies in rats of acute dimethoate poisoning. Toxicol Lett 107: 249–254.

DuToit PW, Muller FO, van Tonder WM, et al. (1981). Experience with the intensive care management of organophosphate insecticide poisoning. S Afr Med J 60: 227–229.

Duysen EG, Li B, Xie W, et al. (2001). Evidence for nonacetylcholinesterase targets of organophosphorus nerve agent: supersensitivity of acetylcholinesterase knockout mouse to VX lethality. J Pharmacol Exp Ther 299: 528–535.

Eccles JC, McFarlane WV (1949). Actions of anticholinesterase on end plate potential of frog muscle. J Neurophysiol 12: 59.

Eddleston M, Karalliedde L, Buckley N, et al. (2002a). Pesticide poisoning in the developing world—a minimum pesticide list. Lancet 360: 1163–1167.

Eddleston M, Szinicz L, Eyer P, et al. (2002b). Oximes in acute organophosphorus pesticide poisoning: a systematic review of clinical trials. QJM 95: 275–283.

Ellman GL, Courtney KD, Andres V, et al. (1961). A new and rapid colorimetric determination of acetylcholinesterase activity. Biochem Pharmacol 7: 88–95.

Engel AG, Lambert EH, Gomez MR (1977). A new myasthenic syndrome with end-plate acetylcholinesterase deficiency, small nerve terminals, and reduced acetylcholine release. Ann Neurol 1: 315–330.

Evans RT (1986). Cholinesterase phenotyping: clinical aspects and laboratory applications. CRC Crit Rev Clin Lab Sci 23: 35–64.

Eyer P (2003). The role of oximes in the management of organophosphorus pesticide poisoning. Toxicol Rev 22: 165–190.

Fenichel GM, Kibler WB, Olson WH, et al. (1972). Chronic inhibition of cholinesterase as a cause of myopathy. Neurology 22: 1026–1033.

Fenichel GM, Dettbarn W-D, Newman TM (1974a). An experimental myopathy secondary to excessive acetylcholine release. Neurology 24: 41–45.

Fenichel GM, Kibler WB, Dettbarn W-D (1974b). The effects of immobilization and exercise on acetylcholine-mediated myopathies. Neurology 24: 1086–1090.

Fenthon JCB (1955). The nature of the paralysis in chickens following organophosphorus poisoning. J Pathol Bacteriol 69: 181–189.

Firemark H, Barlow CF, Roth LJ (1964). The penetration of 2-PAMCl into brain and the effects of cholinesterase inhibitors on its transport. J Pharmacol Exp Ther 145: 252–265.

Food and Agriculture Organization/World Health Organization (1993). WHO/PCS/93.34, Pesticide Residues in Food: 1992 Evaluations. Part II—Toxicology. World Health Organization, Geneva.

Food and Agriculture Organization/World Health Organization (1994). WHO/PCS/94.4, Pesticide Residues in Food: 1993 Evaluations. Part II—Toxicology. World Health Organization, Geneva.

Forbat JN, Skehan JD (1992). Health effects of organophosphate sheep dips. Br Med J 305: 1503.

Frederikssons T (1957). Pharmacological properties of methyl-fluorophosphoryl cholines. Two synthetic cholinergic drugs. Arch Int Pharmacodyn 113: 101–113.

Frederikssons T (1958). Further studies on fluorophosphorylcholines. Pharmacological properties of two new analogues. Arch Int Pharmacodyn 115: 474–482.

Froede HC, Wilson IB (1984). Direct determination of acetyl-enzyme intermediate in the acetylcholinesterase-catalyzed hydrolysis of acetylcholine and acetylthiocholine. J Cell Biochem 259: 11010–11013.

Gadoth N, Fisher A (1978). Late onset of neuromuscular block in organophosphorus poisoning. Ann Intern Med 88: 654–655.

Gan KN, Smolen AL, Eckerson HW, et al. (1991). Purification of human serum paraoxonase/arylesterase. Evidence for one esterase catalyzing both activities. Drug Metab Dispos 19: 100–106.

Glynn P (1999). Neuropathy target esterase. Biochem J 344: 625–631.

Gordon JJ, Leadbeater L, Maidment MP (1978). The protection of animals against organophosphate poisoning by pretreatment with a carbamate. Toxicol Appl Pharmacol 43: 207–216.

Grob D (1963). Anticholinesterase intoxication in man and its treatment. In: GB Koelle (Ed.), Cholinesterases and Anticholinesterase Agents. Springer-Verlag, Berlin, Gottingen, Heidelberg, pp. 989–1027.

Guadarrama-Naveda M, de Cabrera LC, Matos-Bastidas S (2001). Intermediate syndrome secondary to ingestion of chlorpiriphos. Vet Hum Toxicol 43: 34.

Gupta A, Agarwal R, Shukla GS (1999). Functional impairment of blood–brain barrier following pesticide exposure during early development in rats. Hum Exp Toxicol 18: 174–179.

Gupta RC, Patterson G, Dettbarn W-D (1986). Mechanisms of toxicity and tolerance to diisopropylphosphorofluoridate at the neuromuscular junction of the rat. Toxicol Appl Pharmacol 84: 541–550.

Haley RW (2003). Excess incidence of ALS in young Gulf War veterans. Neurology 61: 750–756.

Haley RW, Hom J, Roland PS, et al. (1997a). Evaluation of neurologic function in Gulf War veterans. A blinded case-control study. JAMA 277: 223–230.

Haley RW, Kurt TL, Horn J (1997b). Is there a Gulf War Syndrome? Searching for syndromes by factor analysis of symptoms. JAMA 277: 215–222.

Harel M, Sussman JL, Krejci E, et al. (1992). Conversion of acetylcholinesterase to butyrylcholinesterase, modeling and mutagenesis. Proc Natl Acad Sci U S A 89: 10827–10831.

Harris LW, Talbot BG, Lennox WJ, et al. (1989). The relationship between oxime-induced reactivation of carbamylated acetylcholinesterase and antidotal efficacy against carbamate intoxication. Toxicol Appl Pharmacol 98: 128–133.

Hasin Y, Avidan N, Bercovich D, et al. (2004). A paradigm for single nucleotide polymorphism analysis: the case of the acetylcholinesterase gene. Hum Mutat 24: 408–416.

Hata S, Bernstein E, Davis LE (1986). Atypical ocular bobbing in acute organophosphate poisoning. Arch Neurol 43: 185–186.

He F, Xu H, Qin F, et al. (1998). Intermediate myasthenia syndrome following acute organophosphates poisoning—an analysis of 21 cases. Hum Exp Toxicol 17: 40–45.

Hena S, Finkelman J (1993). De plaguicidas y salud en las Americas Centro Panamericano de Ecologia Humana y Salud, Mexico.

Hierons R, Johnson MK (1978). Clinical and toxicological investigation of a case of delayed neuropathy in man after acute poisoning by an organophosphorus pesticide. Arch Toxicol 40: 279–284.

Hobbiger F (1963). Reactivation of phosphorylated AChE. Handbuch der Experimentellen Pharmakologie. Springer-Verlag, Berlin, pp. 921–988.

Horner RD, Kamins KG, Feussner JR, et al. (2003). Occurrence of amyotrophic lateral sclerosis among Gulf War veterans. Neurology 61: 742–749.

Hudson CS, Foster RE (1984). Presynaptic effects of pyridostigmine on the neuro-muscular junction of the rat diaphragm. J Cell Biochem 99: 29.

Hudson CS, Foster RE, Kahng MW (1985). Neuromuscular toxicity of pyridostigmine-bromide in the diaphragm, extensor digitorum longus, and soleus muscles of the rat. Fund Appl Toxicol 5: 260–269.

Idriss MK, Aguayo LG, Rickett DL, et al. (1986). Organophosphate and carbamate compounds have pre- and postjunctional effects at the insect glutamatergic synapse. J Pharmacol Exp Ther 239: 279–285.

Inns RH, Marrs TC (1992). Prophylaxis against anticholinesterase poisoning. In: B Ballantyne and TC Marrs (Eds.), Clinical and Experimental Toxicology of Organophosphates and Carbamates. Butterworth-Heinemann, Oxford, pp. 602–610.

Inns RH, Tuckwell NJ, Bright JE, et al. (1990). Histochemical demonstration of calcium accumulation in muscle fibres after experimental organophosphate poisoning. Hum Exp Toxicol 9: 245–250.

Inoue N, Fujishiro K, Mori K, et al. (1988). Triorthocresyl phosphate poisoning. A review of human cases. J UOEH 10: 433–442.

Jedrzejowska H, Rowinska-Marcinska K, Hoppe B (1980). Neuropathy due to phytosol (Agritox). Report of a case. Acta Neuropathol 49: 163–168.

Jett DA, Navoa RV, Beckles RA, et al. (2001). Cognitive function and cholinergic neurochemistry in weanling rats exposed to chlorpyrifos. Toxicol Appl Pharmacol 174: 89–98.

Jeyaratnam J, De Alwis Senewiratne RS, Copplestone JF (1982). Survey of pesticide poisoning in Sri Lanka. Bulletin of the World Health Organisation 60: 615–619.

Johnson MK (1975). The delayed neuropathy caused by some organophosphate esters: mechanisms and challenge. Crit Rev Toxicol 3: 289–316.

Johnson MK (1990). Organophosphates and delayed neuropathy. Is NTE alive and well? Toxicol Appl Pharmacol 102: 385–399.

Jortner BS, Hancock SK, Hinckley J, et al. (2005). Neuropathological studies of rats following multiple exposure to tri-ortho-tolyl phosphate, chlorpyrifos and stress. Toxicol Pathol 33: 378–385.

Joubert J, Joubert PH (1988). Chorea and psychiatric changes in organophosphate poisoning. S Afr Med J 74: 32–34.

Joubert J, Joubert PH, van der Spuy M, et al. (1984). Acute organophosphate poisoning presenting with choreoathetosis. J Toxicol Clin Toxicol 22: 187–191.

Karademir M, Ertürk F, Koçak R (1990). Two cases of organophosphate poisoning with development of intermediate syndrome. Hum Exp Toxicol 9: 187–189.

Karalliedde L, Szinicz L (2001). Management of organophosphorus compound poisoning. In: L Karalliedde, S Feldman, J Henry et al. (Eds.), Organophosphates and Health. Imperial College Press, London, pp. 257–293.

Karalliedde L, Senanayake N, Ariaratnam A (1988). Acute organophosphorus insecticide poisoning during pregnancy. Hum Toxicol 7: 363–364.

Kawabuchi M, Boyne AF, Deshpande SS, et al. (1988). Enantiomer (+)physostigmine prevents organophosphate-induced subjunctional damage at the neuromuscular synapse by a mechanism not related to cholinesterase carbamylation. Synapse 2: 139–147.

Kawabuchi M, Boyne AF, Desphande AF, et al. (1989). The reversible carbamate, (−)physostigmine, reduces the size of synaptic end plate lesions induced by sarin, an irreversible organophosphate. Toxicol Appl Pharmacol 97: 98–106.

Kiderlen D, Worek F, Klimmek R, et al. (2000). The phosphoryl oxime-destroying activity of human plasma. Arch Toxicol 74: 27–32.

Kilby BA, Kilby M (1947). The toxicity of alkyl fluorophosphorates in man and animals. Br J Pharmacol 2: 234–240.

Kovarik Z, Radic Z, Berman HA, et al. (2003). Acetylcholinesterase active centre and gorge conformations analysed by combination mutations and enantiomeric phosphonates. Biochem J 373: 33–40.

Kusic R, Jovanovic D, Randjelovic S, et al. (1991). HI-6 in man: efficacy of the oxime in poisoning by organophosphorus insecticides. Hum Exp Toxicol 10: 113–118.

Lai MW, Moen M (2005). Pesticide-like poisoning from a prescription drug. N Engl J Med 353: 317–318.

Laskowski MB, Dettbarn W-D (1979). An electrophysiological analysis of the effects of paraoxon at the neuromuscular junction. J Pharmacol Exp Ther 210: 269–274.

Lekeux P, Kyavu A, Clercx C, et al. (1986). Pulmonary function changes induced by experimental dichlorvos toxicosis in calves. Res Vet Sci 40: 318–321.

Leonard JP, Salpeter MM (1979). Agonist-induced myopathy at the neuromuscular junction is mediated by calcium. J Cell Biol 82: 811–819.

Li B, Stribley JA, Ticu A, et al. (2000). Abundant tissue butyrylcholinesterase and its possible function in the acetylcholinesterase knockout mouse. J Neurochem 75: 1320–1331.

Lockridge O, Masson P (2000). Pesticides and susceptible populations: people with butyrylcholinesterase genetic variants may be at risk. Neurotoxicology 21: 113–126.

Lockridge O, Duysen EG, Voelker T, et al. (2005). Life without acetylcholinesterase: the implications of cholinesterase inhibitor toxicity in AChE-knockout mice. Environ Toxicol Pharmacol 19: 463–469.

Loewenstein-Lichtenstein Y, Schwartz M, Glick D, et al. (1995). Genetic predisposition to adverse conditions of anti-cholinesterases in "atypical" BCHE. Nature Med 1: 1082–1085.

Lotti M (1992). The pathogenesis of organophosphate delayed polyneuropathy. Crit Rev Toxicol 21: 465–487.

Lotti M, Johnson MK (1978). Neurotoxicity of organophosphorus pesticides: predictions can be based on in vitro studies with hen and human enzymes. Arch Toxicol 41: 215–221.

Lotti M, Moretto A (2005). Organophosphate induced delayed polyneuropathy. Toxicol Rev 24: 37–49.

Lotti M, Becker CE, Aminoff MJ (1984). Organophosphate polyneuropathy: pathogenesis and prevention. Neurology 34: 658–662.

Lotti M, Moretto A, Zoppellari R, et al. (1986). Inhibition of lymphocytic neuropathy target esterase predicts the development of organophosphate-induced delayed polyneuropathy. Arch Toxicol 59: 176–179.

Lotti M, Moretto A, Capodicasa E, et al. (1993). Interaction between neuropathy target esterase and its inhibitors and the development of polyneuropathy. Toxicol Appl Pharmacol 122: 165–171.

Luo C, Ashani Y, Doctor BP (1998). Acceleration of oxime-induced reactivation of organophosphate-inhibited fetal bovine serum acetylcholinesterase by monoquaternary and bisquaternary ligands. Mol Pharmacol 53: 718–726.

Luo C, Saxena A, Smith M, et al. (1999). Phosphoryl oxime inhibition of acetylcholinesterase during oxime reactivation is prevented by edrophonium. Biochemistry 38: 9937–9947.

Mackerer CR, Barth ML, Krueger AJ, et al. (1999). Comparison of neurotoxic effects and potential risks from oral administration or ingestion of tricresyl phosphate and jet engine oil containing tricresyl phosphate. J Toxicol Environ Health 57: 293–328.

Mahieu P, Hassoun A, Van Binst R, et al. (1982). Severe and prolonged poisoning by fenthion. Significance of the determination of the anticholinesterase capacity of plasma. Clin Toxicol 19: 425–432.

Marrs TC (1993). Organophosphate poisoning. Pharmacol Ther 58: 51–66.

Martinez-Chuecos J, Jurado MC, Gimenez MP, et al. (1992). Experience with hemoperfusion for organophosphate poisoning. Crit Care Med 20: 1538–1543.

Maselli RA, Soliven BC (1991). Analysis of the organophosphate-induced electromyographic response to repetitive nerve stimulation: paradoxical response to edrophonium and D-tubocurarine. Muscle Nerve 14: 1182–1188.

Mason HJ (2000). The recovery of plasma cholinesterase and erythrocyte acetylcholinesterase activity in workers after overexposure to dichlorvos. Occup Med 50: 343–347.

Mason HJ, Sains C, Stevenson AJ, et al. (2000). Rates of spontaneous reactivation and aging of acetylcholinesterase in human erythrocytes after inhibition by organophosphorus pesticides. Human Exp Toxicol 19: 511–516.

Maxwell DM, Lenz DE, Groff WA, et al. (1987). The effects of blood flow and detoxification on in vivo cholinesterase inhibition by soman in rats. Toxicol Appl Pharmacol 88: 66–76.

McCain WC, Lee R, Johnson MS, et al. (1997). Acute oral toxicity study of pyridostigmine bromide, permethrin and DEET in the laboratory rat. J Toxicol Environ Health 50: 113–124.

McConnell R, Delgado-Tellez E, Caudra R, et al. (1999). Organophosphate neuropathy due to methamidophos: biochemical and neurophysiological markers. Arch Toxicol 73: 296–300.

Meshul CK, Boyne AF, Deshpande SS, et al. (1985). Comparison of the ultrastructural myopathy induced by anticholinesterase agents at the end plates of rat soleus and extensor muscles. Exp Neurol 89: 96–114.

Meshul CK, Kriho V, Kriho N, et al. (1990). Calcium channel blocker influences the density of alpha-actinin labelling at the rat neuromuscular junction. Muscle Nerve 13: 348–354.

Molphy R, Rathus EM (1964). Organic phosphorus poisoning and therapy. Med J Aust 2: 337–340.

Moretto A (1999). Testing for organophosphate delayed polyneuropathy. In: MD Maines, LG Costa, DJ Reed et al. (Eds.), Current Protocols in Toxicology. Wiley, New York, pp. 11.5.1–11.5.14.

Moretto A, Lotti M (1998). Poisoning by organophosphorus insecticides and sensory neuropathy. J Neurol Neurosurg Psychiatry 64: 464–468.

Moretto A, Lotti M, Sabri MI, et al. (1987). Progressive deficit of retrograde axonal transport is associated with the pathogenesis of di-n-butyl dichlorvos axonopathy. J Neurochem 49: 1515–1522.

Moretto A, Capodicasa E, Peraica M, et al. (1991). Age sensitivity to organophosphate-induced delayed polyneuropathy. Biochemical and toxicological studies in developing chicks. Biochem Pharmacol 41: 1497–1504.

Moretto A, Capodicasa E, Lotti M (1992). Clinical expression of organophosphate-induced delayed polyneuropathy in rats. Toxicol Lett 63: 97–102.

Morgan JP, Petrovich P (1978). Jamaica ginger paralysis. Forty-seven-year follow-up. Arch Neurol 35: 530–532.

Moser VC (1995). Comparisons of the acute effects of cholinesterase inhibitors using a neurobehavioral screening battery in rats. Neurotoxicol Teratol 17: 617–625.

Nagata K, Huang C-S, Song J-H, et al. (1997). Direct actions of anticholinesterases on the neuronal nicotinic acetylcholine receptor channels. Brain Res 769: 211–218.

Namba T, Nolte CT, Jackrel J, et al. (1971). Poisoning due to organophosphate insecticides. Am J Med 50: 475–492.

Newmark J (2004). Therapy for nerve agent poisoning. Arch Neurol 61: 649–651.

Nisse P, Forceville X, Cezard CC, et al. (1998). Intermediate syndrome with delayed distal polyneuropathy from ethyl parathion poisoning. Vet Hum Toxicol 40: 166–168.

Norman J (1990). Neuromuscular blockade. In: AR Aitkenhead, G Smith (Eds.), A Textbook of Anaesthesia. Churchill Livingstone, London, pp. 211–224.

Ohno K, Brengman JM, Tsujino A, et al. (1998). Human endplate acetylcholinesterase deficiency caused by mutations in the collagen-like tail subunit (ColQ) of the asymmetric enzyme. Proc Natl Acad Sci U S A 95: 9654–9659.

Okumura A, Kato T, Hayakawa F, et al. (2004). Nonepileptic pedaling-like movement induced by triclofos. Brain Dev 26: 487–489.

Ordentlich A, Barak D, Kronman C, et al. (1996). The architecture of human acetylcholinesterase active center probed by interactions with selected organophosphate inhibitors. J Biol Chem 271: 11953–11962.

Ordentlich A, Barak D, Kronman C, et al. (1998). Functional characteristics of the oxyanion hole in human acetylcholinesterase. J Biol Chem 273: 19509–19517.

Ordentlich A, Barak D, Sod-Moriah G, et al. (2004). Stereoselectivity toward VX is determined by interactions with residues of the acyl pocket as well as of the peripheral anionic site of AChE. Biochemistry 43: 11255–11265.

Peeples ES, Schopfer LM, Duysen EG, et al. (2005). Albumine, a new biomarker of organophosphorus toxicant exposure, identified by mass spectrometry. Toxicol Sci 83: 303–312.

Perron R, Johnson BB (1969). Insecticide poisoning. N Engl J Med 281: 274–275.

Petroianu GA, Missler A, Zuleger K, et al. (2004). Enzyme reactivator treatment in organophosphate exposure: clinical relevance of thiocholinesteratic activity of pralidoxime. Appl Toxicol 24: 429–435.

Pope CN (1999). Organophosphorus pesticides: do they all have the same mechanism of toxicity? J Toxicol Environ Health B Crit Rev 2: 161–181.

Prineas J (1969). The pathogenesis of dying-back polyneuropathies. Part I. An ultrastructural study of experimental tri-ortho-cresyl phosphate intoxication in the cat. J Neuropathol Exp Neurol 28: 571–597.

Prody CA, Dreyfus P, Zamir R, et al. (1989). De novo amplification within a "silent" human cholinesterase gene in a family subjected to prolonged exposure to organophosphorous insecticides. Proc Natl Acad Sci U S A 86: 690–694.

Quinn DM (1987). Acetylcholinesterase: enzyme structure, reaction dynamics, and virtual transition states. Chem Rev 87: 955–979.

Rantanen J, Lehtinen S, Savolainen K (2004). The opportunities and obstacles to collaboration between the developing and developed countries in the field of occupational health. Toxicology 198: 63–74.

Richards P, Johnson M, Ray D, et al. (1999). Novel protein targets for organophosphorus compounds. Chem-Biol Interact 119–120: 503–511.

Rose MR (2003). Gulf War service is an uncertain trigger for ALS. Neurology 61: 730–731.

Rose MR, Sharief MK, Priddin J, et al. (2004). Evaluation of neuromuscular symptoms in UK Gulf War veterans. Neurology 63: 1681–1687.

Rousseaux CG, Dua AK (1989). Pharmacology of HI-6, an H-series oxime. Can J Physiol Pharmacol 67: 1183–1189.

Sanderson DM (1961). Treatment of poisoning by anticholinesterase insecticides in the rat. J Pharm Pharmacol 13: 435–442.

Sedgwick ME, Senanayake N (1997). Pathophysiology of the intermediate syndrome of organophosphorus poisoning. J Neurol Neurosurg Psychiatry 62: 201–202.

Senanayake N (1981). Tri-cresyl phosphate neuropathy in Sri Lanka: a clinical and neurophysiological study with a three year follow up. J Neurol Neurosurg Psychiatry 44: 775–780.

Senanayake N (1998). Organophosphorus insecticide poisoning. Ceylon Med J 43: 22–29.

Senanayake N, Johnson MK (1982). Acute polyneuropathy after poisoning by a new organophosphate insecticide. N Engl J Med 306: 155–157.

Senanayake N, Karalliedde L (1987). Neurotoxic effects of organophosphorus insecticides. An intermediate syndrome. N Engl J Med 316: 761–763.

Senanayake N, Sanmuganathan PS (1995). Extrapyramidal manifestations complicating organophosphorus insecticide poisoning. Hum Exp Toxicol 14: 600–604.

Sevim S, Aktekin M, Dogu O, et al. (2003). Late onset polyneuropathy due to organophosphate (DDVP) intoxication. Can J Neurol Sci 30: 75–78.

Sharief MK, Priddin J, Delamont RS, et al. (2002). Neurophysiologic analysis of neuromuscular symptoms in UK Gulf War veterans. Neurology 59: 1518–1525.

Shaw K-P, Aracava Y, Akaike A, et al. (1985). The reversible cholinesterase inhibitor physostigmine has channel-blocking and agonist effects on the acetylcholine receptor–ion channel complex. Mol Pharmacol 28: 527–538.

Shiraishi S, Inoue N, Murai Y, et al. (1983). Dipterex (trichlorfon) poisoning—clinical and pathological studies in human and monkeys. J UOEH Suppl 5: 125–132.

Singh G, Avasthi G, Khurana D (1998a). Neurophysiological monitoring of pharmacological manipulation in acute organophosphate poisoning. The effects of pralidoxime, magnesium sulphate and pancuronium. Electroencephalogr Clin Neurophysiol 107: 140–148.

Singh G, Mahajan R, Whig J (1998b). The importance of electrodiagnostic studies in acute organophosphate poisoning. J Neurol Sci 157: 191–200.

Smith DM (1977). Organophosphorus poisoning from emergency use of a handsprayer. Practitioner 218: 877–883.

Smulders C, Bueters T, Vailati S, et al. (2004). Block of neuronal nicotinic acetylcholine receptors by organophosphate insecticides. Toxicol Sci 82: 545–554.

Soreq H, Seidman S (2001). Acetylcholinesterase—new roles for an old actor. Nat Rev Neurosci 2: 294–301.

Spencer PS, McCauley LA, Lapidus JA, et al. (2001). Self-reported exposures and their association with unexplained illness in a population-based case—control study of Gulf War veterans. J Occup Environ Med 43: 1041–1056.

Stephens R, Spurgeon A, Calvert IA, et al. (1995). Neuropsychological effects of long-term exposure to organophosphates in sheep dip. Lancet 345: 1135–1139.

Sudakin DL, Mullins ME, Horowitz BZ, et al. (2000). Intermediate syndrome after malathion ingestion despite continuous infusion of pralidoxime. J Toxicol Clin Toxicol 38: 47–50.

Susser M, Stein Z (1957). An outbreak of tri-ortho-cresyl phosphate (T.O.C.P.) poisoning in Durban. Br J Ind Med 14: 111–120.

Suzuki T, Morita H, Ono K, et al. (1995). Sarin poisoning in Tokyo subway. Lancet 345: 980.

Talbot BG, Anderson DR, Harris LW, et al. (1988). A comparison of in vivo and in vitro rates of aging of soman-inhibited erythrocyte acetylcholinesterase in different animal species. Drug Chem Toxicol 11: 289–305.

Taylor P (2001). Anticholinesterase agents. In: JG Hardman, LE Limbird (Eds.), Goodman & Gilman's the Pharmacological Basis of Therapeutics. McGraw-Hill, New York, pp. 175–191.

Thiermann H, Mast U, Klimmek R, et al. (1997). Cholinesterase status, pharmacokinetics and laboratory findings during obidoxime therapy in organophosphate poisoned patients. Hum Exp Toxicol 16: 473–480.

Thiermann H, Szinicz L, Eyer F, et al. (1999). Modern strategies in therapy of organophosphate poisoning. Toxicol Lett 107: 233–239.

Tracy JA, Gallagher H (1990). Use of glycopyrrolate and atropine in acute organophosphorus poisoning. Hum Exp Toxicol 9: 99–100.

Tush GM, Anstead MI (1997). Pralidoxime continuous infusion in the treatment of organophosphate poisoning. Ann Pharmacother 31: 441–444.

Umehara F, Izumo S, Arimura K, et al. (1991). Polyneuropathy induced by m-tolyl methyl carbamate intoxication. J Neurol 238: 47–48.

Van Dijk JG, Lammers GJ, Wintzen AR, et al. (1996). Repetitive CMAPs: mechanisms of neural and synaptic genesis. Muscle Nerve 19: 1127–1133.

van Helden HPM, Busker RW, Melchers BPC, et al. (1996). Pharmacological effects of oximes: how relevant are they? Arch Toxicol 70: 779–786.

Vasconcellos LF, Leite AC, Nascimento OM (2002). Organophosphate-induced delayed neuropathy. Arq Neuropsiquiatr 60: 1003–1007.

Vasilescu C, Florescu A (1980). Clinical and electrophysiological study of neuropathy after organophosphorus compounds poisoning. Arch Toxicol 43: 305–315.

Vasilescu C, Alexianu M, Dan A (1984). Delayed neuropathy after organophosphorus insecticide (Dipterex) poisoning: a clinical, electrophysiological and nerve biopsy study. J Neurol Neurosurg Psychiatry 47: 543–548.

Veronesi B (1984). A rodent model of organophosphorus-induced delayed neuropathy: distribution of central (spinal cord) and peripheral nerve damage. Neuropathol Appl Neurobiol 10: 357–368.

Wadia RS, Sadagopan C, Amin RB, et al. (1974). Neurological manifestations of organophosphorus insecticide poisoning. J Neurol Neurosurg Psychiatry 37: 841–847.

Walsh C (1979). Enzymatic Reaction Mechanisms. Freeman, San Francisco.

Wecker L, Kiauta T, Dettbarn W-D (1978a). Relationship between acetylcholinesterase inhibition and the development of a myopathy. J Pharmacol Exp Ther 206: 97–104.

Wecker L, Laskowski MB, Dettbarn W-D (1978b). Neuromuscular dysfunction induced by acetylcholinesterase inhibition. Fed Proc 37: 2818–2822.

Wecker L, Mark RE, Dettbarn W-D (1985). Evidence of necrosis in human intercostal muscle following inhalation of an organophosphate insecticide. J Environ Path Toxicol Oncol 6: 171–175.

Wecker L, Mark RE, Dettbarn W (1986). Evidence of necrosis in human intercostal muscle following inhalation of an organophosphate insecticide. Fundam Appl Toxicol 6: 172–174.

Wehner JM, Smolen A, Smolen TN, et al. (1985). Recovery of acetylcholinesterase activity after acute organophosphate treatment of CNS reaggregate cultures. Fundam Appl Toxicol 5: 1104–1109.

Weinbroum AA (2005). Pathophysiological and clinical aspects of combat anticholinesterase poisoning. Br Med Bull 72: 119–133.

Weisskopf MG, O'Reilly EJ, McCullough ML, et al. (2005). Prospective study of military service and mortality from ALS. Neurology 64: 32–37.

Whittaker M (1986). Cholinesterase. In: L Beckman (Ed.), Monographs in Human Genetics. Vol. 11. Karger, Basel.

Willems JL (1981). Poisoning by organophosphate insecticides: analysis of 53 human cases with regard to management and drug treatment. Acta Med Milit Belg 134: 7–15.

Willems J, Belpaire F (1991). Anticholinesterase poisoning: an overview of pharmacotherapy and clinical management. In:In: B Ballantyne, T Marrs (Eds.), Clinical and Experimental Toxicology of Anticholinesterases. Butterworths, Guildford, pp. 536–542.

Willems JL, Belpaire FM (1992). Anticholinergic poisoning: an overview of pharmacotherapy. In: B Ballantyne, TC Marrs (Eds.), Clinical and Experimental Toxicology of Organophosphates and Carbamates. Butterworth-Heinemann, Oxford, pp. 536–542.

Willems JL, Langenberg JP, Verstraete AG, et al. (1992). Plasma concentrations of pralidoxime methylsulphate in organophosphorus poisoned patients. Arch Toxicol 66: 260–266.

Willems JL, De Bisschop HC, Verstraete AG, et al. (1993). Cholinesterase reactivation in organophosphorus poisoned patients depends on the plasma concentrations of the oxime pralidoxime methylsulphate and of the organophosphate. Arch Toxicol 67: 79–84.

Wilson BH, Hooper MJ, Hansen ME, et al. (1992). Reactivation of organophosphorus inhibited AChE with oximes. In: JE Chambers, PE Levi (Eds.), Organophosphates—Chemistry, Fate and Effects. Academic Press, San Diego, pp. 107–137.

Wilson BW (2001). Cholinesterases. In: RI Krieger (Ed.), Handbook of Pesticide Toxicology. Academic Press, San Diego, pp. 967–985.

Wilson IB, Ginsburg S (1955). A powerful reactivator of alkyl phosphate-inhibited acetylcholinesterase. Biochem Biophys Acta 18: 168–170.

Wong L, Radic Z, Bruggermann RJM, et al. (2000). Mechanism of oxime reactivation of acetylcholinesterase analyzed by chirality and mutagenesis. Biochemistry 39: 5750–5757.

Worek F, Kirchner T, Bäcker M, et al. (1996). Reactivation by various oximes of human erythrocytes acetylcholinesterase inhibited by different organophosphorus compounds. Arch Toxicol 70: 497–503.

Worek F, Diepold C, Eyer P (1999). Dimethylphosphoryl-inhibited human cholinesterase: inhibition, reactivation, and aging kinetics. Arch Toxicol 73: 7–14.

World Health Organization (1990). Public Health Impact of Pesticides Used in Agriculture. World Health Organization, Geneva.

Xie W, Stribley JA, Chatonnet A, et al. (2000). Postnatal developmental delay and supersensitivity to organophosphate in gene-targeted mice lacking acetylcholinesterase. J Pharmacol Exp Ther 293: 896–902.

Yang PY, Tsao TCY, Lin JL, et al. (2000). Carbofuran-induced delayed neuropathy. Clin Toxicol 38: 43–46.

Zilker T, Hibler A (1996). Treatment of severe parathion poisoning: clinical aspects. In: L Szinicz, P Eyer, R Klimmek (Eds.), Role of Oximes in the Treatment of Anticholinesterase Agent Poisoning. Spectrum Akademischer Verlag, Heidelberg, pp. 9–17.

Zwiener RJ, Ginsburg M (1988). Organophosphate and carbamate poisoning in infants and children. Pediatrics 81: 121–126.

Handbook of Clinical Neurology, Vol. 91 (3rd series)
Neuromuscular junction disorders
A.G. Engel, Editor

Chapter 14

Peripheral nerve hyperexcitability and the neuromuscular junction

STEVEN VERNINO*

University of Texas Southwestern Medical Center, Dallas, TX, USA

14.1. Background

The terms neuromyotonia, myokymia, neuromuscular hyperexcitability, peripheral nerve hyperexcitability, continuous muscle fiber activity, quantal squander, cramp-fasciculation syndrome, Armadillo syndrome, rippling muscles and the eponyms "Isaacs syndrome" and "Morvan syndrome" describe a heterogeneous group of neuromuscular disorders characterized by spontaneous and continuous muscle activity (Auger, 1994; Hart et al., 2002). The term peripheral nerve hyperexcitability (PNH) will be arbitrarily used here to encompass this topic. Current evidence indicates that a majority of these disorders result from hyperexcitability of the distal motor nerve or motor nerve terminal, so these conditions are appropriately considered in this section on neuromuscular junction disorders. Additionally, features of PNH can result from agents that inhibit acetylcholinesterase at the neuromuscular junction (as discussed below).

A syndrome of acquired PNH was recognized as early as 1870 by the French physician Augustin Morvan who used the term "la chorée fibrillaire" to describe a syndrome characterized by involuntary muscle twitching, dysautonomia, insomnia, and fluctuating delirium (Morvan, 1890). This rare syndrome is now known as Morvan syndrome. The clinical and electrophysiological abnormalities in two patients with PNH without central nervous system (CNS) manifestations were characterized first in the English language literature by Denny-Brown and Foley in 1948 who described two patients with undulating myokymia. Both patients had increased sweating and other typical features of the disorder that would later be known as acquired neuromyotonia, or Isaacs syndrome.

In 1961, Isaacs demonstrated in two cases that the spontaneous motor activity was not eliminated by blockade of the peripheral nerve but could be eliminated by curare. He concluded that the hyperexcitability originated in the distal peripheral nerve or motor nerve terminal (Isaacs, 1961). Mertens and Zschocke coined the term "neuromyotonia" in 1965 to describe the high frequency electrical discharges in muscle and differentiate this disorder from myotonia (Mertens and Zschocke, 1965). Our understanding of this disorder and related ones has increased recently. Mutations in ion channel genes have been described in some inherited forms of PNH, and antibodies against voltage-gated potassium channels have been identified in many patients with acquired PNH.

14.2. Clinical and electromyographic features

The clinical and electromyographic features of PNH are quite varied and reflect a continuous spectrum of manifestations ranging from frequent fasciculations to high-frequency bursts of motor unit discharges (neuromyotonia). Additionally, these manifestations can be generalized or limited to one muscle or group of muscles. Clinically, fasciculations appear as localized rapid twitches of a small area of muscle. Recurrent groups of fasciculations or multiple continuous fasciculations appear as random, undulating, "worm-like" movements of the muscle (myokymia, from the Greek word for "muscle wave"). When myokymia is generalized and associated with muscle stiffness and delayed relaxation, the term neuromyotonia is used. These clinical definitions for fasciculation, myokymia and neuromyotonia must be distinguished from the electromyographic definitions (Gutmann, 2001).

*Correspondence to: Steven Vernino, MD, PhD, University of Texas Southwestern Medical Center, 5323 Harry Hines Blvd, Dallas, TX 75390-9036, USA. E-mail: steven.vernino@utsouthwestern.edu, Tel: 1-214-648-8816, Fax: 1-214-648-9129.

Some cases of PNH may be so mild that the patient is unaware of the spontaneous activity or considers it only a curiosity. With more vigorous muscle activity, the sensation of movement may become bothersome but not disabling. In the most severe cases (neuromyotonia), affected muscles do not relax fully, and patients have difficulty using the affected muscles. Clinical neuromyotonia is often also associated with increased sweating (hyperhidrosis), weight loss and muscle hypertrophy due to the excess muscle activity.

Electrically, fasciculations appear as spontaneous motor unit potentials. When a single identified fasciculation potential appears repetitively, the firing is usually random, and the morphology of the motor unit often varies (Fig. 14.1A). This variation is one piece of evidence that fasciculations may be generated near a single motor nerve terminal rather than in the more proximal motor axon. In PNH, fasciculations often appear in groups of doublets, triplets and multiplets with interpotential intervals that vary widely but may be quite short (10–20 ms) (Denny-Brown and Foley, 1948; Gutmann, 2001).

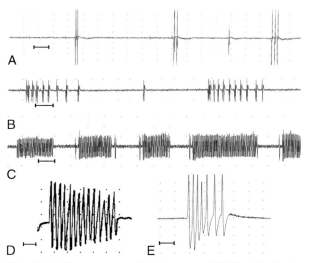

Fig. 14.1. Electromyographic features of PNH. (A) Single and groups of doublet or triplet fasciculations in a patient with cramp-fasciculation syndrome (first dorsal interosseous muscle, scale bar = 200 ms). (B) Repetitive spontaneous firing of a motor unit potential (myokymic discharges) in a patient with Isaacs syndrome (deltoid muscle, scale bar = 100 ms). The initial intraburst frequency is 40 Hz. The interpotential interval gradually increases within the burst. (C) Slower and more prolonged myokymic discharges in a patient with radiation plexopathy (triceps muscle, scale bar = 1 s). Within a burst, the motor unit fires at 12–15 Hz. D, E Neuromyotonic discharges in patients with acquired neuromyotonia. (D, first dorsal interosseous muscle and E, gastrocnemius muscle, scale bar = 20 ms). Initial intraburst frequency in these examples is 200 Hz.

Myokymic discharges are similar bursts of motor unit potentials (grouped fasciculations) that occur repeatedly at regular intervals (Fig. 14.1A and B). Each burst may contain 2, 3 or up to 100 potentials. These bursts fire recurrently up to several times per second. The inter-burst interval (time between successive bursts) can range from 0.3 s to 120 s. Typically, longer bursts fire less frequently. The discharges continue during voluntary contraction and may transiently increase in frequency following exercise. The intraburst frequency (of potentials within an individual burst) can range from 5 Hz to 100 Hz with typical frequencies within myokymic discharges of 40 Hz to 60 Hz. Within a single burst, the interval between successive motor unit potentials becomes slightly longer.

Neuromyotonic discharges are similar to myokymic discharges but have higher intra-burst frequency and longer burst duration (Fig. 14.1C). The precise frequency that differentiates myokymic from neuromyotonic discharges is somewhat arbitrary. Neuromyotonic discharges often have an intra-burst frequency of 150 Hz or greater, and initial inter-spike intervals may be as short as 3–5 ms (200–300 Hz; Fig. 14.1D). Neuromyotonic bursts tend to occur irregularly. Within longer neuromyotonic bursts, the frequency and amplitude of the potentials often decrease with time. These features give neuromyotonic discharges a characteristic high-frequency sound variably described as a "race car" or "ping" (Torbergsen et al., 1996).

The clinical and electromyographic characteristics may be discordant. Clinical myokymia and neuromyotonia may be associated with electromyography (EMG) findings of dense fasciculations, myokymic discharges, neuromyotonic discharges, or some combination of these. In other cases, muscles that visually appear normal may prove to be quite active on needle EMG.

On nerve conduction studies, PNH may be associated with multiple compound muscle action potentials after a single nerve stimulus (Fig. 14.2). These have been called "after discharges" or repetitive F-waves, depending on their latency. Recurrent discharges may be provoked more readily by repetitive nerve stimulation.

The clinical and electromyographic features of PNH are associated with various nerve disorders (Table 14.1) (Auger, 1994; Hart et al., 2002). It is also important to distinguish PNH from disorders that are associated with increased muscle activity but not due to nerve hyperexcitability (Table 14.2). Some myopathic disorders are associated with myotonia, electrically silent muscle contractures or muscle rippling. The spontaneous activity in these disorders may resemble PNH clinically but is generally easy to distinguish by EMG examination. Central causes of increased muscle activity (spasticity, rigidity, spasms or tremor) may enter into the

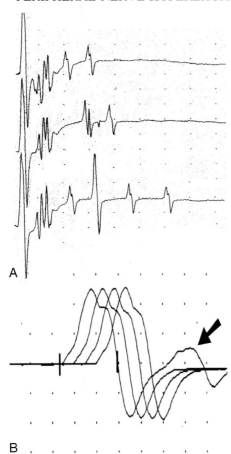

Fig. 14.2. Motor nerve conduction studies in PNH. (A) Peroneal nerve motor response in a patient with Isaacs syndrome (recorded over the extensor digitorum brevis muscle with stimulation at the ankle, scale = 500 μV and 10 ms per division). The initial M wave is followed by multiple after discharges, some of which have the same morphology. The after discharges may vary in timing and appearance with each stimulation. (B) Peroneal motor response (4 repetitive stimuli at 2 Hz) in a patient with fasciculations associated with the use of pyridostigmine (scale = 2 mV and 2 ms per division). The initial CMAP is followed by a single smaller second response (arrow). The main component shows no decrement to repetitive stimulation, while the extra component is absent in subsequent discharges (van Dijk et al., 1996). This type of single after discharge may also be seen in patients with congenital myasthenia due to slow channel mutations of the AChR.

Table 14.1

Causes of peripheral nerve hyperexcitability

Inherited disorders
  Episodic ataxia type 1 with myokymia (Kv1.1; KCNA1)
  Benign familial neonatal epilepsy and myokymia (KCNQ2)
  Hereditary myokymia without central nervous system features
  Familial cramp syndrome
Toxins
  Acetylcholinesterase inhibitors
  Gold
  Toluene
  Oxaliplatin (Wilson et al., 2002)
  Timber rattle snake venom
  Black widow spider venom (α-latrotoxin)
  Green mamba venom (α-dendrotoxin)
Nerve injury
  Radiation toxicity
  Inherited neuropathies (CMT II)
  Inflammatory demyelinating neuropathies
  Multiple sclerosis (facial myokymia)
  Conduction block neuropathy
  Focal compression neuropathy
  Chronic motor nerve disorders (ALS)
  Amyloidosis
  Uremia
Autoimmune disorders
  Acquired neuromyotonia (Isaacs syndrome)
  Morvan syndrome
  Cramp-fasciculation syndrome
  Paraneoplastic neuromyotonia
    Thymoma (with or without myasthenia gravis)
    Small-cell lung carcinoma
Associated with other autoimmune conditions
  Myasthenia gravis
  Guillain–Barré syndrome or Chronic Inflammatory Demyelinating Polyneuropathy (CIDP)
  Systemic lupus
  Multiple sclerosis
  Penicillamine
Other disorders
  Benign fasciculation syndrome
  Benign focal myokymia

differential diagnosis of PNH. Muscles may show poor relaxation and episodic contraction but do not have the appearance of twitching or myokymia. Central nervous system disorders are associated with motor units firing in a physiological pattern.

Diffuse PNH can usually be attributed to genetic, toxic or immune-mediated causes. Focal PNH can occur in the distribution of an injured nerve, especially in nerves affected by conduction block or radiation injury.

14.3. Inherited myokymia (potassium channel mutations)

Several genetic disorders are associated with myokymia. Episodic ataxia type 1 (EA1) is a rare autosomal dominant disorder characterized by sudden brief

Table 14.2

Disorders mimicking peripheral nerve hyperexcitability

Muscle disorders
  Myotonia
  Myotonic dystrophy
  Non-dystrophic myotonia
  Periodic paralysis
  Toxic myopathies
  Contracture (electrically silent) metabolic myopathies
  Rippling muscle disease (electrically silent)
  Autosomal dominant, type 1 and type 2
Central nervous system disorders
  Stiff-man syndrome
  Tetanus
  Spasticity

episodes of ataxia (Zuberi et al., 1999). The ataxia may be precipitated by movement or emotion and lasts for seconds to minutes. Some patients with EA1 have partial epilepsy. The clinical presentation can be varied, even within family members. Infants may present with severe postural deformities while other patients present with minimal symptoms in adulthood. The clinical variability can be attributed in part to different identified mutations. Continuous myokymia appears to be a consistent feature in EA1. Although it may or may not be clinically evident, it can be detected by EMG in most muscles. It appears as a fine twitching or rippling of muscles. The spontaneous activity is often most clinically apparent as fine finger tremor or periorbital quivering. Autonomic disturbances have not been reported in patients with EA1. Acetazolamide, a carbonic anhydrase inhibitor, may be effective in reducing ataxic episodes in some individuals but does not appear to reduce myokymia. This disorder is distinguished from episodic ataxia type 2, which presents with longer episodes of ataxia and no myokymia.

EA1 is associated with point mutations in a voltage-gated potassium channel gene (KCNA1 or Kv1.1) on chromosome 12. More than 10 different point mutations have been described (Zuberi et al., 1999). Kv1.1 potassium channels are present in juxtaparanodal zones of myelinated nerves and are expressed by cortical neurons (especially in hippocampus). These channels probably contribute to regulating excitability (particularly in the terminal motor branches of nerves as described below). Experimental mice with deletion of the Kv1.1 gene have hyperexcitable motor nerve terminals and seizures (Zhou et al., 1999). Some patients with EA1 mutations have been reported with myokymia but without ataxic episodes.

Mutations in genes encoding a different class of voltage-gated potassium channel (KCNQ2 or KCNQ3) are associated with benign familial neonatal epilepsy. Most of these mutations are not associated with PNH although one KCNQ2 mutation kindred showed both neonatal convulsions and later onset continuous generalized myokymia (Dedek et al., 2001).

Other inherited forms of PNH have been reported without identified gene mutation. These include families with isolated neuromyotonia or myokymia, which could represent as yet unidentified potassium channel disorders (Auger et al., 1984). Other families with autosomal dominant episodic ataxia and myokymia have been reported that do not have mutations in the EA1 or EA2 loci (these were designated episodic ataxia type 4 in one report) (Steckley et al., 2001). Families with excessive cramps or fasciculations have been described, but these probably do not represent a simple genetic syndrome.

14.4. PNH secondary to toxins

A number of toxins can affect the neuromuscular junction or motor nerve terminal. Timber rattlesnake envenomation is associated with generalized myokymia. The underlying spontaneous activity consists of grouped fasciculations and myokymic and neuromyotonic discharges. Some snake venom toxins, notably dendrotoxin from the African mamba, are potent inhibitors of voltage-gated potassium channels. Alpha-dendrotoxin acts on Kv1.1, Kv1.2 and Kv1.6 channels. Envenomation leads to seizures as well as diffuse myokymia.

Drugs and toxins, which increase acetylcholine levels at the neuromuscular junction, can also produce motor nerve hyperexcitability. Excessive amounts of acetylcholinesterase inhibitors (such as those used for treatment of myasthenia gravis or dementia) or exposure to organophosphates can produce a variety of symptoms, including abundant fasciculations or even myokymia. The increase in acetylcholine appears to evoke spontaneous activity in the motor nerve, perhaps through an action on presynaptic neuronal acetylcholine receptors. PNH is commonly seen with high doses of these drugs, but is not usually clinically significant. Autonomic hyperactivity is the more serious clinical side effect of acetylcholinesterase inhibition.

Other nerve toxins have been associated with features of PNH (Table 14.1). Black widow spider venom (α-latrotoxin) has numerous effects including a stimulation of neurotransmitter release and will cause a period of autonomic and neuromuscular hyperactivity. Some other toxins associated with PNH probably act by causing nerve injury (e.g., gold, toluene) and nerve irritability.

14.5. Hyperexcitability due to peripheral nerve disorders

Demyelination or radiation injury of peripheral nerves can produce focal PNH. Facial myokymia may be seen in patients with pontine glioma, Guillain–Barré syndrome, or multiple sclerosis. High frequency discharges are seen in cases of hemifacial spasm, which is often related to proximal nerve injury due to compression of the facial nerve near the brainstem. The mechanism of hyperexcitability in these disorders may be quite different from those leading to generalized PNH since the site of hyperexcitability is likely in a very proximal abnormal part of the nerve.

Abundant fasciculations or even myokymia can be seen associated with lesions in intermediate segments of the motor nerve, especially those associated with prolonged or complete conduction block (Roth and Magistris, 1987). The spontaneous activity is restricted to affected nerves. Acute demyelination appears to result in redistribution of ion channels, which may be relevant to axon excitability (Arroyo et al., 2004). Action potentials may fail to propagate across these lesions resulting in conduction block. At the same time, depolarization near the distal end of the demyelinated segment may produce recurrent action potentials in the nerve distal to the lesion. Inflammation at the site of demyelination may also contribute to nerve hyperexcitability.

Although it is attractive to think of hyperexcitability generated at the site of the nerve injury, it appears that spontaneous discharges in nerve fibers with proximal conduction block may often arise in the terminal motor nerve branches (Roth and Magistris, 1987). The mechanism is unknown, but may relate to compensatory redistribution of ion channels leading to changes in excitability in the terminal myelinated segments of the motor nerve. Experimentally, mice with hereditary myelinopathies

may show PNH, which seems to be generated in the terminal parts of the motor axon (Zielasek et al., 2000).

Spontaneous discharges, in the form of fasciculations or less commonly myokymia, can be seen in a variety of axonal degenerations as well. Motor nerves, which have undergone sprouting of terminal axons, appear to be more unstable. The fasciculations associated with amyotrophic lateral sclerosis, for example, have been extensively studied. The preponderance of evidence points to a distal origin of this activity (Layzer, 1994). The spontaneous activity persists and even increases for several days following proximal nerve transection (Forster et al., 1946). Electromyographic studies reveal that the shape of successive single or grouped fasciculations often varies. This variability suggests that the spontaneous discharge originates within single motor nerve terminals and then propagates to the entire motor unit by an axon reflex (Layzer, 1994; Torbergsen et al., 1996).

14.6. Autoimmune PNH

14.6.1. Neuromyotonia (Isaacs syndrome)

Many acquired cases of generalized PNH appear to have an autoimmune basis. This concept was originally based on the observation that acquired myokymia or neuromyotonia could coexist with myasthenia gravis or other autoimmune disorders (Tables 14.1 and 14.3). PNH can occur in patients with thymoma or small-cell lung carcinoma as part of a paraneoplastic syndrome (Newsom-Davis and Mills, 1993; Hart et al., 2002; Vernino and Lennon, 2002). Further evidence for an autoimmune cause include clinical improvement after therapeutic plasmapheresis or immunosuppression (Newsom-Davis and Mills, 1993; Riche et al., 1995; Madrid et al., 1996a) and the identification of voltage-gated potassium channel (VGKC) autoantibodies in many cases of neuromyotonia.

Table 14.3

Autoimmune peripheral nerve hyperexcitability

Diagnosis	VGKC antibody (%)*	Ganglionic AChR Ab (%)	MG (%)	Cancer (%)
Neuromyotonia or myokymia	47	10	15	27 (thymoma or SCLC)
Cramp-fasciculation syndrome	23	5	11	7 (thymoma)
Acquired rippling muscle syndrome	20	20	75	25 (thymoma)
Normal controls	2	0		
Thymoma (without PNH)	14	10	~35	

*Voltage-gated potassium channel antibodies detected using dendrotoxin receptor immunoprecipitation assay.
PNH, peripheral nerve hyperexcitability.
Data compiled from Vernino and Lennon, 2002; Hart et al., 2002.

Classical Isaacs syndrome is an acquired disorder characterized by insidious onset of generalized muscle stiffness. This is associated with continuous muscle twitching and undulation (myokymia), muscle hypertrophy and stiffness, weight loss and hyperhidrosis. The continuous muscle activity results in slowness of movement or can affect bulbar muscles leading to dysarthria and dysphagia. The disease presents at any age. The clinical symptoms may fluctuate, and most cases progress slowly over time. Some patients have evidence of a mild peripheral neuropathy and frequently have modest elevation of serum creatine kinase (Vernino et al., 1999; Hart et al., 2002).

Autonomic symptoms are common and may reflect hyperactivity of autonomic motor nerves. Excessive sweating is common and may be so severe that patients need to change clothes several times per day. The hyperhidrosis may be due in part to increased metabolic activity and increased heat production from continuously active muscles. However, hyperactivity of autonomic nerves is more likely since abundant sweating occurs even with a low core body temperature (Josephs et al., 2004). Increased salivation, piloerection (goose flesh), and abdominal distress are other signs of autonomic involvement (Viallard et al., 2005). Many patients describe sensory symptoms, especially transient migratory paresthesias or less commonly neuropathic pain (Josephs et al., 2004; Herskovitz et al., 2005). The sensory manifestations may represent hyperexcitability of the sensory nerves. Many patients have associated CNS features, such as mood changes, sleep disturbances, or hallucinations. When the behavioral manifestations are severe, the patients may be designated as having Morvan syndrome (see below).

Electrophysiological studies show repetitive after discharges following the CMAP, repetitive firing of F waves, and high frequency activity induced by repetitive nerve stimulation (Fig. 14.2) (Auger et al., 1984; van Dijk et al., 1996). On the needle EMG examination, a wide variety of spontaneous motor unit activity is seen, including abundant fasciculations, myokymic discharges, neuromyotonic discharges, and voluntary motor units firing as doublets and triplets (Fig. 14.1). The activity persists during sleep. Single fiber EMG studies often show mild abnormalities (increased jitter) in PNH patients and should not be interpreted as definitive evidence of subclinical myasthenia gravis. Instead, these abnormalities may reflect the instability of motor nerve terminal excitability.

Diffuse neuromyotonia is usually disabling and warrants treatment. Symptomatic treatments with membrane stabilizing drugs (such as phenytoin, carbamazepine, gabapentin) are often effective and sufficient in milder cases. In more severe cases of autoimmune PNH (especially those with VGKC autoantibodies), immunomodulatory treatment is appropriate. Plasma exchange or infusion of intravenous immunoglobulin have been reported to produce improvement (Sinha et al., 1991; Shillito et al., 1995). Many patients require some form of maintenance therapy, and immunosuppressants (e.g., azathioprine, cyclophosphamide) have been used.

14.6.2. Morvan syndrome

The typical presentation of Morvan syndrome includes the progressive onset of muscle twitching, stiffness, and hyperhidrosis, as seen in cases of acquired neuromyotonia. Autonomic dysfunction and sensory symptoms may be more prominent than in Isaacs syndrome (Liguori et al., 2001). Additionally, patients with Morvan syndrome have a fluctuating encephalopathy and severe insomnia. Among the cases described in English literature, over 90% of patients are male. Abnormal cognition may be characterized by episodes of disorientation with prominent hallucinations and severe short term memory dysfunction. The electroencephalogram typically shows diffuse slowing, but does not show epileptiform activity. Cranial CT and MRI show no significant abnormalities. These features help differentiate Morvan syndrome from limbic encephalitis (Lawn et al., 2003; Josephs et al., 2004). The sleep disturbance is quite severe. In some cases, formal sleep studies document a complete absence of sleep (sometimes leading to a misdiagnosis of fatal familial insomnia). When sleep does occur, dramatic dream enactment behavior may be seen along with significant abnormalities of sleep architecture.

Like neuromyotonia, Morvan syndrome is seen in association with myasthenia gravis, thymoma, or small cell lung carcinoma. In about 20%, the CSF shows increased protein, and oligoclonal bands. Most patients have VGKC antibodies (Barber et al., 2000; Liguori et al., 2001). Both the central and the neuromuscular symptoms improve with immunomodulatory treatments including plasma exchange (Madrid et al., 1996b; Josephs et al., 2004).

14.6.3. Cramp-fasciculation syndrome

The characteristic presentation of acquired neuromyotonia is quite rare. More frequently, one encounters patients with less severe forms of PNH without neuromyotonic discharges. These patients may have fasciculations, cramps, or focal intermittent myokymia. Recent evidence indicates that at least some of these patients have an autoimmune basis for their symptoms.

Cramp-fasciculation syndrome is an acquired disorder of peripheral nerve hyperexcitability characterized by muscle aching, cramps, exercise intolerance, and visible fasciculations (Tahmoush et al., 1991). Painful cramps characteristically develop during rest after a period of exercise and may involve unusual muscles, such as the abdominal muscles or intrinsic foot muscles. Similar to neuromyotonia, motor nerve conduction studies may show after discharges in a minority of cases, and repetitive nerve stimulation may induce repetitive discharges, sometimes associated with cramps. A typical testing protocol is stimulation of the tibial nerve (4 stimuli at 10 Hz) while recording over the abductor hallucis muscle. In our experience, however, inducing a muscle cramp with this provocative electrophysiological test is neither sensitive nor specific for a particular diagnosis. Like neuromyotonia, cramp-fasciculation syndrome may be associated with myasthenia gravis, thymoma or cognitive and behavioral changes (Table 14.3) (Hart et al., 2002; Vernino and Lennon, 2002). The cramp-fasciculation syndrome is heterogeneous, but about 20% of patients have VGKC antibodies indicating an autoimmune disorder in those cases (Table 14.3) (Hart et al., 2002; Vernino and Lennon, 2002). The syndrome in such cases could be considered a mild phenotypic variant of neuromyotonia. In patients without antibodies, it may be difficult to distinguish this disorder from benign fasciculations and physiologic cramps.

Many patients do not require treatment and are reassured that they do not have a progressive neurological disorder (like amyotrophic lateral sclerosis). If cramps and muscle twitching is problematic, symptomatic therapy with carbamazepine (or other membrane stabilizing drugs) is often effective. Immunomodulatory treatment is seldom needed but may be effective in severe cases. Such treatment is probably best reserved for those with evidence of an autoimmune disorder (i.e., seropositive for antibodies or associated with known autoimmune disease).

14.6.4. Voltage-gated potassium channel antibodies

Voltage-gated potassium channels are important for the regulation of neuronal excitability. Over 70 genes encoding mammalian potassium channels have been identified, including eight members of the Kv1 (Shaker-type) voltage-dependent potassium channel family. Antibodies specific for voltage-gated potassium channels can be detected with an immunoprecipitation assay using membranes solubilized from human cerebral cortex and complexed with radio-labeled α-dendrotoxin. Using this assay, elevated levels of VGKC antibody are found in about 50% of patients with idiopathic neuromyotonia or myokymia (Table 14.3) (Hart et al., 1997, 2002; Vernino and Lennon, 2004). This method for detecting VGKC antibody has some shortcomings that may account, in part, for the failure to detect VGKC antibodies in all patients with neuromyotonia. The radioligand used in the assay, α-dendrotoxin, is known to bind to Kv1.1, 1.2 and 1.6 type VGKCs but not to other VGKC subtypes and may not bind to some native conformational variants. Hart et al. (1997) used a different approach to detect VGKC antibodies. They expressed individual VGKC subtypes in Xenopus oocytes and then made either frozen sections of the oocytes or detergent extractions of the oocyte membranes. Antibodies specific for individual VGKC subtypes were detected by binding to the oocyte material. Using this assay, VGKC antibodies were found in nearly all patients with neuromyotonia, but the antibodies did not consistently recognize one VGKC type. Some patient sera bound to all three types of dendrotoxin-sensitive VGKC while others recognized mainly Kv1.2 or Kv1.6. While apparently more sensitive, this detection method is not practical for clinical diagnostic use.

In the absence of nerve injury or toxic exposure, acquired neuromyotonia (defined by the presence of spontaneous diffuse myokymic or neuromyotonic discharges on EMG examination) should be considered an antibody-mediated disorder. The clinical response to plasma exchange in many patients supports this concept. Antibodies from patients have been shown to cause a reduction in potassium currents in cultured cells (Arimura, 1999; Tomimitsu et al., 2004) and can promote repetitive firing of action potentials in cultured dorsal root ganglia neurons (similar to the effects of potassium channel antagonists) (Shillito et al., 1995). Additionally, conventional passive transfer (administration of antibodies to mice) produces several effects that are subtle but consistent with nerve hyperexcitability due to potassium channel inhibition. Neuromuscular diaphragm preparations from mice injected repeatedly with VGKC antibodies show relative resistance to d-tubocurarine (Sinha et al., 1991) and slightly increased quantal content of endplate potentials (Shillito et al., 1995). Although antibody-treated mice do not develop clinical or electromyographic PNH, these data show a pathophysiological role for VGKC antibodies.

VGKC antibodies are also found in patients with autoimmune limbic encephalitis without PNH (Thieben et al., 2004; Vincent et al., 2004). It is very likely that different specificities of VGKC antibodies are responsible for the different clinical presentations. For example, antibodies specific for Kv1.1 (VGKC expressed in high levels in hippocampus) may be more associated with encephalitis, while antibodies against Kv1.2 (which are expressed highly in the juxtaparanodal region of myelinated nerves) may be more important in PNH.

14.6.5. Other antibodies

Other autoantibodies can be found in patients with PNH. Antibodies against ganglionic neuronal nicotinic acetylcholine receptors (which are typically associated with an autoimmune form of autonomic failure) are found in some patients with neuromyotonia who do not have VGKC antibodies (Vernino et al., 1998; Vernino and Lennon, 2002). Ganglionic AChR antibodies are much less common in these patients (Table 14.3), and may be non-specific or may interact with presynaptic neuronal AChR on the motor nerve terminal that regulates transmitter release (Tsuneki et al., 1995).

Muscle acetylcholine receptor antibodies or striational antibodies are also found in patients with PNH especially when there is coexisting myasthenia gravis or thymoma (Table 14.3).

14.7. Other forms of hyperexcitability

Rippling muscle syndrome is another unusual neuromuscular hyperexcitability disorder characterized by waves of rippling or rolling muscle movements following muscle percussion or stretching. Inherited forms of muscle rippling are due to intrinsic muscle abnormality (mutation in caveolin-3 in some cases). Several sporadic cases have been reported in association with myasthenia gravis suggesting an autoimmune cause (Ansevin and Agamanolis, 1996; Vernino et al., 1999). In some reported acquired cases, the muscle rippling is electrically silent (i.e., no electromyographic activity is detected despite the visible waves of contraction in the muscle) suggesting a disorder of intrinsic muscle contractility (Schulte-Mattler et al., 2005). In other reports, muscle rippling was associated with bursts of high frequency discharges (suggesting an origin in the peripheral nerve or motor nerve terminal). Those with electrically active rippling may have a variant of autoimmune PNH since some have VGKC antibodies (Vernino and Lennon, 2002).

Although Isaacs syndrome, cramp-fasciculation syndrome and rippling muscle syndrome are distinct clinical entities, they have some overlap clinically and serologically. The spectrum of autoimmune peripheral nerve hyperexcitability also includes clinical presentations that do not fit into these three diagnoses, idiopathic facial myokymia (Gutmann et al., 2001) and focal cramps with high frequency discharges (Modarres

et al., 2000; Vernino and Lennon, 2002). These may or may not be associated with VGKC antibodies.

The signs and symptoms of milder forms of peripheral nerve hyperexcitability are fairly non-specific. For example, fasciculations and cramps, which are the hallmark of the cramp-fasciculation syndrome, are prominent in amyotrophic lateral sclerosis and other degenerative neuromuscular disorders. Fasciculations may also occur in healthy individuals (Blexrud et al., 1993) and may develop during treatment with acetylcholinesterase inhibitors (Heijnsbroek and van Gijn, 1983).

14.8. Pathophysiology

14.8.1. Hyperexcitability of the motor nerve terminal

Ectopic excitability may originate at one or more different sites along the motor unit depending on the underlying etiology. In the absence of a focal nerve injury, the site of origin of spontaneous motor unit discharges in most cases appears to be near the motor nerve terminal in the terminal intramuscular nerve branches. Some have suggested that the motor nerve terminal is not protected by a blood–nerve barrier and is therefore more accessible to pathogenic antibodies and toxins. However, the intrinsic electrical properties of the terminal intramuscular axons are a more likely explanation for the generation of PNH (Zhou et al., 1999). Along the main myelinated motor axon, voltage-gated sodium channels are clustered at the nodes of Ranvier. Fast Shaker-type voltage-gated potassium channels (Kv1.1 and Kv1.2) are not found at the node but are present in internodal regions and cluster in the juxtaparanodal zones (Arroyo et al., 1999). These fast potassium currents appear to contribute little to nodal repolarization in adult myelinated nerve but may have a role during development (Vabnick et al., 1999). However, these channels appear to prevent re-entrant depolarization and nerve backfiring especially near the terminal heminode and in abnormal nerve regions with short internodes (Zhou et al., 1999). Nodal slow potassium currents (possibly generated by KCNQ2) may be more important for normal action potential repolarization (Devaux et al., 2004). Thus, spontaneous action potentials or recurrent evoked action potentials are unlikely to be generated along the intact myelinated motor axon.

The transition zone near the motor nerve terminal (where myelin ends and the distal unmyelinated intramuscular terminal nerve branches begin) is an important area for nerve excitability. After this point, the axons no longer have compact myelin but continue to be surrounded by Schwann cell processes.

The transition zone consists of several shortened myelin internodes prior to the terminal heminode. This configuration is required to allow the action potential to effectively propagate into the unmyelinated terminal nerve segments. The transition zone, as a result, is somewhat unstable and prone to abnormal hyperexcitability due to backfiring of the last few short internodes (Fig. 14.3). Fast potassium currents are important to prevent repetitive discharges in this region. Nerves from young Kv1.1-deficient mice show after discharges originating from the transition zone. Nerves from older mice display spontaneous activity, which originates in the terminal myelinated nodes and propagates to the entire motor unit. An inhibitor of slow potassium currents (TEA) amplifies the spontaneous activity in the knockout mice. In wild-type mice, TEA does not cause nerve hyperexcitability. However, 4-aminopyridine (an inhibitor of fast potassium currents) can produce spontaneous nerve hyperexcitability, especially in nerves pretreated with TEA (Vabnick et al., 1999; Zhou et al., 1999).

These observations in experimental animals correlate well with data from patients with acquired neuromyotonia. In these patients, hyperexcitability is abolished by neuromuscular blockade, but not by peripheral nerve block indicating a distal site of origin for the spontaneous discharges. Antibody-mediated inhibition of fast potassium currents would produce spontaneous and evoked repetitive discharges from the distal nerve terminal transition zone (similar to the effects of 4-aminopyridine or dendrotoxin). Computer simulation of fast potassium current deficiency predicts high frequency repetitive discharges originating in the transition zone (and predicts bursts of discharges with inter-potential interval less than 5 ms) (Zhou et al., 1999). Generation of spontaneous discharges in patients with inherited myokymia (associated with potassium channel mutations) or in those exposed to potassium channel toxins likely also occurs in the motor nerve terminal.

14.8.2. Hyperexcitability of neuromuscular junction

An early model of motor nerve hyperexcitability was produced by treatment with acetylcholinesterase inhibitors (Riker and Standaert, 1966). These drugs enhance neuromuscular junction transmission, but also promote the appearance of spontaneous motor unit fasciculations (Heijnsbroek and van Gijn, 1983). Patients who receive excess amounts of these drugs or who are exposed to organophosphates develop fasciculations or even clinical myokymia (as well as autonomic hyperactivity). The appearance of fasciculations cannot be explained on the basis of single motor endplate stimulation. Acetylcholinesterase inhibitors produce discharges of the whole motor unit and antidromic discharges of the motor axon indicating stimulation near the motor nerve terminal (Riker and Standaert, 1966). This phenomenon is abolished by low doses of curare, which are insufficient to block neuromuscular junction transmission. Nerve conduction studies may show a single after discharge, but do not show repetitive after discharges that are commonly seen in acquired neuromyotonia (Fig. 14.2) (van Dijk et al., 1996). Neuronal acetylcholine are receptors present on the motor nerve terminal and may explain this type of nerve hyperexcitability caused by acetylcholine (Tsuneki et al., 1995).

14.9. Summary

Neuromytonia is a rare, but dramatic, disorder resulting from high frequency spontaneous repetitive discharges arising at or near the motor nerve terminal. This along with myokymia, cramp-fasciculation syndrome and other forms of PNH are characterized by abnormal muscle twitching. PNH can result from genetic causes, especially mutations in voltage-gated potassium channels such as episodic ataxia type 1. Focal nerve injury or toxins that alter nerve excitability can produce PNH. Recent evidence indicates that many cases of acquired generalized PNH have an autoimmune etiology. Antibodies against voltage-gated potassium channels (VGKC, specifically α-dendrotoxin sensitive Kv1 channels found in juxtaparanodal regions of myelinated peripheral nerves) are found in many patients and appear to alter VGKC function directly.

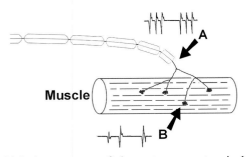

Fig. 14.3. Arrangement of the motor nerve terminal. The last few myelin internodes are progressively shortened to compensate for the impedance mismatch at the transition between the myelinated and unmyelinated axon. High frequency aberrant multiplet discharges of the motor unit can originate at this transition zone (A). Alternatively, spontaneous discharges may originate more distally in the prejunctional nerve terminal (B) and then propagate to the entire motor unit. This latter mechanism appears to be important for simple fasciculations and those induced by acetylcholinesterase inhibitors.

Neuromyotonia may occur in association with other autoimmune disorders or with cancer (especially thymoma or small-cell lung carcinoma). Encephalopathy, seizures or behavioral changes may co-exist with PNH and may represent the effects of VGKC antibodies on neuronal excitability in the CNS. Autoimmune neuromyotonia represents one of several antibody-mediated disorders of the neuromuscular junction.

References

Ansevin C, Agamanolis D (1996). Rippling muscles and myasthenia gravis with rippling muscles. Arch Neurol 53: 197–199.

Arimura K (1999). Antibodies directed to voltage-gated potassium channels in sera from acquired neuromyotonia and related disorders. Rinsho Shinkeigaku—Clin Neurol 39: 1235–1236.

Arroyo EJ, Xu YT, Zhou L, et al. (1999). Myelinating Schwann cells determine the internodal localization of Kv1.1, Kv1.2, Kvbeta2, and Caspr. J Neurocytol 28: 333–347.

Arroyo EJ, Sirkowski EE, Chitale R, et al. (2004). Acute demyelination disrupts the molecular organization of peripheral nervous system nodes. J Comp Neurol 479: 424–434.

Auger RG (1994). AAEM Minimonograph #44: diseases associated with excess motor unit activity. Muscle Nerve 17: 1250–1263.

Auger RG, Daube JR, Gomez MR, et al. (1984). Hereditary form of sustained muscle activity of peripheral nerve origin causing generalized myokymia and muscle stiffness. Ann Neurol 15: 13–21.

Barber PA, Anderson NE, Vincent A (2000). Morvan's syndrome associated with voltage-gated K+ channel antibodies. Neurology 54: 771–772.

Blexrud MD, Windebank AJ, Daube JR (1993). Long-term follow-up of 121 patients with benign fasciculations. Ann Neurol 34: 622–625.

Dedek K, Kunath B, Kananura C, et al. (2001). Myokymia and neonatal epilepsy caused by a mutation in the voltage sensor of the KCNQ2 K+ channel. Proc Natl Acad Sci U S A 98: 12272–12277.

Denny-Brown D, Foley J (1948). Myokymia and the benign fasciculation of muscular cramps. Trans Assoc Am Physicians 61: 88–96.

Devaux JJ, Kleopa KA, Cooper EC, et al. (2004). KCNQ2 is a nodal K+ channel. J Neurosci 24: 1236–1244.

Forster FM, Borkowski WJ, Alpers BJ (1946). Effects of denervation on fasciculations in human muscle. Arch Neurol Psychiatry 56: 276–283.

Gutmann L (2001). When is myokymia neuromyotonia? Muscle Nerve 24: 151–153.

Gutmann L, Tellers JG, Vernino S (2001). Persistent facial myokymia associated with K(+) channel antibodies. Neurology 57: 1707–1708.

Hart IK, Waters C, Vincent A, et al. (1997). Autoantibodies detected to expressed potassium channels are implicated in neuromyotonia. Ann Neurol 41: 238–246.

Hart IK, Maddison P, Newsom-Davis J, et al. (2002). Phenotypic variants of autoimmune peripheral nerve hyperexcitability. Brain 125: 1887–1895.

Heijnsbroek GJ, van Gijn J (1983). Neostigmine-induced fasciculations—a useful diagnostic test? Clin Neurol Neurosurg 85: 231–234.

Herskovitz S, Song H, Cozien D, et al. (2005). Sensory symptoms in acquired neuromyotonia. Neurology 65: 1330–1331.

Isaacs H (1961). A syndrome of continuous muscle-fibre activity. J Neurol Neurosurg Psychiatry 24: 319–325.

Josephs KA, Silber MH, Fealey RD, et al. (2004). Neurophysiologic studies in Morvan syndrome. J Clin Neurophysiol 21: 440–445.

Lawn ND, Westmoreland BF, Kiely MJ, et al. (2003). Clinical, magnetic resonance imaging, and electroencephalographic findings in paraneoplastic limbic encephalitis. Mayo Clin Proc 78: 1363–1368.

Layzer RB (1994). The origin of muscle fasciculations and cramps. Muscle Nerve 17: 1243–1249.

Liguori R, Vincent A, Clover L, et al. (2001). Morvan's syndrome: peripheral and central nervous system and cardiac involvement with antibodies to voltage-gated potassium channels. Brain 124: 2417–2426.

Madrid A, Gil-Peralta A, Gil-Neciga E, et al. (1996). Morvan's fibrillary chorea: remission after plasmapheresis. J Neurol 243: 350–353.

Mertens HG, Zschocke S (1965). [Neuromyotonia]. Klin Wochenschr 43: 917–925.

Modarres H, Samuel M, Schon F (2000). Isolated finger flexion: a novel form of focal neuromyotonia. J Neurol Neurosurg Psychiatry 69: 110–113.

Morvan A (1890). De la choree fibrillaire. Gazette hebdomadaire de médecine et de chirurgie 27: 173–176.

Newsom-Davis J, Mills KR (1993). Immunological associations of acquired neuromyotonia (Isaacs' syndrome). Report of five cases and literature review. Brain 116: 453–469.

Riche G, Trouillas P, Bady B (1995). Improvement of Isaacs' syndrome after treatment with azathioprine. J Neurol Neurosurg Psychiatry 59: 448.

Riker WF Jr, Standaert FG (1966). The action of facilitatory drugs and acetylcholine on neuromuscular transmission. Ann N Y Acad Sci 135: 163–176.

Roth G, Magistris MR (1987). Neuropathies with prolonged conduction block, single and grouped fasciculations, localized limb myokymia. Electroencephalogr Clin Neurophysiol 67: 428–438.

Schulte-Mattler WJ, Kley RA, Rothenfusser-Korber E, et al. (2005). Immune-mediated rippling muscle disease. Neurology 64: 364–367.

Shillito P, Molenaar PC, Vincent A, et al. (1995). Acquired neuromyotonia: evidence for autoantibodies directed against K+ channels of peripheral nerves. Ann Neurol 38: 714–722.

Sinha S, Newsom-Davis J, Mills K, et al. (1991). Autoimmune aetiology for acquired neuromyotonia (Isaacs' syndrome). Lancet 338: 75–77.

Steckley JL, Ebers GC, Cader MZ, et al. (2001). An autosomal dominant disorder with episodic ataxia, vertigo, and tinnitus. Neurology 57: 1499–1502.

Tahmoush A, Alonso R, Tahmoush G, et al. (1991). Cramp-fasciculation syndrome: a treatable hyperexcitable peripheral nerve disorder. Neurology 41: 1021–1024.

Thieben MJ, Lennon VA, Boeve BF, et al. (2004). Potentially reversible autoimmune limbic encephalitis with neuronal potassium channel antibody. Neurology 62: 1177–1182.

Tomimitsu H, Arimura K, Nagado T, et al. (2004). Mechanism of action of voltage-gated K+ channel antibodies in acquired neuromyotonia. Ann Neurol 56: 440–444.

Torbergsen T, Stalberg E, Brautaset NJ (1996). Generator sites for spontaneous activity in neuromyotonia. An EMG study. Electroencephalogr Clin Neurophysiol 101: 69–78.

Tsuneki H, Kimura I, Dezaki K (1995). Immunohistochemical localization of neuronal nicotinic receptor subtypes at the pre- and postjunctional sites in mouse diaphragm muscle. Neurosci Lett 196: 13–16.

Vabnick I, Trimmer JS, Schwarz TL, et al. (1999). Dynamic potassium channel distributions during axonal development prevent aberrant firing patterns. J Neurosci 19: 747–758.

van Dijk JG, Lammers GJ, Wintzen AR, et al. (1996). Repetitive CMAPs: mechanisms of neural and synaptic genesis. Muscle Nerve 19: 1127–1133.

Vernino S, Lennon VA (2002). Ion channel and striational antibodies define a continuum of autoimmune neuromuscular hyperexcitability. Muscle Nerve 26: 702–707.

Vernino S, Lennon VA (2004). Autoantibody profiles and neurological correlations of thymoma. Clin Cancer Res 10: 7270–7275.

Vernino S, Adamski J, Kryzer TJ, et al. (1998). Neuronal nicotinic ACh receptor antibody in subacute autonomic neuropathy and cancer-related syndromes. Neurology 50: 1806–1813.

Vernino S, Auger RG, Emslie-Smith AM, et al. (1999). Myasthenia, thymoma, presynaptic antibodies, and a continuum of neuromuscular hyperexcitability. Neurology 53: 1233–1239.

Viallard J-F, Vincent A, Moreau J-F, et al. (2005). Thymoma-associated neuromyotonia with antibodies against voltage-gated potassium channels presenting as chronic intestinal pseudo-obstruction. Eur Neurol 53: 60–63.

Vincent A, Buckley C, Schott JM, et al. (2004). Potassium channel antibody-associated encephalopathy: a potentially immunotherapy-responsive form of limbic encephalitis. Brain 127: 701–712.

Wilson RH, Lehky T, Thomas RR, et al. (2002). Acute oxaliplatin-induced peripheral nerve hyperexcitability. J Clin Oncol 20: 1767–1774.

Zhou L, Messing A, Chiu SY (1999). Determinants of excitability at transition zones in Kv1.1-deficient myelinated nerves. J Neurosci 19: 5768–5781.

Zielasek J, Martini R, Suter U, et al. (2000). Neuromyotonia in mice with hereditary myelinopathies. Muscle Nerve 23: 696–701.

Zuberi SM, Eunson LH, Spauschus A, et al. (1999). A novel mutation in the human voltage-gated potassium channel gene (Kv1.1) associates with episodic ataxia type 1 and sometimes with partial epilepsy. Brain 122: 817–825.

Index

Page numbers in italic, e.g. *65*, refer to figures. Page numbers in bold, e.g. **64**, denote tables.